Endotoxins

DRUGS AND THE PHARMACEUTICAL SCIENCES
A Series of Textbooks and Monographs

Executive Editor
James Swarbrick
PharmaceuTech, Inc.
Pinehurst, North Carolina

Advisory Board

Endotoxins

Pyrogens, LAL Testing and Depyrogenation

Third Edition

edited by

Kevin L. Williams
Eli Lilly & Company
Indianapolis, Indiana, U.S.A.

informa
healthcare

New York   London

Informa Healthcare USA, Inc.
270 Madison Avenue
New York, NY 10016

© 2007 by Informa Healthcare USA, Inc.
Informa Healthcare is an Informa business

No claim to original U.S. Government works
Printed in the United States of America on acid-free paper
10 9 8 7 6 5 4 3 2 1

International Standard Book Number-10: 0-8493-9372-8 (Hardcover)
International Standard Book Number-13: 978-0-8493-9372-3 (Hardcover)

Visit the Informa Web site at
www.informa.com

and the Informa Healthcare Web site at
www.informahealthcare.com

Preface

This book deals with the discovery, control, and continued elucidation of endotoxin as a bacterial artifact and parenteral contaminant, and the discovery, application, and regulation of *Limulus* amebocyte lysate (LAL) as the primary means of detection and quantification of endotoxin. It is intended to provide detailed information to a wide variety of healthcare professionals, including quality control personnel, pharmacists, and researchers, as well as clinicians, microbiologists, and academics. The book may serve as an introductory text to graduate and undergraduate courses intended to thoroughly treat the nature, detection, and control of endotoxins as well as a broad spectrum of microbiological knowledge applicable to the pharmaceutical manufacturing environment. While all endotoxins are pyrogens, not all pyrogens are endotoxins. The concept of "pyrogenicity" as a systemic host response has given way to cellular and molecular descriptions of the interactions that occur and are now known to include virtually the entire spectrum of microbial cellular envelope constituents.

It has been five years since I penned the second edition of this book and seemingly the world of endotoxin testing remained fairly static; however, the changes occurring all around the discipline have been overwhelming. The entire context of microbiology of which endotoxin testing is a subset has shifted in a paradigm fashion.[a] Can we understand our test subject and ignore the changes occurring in the understanding of the organisms that generate it, the host effects that it produces, or the changes in the media from which it is to be precluded? It becomes more and more rare to design and perform a simple test without a host of mitigating factors, for example, considering the context of the drug product method of manufacture, indication, consideration of potential alternate contaminants, and other lurking factors. The knowledge necessary to apply the technology has become increasingly specific. Endotoxin has always had a phantom nature; it hides and clings to itself, containers, and hydrophobic surfaces in general, and can be masked by the products themselves. There are a myriad of ways to "go wrong" in applying the technology.

Consider if you will, endotoxin as a constant marker, a buoy, in a sea of microbiological change. *Changed* is the classification and nomenclature of microbes, now grouped according to their genetic relatedness. *Changed* are pharmaceutical manufacturing processes and associated control points. *Changed* are the delivery methods of many drugs, split as a hydra's head into a myriad of novel routes. *Changed* are the requirements for the validation of computerized kinetic tests. *Changed* is the FDA's broad method of regulation. *Changed* is the application of

---

[a] "... associated with a fundamental belief system or map of reality: the lenses through which one sees everything" (1).

iii

regulations regarding new methods of LAL testing (rFC). *Changed* is the detail of the endotoxic principle in the discovery and elucidation of Toll-like receptors. This 3rd edition seeks to provide a necessary update, an expanded *a priori* context, for what Woese has called "A New Biology for a New Century" (2) and posits that endotoxin does not exist in a microbiological vacuum. Though endotoxin is the most studied and best elucidated pathogen-associated molecular pattern (PAMP), it remains as elusive as ever in regard to treating and overcoming its effects in man.

Included in this edition is the history of the fever response, the discovery of the mechanism of interaction of the causative agent (microbial pyrogen or endotoxin) and LAL by Levin and Bang. This is then put into the historical context of the development of parenteral dosage forms and federal regulations governing them. The shift in industry and medicinal focus from pyrogens to endotoxin, the refining and automation of LAL assays including the development and proliferation of semi-automated kinetic assays and the associated necessity of computer validation, the ever-changing regulation of the pharmaceutical industry as pertains to endotoxin control, and the clinical advances in understanding sepsis are all covered herein.

In addition to the changes in content and context throughout the book, several new chapters have been added or changed significantly:

- A new BET risk-assessment/contamination control chapter by Edward Tidswell
- A new medical device chapter by industry expert Peter S. Lee
- A new chapter on *Limulus's* (and other arthropod's) contribution and relevance to medical science including the more recent detail of Toll-like receptor activation via endotoxin as a PAMP
- A new chapter on LPS heterogeneity provides texture to our understanding of the occurrence of endogenous endotoxin
- An overview of computer validation in regard to kinetic testing has been added to the validation chapter
- A new chapter has been written with James F. Cooper, an LAL pioneer, with case studies involving pyrogenic reactions to medicines
- A discussion of PAT and the new recombinant LAL method (rFC) has been added
- The chapter on LAL test method development has been expanded to include novel methods of testing difficult compounds (e.g., liposomes, testing proteins via protease digestion) with case studies of significant efforts
- A completely revised chapter on automation concentrates on instruments that are available commercially including fully automated systems and a handheld, point-of-use system
- A new chapter on sepsis has been included by Edwin S. Van Amersfoort and Johan Kuiper

Thanks are due to many people for their contribution to this edition, including the first edition authors Frederick Pearson III and Marlys Weary. Each reference in the book is an acknowledgment of an expert that has toiled in the field, sometimes for a lifetime, to produce the knowledge that the book attempts to reflect. I am grateful to the publisher, Informa Healthcare, for the opportunity to update the work and to the co-authors for their chapter contributions. Special thanks are due to Dr. Thalia Nicas for her review of the entire manuscript. I'd also like to thank my Lilly management, co-workers, and family.

Kevin L. Williams

REFERENCES

1. Molin and Molin. CASE: Complex Adaptive Systems Ecology. Adv Microb Ecol 1997; 15:27–53.
2. Woese C.R. A new biology for a new century. Microbiol Mol Biol Rev 2004; 68(2): 173–186.

Contents

Contributors

James F. Cooper   Endotoxin Consulting Services, Greensboro, North Carolina, U.S.A.

Johan Kuiper   Division of Biopharmaceutics, Leiden/Amsterdam Center of Drug Research, Leiden University, Leiden, The Netherlands

Peter S. Lee   Baxter Healthcare Corporation, Round Lake, Illinois, U.S.A.

Karen J. Roberts   Eli Lilly & Company, Indianapolis, Indiana, U.S.A

Edward Tidswell   Eli Lilly & Company, Indianapolis, Indiana, U.S.A.

Edwin S. Van Amersfoort   Division of Biopharmaceutics, Leiden/Amsterdam Center of Drug Research, Leiden University, Leiden, The Netherlands

Kevin L. Williams   Eli Lilly & Company, Indianapolis, Indiana, U.S.A.

1 Historical and Emerging Themes

Kevin L. Williams

Eli Lilly & Company, Indianapolis, Indiana, U.S.A.

Parenteral manufacturing occurs at an interface of science and regulatory compliance. Change, of necessity, must occur together, in lockstep, to balance the risks of life-saving technological advancements with the safety of traditional methods.

INTRODUCTION

Man has been described as an obligate aerobe. Oxygen floods the lungs, dissolves in the blood, and spills into a thousand capillaries as a great waterfall aerates a mighty river. The same blood that brings oxygen is the route of choice for many pharmaceuticals that can only reach the inner most depths of the body via this route to dispense their therapeutic properties. The word "parenteral" is derived from the Greek "para" (beyond) and "enteral" (gut)[a] because it bypasses the digestive system. The effectiveness of this route necessitates a level of cleanliness approaching the absolute. Therefore, a single viable organism, bacteria or virus, introduced into the body evades all but the final mechanism of defense and thus the medicine designed to bring life could bring infection, fever, shock, or death.

It is desirous to step back and view the scientific, regulatory, and technological events (historical and contemporary) that contribute to the current state of complexity encompassing the control of contaminants, particularly endotoxin, in the manufacture of parenteral drugs. Such an endeavor occurs in sharp contrast to almost all other earthly activities. Amazingly, perhaps uniquely, this planet teems, festers, even boils with life. To carve a sterile niche free of microbes and their residues even briefly in the biosphere is no small task. Once a given biomolecule is in hand, the daunting task of large-scale production, separation, and purification amid a myriad of other by-products begins, all the while repelling repeated attempts by microbes to reclaim Nature's substance. The breaking of the genetic code to produce complex biomolecules, the dedication of facilities, the active and passive methods used to exclude contaminants from processes, and the delicate twists and turns of engineering necessary to mass-produce a final drug can be counted as among man's most prized achievements.

THE BIRTH OF MICROBIOLOGICAL THEORY

The birth of modern microbiology in the later nineteenth century, heralded by Louis Pasteur, Robert Koch, Joseph Lister, and others, began the quest to clarify the bacterial causation and mechanisms of infection. Though Anton van Leeuwenhock, the "uneducated" Dutch merchant and amateur microscope maker, made detailed

---

[a]Note that much of this chapter is derived from Ref. 1.

observations of microorganisms, even proposing a role in disease causation in letters to the Royal Society in London between 1675 and 1685, the new paradigm of microscopic life was not generally accepted as fact for at least the following two hundred years (2). Pasteur's refutation of spontaneous generation, description of fermentation as a by-product of microorganisms, ideas on putrification, and invention of pasteurization (3) dispelled many of the prevalent myths of the day, sometimes in dramatic fashion (e.g., the swan-necked flask). Lister, meanwhile elaborated his "germ theory" from Glasgow and performed the first successful antiseptic operation using carbolic acid (phenol) to steam sterilize medical instruments. Pasteur's and Lister's work served to dispel the thought that vapors ("miasma" or "bad air" as it was called) and other vague forms of suspected "contagion" by gases held any role in disease causation (4).[b] Though Edward Jenner developed the first vaccine using the cowpox virus 100 years before Pasteur, it was Pasteur who knowingly manipulated living microbes to alter the course of disease. He heated anthrax bacilli and dried the spinal cords of rabies-infected rabbits to develop vaccines against anthrax in sheep (1881) and rabies in man (1885), respectively (5).

In the late 1870s, Robert Koch established that individual types of microbes were associated with specific diseases including anthrax and tuberculosis (6). Koch laid out postulates purporting the conditions that must be met prior to regarding an organism as the cause of a given disease: (*i*) The organism must be present in every case under conditions explaining the pathological changes and clinical symptoms, (*ii*) the organism must not be associated causally with other diseases, and (*iii*) after isolation from the body and cultivation in pure culture, the organism must be able to produce the disease in animals. Koch refined tools and techniques needed to prove his postulates including solid agar and a method of isolating singular bacterial colonies by means of a heated inoculating loop, both of which remain staples of the microbiological trade today. Koch's methods led to the rapid identification of the specific bacteria associated with many of the infectious diseases of the late 1800s and early 1900s. The Gram stain, invented by Hans Christian Joachim Gram in 1884, proved to be a most useful tool in the study of fever causation; it splits the newly discovered bacterial world into two distinct groups that, unknown at the time, included those containing endotoxin and those that did not (7). Since the cellular wall contents determined the amount of stain retained in the staining process, subsequent observations were based on cellular morphology and were not merely an arbitrary classification technique. These new theories and methods provided the *a priori* background for further research into the newly discovered microbial world, established the ubiquity of microorganisms as causative agents of disease, and underscored the rationale and processes on which to base research into aseptic technology and disease prevention and cure.

HISTORICAL FOUNDATIONS OF PYROGEN RESEARCH

Many notable ancient physicians beginning with the Greeks believed that fever should be promoted as a means of combating disease. Hippocrates believed that fever served to cook excess "humors" (the purported cause of disease in that day) and therefore remove them from the body (8). It was not until the early eighteenth century that serious inroads were made in the study of fever causation. Early studies arose from observations associating the onset of fever in man and animals

---

[b]Ref. 4 is a definitive account of pyrogen research.

with contact with putrid organic materials. Between 1809 and 1822 Gaspard injected putrid fluid extracts into dogs and showed them to be a cause of fever and disease (9). In 1823 Francois Magendie noted the putrid conditions in and around many harbors (10) and reasoned that the putrid waters were common to the occurrence of many severe illnesses, including typhoid fever, plague, intermittent fever, dysentery, yellow fever, cholera, and so on. He followed Gaspard's experimental lead and found putrid fish water to be a particularly potent fever inducer. He demonstrated that without putrid decomposition of organic matter, no fever could be induced and that to be effective it must be absorbed through the veins. Concurrent with Magendie's observations, the French pharmacists Pelletier and Caventue isolated quinine as a pure antipyretic drug from cinchona bark. Thus, pyresis and antipyresis (from the Greek "pyreto" for fever) could be artificially produced and studied (4). The quest to clarify the fever mechanism and the role that bacteria play in its causation were aided greatly by the birth of modern microbiological theory and methods and was pursued along several overlapping lines of inquiry including (*i*) general medical hygiene and wound (or septic) infection, (*ii*) bacterial toxins, (*iii*) injection fever, (*iv*) fever therapy, (*v*) the chemical purification and structural elucidation of endotoxin, and (*vi*) modern molecular characterization of lipopolysaccharide (LPS).

MEDICINAL HYGIENE AND WOUND INFECTION

It was not until the mid to late 1800s that even the most basic practices of hygiene were applied to medical procedures. In a Paris hospital between 1861 and 1864, 1226 of 9886 pregnant women died a few days after childbirth. The deaths were attributed to "puerperal fever." The situation was similar the world over. In Boston in 1843, Oliver Wendall Holmes taught that germs on physicians' and midwives' hands caused puerperal fever (4). Other doctors largely dismissed his ideas. Ignaz Semmelweiss taught the same hygienic concepts in Vienna (11). He realized the dangers of many of the current practices including that of medical students performing post mortem dissections and then assisting in childbirth without so much as breaking to wash their hands. He instituted a strict rule requiring doctors, midwives, and medical students to hand wash in a chloride of lime solution prior to examining expectant women. Mortality fell from 18% to 1%. In 1861 he published *The Cause and Prevention of Puerperal Fever*. Nevertheless, his ideas were largely scorned, which contributed to his own mental decline. He died, ironically, of a septic wound of the hand.

    In the mid nineteenth century, the study of wound or septic infection was clarified by several notable publications including Theodor Billroth's "Observations on Fever Caused by Wounds and Accidental Wound Diseases" (12) in which he uses the terms "pyrogen" and "pyrogenic" for the first time. He isolated a bacterium he called *Coccobacteria septica* and declared it to be the causative agent of wound infection. In 1868 the eminent German surgeon Ernst Von Bergmann, head of the Surgical Hospital of the University of Berlin, published *The Putrid Poison and the Putrid Intoxication* (13) followed by *On Sepsin, the Poison of Putrid Substances* (14) and *On Fever Caused by Products of Putrefaction and Inflammation* (15). Bergmann believed pyrogen, or sepsin as he called it, was a chemically defined substance and he produced it in a semi-purified form from putrefying yeast. In 1865 Joseph Lister, an Englishman, was impressed by Pasteur's writings on the ubiquity of microorganisms (16). Lister postulated that infection may be caused by pollen-like particles and began the practice of aseptic technique in his clinics using carbolic acid (phenol) steam spray for sterilization of medical instruments. Lister became renowned for his "germ theory," which, though still not wholly accepted, added to the growing view of the importance of the microscopic world. Bergmann later applied Lister's techniques to the battlefield setting in the Franco-Prussian War (1870–1871) with great success (4). Both men demonstrated a reduction in wound infections when precautions were taken to exclude organisms from patient contact and/or to eradicate microorganisms associated with surgical implements. In 1876, Sir John Burdon-Sanderson, an Oxford physiology professor, summarized the views on the state of understanding of fever causation at that time in a review called "On the Process of Fever" (17). Specifically and prophetically, in answer to whether the cause of fever resided in the microbes or the tissue itself, he stated: "At bottom we are all humoralists, and believe in infection. It is not until we have to say where and how infection acts that questions arise" (18). In 1880, Koch contributed to the understanding of wound sepsis by writing *Investigations on the Aetiology of Infectious Wound Diseases* (19). He drew on his own war-time experience with thousands of soldiers, as well as with his animal experiments using injections of pure bacterial cultures. From this period forward, the study of fever causation focused on its bacterial origin.

STUDY OF MICROBIAL TOXINS

Expanding on the characterization of microbial pyrogen in 1892 were two European scientists who were independently studying bacterial toxins: Richard Pfeiffer and Eugenio Centanni. Richard Pfeiffer, one of Koch's students in Berlin, discovered that the *Vibrio cholerae* bacterium produced two distinct types of toxins: a heat-labile exotoxin and a heat-resistant substance that were not secreted by the cell but released upon cellular disintegration. This had been previously studied by Panum (20), whose work remained unknown for many years. Pfeiffer first used the word "endotoxin" to describe this "within toxin," which actually turned out to be somewhat of a misnomer as it resides on the surface of the cells. He was correct in that it is part of the organism and not a secretion as are exotoxins (21). Centanni at the University of Bologna extracted a heat-stable toxin from *Salmonella typhi*, the causative agent of typhoid fever. Centanni called it "pyrotoxina" (22). It is now known that Pfeiffer's and Centanni's heat stable toxins were both endotoxin, common to gram-negative bacteria. Centanni's series of papers in 1894 began with: "Investigations on Fever Infections—The Fever Toxin of Bacteria" (23) in which he described the preparation of "pyrotoxina bacterica." He prepared a bacterial endo-toxin preparation by growing pure bacterial cultures, collecting a sterile filtrate. After alcoholic fractionation he ended up with a sterile white powder. He produced the same material from several starting bacteria, including *Escherichia coli*. He believed that "the whole family of bacteria possess essentially the same toxin, a poison which is tied inseparably to their existence and upon which depends the typical picture of the general disturbances caused by bacterial infections" (4). Though now known to be limited to gram-negative bacteria, Centanni had correctly described the nature of endotoxin. Unfortunately, much of Centanni's work remained unheralded, hidden away in specialized Italian journals.

FEVER THERAPY AND INJECTION FEVER

Given the new-found tools of inducing and relieving fever in a controlled manner, physicians began to experiment with provoking the fever response as a form of therapy for given indications in which alternative remedies were ineffective. Rosenblum in Odessa (1876) used artificial fever for psychiatric disorders (4). Julius Wagner von Jauregg, a Vienna neuropathologist, received the 1927 Nobel prize in medicine for his systematic studies of fever as a therapy for paralytic patients (4). Fever therapy was applied extensively in the field of cancer treatment. In 1881 Fehleisen, an assistant to von Bergmann, used streptococcal cultures and found that the fever and chills produced were very consistent (24). William Bradley Coley discontinued the risky use of induced infection via living organisms and used instead a killed mixture of *Serratia marcescens*. Since the 1890s "Coley's toxin," as it came to be known, has been used in thousands of cancer cases in the United States. Prior to the use of antibiotics, chemotherapy, and corticosteroids, fever therapy became popular in Germany, Austria, and Russia as a nonspecific treatment where specific treatment had failed (4).

With the development of parenteral (injectable) pharmaceutical solutions, such as glucose for infusion, in the early 1900s, a common associated problem arose called "injection fever." In 1912 Hort and Penfold published several conclusive studies including, *Microorganisms and Their Relation to Fever* (25). The pair demonstrated that the toxic material originated from only gram-negative bacteria, that the pyrogenic activity in distilled water correlated to the microbial count, and that dead bacteria were as pyrogenic as living ones. Hort and Penfold were the first to design and standardize a rabbit pyrogen test with which they were able to classify bacteria into pyrogenic and nonpyrogenic types. They concluded that a heat stable bacterial substance was most likely the cause of injection fevers.

The work of Hort and Penfold was largely overlooked until 1923 when Florence Seibert in the United States explored the causes of pyrogenicity of distilled water (26). She demonstrated conclusively that bacterial contamination was indeed the cause of what had become known as "fever shots" (27). She determined that even miniscule, unweighable amounts were biologically very active (28). During this time it became obvious to numerous investigators that gram-negative bacteria possessed a high molecular weight complex as part of their outer cell wall. The complex came to be called the "endotoxic complex," which as a whole was thought to be responsible for the toxic, pyrogenic, and immunological responses induced by gram-negative bacteria. Furthermore, it became clear that various factors affected the severity of the response including the dose, the host species infected, the species of bacteria from which the infection or endotoxin was derived, as well as the mode of entry. Rademaker (29) confirmed Seibert's findings and stressed the importance of avoiding bacterial contamination at each stage of pharmaceutical production, pointing out that sterility is no guarantee of apyrogenicity. Nearly two decades elapsed before a collaborative study was undertaken by the United States National Institutes of Health and 14 pharmaceutical manufacturers to establish an animal system to be used to assess the pyrogenicity of parenteral solutions. This study resulted in the development of the first official rabbit pyrogen test, which was incorporated into the twelfth edition of the *United States Pharmacopeia* (USP) in 1942.

CHEMICAL PURIFICATION AND STRUCTURAL CHARACTERIZATION

The next area of endotoxin study centered on the chemical purification, standardization, structural characterization, and revelation of the mode of action of the endotoxin complex. This phase (if it can be viewed as such) began in 1932 with

French microbiologist Andre Boivin and Romanian Lydia Mesrobeanu at the Pasteur Institute in Paris (30). They devised a broadly applicable method for extracting the endotoxin complex from gram-negative bacteria using trichloroacetic acid. Boivin called the extract "antigenes glycido-lipidiques," thus correctly defining the main constituents as polysaccharide and lipid with small amounts of protein. In the 1930s and 1940s Walter Morgan at the Lister Institute in London and Walther Goebel at the Rockefeller Institute in New York refined the endotoxin extraction (purification) procedure using organic solvents and water (4). Morgan's extractions from *Salmonella* and *Shigella* resulted in a more refined substance than previous extractions. Murray Shear and others at the National Institutes of Health demonstrated that the tumor necrosis activity of *Serratia marcessens* endotoxin (*S. marcessens* commonly caused hospital acquired infections), sometimes used in inducing cancer remissions resided in the endotoxin complex. He called it "LPS" to describe the general behavior of the overall compound (31).

THE MODERN ERA

Given that endotoxin was known to be a complex molecule, researchers sought to determine the relationship between the structure of endotoxin and its function as a toxin. The modern era is one in which the central character in the endotoxin drama, namely LPS, is chemically manipulated via modern chemical techniques devised, beginning with the extraction method of Westphal and Luderitz, at the Wander Research Institute, which later became the Max Planck Institute for Immunology (32) in the late 1940s (33). They used hot phenol/water extraction on several members of the *Enterobacteriaceae* family to produce pure, protein free LPS. These preparations were pyrogenic in rabbits in doses of as little as 1 nanogram per kilogram when administered intravenously. Their extraction method allowed for the production of large amounts of pure LPS suitable for research. The same team in 1954 precipitated the lipid fragment of LPS with 1 N HCl by heating it at $100°C$ for thirty minutes (34). They called it "lipid A" in contrast to the more easily removed lipid layer, which they called "lipid B" (35).

Nikaido characterized the so-called deep rough mutants of *Salmonella minnesota*, which gave researchers a new characterization method to help define the role of the lipid A moiety in the biological activity of LPS (36). Attempting to prove the assumption that the endotoxic principle was borne by lipid A, several teams of researchers in the 1960s began generating mutants containing a range of associated polysaccharide. Luderitz et al. chemically induced and otherwise isolated mutant endotoxins from "rough" (called R) strains of *Salmonella minnesota* that lacked varying degrees of the O-antigenic polysaccharide (37). These R mutants known for their wrinkled visible colony morphology and agglutination and sedimentation in liquid culture (as opposed to their naturally smooth counterparts—called S strains—possessing the attached O-antigen that remained uniformly turbid in liquid culture) have been used extensively to characterize the structural and functional relationship of the LPS molecule (Chapter 3) since free lipid A does not occur naturally. Galanos, Luderitz, and Westphal later used phenol-chloroform-petroleum-ether to select and isolate various R- and S-forms of bacterial endotoxin as well as lipid A partial structures (38). It was rightly believed, though unprovable, for many years that lipid A contained the biologically active or endotoxic portion of the LPS molecule, largely because it was shown to maintain a fairly constant structure among a wide range of species, while the O-antigen varied greatly even within species.

Given that the biological activity of LPS (and therefore the study of structures producing such activity) is dependent upon water solubility, devising soluble LPS and lipid A forms was another important technique to further the on-going studies of the relationship of LPS structure to function. Electrodialysis of LPSs, developed in the mid 1970s by Galanos and Luderitz, allowed for the removal of mono- and divalent metal cations and polyamines, which neutralize the negative charges of the core and lipid A regions (39). In this manner the R and S forms of LPS (and free lipid A) could be converted to the acid forms and uniform salts when neutralized with a base. In 1973 Rietschel et al. bound lipid A noncovalently to serum albumin to achieve increased solubility, and demonstrated a concomitant increase in associated biological activity (40).

Though now long suspected, the final proof that the endotoxicity of LPS resides in the lipid A moiety was readied in the early 1980s by Tesuo Shiba et al. by their chemical synthesis of the lipid A molecule (41). This was finished shortly thereafter by Galanos et al. (at the Borstel Institute, the Max who, Planck Institute, and Osaka University) employed in vitro and in vivo methods (including lethal toxicity, pyrogenicity, local Shwartzman reactivity, LAL gelation capacity, tumor necrotizing activity, B-cell mitogenicity, induction of prostaglandin synthesis in macrophages, and antigenic specificity) to demonstrate that solubilized, synthetic lipid A was a fully biologically active component and was indistinguishable from natural endotoxin (42). Thus, after over 20 years of work, the Max Planck group was able to prove that the bound, lipid part of the LPS complex they first called "lipid A" was responsible for the majority of the diverse biological properties induced by bacterial endotoxin (44).

More recently, the study of substructures of various lipid A portions of LPS has been aided by the isolation of so-called "unusual" LPS as well as synthetic structures. Such isolates have aided in the clarification of the minimal structures necessary to elicit host responses that can be characterized as "endotoxic" (45). Such "unusual" lipid As provide a distinct advantage over the use of mutants by providing more homogeneous materials than those that occur naturally due to the fact that they may be grown in pure culture and harvested for such studies. Unusual lipid As from diverse gram-negative bacteria (and rarely a non-gram-negative LPS and even more rarely an endotoxin of nonbacterial origin, for example, algae) are still being studied to reveal the minute changes in lipid A substructures. This can spell the difference between highly lethal and pyrogenic endotoxins from inactive LPS structures and structures with endotoxic antagonistic activity (such as that from *Rhodopseudomonas sphaeroides*) (46). Mayer and Weckesser (45) point out that too few bacteria have been investigated to date to truly label *Salmonella* and *E. coli* lipid A as "usual" in their frequency of occurrence and other (nonenteric) lipid As as "unusual." It may well turn out that the latter is more frequent in a wider variety of species than the former.

Study of the submolecular structures of lipid A has resulted in the definition of an endotoxic prerequisite structure or "endotoxic conformation" of individual submolecular and resultant supramolecular aggregates of LPS (47). In what might be called the "ultra-modern era," today's endotoxin research has ballooned to touch the core of almost every biological discipline in some fashion, including the interface of cellular host defense mechanisms, infection, and inflammation. The scope of research into cytokine action (the mediators of endotoxicity) today ranges from arthritis and adult respiratory distress syndrome (ARDS) to the interplay of endo-toxin, superantigens, and resultant cytokine profiles in septic disease causation.

HISTORICAL DEVELOPMENT AND REGULATION OF PARENTERAL DOSAGE FORMS

The manner of origin of most dosage forms is largely unknown. Early man may have fashioned primitive injections modeled after venomous snakes or insect bites and stings (natural puncture injections). East Asians were inoculated for the prevention of small pox by pricking with needles dipped in pus centuries before the technique was used in Western cultures. Jenner used the same technique in 1796 using a cowpox sore (48). Sir Christopher Wren was the first to inject a drug in 1657, a process later used routinely by the English practitioner Johan Major in 1662. At this time it was referred to as "chirurgica infusoria" (49). In the early 1800s Gaspard experimented by injecting putrid extracts into dogs (9). Doctors experimented with injecting some potentially useful compounds and some bizarre and even fatal substances. Stanislas Limousin invented the ampoule in 1886 and Charles Pravex of Lyons proposed the hypodermic syringe in 1853. The Royal Medical and Chirurgical Society of London approved hypodermic injections in 1867 concurrently with the first official injection (Injectio Morphine Hypoder-mica) published in a monograph in the *British Pharmacopoeia* (BP) (50). Early progress in injectable therapy was slowed by fever occurrences and other symptoms associated with the crude state of early parenteral manufacturing. Exceptions existed that allowed progress, notably Ehrlich's use of hypeodermic injections of salvarsan for syphilis in 1910 (48). Martindale and Wynn proposed active manufacturing techniques to produce aseptic salvarsan in the same year that Hort and Penfold were describing the active agent in producing fevers (bacterial endotoxin) (25).

It is interesting to note that the very first parenteral applications, vaccines, were in effect contaminated solutions used to trigger the body's immune response (rabies, tetanus, tuberculosis, small pox). The concept of sterility was introduced at the beginning of parenteral manufacturing and was first required in the ninth revision of the USP in 1916, accompanied by an introductory chapter on achieving steri-lity. The only parenteral solutions included at that time were distilled water, solution of hypophysis, and solution of sodium chloride (49). The fever that accompanied early injections was believed to be due to the route of administration (i.e., the body's response to being pricked by a needle) rather than being viewed as a drug contaminant and was therefore referred to as "injection fever."

A test for parenteral sterility (to support the 1916 contention that they should be sterile) originated in the BP in 1932 and in the USP in 1936 (49). By 1936 there were 26 parenteral drug monographs in the sixth edition of the *National Formulary* (NF VI), many of which were packaged in ampoules (50). The methods of gauging sterility have been modified repeatedly since, but the basic concept of what sterility means has not changed. Halls lists some major limitations of the very first sterility test (51). Limitations associated with the necessity of demonstrating the lack of sterility from a quality perspective still exists in today's test 70 years later:

1. The test presumed sterility. Even with the limitations of the sterilization tech-nology of the 1930s, the USP was presuming sterility unless nonsterility could be convincingly and conclusively demonstrated. This is rather unusual because it goes against the grain of scientific criticality to assume that a

hypothesis is valid unless it can be proven otherwise. The test was far less a critical test for sterility, as one might suppose it was intended to be, than a test for nonsterility; that is, false nonsterile results were thought to be more likely than false sterile results. (The USP had more faith in the potential of the recommended media to recover microorganisms than it had in the ability of the laboratories to perform successful aseptic manipulations.)

2. The test did not address total freedom from microorganisms for preparations in 2 mL volumes or greater. For these larger volumes it was really a microbial limit test with a lower sensitivity of detection of one microorganism per mL.
3. The test gave no guidance on interpretation of data from replicate recovery conditions (51).

The dawn of drug manufacturing as a means of disease prevention (vaccination) and treatment (antibiotics, insulin, etc.) brought about the concurrent need to both harness microbes to manufacture cures and to eliminate them from contaminating medicine-producing processes. Concomitant with the medical necessity of providing safe and effective drugs was the political necessity of ensuring that manufacturers would not violate the accumulating regulations of manufacture. The laws governing pharmaceutical manufacturing have come about in stair-step fashion side by side with tragic events. To add insult to injury, commercial opportunists blatantly hawked unproven "cures" thus diluting out the few serious medicines that were available in the early twentieth century. Few companies at the time limited their sales directly to physicians (so-called ethical drugs) but instead appealed to the hopes of consumers seeking easy and inexpensive cures for every ailment.

> Voluminous newspaper advertisements (sometimes one-fourth of the space), traveling "doctors" and pitch men with or without their slide shows, druggists, and general storekeepers proclaimed loudly and constantly the merits of various panaceas. So powerful was the influence that millions of people had come to expect, all in one remedy (at a dollar or two the bottle), certain cure for consumption, cholera morbus, dyspepsia, fevers, ague, indigestion, diseases of the liver, gout, rheumatism, dropsy, St. Vitus's dance, epilepsy, apoplexy, paralysis, greensickness, smallpox, measles, whooping cough, and syphilis (52).

Parenteral manufacturing occurs at an interface of science and regulatory compliance. Change, of necessity, must occur together, in lockstep, to balance the risks of life-saving technological advancements with the safety of traditional methods. Given that every risk of process failure, human error, or act of maliciousness could not be precluded and addressed by laws governing the manufacture of drugs, broad and general requirements were enacted initially in the 1906 Pure Food and Drug Act (the Act) and revised notably in 1938 and 1962. The 1962 amendment to the Act expanded the Food and Drug Administration (FDA) definition of adulteration to include "conformance with current good manufacturing practice" (53). A drug could be considered adulterated if:

> ... the methods used in, or the facilities, or controls used for its manufacture, processing or holding do not conform to or are not operated or administered in conformity with current good manufacturing practice to assure that such drug meets the requirements of this Act as to the safety and has the identity and strength, and meets the quality and purity characteristics which it purports to possess [Section 501(a)(2)(B)] (53).

The "c" in cGMP ("current" Good Manufacturing Practices) allowed the law to live and the regulatory expectations to grow to meet improvements in technology and/or changing hazards. Regulations still favor the most cautious of manufacturers and act as a failsafe for those who seek to form the lowest denominator of industry practice. Without strict regulatory oversight safety, identity, strength, purity, quality (SISPQ) might not be the overriding manufacturing concern. Table 1 is a sampling of U.S. government regulations governing the drug industry along with the corresponding, often tragic, precipitating events. The use of thalidomide as a prescription for morning sickness is a particularly gruesome example of an adverse event that brought about positive, wholesale change even though the existing FDA regulations prevented the approval of the drug in the United States (due to the efforts of Frances Kelsey who assigned the application at the FDA) in 1960 (54).

FROM ANTIBIOTICS TO BIOLOGICS

Drug discovery began in ancient times with the use of plants as medicinal treatments and centered more recently on the isolation and purification of their bioactive ingredients. Fermentation processes have been used since antiquity to produce a multitude of food products (cheese, yogurt, vinegar, wine, beer, and bread) but the scientific basis of fermentation was unknown and became a topic of contention between chemists and microbiologists as to the underlying cause, chemical or microbial. Pasteur's publication on fermentation in 1857 largely laid the matter to rest by not only associating organisms with fermentation in every case but by describing the specific organisms associated with each (alcohol by yeasts, lactic acid by nonmotile bacteria, and butyric acid by motile rods) (58). Fermentation, when combined with microbial strain improvement (via mutant screening), was an important technological platform that served to produce everything from food for man and animals to acetone and butanol (needed for war materials) as prototypes for modern manufacturing processes, which clearly remain analogous.

The extraction and use of animal proteins as roughly human equivalents came next (first bovine insulin from the animal pancreas and then growth hormone from the animal pituitary gland) to treat diseases of deficiency. The discovery of insulin in 1921 by Dr. Banting of Toronto (for which he shared the Nobel prize) set the stage for the mass production of insulin (Lilly Iletin™), which by the spring of 1923 became available to doctors for general administration (52). The widely visible "miracle cure" that insulin provided to critically ill diabetics solidified the budding disciplines of drug development and parenteral manufacturing. The discovery of penicillin by Alexander Fleming[c] in the 1920s resulted in the use of microbial fermentation by-products (antibiotics) to treat infection followed by the development of fermentation processes for steroids and was accompanied by the introduction of the concept of "randomization" in drug clinical trials (59). The control of infectious disease is credited with much of the increased lifespan from the beginning of the 20th century to 1950, rising from below 50 years to the mid 70s where it remains today (60). Interestingly, the chart is punctuated with epidemics such as the 1918 outbreak of Spanish flu that reduced the life expectancy for that year to below 40.

---

[c]The discovery of penicillin from a random *Penicillium* mold growing in Fleming's *Staphylococcus* culture (agar plate) typified the serendipity associated with the discovery of early drugs.

TABLE 1 Chronology of U.S. Drug Regulation and Related or Precipitating Tragic Events

Year(s)	Event(s)	Subsequent regulation
1902	Diphtheria antitoxin contaminated with live tetanus bacilli, resulting in the death of 12 by lockjaw	Biologics Control Act of 1902 required inspections of biological manufacturing
1906	Upton Sinclair's *The Jungle* rallied against the unsanitary practices of the food industry and aided passage of stalled legislation championed for over two decades by Dr. Harvey Watson (chemist, Purdue professor, FDA commissioner)	Federal FDC created the Bureau of Chemistry, forerunner of the FDA
1935	Elixir of sulfanilamide killed 107 due to its formulation in diethylene glycol at toxic concentrations	FDC Act of 1938 required proof of safety prior to marketing
1941	Sulfathiazole tainted with phenobarbital; 300 died due to ineffective recall efforts by Winthrop. One lot contained on average 0 mg of sulfathiazole and 350 mg of phenobarbital; 100–150 mg dose being hypnotic	Manufacturing and quality control requirements precursors to GMPs
1940	Yellow fever vaccine contaminated with hepatitis virus	
1955	Virus not killed in polio vaccine; 150 contract polio directly or via those infected	
1955–1963	Polio and adenovirus vaccines contaminated with SV40 (simian virus)	
1960	Thalidomide marketed in Europe for morning sickness results in 10,000 severe birth defects	Kefauver-Harris Act of 1962 strengthened animal toxicity and teratogenic requirement established by 1938 FD&CA made mention of cGMPs for the first time
Early 1960	Blood products contaminated with hepatitis virus	
1978	GMPs made final	21 CFR part 210 and 211
1980	TSS outbreak; 314 cases, 38 died	FDA required tampon package inserts to educate on TSS hazards
1982/83	Tylenol cyanide tampering killed 7	Federal Anti-Tampering Act
1980–1990[a]	Iatrogenic prior disease infections (medically induced); dura matter (brain) grafts (>60 cases), human growth hormone (animal sourced, not t-HGH, >90 cases), corneal transplants, and gonadatropin from cadavers—all contaminated with Creutzfeldt–Jakob prion	Industry acts to limit use of animal-sourced raw materials; CBER requires BSE testing of raw materials derived from animal sources
1998	Gentamicin fever reactions; investigations find the bulk from China borderline futures based on off-label use 3× daily dose	Drug Modernization Act allowed for off-label dosing of drugs

[a]Time from infection to symptoms may be ≥10 years.

Abbreviations: BSE, bovine spongiform encephalopathy (mad cow disease); CBER, Center for Biologics Evaluation and Research; CFR, Code of Federal Regulations; cGMP, Current Good Manufacturing Practices; FDA, Food and Drug Administration; FDC Act, Food, Drug, and Cosmetic act.

Source: From Refs. 20–23.

Tools developed in the early 1970s (restriction enzymes and plasmids) allowed the development of recombinant DNA technology whereby the genes encoding human proteins (insulin and growth hormone) could be inserted into *E. coli* followed by their over-expression via fermentation (i.e., the combination of two previous technologies with the new technology). The first product of biotechnology, in the modern sense of the word, was recombinant human insulin in 1982 (Lilly's Humulin™). The origin of the term "biotechnology" is said to have been coined in Karl Ereky's 1917 to 1919 publications, in which he dealt with the concept of the "animal-machine" that he envisioned could help supply foodstuff for war-torn Europe (61).

The new recombinant drugs not only replaced the need for using animal sourced proteins and all the associated contamination problems (i.e., viruses and prions), but also resulted in very efficient and economical manufacturing processes.

It became clear that recombinant DNA technology yielded purer proteins and was much more economical than conventional techniques. As a result, a large number of mammalian peptide genes were cloned and expressed in *E. coli, B. subtilis* and other bacilli, *Saccharomyces cerevisiae* and other yeasts, *Aspergillus niger*, insect cells and mammalian cells. The benefits of *E. coli* as a recombinant host included (*i*) ease of quickly and precisely modifying the genome, (*ii*) rapid growth, (*iii*) ease of fermentation, (*iv*) ease of reduction of protease activity, (*v*) ease of avoidance of incorporation of amino acid analogs, (*vi*) ease of promoter control, (*vii*) ease of alteration of plasmid copy number, (*viii*) ease of alteration of metabolic carbon flow, (*ix*) ease of formation of intracellular disulfide bonds, (*x*) growth to very high cell densities, (*xi*) accumulation of heterologous proteins up to 50% of dry cell weight, (*xii*) survival in a wide variety of environmental conditions, (*xiii*) inexpensive medium ingredients, (*xiv*) reproducible performance especially with computer control, and (*xv*) high product yields (Swartz, 1996). Many benefits to society have resulted from proteins made in *E. coli* (Swartz, 1996). (*i*) Diabetics do not have to fear producing antibodies to animal insulin. (*ii*) Children deficient in growth hormone no longer have to suffer from dwarfism or fear the risk of contracting Creutzfeldt-Jakob syndrome. (*iii*) Children who have chronic granulomatous disease can have a normal life by taking interferon gamma therapy. (*iv*) Patients undergoing cancer chemotherapy or radiation therapy can recover more quickly with fewer infections when they use G-CSF (62).

The 1984 Nobel Prize in medicine was awarded to two scientists, Koehler in Germany and Milstein in England, for their efforts to develop a method for producing monoclonal antibodies (mAb) (63). With this discovery, highly specific antibodies, products of individual lymphocytes, could be generated against specific antigens. Initially, mAbs were made by inoculating mice with an antigen and isolating and purifying the resulting antibodies or antibody-producing cells. For large-scale production the utilization of recombinant methods and fermentation with specialized cell lines have been employed to produce human antibodies to various antigenic disease targets (e.g., tumor cells targeted by Genentech's Herceptin™, etc.).

Current methods of drug discovery and production are invariably based on genomics and proteomics, which have flowed from the sequencing of over 297 microbial genomes[d] (up from 60 for the 2nd edition of this book in 2001) (64) and more recently the entire human genome (65). Thomas Roderick is credited with

---

[d]See the NCBI microbial database for prokaryotic and eukaryotic (completed and on-going) sequencing projects. http://www.ncbi.nlm.nih.gov/.

coining the word "genomics" in 1986 which has been defined as the "scientific discipline of mapping, sequencing, and analyzing genomes" and as a tag for a new journal (66). There are two areas of genomics, functional and structural. Structural genomics is the construction of high-resolution genetic maps for specific organisms, and functional genomics involves mining the data generated in the structural genome to explore how it functions, particularly from a disease causation vantage. The term "proteomics" was first used in 1995 to describe the characterization of all the proteins of a cell or organism, referred to as the proteome (67).

Biologics are macromolecular (>500 kd) substances either composed of, or extracted from, a living organism.[e] Biologics bring with them increasing complexity, including glycosylation[f] that often cannot be manufactured by older technologies employing single-celled organisms as expression systems (i.e., bacteria and yeasts). Biologics, considered by USP 26 as predominately recombinants and monoclonals, tend to be less well defined analytically (68). While biologics as a group are not new (the Biologics Control Act of 1902 covered vaccines, anti-toxins, blood, and blood derivatives), the ones that are new *are* often derived from new technologies, are very different in their method of manufacture, and are susceptible to nontraditional contaminants. As the complexity of manufactured biomolecules (biologics) has increased, so too have the processes for producing them. Changes in manufacturing processes that have the capability to affect the control of contaminants include:

1. the use of new expression systems
2. the use of new media, cell cultures and transgenics that do not subscribe to previous limitations of potential contaminant types[g]
3. the development of altogether new classes of drugs and drug excipients to be parenterally administered.

A simple diagram of the process flow typical of manufacturing a biologic is shown in Figure 1.

Perhaps of greatest relevance from a contamination control perspective associated with the manufacture of biologics and biotechnology-derived materials is the careful analytical monitoring required (in addition to that already required for injectable drugs) including: expression system genetic content, viral particles, expression of endogenous retrovirus genes, and other adventitious microbial agents (mycoplasma as per 21 CFR 610.12), to name a few. The regulations governing biologics are necessarily stringent, requiring the FDA's permission to release every lot manufactured. The types of concerns involved in the manufacturing processes can be surveyed by observing the CBER-issued "Points to Consider" documents (http://www.fda.gov/cber/guidelines.htm), especially those referenced later in this section contained within the Points to Consider on the Manufacture and Testing of Monoclonal Antibody Products for Human Use (69).

---

[e]"For pharmacopeial purposes, the term 'biologics' refers to those products that must be licensed under the Act (1944 Public Health Service Act) and comply with Food and Drug Regulations-Code of Federal Regulations, Title 21 Parts 600-680, as administered by the Center for Biologics Evaluation and Research...." USP 26, <1041>

[f]The attachment of carbohydrates that affects the configuration of the molecule (usually a protein) to which they are attached.

[g]Recently the first animal vaccine to be produced in a plant cell culture was approved by the FDA (March 2006, BioPharm International).

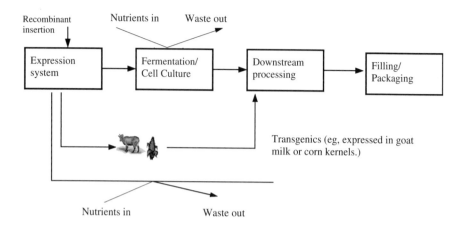

Addition of gene encoding therapeutic molecule (protein, antibody) into the genome of the desired expression organism: *E. coli, S. cerevisieae* Chinese Hamster Ovary cells (CHO), transgenic animal or plant.	Suitable environment for host organism's growth and production of desired molecule. Suspended in a medium or anchored to a base. Stirred container, continuous growth, batch fermentation, etc. Culture is fed and growth is monitored.	Separation and Purification: removal of host cells, by-products that are not the desired drug and virus or other adventitious contaminants.	Purified product is aseptically filled as per traditional drugs, packaged and sampled for analytical testing.

FIGURE 1   Simplified process flow diagram for a biological molecule. *Source*: From Ref. 1.

Sponsors are encouraged to consult the most recent available versions of the Points to Consider in the Characterization of Cell Lines Used to Produce Biologicals, Points to Consider in the Production and Testing of New Drugs and Biologicals Produced by Recombinant DNA Technology, or Points to Consider in the Manufacture and Testing of Therapeutic Products for Human Use Derived from Transgenic Animals (1,2,5), the 1996 CBER/CDER Guidance Document on the Submission of Chemistry, Manufacturing and Controls Information for a Therapeutic Recombinant DNA-Derived Product, or a Monoclonal Antibody Product for In Vivo Use (4), as well as relevant International Conference on Harmonization documents (6,7), if applicable to their expression systems. Sponsors considering novel expression systems not specifically covered by guidance documents are encouraged to consult with CBER.[h]

The task of excluding microbes from drug manufacturing processes contrasts sharply with their ever-expanding utility in producing medicines. Expression systems for generating unique biochemical entities include single-celled organisms such as *E. coli* and *S. cerevisiae*, mammalian cells, insect cells, and hybridomas (immortalized cell lines). The fermentation and cell culture steps of biologics manufacture are distinguished in that fermentation refers to the process that utilizes single-cell organisms, and cell cultures utilize cells derived from higher multicellular organisms. A third type is both an expression system and a "bioreactor" and is referred to as transgenic. The increasing costs associated with greater product complexity[i] is driving the use of transgenics including (*i*) transgenic mammals that produce proteins in their milk (cows and goats), (*ii*) transgenic hens that lay eggs containing recombinant proteins, (*iii*) a slime mold (*Dictyostelium discoideum*) that secretes recombinant proteins, (*iv*) the use of plants such as corn or tobacco, (*v*) the use of insect cells inoculated with viruses specific to insects (Baculovirus) that have been genetically modified to encode for therapeutic proteins instead of viral proteins (70), and (*vi*) the recent similar utilization of the silk worm (71). Each drug discovered eventually presents a preferred method of production and each production method has an associated set of benefits as well as constraints.

Parenteral drug presentations include new classes, some of which are still being defined.[k] Biologicals may bring with them unknowns as to their ability to contain and/or mask microbial contaminants and/or associated artifacts, and the possible effects of unique therapeutic activities on potential contaminant interactions with host systems [i.e., endotoxin liberation was found to be associated with the use of some antibiotics (72)]. Some contain ingredients that are not typically associated with parenterals, many of them of natural origin, that are not readily soluble or contain ingredients not historically used, and, therefore, that may bring with them new potential contaminants (73). Some, such as sustained-release, liposome-contained, and bone-paste drugs may contain polymers, plastics, or adhesives intended to delay degradation or support their therapeutic function (73). "Furthermore, many emerging delivery systems use a drug or gene covalently linked to the molecules, polymers, antibody, or chimera responsible for drug targeting, internalization, or transfection" (74). To demonstrate the uncertainty and novelty of some presentations, the FDA has recently reclassified a paste injected into bone from a parenteral to a device due to its relative inertness. There is also research into delivering toxic substances directly to diseased or infected tissues to bypass toxicity associated with systemic administration. Additionally, there are on-going attempts to combine the convenience of nonparenteral administration with the benefits associated with parenteral drugs such as those designed for

---

[i]Consider the initial average cost of treating Gaucher's disease using human glucocerebrosidase: $160,000 (70).

[j]CropTech introduced the gene that produced glucocerebrosidase into the tobacco plant.

[k]"The novel approaches permitted by biotechnology can make it difficult to apply classic definitions of these (drug biologic or diagnostic) categories and FDA has advised manufacturers to seek clarification in the early stages of development for how a product will be regulated when classification is not obvious" USP 26 <1045>.

inhalation or those presented as oral tablets intended to pass directly from the small intestine to the bloodstream. The concern for the characterization of biologics revolves around more than the finished product:

> Given the importance of biopharmaceuticals, regulatory authorities are emphasizing the requirements of well-characterized biologicals[1]. . . . This has focused particular attention on the composition not only of the final biological product, but also of the processing materials in contact with that product. In the downstream processing system, contaminants may be carried through to the final product either through the feedstock or through components of the processing media (75).

Indeed, the beginning of concern for product contamination begins before downstream processing with the characterization of the cell bank used:

> The production of biologics requires the use of raw materials derived from human or animal sources, and that poses a threat of pathogen transmission. Potential contamination may arise from the source material (such as cell bank of animal origin) or as adventitious agents introduced by the manufacturing process (such as murine monoclonal antibodies used in affinity chromatography). Evaluating the safety of a biological product begins at the level of the source material, such as the manufacturer's working cell bank (WCB) or, in our case, the master cell bank (MCB) (76).

One can speculate that for every niche man finds to manufacture and administer drugs, microbes (or their genetic insertions, byproducts, artifacts, toxins, etc.) will seek to hitch a ride [i.e., invasins, adhesins, etc. (77)] via that particular endeavor, thus providing unique challenges in contamination control.

CHANGING PERSPECTIVES ON CONTAMINANTS

Microbiology and genetics are in the midst of unprecedented historical change. Changes occurring that affect the way that microbial "contaminants" are viewed include (*i*) the recent explosion of knowledge in microbial genetics that has brought about the wholesale change in microbial classification[m] as evidenced by the on-going retooling of classification from historical phenotypic to genotypic based approaches, (*ii*) the realization that most organisms remain unculturable by standard methods (*iii*) the discovery of emerging microbial pathogens in the form of genetic insertions (free of associated microbes) into human and animal genomes, and (*iv*) the discovery of a previously inconceivable form of infectious disease causing agent: the prion.

Historically, bacteria and other microbes have been classified by "what they do" (i.e., ferment various sugars, retain crystal violet in the Gram stain, etc.) but are now beginning to be reclassified by "what they are" or "who they are" (i.e., their genetic relatedness). The most widely used genetic classification system as proposed by Woese (78–80) can be briefly described as centered around the similarity or dissimilarity in ribosomal RNA (rRNA) sequences, which are conserved genetically across species barriers (and significantly in all life forms). The use of the rRNA avoids a caveat that exists in the characterization of genomes in that they contain errant or wandering sequences (horizontal transmission) associated with insertions from plasmids, phage, pieces of phage, etc. that may confound

---

[1]Embedded Refs. 116,117.
[m]Note that classification does not equal identification (78).

attempts toward classification, whereas rRNA is not shared. As an example, the 16S rRNAs for *E. coli* and *P. aeruginosa* are members of Proteobacteria and differ by about 15% whereas *E. coli* differs from *B. subtilis* by about 23% (81).

The realization that most of Nature's microbes (by some estimates 99%) cannot be cultivated by standard methods has supported genomics-based reclassification efforts. Genetic methods have allowed for the classification of unknown organisms that cannot be cultured and have the ability to place such organisms between known species within a genetic-based continuum. Amann et al. point out that the 5,000 known species of Bacteria and Archaea must represent a tiny fraction of species existing in nature (82). They note that there are 800,000 species of insects and each insect harbors millions to billions of bacteria and "thus, consideration of insect symbionts alone could increase the number of extant bacterial species by several orders of magnitude" (82). While the relevance to parenteral manufacturing is not known, it supports the contention that there are most certainly forms of contamination that are invisible to current methods of detection, particularly in water, air, and naturally sourced raw materials and culture media. Some[n] maintain that: "The Petri dish and traditional tissue stains have been supplanted by nucleic acid amplification technology and in situ oligonucleotide hybridization for 'growing' and 'seeing' some microorganisms."

The lines of disease causation have become blurred at the genetic level by the discovery of microbe-induced disease processes not originally associated with microbial causes and only recently identified by genotypic approaches. The latter include viral-induced cancers[o] (83–85), schizophrenia (86), and diabetes mellitus (87). *Borrelia burgdorferi* DNA incorporated in the genome of arthritic mice (88) [and detected in humans (89)] and a list of organisms referenced by Relman (87) have been found using genotypic approaches to detect microbial genes inserted into the genome of man and animals and therefore associated with specific diseases. These include: *Helicobacter pylori* (peptic ulcer disease), hepatitis C virus (non-A, non-B hepatitis), *bartonella henselae* (Bacillary angiomatosis), *Tropheryma whippelii* (Whipple's disease), sin nombre virus (Hantavirus pulmonary syndrome), and Kaposi's sarcoma-associated herpes virus (Kaposi sarcoma). In this context Fredricks and Relman have called for the modernization of Koch's postulates of disease causation.

The discovery of emerging pathogens brings with it the implication of precluding organisms that may be only vaguely associated with disease and that are very difficult to detect and cultivate. Relman maintains that the human intestinal tract harbors Archaea but there are no known pathogens from this group: "in vitro cultivation methods for many Archaea are unavailable, so how would we know if archaeal pathogens existed?" (87). Archaea represent an entire domain as defined by Woese (the other two being Bacteria and Eucarya). The limitations of microbial sampling have not been lost on some in the parenteral industry: "Our industry has conventionally defined sterility in aseptic processing only in terms

---

[n]see Chapter 6, p. 112.
[o]The discovery of SV40 and subsequent detection in polio vaccines administered to an estimated 100 million people (1953–1960) is an interesting detective story. The vaccines were made from viruses grown in Rhesus monkey kidney cells that harbored SV40 and researchers now wonder if SV40 infection in man originated from those early polio inoculations to now cause specific cancers (brain, bone, lymphomas, and mesotheliomas) that mirror those occurring in hamsters infected with SV40 (83).

of bacteria, yeasts, and molds because of technical limitations in detection, growth and measurement rather than scientific realities" (90).

The change in microbial classification and new microbial-host disease associations comes at a unique time in microbiological history concurrent with a new type of infectious agent that is being elucidated: the prion. Dr. Prusiner proposed the existence of prions, or proteinecious infectious agents in 1997 for which he received the Nobel Prize in Medicine (57). These agents of disease are not alive; indeed they do not contain DNA or RNA, but propagate within living hosts (with resulting neurological damage) by a domino effect of altering the three-dimensional protein conformation of the normal prion protein (PrP^c) in the neurological systems of several mammals including humans, sheep, cattle[P], mink, deer, elk, and cats[q] (91). The body can break down the normal form of PrP^c but not the abnormal form (PrP^{Sc}) (92). The prion concept as elucidated by Prusiner, demonstrates how prion-generated disease may be manifested by spontaneous mutation, heredity, as well as infection (by ingestion, injection, transfusion, and transplantation[r]) (93). The existence of prions has affected the parenteral manufacturing industry by necessitating the exclusion of certain animal-sourced raw materials and requiring additional testing for those that cannot be replaced. Furthermore, traditional methods of detection[s] and decontamination have little or no effect on prions, which have been described as virtually indestructible[t] by heat, chemical treatment, or desiccation. Iatrogenic (medically induced) passage of prions has been documented in several instances and point to the tenacity of the prion molecule:

> An electrode that had been inserted into the cortex of an unrecognized Creutzfeldt-Jakob Disease (CJD) patient was subjected to a decontamination procedure involving treatment with benzene, 70% ethanol, and formaldehyde vapor. It was then used in succession on two young patients and cleaned as explained earlier in this chapter after each use. Within two years, both patients came down with CJD. After these events, the tip of the electrode was implanted into the brain of a chimpanzee where it too caused lethal spongiform encephalopathy, proving that the electrode had retained infectious prions over several years and despite repeated attempts at sterilization (94).

Lastly, relevant to paradigm changes in the view of contaminants, consider current speculation that the prion concept of infection may apply to other disease processes:

> Ongoing research may also help determine whether prions consisting of other proteins play a part in more common neurodegenerative conditions, including Alzheimer's disease, Parkinson's disease, and amyotrophic lateral sclerosis. There are some marked similarities in all these disorders. As is true of the known prion diseases, the more widespread ills mostly occur sporadically but sometimes "run" in families. All

---

[P]And other ruminants in UK zoos between 1986–1992: bison, nyala, gemsbok, oryx, greater kudu, and eland (93).

[q]Including puma, cheetah, ocelot, and a tiger in the same zoos and period noted earlier (93).

[r]The normal prion protein is coded by mammalian genomes and occurs predominately in white blood cells and brain cells.

[s]RNA/DNA methods cannot be used since they contain no nucleic acid and infectivity assays are costly and inexact.

[t]"… sheep were imported from Belgium and the Netherlands and may have consumed tainted feed. The sheep were euthanized and their carcasses dissolved in boiling lye. Barn surfaces and implements were disinfected with sodium hypochlorite or incinerated, and the pastures have been put off limits for five years to allow residual infectivity to diminish" (95).

are also usually diseases of middle to later life and are marked by similar pathology: neurons degenerate, protein deposits can accumulate as plaques, and glial cells (which support and nourish nerve cells) grow larger in reaction to do damage to neurons. Strikingly, in none of these disorders do white blood cells—those ever present warriors of the immune system—infiltrate the brain. If a virus were involved in these illnesses, white cells would be expected to appear (57).

This begs the question: Will discoveries follow of additional infectious proteins and, if so, how might this be relevant to the use of transgenics, given that the crossover of pathogenic contaminants has in the past gone unrecognized[u]? The degree of similarity or dissimilarity in the mammalian gene that encodes the PrP has been found to explain the mechanism of barrier between animals that can and cannot contract the disease in terms of protein conformation similarity (and susceptibility to being converted) relative to the gene that encodes it (the PrP genes of cows, sheep, and humans are very similar). It is not known at what levels of concentration prions are infective or the cause(s) of variability in the time of onset of symptoms. Governments around the world have enacted precautions in food, medical (including blood collection and handling), and drug regulation to contain the spread of known prion diseases (95–97).

It is frightening to see that CJD does occur on a "normal" basis and somewhat reassuring that the CDC is monitoring any suspected outbreaks to determine if they may be due to vCJD, such as the 14 deaths related to CJD that occurred at a New Jersey racetrack over the course of approximately 9 years:

> In 2001, Garden State Racetrack was closed permanently. The number and ages of all persons visiting or dining at the racetrack is unknown, however, according to New Jersey Racing Commission records, attendance at the racetrack during 1988–1992 was approximately 4.1 million. Based on an annual CJD rate of 3.4 cases per 1 million persons (CDC, unpublished data, 2004) and an overall death rate from all causes of 2.9% for persons aged >50 years, the occurrence over approximately 9.25 years (1995–2004) of at least 14 CJD related deaths among as few as 300,000 persons aged >50 years would not be unusual. This number is within the estimated range of the number of persons attending (98).

EMERGING APPROACHES TO FINDING AND IDENTIFYING CONTAMINANTS

From a less theoretical vantage, the processes used to manufacture parenteral drugs can be separated into two broad categories: those that manufacture, fill, package, and end in terminal sterilization and those that manufacture and fill aseptically without terminal sterilization. The former category is possible only for those drugs capable of withstanding the protracted heating cycle associated with steam sterilization (or alternatively chemical or radiation treatment), whereas the aseptically filled category encompasses a greater variety and more problematic route of production from a contamination control perspective. The "problems" associated with aseptic manufacturing have multifaceted aspects but the FDA has noticed a common theme as summarized in this PDA Letter excerpt:

> The Agency (FDA) has also looked at 10-year nonsterility trends. Nonsterility in the recall context means the distributed drug was found to be nonsterile by FDA or another

---

[u]This is somewhat analogous to the issues facing xenotransplantation (118).

government laboratory, or by the manufacturer's own laboratory. When the FDA looked closely at these data trends, they distilled one overwhelming fact from it: all drugs recalled due to nonsterility over the last 10 years were produced by aseptic processing (99).

The numbers associated with such recalls include 135 drugs (in some cases multiple lots) in the years 1999, 2000, and 2001 (99). Many of the tasks associated with contamination are brought about by the interaction of humans with the drug material during aseptic processing. The causes in order of occurrence listed by survey respondents (99) include:

1. Personnel borne contaminants
2. Human error
3. Nonroutine operations
4. Assembly of sterile equipment prior to use
5. Mechanical failure
6. Inadequate or improper sanitization
7. Transfer of materials within aseptic processing area (APA)
8. Routine operations
9. Airborne contaminants
10. Surface contaminants
11. Failure of sterilizing filter
12. Failure of high efficiency particulate air (HEPA) filters
13. Inadequate or improper sterilization

Halls (51) condenses the sources of contamination into five overarching routes: (*i*) environmental air, (*ii*) manufacturing equipment facilities and services, (*iii*) dosage form with product containers and closures, (*iv*) personnel operating the manufacturing equipment, and (*v*) water and drainage.

Issues in parenteral manufacturing contamination control often revolve around the implausibility (from a statistical vantage) of finding microbiological contamination by way of quality testing without exhaustive sampling schemes. Since the absence of contamination (sterility) is only a statistical likelihood of occurrence and can never be proven absolutely without consuming (testing) an entire manufactured drug lot, the industry-regulatory tension always exists to prove the unprovable (i.e., that a given lot is in fact sterile by a number of criteria including, but not limited to, end product testing). Furthermore, since the likelihood of the occurrence of artifacts (false-positives) arising during analytical testing is not negligible, it creates an additional layer of tension between manufacturers and their own quality processes.

The 1978 case of *Northern District of New York v Morton-Norwich Products, Inc.* involved the sterility of gauze pads containing an antibacterial dressing (53). Sterility testing by the FDA determined that units of the gauze were adulterated. The defendants argued that sterility is a probabilistic and not an absolute concept and that by passing the in-house sterility test the article was in fact sterile by definition.

> The importance of the court's finding to persons involved in the manufacturing and testing of injectable drug products is immense. The court, knowing that an absolute cannot be measured, insisted that the absolute situation must prevail. Every single unit in every single manufacturing batch is required by the Act to be sterile if the product purports to be sterile or is represented in its labeling to be sterile (53).

The advance of genetic-based identification [DNA fingerprinting (100)] may come to aid the resolution of sterility-test failure ambiguity in that genomic characterization makes it possible, in theory, to determine the origin of contaminants (i.e., a true product contaminant or an artifact of testing) based on an organism's genetic relatedness to environmental isolates, either of production or lab origin. Genetic methods are being developed for analogous epidemiological purposes in other disciplines including diagnosing, identifying, and tracking the origin and progress of infectious agents (101) and food-borne disease without the concomitant need for microbial enrichment (102), in some cases supplanting traditional, culture dependent serotyping (103); tracking antibiotic resistance genes (104); and tracking the origin of organisms used for bioterrorism (i.e., anthrax) (105,106). This latter field has been referred to as "microbial forensics" (107).

The PDA *Journal of Pharmaceutical Science and Technology* technical report No. 33 (108) describes three broad categories of microbiological testing technologies including (*i*) viability-based, (*ii*) artifact-based, and (*iii*) nucleic acid-based technologies. Clearly, the latter category is primed to have a profound effect on pharmaceutical analytical testing for contaminants given the genesis of microarrays[v] (oligonucleotide arrays) (109–111), instrumental biosensors (112–113), and DNA probes (PCR) (114–115) that are capable of detecting femtogram levels (10^{-15}) of DNA or mRNA (or ribosomal RNA). Some have noted a paradigm shift from the detection of gene products [such as proteins and contaminating antigens (endotoxin)] to genome fragments especially, given the sequencing of the whole genomes of numerous organisms (114). DiPaolo et al. (115) describe the importance of monitoring for potential host cell DNA contamination in the production of drugs using recombinant methods:

> The use of recombinant DNA technology and continuous cell lines in the manufacture of biopharmaceuticals has raised the possibility of introducing potentially oncogenic or transforming DNA into the product as an impurity. Although the actual risk of incorporating tumorigenic sequences into the recipient's DNA is negligible, the FDA continues to require lot-to-lot testing for residual host cell DNA, recommending that the final product should contain no more than 100 pg cellular DNA per dose, as determined by a method with a sensitivity of 10 pg (69). These recommendations have resulted in a significant scientific challenge to develop sensitive and robuts assays that can meet the criteria with samples typically containing milligram amounts of biotherapeutic protein.

REFERENCES

1. Williams KL ed. Microbial Contamination Control in Parenteral Manufacturing. New York: Marcel Dekker, 2004.
2. De Kruif P. Microbe Hunters. 4th ed. New York: Harcourt, Brace and Company, 1940:350.
3. Demain AL, Solomon NA. Industrial microbiology. Sci Am 1981; 245(3):67–75.
4. Westphal O, Westphal U, Sommer T. History of pyrogen research. In: Schlessinger D, ed. Microbiology. Washington: American Society for Microbiology, 1977:221–238.
5. Roitt I, Brostoff J, Male D. Immunology. 4th ed. London: Mosby, 1996.

---

[v]"When gene sequence information is available, oligonucleotides can be synthesized to hybridize specifically to each gene. Oligonucleotides can be sysnthesized in situ, directly on the surface of a chip, or can be pre-synthesized and then deposited on to the chip" (109).

61. Bud R. History of Biotechnology. Encyclopedia of Life Sciences. London: Nature Publishing Group, 2001. http://www.els.net

62. Demain AL, Lancini G. Bacterial pharmaceutical products. In: Dworkin M et al., eds. The Prokaryotes: An Evolving Electronic Resource for the Microbiological Community. 3rd ed. New York: Springer-Verlag, 2001. http://link.springer-ny.com/link/service/books/10125/

63. The BioPharm Guide to Biopharmaceutical Development. Supplement to BioPharm. 2nd ed, 2002.

64. http://www.ncbi.nlm.nih.gov/genomes/lproks.cgi?view=1.

65. Venter JC et al. The sequence of the human genome. Science 2001; 291(16):1304–1351.

66. Hieter P, Boguski M. Functional genomics: its all how you read it. Science 1997; 278(24):601–602.

67. Graves PR, Haystead T. Molecular biologist's guide to proteomics. Micro Mol Biol Rev 2002; (66):39–63.

68. US Pharmacopoeia, 26, 2002.

69. Points to Consider in the Manufacture and Testing of Monoclonal Antibody Products for Human Use. U. S. Department of Health and Human Services, Food and Drug Administration, Center for Biologics Evaluation and Research, Feb 28, 1997.

70. The BioPharm International Guide to Fermentation and Cell Culture. Supplement to BioPharm. 2nd ed, 2003.

71. Tomita M et al. Transgenic silkworms produce recombinant human type III procollagen in cocoons. Nature 2003; 21(1):52–56.

72. Kirikae T et al. Biological characterization of endotoxins released from antibiotic-treated *Pseudomonas aeruginosa* and *Escherichia coli*. Antimicrob Agents Chemother 1998; 42:1015–1021.

73. Apte SP, Ugwu SO. A Review and classification of emerging excipients in parenteral medications. Pharm Technol 2003:46–60.

74. Kannan V, Kandarapu R, Garg S. Optimization techniques for the design and development of novel drug delivery systems, Part I. Pharm Technol 2003; 27(2):74–90.

75. Behizad M, Curling JM. Comparing the safety of synthetic and biological ligands used for purification of therapeutic proteins. BioPharm 2000; 13(7):42–46.

76. del Rosario M et al. Some methods for contamination testing of a master cell bank. BioPharm 2000; 48–52.

77. Finlay BB, Falkow S. Common themes in microbial pathogenicity revisited. Micro Mol Biol Rev 1997; 61(2):136–169.

78. Woese CR. Prokaryote systematics: the evolution of a science. In: Dworkin M et al., eds. The Prokaryotes: An Evolving Electronic Resource for the Microbiological Community. 3rd ed. New York: Springer-Verlag, 2001. http://link.springer-ny.com/link/service/books/10125/

79. Woese CR et al. Towards a natural system of organisms: proposal for the domains archaea, bacteria, and eucarya. Proc Natl Acad Sci USA 1990; 87:4576–4579.

80. Woese CR. Interpreting the universal phylogenetic tree. Proc Natl Acad Sci 2000; 97(15):8392–8396.

81. Hugenholtz P et al. Impact of culture-independent studies on the emerging phylogenetic view of diversity. J Bact 1998; 4765–4774.

82. Amann RI et al. Phylogenetic identification and in situ detection of individual microbial cels without cultivation. Microbiol Rev 1995; 59(1):143–169.

83. Garcea RI, Imperiale MJ. Simion virus 40 infection. J Virol 2003; 77(9):5039–5045.

84. Urnovitz HB, Murphy WH. Human endogenous retroviruses: nature, occurrence, and clinical implications in human disease. Clin Microbiol Rev 1996; 9:72–99.

85. Lower R et al. The viruses in all of us: characteristics and biological significance of human endogenous retroviral sequences. Proc Nat Acad Sci USA 1996; 93:5177–5184.

86. Karlsson H, Bachmann S, Schroder J, McArthur J, Torrey EF, Yolken RH. From the cover: retroviral RNA identified in the cerebrospinal fluids and brains of individuals with schizophrenia. Proc Natl Acad Sci USA 2001; 98:4634–4639.

87. Relman DA. Detection and identification of previously unrecognized microbial pathogens. Emerg Infect Dis 1998; 4(3):

88. Yang L et al. Heritable susceptibility to severe borrelia burgdorferi-induced arthritis is dominant and is associated with persistence of large numbers of spirochetes in tissues. Infect Immun 1994; 64:492–500.

89. Schmidt BL. PCR in laboratory diagnosis of human *Borrelia burgdorferi* infections. Clin Microbiol Rev 1997; 10:185–201.

90. Akers J, Agalloco J. Sterility and sterility assurance. PDA J Pharm Sci Technol 1997; 51(2):72–77.

91. Pattison J. The emergence of bovine spongiform encephalopathy and related diseases. Emerg Infect Dis 1998; 4(3).

92. Aranha H, Larson R. Prions: Mayhem and Management, part I, general considerations in mayhem and management BioPharm 2002; (suppl):11–17.

93. Yam P. Keeping mad cows at bay. Sci Am 2002; (59).

94. Weissmann C et al. Transmission of prions. PnAS early ed. www.pnas.org/cgi/doi/10.1073/pnas.172403799, pg. 1–6.

95. ASM Comments on Docket No. 02D-0266. FDA Draft Guidance Document for Industry: Preventive Measures to Reduce the Possible Risk of Transmission of Creutzfeldt-Jakob Disease (CJD) and Variant Creutzfeldt-Jakob Disease (vCJD) by Human Cells, Tissues, and Cellular and Tissue-Based Products (HCT/Ps). http://dev.asmusa.org/pasrc/CJDvCJD.htm, last modified January 21, 2003 (ASM).

96. Coulthart MB, Cashman NR. Variant Creutzfeld-Jakob disease: a summary of current scientific knowledge in relation to public health. CMAJ 2001; 165(1).

97. Aranha H, Larson R. Part Four, Due diligence in the manufacture of biologicals. BioPharm 2002; (May Suppl):36–40.

98. Creutzfeldt-Jakob Disease Not Related to a Common Venue - New Jersey, 1995–2004. Morbidity and Mortality Weekly Report, CDC, May 14, 2004; 53(18).

99. PDA Letter, Regulatory News: Aseptic Processing: How Good Science and Good Manufacturing Practices Can Prevent Contamination. 2002:10–11.

100. van Belkum A. DNA fingerprinting of medically important microorganisms by use of PCR. Clin Microbiol Rev 1994; 7:174–184.

101. Cunningham MW. Pathogenesis of group A streptococcal infections. Clin Microbiol Rev 2000; 13:470–511.

102. Cocolin L et al. Direct identification in food samples of *Listeria* spp. and *Listeria monocytogenes* by molecular methods. Appl Envir Microbiol 2002; 68:6273–6282.

103. Muir P et al. Molecular typing of enteroviruses: current status and future requirements. Clin Microbiol Rev 1998; 11:202–227.

104. Chopra I, Roberts M. Tetracycline antibiotics: mode of action, applications, molecular biology, and epidemiology of bacterial resistance. Microbiol Mol Biol Rev 2001; 65:232–260.

105. Sacchi CT et al. Sequencing of 16S rRNA gene: a rapid tool for identification of *Bacillus anthracis*. Emerg Infect Dis 2002:8. Available from: URL: http://www.cdc.gov/ncidod/EID/vol8no10/02-0391.htm

106. Hoffmaster AR et al. Molecular subtyping of *Bacillus anthracis* and the 2001 bioterrorism-associated anthrax outbreak, United States. Emerg Infect Dis [serial online] 2002:8. Available from: URL: http://www.cdc.gov/ncidod/EID/vol8no10/02-0394.htm.

107. Cummings CA, Relman DA. Microbial forensics- cross-examining pathogens. Science 2002; 296:1976–1978.

108. PDA, evaluation, validation and implementation of new microbiological testing methods. PDA Jf Pharm Sci Technol 2000; 54:1–39.

109. Watson A et al. Technology for microarray analysis of gene expression. Curr Opin Biotechnol 1998; 9:609–614.

110. Braxton S, Bedilion T. The Integration of microarray information in the drug development process. Curr Opin Biotechnol 1998; 9:643–649.

111. Gingeras TR. Studying microbial genomes with high-density oligonucleotide Ar-rays. ASM News 2000; 66(8):463–469.

112. Nice EC, Catimel B. Instrumental biosensors: new perspectives for the analysis of biomolecular ineractions. BioEssays 1999; 21:339–352.

113. Briggs J. Sensor-based system for rapid and sensitive measurement of contaminating dna and other analytes in biopharmaceutical development and manufacturing. J Parenter Sci Technol 1991; 45(1):7–12.
114. Swarbrick J, Boyan JC, eds. DNA Probes for the Identification of Microbes. Encyclopedia of Pharmaceutical Technology. Vol. 19.
115. DiPaolo B et al. Monitoring impurities in biopharmaceuticals produced by recombinant technology. PSTT 1999; 2(2):70–82.
116. Little L. Current trends: impact of the well-characterized regulatory paradigm. BioPharm 1997; 10(8):8–12.
117. Seely RJ et al. Defining critical variables in well-characterized biotechnology processes. BioPharm 1999; 12(4):33–36.
118. Boneva RS, Folks TM, Chapman LE. Infectious disease issues in Xenotransplantation. Clin Microbiol Rev 2001; 14(1):1–14.

2

Endotoxin Relevance and Control Overview

Kevin L. Williams

Eli Lilly & Company, Indianapolis, Indiana, U.S.A.

The importance of endotoxin contamination control in parenteral manufacturing becomes apparent when confronted with four aspects of its existence. The first is its ubiquity in nature, the second is the potent toxicity it displays relative to other pyrogens, the third is its stability . . . and the fourth is the relative likelihood of its occurrence in parenteral solutions.

NOMENCLATURE/CLASSIFICATION OF PYROGENS AND ENDOTOXIN

The first order of business in any study of endotoxin is to define its relative position as one of many pyrogens. Some confusing nomenclature must be sorted through. Pyrogens include any substance capable of eliciting a febrile (or fever) response upon injection or infection (as in endotoxin released in vivo by infecting gram-negative bacteria). Endotoxin is a subset of pyrogens that are strictly of gram-negative bacterial origin; they occur (virtually) nowhere else in nature. The terms lipopolysaccharide (LPS) and endotoxin are often used interchangeably (as they will be throughout this book). To be more precise, endotoxin is the natural complex of LPS occurring in the outer layer of the bilayered gram-negative bacterial cell, and LPS is the purified form used as a standard in the pharmaceutical industry for quality control or research purposes. The definition of endotoxin as "lipopolysaccharide-protein complexes contained in cell walls of gram-negative bacteria, including non-infectious gram-negatives" has been used to denote their heterogenous nature (1).

Pyrogens are separated into exogenous and endogenous pyrogens based upon their origin from outside or inside the body, respectively. The term "endogenous endotoxin" is used to denote natural or environmental endotoxin and should not be confused with "endogenous pyrogen" (EP) and "endogenous mediator," which describe substances produced by the body and which are responsible for mediating the body's inflammatory, coagulation, and fever mechanisms. The latter term is used generically to refer to the group of host responder proteins now called cytokines. Exogenous pyrogen is any substance foreign to the body capable of inducing a febrile response upon injection or infection and would, of course, include microbial pyrogen, the most potent of which is endotoxin. Nonmicrobial exogenous pyrogen includes certain pharmacological agents or, for a sensitized host, antigens such as human serum albumin (2).

The term "pyrogen" has diminished both in terms of popularity[a] and accuracy of use. The popularity of the term has been eroded by (*i*) the replacement of the pyrogen assay with the *Limulus* amebocyte lysate (LAL) test, (*ii*) the

---

[a]As an unscientific example, consider the following web query responses for "pyrogen" and "endotoxin," respectively: ASM.org (12 vs. 408), CDC.gov (8 vs. 220), and FDA.gov (975 vs. 1550) (February 2006).

characterization of a number of analogous microbial host-active by-products, (*iii*) the identification of deleterious host responses that do not include fever, (*iv*) the discovery of LAL reactive materials some of which may be host reactive but nonpyrogenic, and (*v*) perhaps that most significantly, the modern focus on cellular and molecular mechanisms that are not particularly concerned with fever as a measure of biological response. Concerning the loss of accuracy implied by the term, there are now so many host active compounds recognized, with various potencies, and sometimes acting in concert (Chapter 6) that the term pyrogen now requires various qualifiers and descriptors if it is to be used meaningfully. Dozens of microbial compounds have been found to either induce fever or activate host events that may lead to fever, especially in combination with endotoxin, but many do so only weakly by themselves or at very high doses. Figure 1 shows a list of significant microbial and nonmicrobial pyrogens and/or otherwise biologically active microbial by-products and compounds. The figure does not distinguish the relative levels of each pyrogen required to bring about a host response or if fever, LAL reactivity, or other biological activation measure is typically associated with it.

Fever is now known to be one of the less physiologically significant aspects of the overall proinflammatory events that occur in response to infection, trauma, and disease progression. Many forms of infection and inflammation progress without the occurrence of fever. Some microbial components can be considered "pyrogens" only in synergy with other factors or in predisposed or specific hosts. LAL activation is considered analogous to the response that is considered to be pyrogenic but is more specific for bacterial endotoxin and at much lower levels of detection. Figure 2 lists some various means of measuring the activation of host defense mechanisms. As more specific methods have become available, the general methods

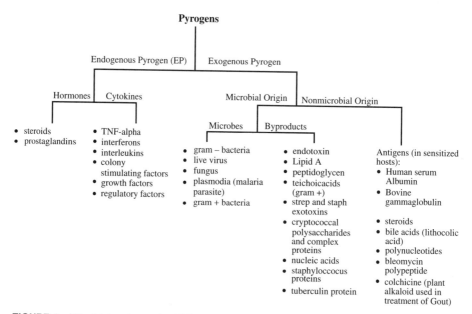

FIGURE 1 Microbial and nonmicrobial pyrogens and associated host active microbial products.

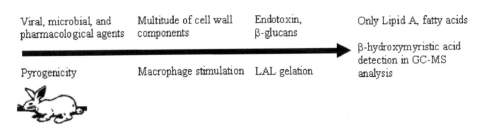

| Viral, microbial, and pharmacological agents | Multitude of cell wall components | Endotoxin, β-glucans | Only Lipid A, fatty acids |

β-hydroxymyristic acid detection in GC-MS analysis

| Pyrogenicity | Macrophage stimulation | LAL gelation |

FIGURE 2 Increasing specificity of host response recognition by various methods. *Abbreviations*: LAL, *Limulus* amebocyte lysate; GC-MS, gas chromatography-mass spectroscopy.

have diminished and may no longer provide the desired level of detail as descriptors. The label pyrogen is less significant today than it was previously when it was the primary method for the recognition of host defense activation.

WHY THE FOCUS ON ENDOTOXIN?

The importance of endotoxin contamination control in parenteral manufacturing becomes apparent when confronted with four aspects of its existence. The first is its ubiquity in nature; the second is the potent toxicity it displays relative to other pyrogens, the third is its stability or ability to retain its endotoxic nature after being subjected to extreme conditions; and the fourth is the relative likelihood of its occurrence in parenteral solutions. The concern for endotoxin from a parenteral manufacturing contamination control perspective has overtaken concerns for guarding against "all pyrogens" that predominated the second half of almost a century of parenteral manufacturing (the first half experiencing little or no quality control at all). The paradigm shift of concern from pyrogens in general to endotoxin specifically began with the testing of pharmaceutical waters and in-process materials and culminated in the availability of the LAL test for most end product items as an alternative to the *United States Pharmacopeia* (USP) pyrogen test in 1980 (3).

Ubiquity of Endotoxin

Endotoxin occurs in the outer membrane of a dual layered, asymmetrical shell that protects gram-negative bacteria from their environment. In the gram-negative organism, the two layers are separated by a thin layer of peptidoglycan (PG). The structure of the endotoxin complex has a number of unique properties tied inseparably with its potent ability to elicit host defense mechanisms. A single bacterial cell has been estimated to contain about 3.5 million LPS molecules occupying an area of 4.9 μm^2 of an estimated 6.7 μm^2 of total outer surface area (4). Thus, the outer membrane consists of three-quarters LPS and one-quarter protein. Endotoxin molecules are crucial to the survival of the gram-negative bacterium, providing structural integrity, physiological, pathogenic, immunologic, and nutrient transport functions. No gram-negative organisms lacking LPS entirely have been found to survive (5).

LPS molecules are freed from bacteria by the multiplication, death, and lysis of whole cells as well as from the constant sloughing off of endotoxin in a manner analogous to the body shedding small pieces of skin or hair. LPS builds up in solution as the skeletons of dead bacteria accumulate. When such solutions rich in gram-negative cellular residues find their way into mammalian blood, they retain their ability to activate host defense mechanisms in nanogram per kilogram amounts. The occurrence of gram-negative organisms in virtually every environment on the earth makes LPS one of the most prevalent complex organic molecules occurring in nature. Gram-negative bacteria have been isolated and are being isolated still (6) wherever man has gone, in soil, fresh and salt water, frigid oceans and hot springs, as well as in significant amounts in ocean sediment. Some gram-negative organisms are able to grow in the lowest temperatures known (<10°C) (7). The gram-negative bacterial count of seawater was taken at Woods Hole Oceanographic Institute and found to be in excess of one million organisms per milliliter and the sand from the shore contained almost a billion organisms per gram (8).

Given its ubiquity, one may wonder at the mammalian host's exaggerated response to the presence of LPS in the blood stream. It is as though a war were being waged between the mammalian [and virtually all multicellular organisms (9,10)] and prokaryotic systems with the mammals always on the defensive, living in fear, and shouting "barbarian at the gates" at the first sight of this invader. It is as though something far larger loomed, ready to squash the mammals; as if the body fears another plague or typhoid (gram-negative invaders) lies ready to threaten the larger society and, therefore, reacts accordingly. Viewed in this context, perhaps the mammalian response to endotoxin is not as exaggerated as it would seem at first glance. The spectrum of organisms induced to fever by endotoxin is extensive including reptiles, amphibians, fish, and even insects such as cockroaches, grasshoppers, and beetles (11). Some animals that were initially believed to be insensitive to LPS, such as rats, mice, and hamsters, have subsequently been shown to respond (12). A study of bacterial infection in the horseshoe crab lead to the discovery and use of a derivative of the crab's blood (LAL) as a reagent for endotoxin detection.

Stability of Endotoxin

Beveridge describes the enduring nature of the gram-negative cell wall as "strong enough to withstand ~3 atm of turgor pressure, tough enough to endure extreme temperatures and pHs (e.g., *Thiobacillus ferrooxidans* grows at a pH of ~1.5), and elastic enough to be capable of expanding several times their normal surface area. Strong, tough, and elastic . . ." (13). Endotoxin, largely responsible for the properties of the gram-negative cell wall, is extremely heat-stable and remains active after ordinary steam sterilization and normal desiccation, and easily passes through filters intended to remove whole bacteria from parenteral solutions. Only at dry temperatures exceeding 200°C for up to an hour do they relent. The ampiphilic nature of the LPS molecule also serves as a resilient structure in solution with the hydrophobic lipid ends adhering tenaciously to hydrophobic surfaces such as glass, plastic, and charcoal (14) as well as to one another. Many of the most basic properties of LPS are those shared with lipid bilayers in general, which form the universal basis for all cell-membrane structures (15). In aqueous solutions, LPS spontaneously forms bilayers in which the hydrophobic lipid A ends with fatty acid tails are hidden in the interior of the supramolecular aggregate as the opposite hydrophilic polysaccharide ends are exposed to and subject to solubilization in the aqueous environment. A property adding to the stability of LPS as a lipid bilayer is its propensity to reseal when disrupted, thus preserving the structure's defense against the environment.

Relative Pyrogenicity

Endotoxin achieves greater leverage in eliciting deleterious host effects than any other microbial pyrogen as is seen in the relative amount of endotoxin needed to provoke a response, which is in the nanogram per kilogram range. If endotoxin is considered to be one of many alarm markers for hosts in recognizing microbial invasion (16), then it elicits the loudest and most variable response of the group. The great leverage of endotoxin can be seen in the wide variety of endogenous mediators elicited, which are active in the picogram (even femtogram) per kilogram range. Therefore, a small amount of endotoxin generates a very large host response in terms of both severity and variety. The complexity of the host response has frustrated efforts to devise treatments against it. The complexity arises from the interplay of the various mediators produced that may have proinflammatory and anti-inflammatory host effects as well as synergistic effects on their own kind. A few nanograms of endotoxin translate into the production of a myriad of manu-factured endogenous pyrogens that are extremely bioactive. Arguably, the closest exogenous pyrogenic mediator analogous to endotoxin is prostaglandin (PG), a significant constituent of the cell wall of gram-positive bacteria (and present in lesser amounts in gram-negative bacteria). The pyrogenicity and endotoxin-like characteristics of PG were demonstrated by Roberson and Schwab in 1961 by using *Streptococcus pyogenes* cellular walls to induce fever in rabbits. Importantly though, the relative pyrogenicity of PG was shown to be on the order of 50,000 times less than the minimum pyrogenic dose of endotoxin (3).

In the early use of the pyrogen assay, no attempt was made to quantitate the amount of endotoxin needed to produce a pyrogenic response in rabbits. Because they are part of one of the most endotoxic families (*Enterobacteriaceae*) of bacteria, *Escherichia coli* and *Salmonella* were later chosen to determine and quantify the amount of endotoxin by weight considered to be pyrogenic. In 1969, Greisman and Hornick (17) performed a study using healthy male inmates (volunteers) and found the threshold pyrogenic response (TPR) level to be about 1 ng/kg[b] for *E. coli* and *Salmonella typhosa* (approximately 0.1–1.0) and 50 to 70 ng/kg for *Pseudomonas*. The same study revealed that the rabbit and human TPRs are approximately the same. Therefore, the amount of purified *E. coli* needed to initiate pyrogenicity in both man and rabbits is approximately 1 ng/kg, which represents about 25,000 *E. coli* bacterial cells (18). In terms of whole cells, the injection of an estimated 1000 organisms per milliliter (10,000/kg) of *E. coli* causes a pyrogenic reaction in rabbits, as compared to 10^7 to 10^8 organisms per kilogram of gram-positive or fungal organisms (19). The pyrogenic dose response curve in man is much steeper than it is in rabbits, although the minimum pyrogenic dose on a weight basis is about the same. Man is the most sensitive creature studied in his response to endo-toxin exposure. It requires 10 times as much *S. typhosa* endotoxin in the rabbit as in man (0.005 µg/kg) to elicit the same degree of relative febrile response (20). Due to the steep response curve in man and the associated dangers, many of the effects of endotoxin exposure at higher doses cannot be studied. It has also been observed that certain illnesses (typhoid fever, hepatic cirrhosis) can increase the host's toxic responsiveness to endotoxin just as other diseases can decrease it (malaria) (17).

Pearson (21) has described that environmental endotoxins are notably less pyrogenic than purified LPS. His study indicated that a given test may fail the

---

[b]See Chapter 9 for a discussion of the relationship of the units: EU versus nanogram.

5.0 EU/kg FDA cutoff [established by the Endotoxin Unit designation as 0.2 ng of FDA RSE EC-2 (3)], but may exhibit a low order of actual pyrogenicity. Thus, the routine use of purified LPS as a control standard serves as a "significant safety factor unwittingly built into LAL endotoxin limits when real-world endotoxins are assayed by LAL" and "the Limulus test 'overpredicts' pyrogenicity." This is due to the high correlation observed between the rabbit pyrogen test and the LAL test using purified LPS, but a much less predictable correlation (biased conservatively) between the pyrogen assay and endogenous endotoxin.[c] Nevertheless, the routine use of worst-case validation philosophy has been borne out as a viable scientific approach for demonstrating the absence of contaminants (in a manner analogous to the use of *Bacillus stearothermophilis* in sterilization validation) and is incorporated into official regulatory requirements the world over.

Relative Likelihood of Endotoxin Occurrence in Parenteral Drugs

A central question that arose upon the proposal to replace the rabbit pyrogen test with the LAL test, and one that deserves serious consideration, is: How can one be sure in testing only for endotoxin that other microbial pyrogens will not be allowed to go undetected in the parenteral manufacturing process? We have answered the question in part by considering the ubiquity, stability, and relative pyrogenicity of gram-negative bacterial endotoxin. But also the minimal growth requirements of gram-negative bacteria allow their growth in the cleanest of water. Conversely, the answer can be found by disqualifying from undue concern each type of non-gram-negative organism that could occur in parenteral manufacturing operations including (*i*) the environmental predisposition of organisms that prevent them from proliferating in largely water-based parenteral manufacturing processes, (*ii*) the relative ease of degradation of their by-products (except heat-stable exotoxins of gram-positive bacteria which have significant growth requirements), and (*iii*) modern aseptic manufacturing procedures and quality control methods required by current good manufacturing practices (cGMPs). A short list of significant organism types rarely encountered in pharmaceutical manufacturing processes are: gram-positive cocci, such as *Staphyloccoccus aureus* and *S. epidermidis*; gram-positive bacilli, such as *B. subtilis*; fungi, such as *Aspergillus niger* and *Candida albicans*; and anaerobes, such as *Clostridium difficile*. When such organisms are found, it is usually in air-borne, spot contamination of aseptic operations or via a human vector and not in significant numbers. A notable exception to the barren manufacturing environment is found in cell culture media, which have requirements for additional testing such as virus and mycoplasma species.

In debating the appropriateness of the replacement of the rabbit pyrogen assay with an assay specific only for endotoxin (LAL), it is often overlooked that although the rabbit pyrogen assay (like the LAL assay) is a good model for the human pyrogenic response, it is not a perfect model. Rabbits are a hundred times less responsive than man to interferon-α, a substance pyrogenic in humans and commercially manufactured as a recombinant parenteral product (9). In 1984, a lot of human growth hormone used in a clinical trial resulted in pyrogenic reactions in human subjects, even though it had passed both LAL and rabbit pyrogen testing

---

[c]Chapter 12 discusses the proposition that nonendotoxin microbial constituents can act synergistically with endotoxin to bring about a lower threshold response.

(22). Subsequent studies determined that the lot was contaminated with endotoxin during manufacture, before lyophilization in glycine phosphate buffer, resulting in a 10- to 20-fold reduction in endotoxin activity in both the in vivo rabbit model and the in vitro LAL model but, obviously, not in the human subjects. Therefore, the idea that the rabbit pyrogen assay (or any assay for that matter) can detect every possible pyrogen in parenteral solutions is a misconception. The FDA Biotechnology Inspection Guide (23) refers to the "EP assay" for use in testing biological pharmaceuticals that may only be pyrogenic in humans.

CONTAMINATION CONTROL PHILOSOPHY IN PARENTERAL MANUFACTURING

Endotoxin is a concern for people only when it comes into contact with the circulatory system. The two relevant mechanisms for such contact involve infection and medically invasive techniques including injection or infusion of parenteral solutions. A notable exception to limiting the concern for endotoxin to blood contact is the effect that minute, almost undetectable, quantities of endotoxin may have upon cell cultures in pharmaceutical manufacturing. Modern methods of manufacturing biologicals make use of complex cell culture media including the addition of fetal bovine serum (FBS) as a growth factor (which has been associated with microbial contamination) to grow mammalian cells for use as recombinant or monoclonal expression systems. Serum has presented manufacturers (and clinicians) difficulties in quantifying and reproducing endotoxin levels due to the presence of little-understood interference factors. This section discusses the philosophy and practicality of preventing the occurrence of microbial contamination in parenteral manufacturing processes.

Often, end product testing is thought to be the absolute determining factor in producing a quality product free of contaminants. However, recent emphasis has been placed on in-process testing and process validation. These have become as integral as end product analytical testing to providing the documented evidence that a product meets predetermined criteria of quality. The FDA guideline on validation of the LAL test as an "end product" test serves to illustrate the contrast between overtly stated requirements and cGMP expectations. The "end product" guideline (24) makes no specific mention of testing requirements for items other than the end products, but clearly a manufacturer would be cited in any FDA inspection for failure to conform to industry expectations for ensuring the suitability of a given manufactured product at each major step of a manufacturing process (CFR reference: 312.23 includes IND requirements for drug substances even at the investigational stage). LAL testing is routinely performed on the active pharmaceutical ingredient (API), bulk products, excipients (particularly those of natural origin), water, cell culture media, and additives, as well as vial and closure components used to contain the end product.

Some definitions of these various drug and in-process forms are in order. The following terms are used in the World Health Organization (WHO) GMP Guide as defined by Kopp-Kubel (25), and a description of the use of excipients is taken from the Handbook of Pharmaceutical Excipients (26):

- *Active pharmaceutical ingredient*: A substance or compound which is intended to be used in the manufacture of a pharmaceutical product as a pharmacologically active compound (ingredient).

- *Batch (or lot)*: A defined quantity of starting material or product processed in one process or series of processes with the expectation that it is homogeneous.
- *Bulk product*: Any product that has completed all processing stages up to, but not including, final packaging.
- *Finished product*: Any product that has undergone all stages of production, including packaging in its final container and labeling.
- *In-process control*: Checks performed during production in order to monitor and if necessary adjust the process to ensure that the product conforms to its specifications. The control of the environment or equipment may also be regarded as a part of in-process control.
- *Intermediate product*: Partly processed material which must undergo further manufacturing steps before it becomes a bulk product.
- *Excipients*: Serve as solvents, solubilizing, suspending, thickening, and chelating agents, antioxidants and reducing agents, antimicrobial preservatives, buffers, pH adjusting agents, bulking agents, and special additives.

Given the statistically low probability of finding a single contaminated vial in a given lot of product (at least for a nonhomogeneous contamination mechanism), the USP chapter on "Sterilization and Sterility Assurance of Compendial Articles" (Chapter 1211) describes the importance of process control in manufacturing. The following was presented in the context of sterility testing in the USP but can be applied to endotoxin sampling and subsequent testing:

> ... this absolute definition (of sterility) cannot currently be applied to an entire lot of finished compendial articles because of limitations in testing. Absolute sterility cannot be practically demonstrated without complete destruction of every finished article. The sterility of a lot purported to be sterile is therefore defined in probabilistic terms, where the likelihood of a contaminated unit or article is acceptably remote. Such a state of sterility assurance can be established only through the use of adequate sterilization cycles and subsequent aseptic processing, if any, under appropriate current good manufacturing practice, and not by reliance solely on sterility testing (27).

The USP chapter continues to outline the basic principles for validation and certification of a sterilizing and subsequent aseptic process. Though sterility is an absolute concept (i.e., contains no viable organisms), endotoxin content is not. There are acceptable, albeit low, levels of bacterial endotoxin allowed in drug products. The FDA (Appendix E) and USP (monograph) publication of tolerance limits (TL) and provision of TL formulae make this distinction. Nevertheless, it does not change the dependence on probabilistic product sampling; hence, the endotoxin test result, like the sterility test result, is not an absolute assurance of the lack of contamination except for the vial(s) consumed in the test.

> It should be recognized that the referee sterility test might not detect microbial contamination if present in only a small percentage of the finished articles in the lot because the specified number of units to be taken imposes a significant statistical limitation on the utility of the test results. This inherent limitation, however, has to be accepted since current knowledge offers no nondestructive alternatives for ascertaining the microbiological quality of every finished article in the lot, and it is not a feasible option to increase the number of specimens significantly (27).

Therefore, even passing the USP gel-clot assay does not provide an absolute guarantee that a drug meets the requirements of the compendia because of the statistical nature of the sampling. The FDA could still declare it adulterated by any number of other inspection criteria and could even obtain a sample, test it in its own laboratory, and determine that the drug is contaminated at the limit. The best way to ensure that a product meets the requirements of the compendia is by using the best test one can develop at levels below the TL at various stages throughout the manufacturing process.

The regulatory precautions set in place are, in many (if not most) cases, due to the poor probabilities associated with finding spot contamination by quality control sampling techniques. The generally accepted sterility acceptance level is often given as 10^{-6} (i.e., one possible survivor in a million units), but according to Akers and Agalloco (28) the value was selected as a convenience. They maintain that 10^{-6} is a minimal sterilization expectation and should be linked "to a specific bioburden model and/or particular biological indicator ... (otherwise) it is a meaningless number that imparts little knowledge on the actual sterilization process."

If the concept of sterility assurance seems somewhat less than rigorously defined when (by necessity) one strays from the absolute definition, then the concept of the bacterial endotoxin TL can also be viewed scientifically (not legally from a compliance point of view) as existing with a range with variability of its own. Values making up the TL calculation include the use of an average patient's weight, a maximum dose (that may be an actual dose subject to volumetric variances), a TPR with a range of its own, and (if present as in the case considering endotoxin content around the tolerance limit) an endogenous endotoxin content that is not *E. coli* LPS and is measured by a control standard endotoxin against a reference standard endotoxin defined by an average potency that sometimes varies widely in different laboratories. In this context, therefore, a passing result that is just under the TL can be viewed as a single sampling point of an endotoxin content that as a whole may be either above or below the TL cutoff. From a legal (compliance) standpoint, a single test may constitute a passing or failing (adulterated) product, which again is a good argument for controlling the endotoxin content of products to levels well below that which creates a dilemma as to whether the product is contaminated at the TL or not.

Bruch (29) relates that the PSI (probability of a survivor per item) for a can of chicken soup is 10^{-11} whereas the assurance provided by the USP sterility test alone is not much better than 10^{-2} given a 20 item sampling and is, as Bruch says, due to the rigorous heating cycles developed by the canning industry to prevent the possibility of survival of *Clostridium botulinum*. Bruch maintains that the industry has "never relied on a USP-type finished product sterility test to assess the quality of its canned goods ... (because) the statistics of detecting survivors are so poor that the public confidence ... would be severely compromised through outbreaks of botulism." He cites the generally accepted sterility assurance for a large volume parenteral item as 10^{-9}, and 10^{-4} for a small volume parenteral that has been aseptically filled and sterile filtered as opposed to terminally sterilized. The apparent contradiction in the necessity of more stringent sterility assurance for a can of soup than for a parenteral drug is due to the ability of organisms to grow in soup as opposed to the likelihood of such growth in the parenteral manufacturing environment (Table 1).

Validation has been defined as "establishing documented evidence which provides a high degree of assurance that a specific process will consistently produce a product meeting its predetermined specifications and quality attributes" (30). Sharp (31) has advocated a common-sense approach to validation while

TABLE 1 Probability of Survivor Estimates for Sterilized Items

Item	Probability of survivor/unit
Canned chicken soup[a]	10^{-11}
Large volume parenteral fluid	10^{-9}
Intravenous catheter and delivery set[a]	10^{-6}
Syringe and needle[a]	10^{-6}
Urinary catheters[a]	10^{-3}
Surgical drape kit[a]	10^{-3}
Small volume parenteral drug (sterile fill)	10^{-3}
Laparoscopic instruments processed with liquid chemical sterilants[b]	10^{-2}

[a]Dosimetric release: no sterility test.
[b]Limits of USP sterility test: $10^{-1.3}$ (with 95% confidence).
Source: From Ref. 29.

lambasting much of the specialized jargon that has grown up around the endeavor: "This, then, is validation. The action of proving (and in the more formal context, documenting the proof) that something 'works.'" Regulation is (of necessity) a function layered over acceptable and sound scientific and business practices to ensure that the lowest denominator manufacturers and/or manufacturing processes produce safe products. Although regulation is necessarily backward looking, validation should be a forward-looking exercise that meets or exceeds regulatory, scientific, and business requirements. If a process involves endotoxin removal, for example, then it is a good business practice to properly validate the process to avoid not only marketing a potentially contaminated product (the major concern), but also from having to destroy a costly drug product that has later been found to be contaminated (a major business concern). It is with this view that many excipient materials are today being tested. As the costs of drugs derived from biotechnology increase, so do the business-related requirements for ensuring that the raw materials that go into making the intermediates of the manufacturing process as well as end products meet appropriate and stringent predetermined specifications.

The concept of adulteration in drug and device manufacture stems from the Federal Food, Drug, and Cosmetic Act, which considers that a drug or device is adulterated if it does not comply with the provisions outlined in the Act (32). A drug is considered adulterated if it is "filthy, putrid or decomposed in whole or in part" (31), if its strength differs from that claimed, or if impurities are present. Though endotoxin content is not required to be absolutely absent as in sterility testing, the definition of "adulteration" cannot leave room for legal disagreement. Ultimately, the method listed in the USP monograph for a specific method serves as the final arbitrator of contamination from a legal standpoint. If the drug is listed in the "official compendium" (the USP in the United States) and the strength, purity, or quality is below the specific requirements listed in the monograph for that item, then it is considered adulterated by the FDA. According to Avallone (33), the FDA does recognize different levels of risk associated with different types of violations. He sites the situation of a sterility test failure as a very serious health hazard worthy of a Class I recall classification. The citation of a more general lack of sterility assurance (i.e., observations but not a direct analytical failure) due to the lack of cGMP conformance is considered a Class II recall classification (a less serious health hazard). Avallone gives three levels of philosophical compliance relating to the retesting and resolution of sterility failures exemplified by manufacturers (33,34):

(i) ... those who recognize the many limitations of aseptic processing and of the sterility test (when an initial positive test result occurs, they reject the batch);

(ii) ... others have this same concern when only gram-negative microorganisms show up on the initial test due to the virulence of the organism and because the organism would be more indicative of a process problem than one which might occur during testing (i.e., lab contamination)

(iii) ... other manufacturers have still another level of GMP philosophy and will do everything to justify the release of a product failing an initial sterility test (33).

It is not the FDA's responsibility to develop and promulgate the best methods for each specific type of analytical testing required to demonstrate the safety, identity, strength, purity, and quality of drugs. The USP (in the United States) serves as a repository for this purpose to a large extent and is an interface between government regulators and industry. The USP is cautious in the unique role that Congress has allowed it; change as a result of consensus often occurs slowly (35). Guidance has from time to time been felt by manufacturers to be lacking, whereas from a regulatory perspective it is perhaps just as well (from the vantage of protecting public safety) to make manufacturers aware of their general obligations and even to let them worry if they are meeting them, but not to dictate the best scientific solution for each situation. It is in these areas that specific manufacturers' scientific and validation proficiency will determine their compliance success. It is conceivable that good science can be lost in bureaucracy because of the elaborate internal requirements that have accumulated over the years. In such cases, the critical science that the regulations were formed to ensure can be neglected. Does the method make sense? Does it really prove what it purports to prove? Has a worst-case validation philosophy been applied? What can go wrong in the test? What is the worst that can happen? The manufacturer should be the expert in the manufacture of pharmaceuticals and contamination control with the appropriate regulatory body overseeing that the valid requirements that have accumulated over time (i.e., the "current" in cGMP requirements) are applied appropriately to ensure that the public will receive safe and effective medicines.

RETEST PHILOSOPHY

Relevant here is a discussion of the retest philosophy of any kind of (statistically gathered) out-of-specification (OOS) analytical result. The U.S. District Court of New Jersey (*U.S. v Barr Laboratories*) ruled that the FDA may not necessarily consider an OOS result automatically to be a test "failure" (36). The court ruled that an OOS due to a laboratory error [as opposed to manufacuturing process and nonprocess (operator) errors] may not be due to the sample itself. Such a result would bring about a laboratory failure investigation, which must be documented and completed in a timely manner. Furthermore, according to Madsen (36):

... the Court ruled that retesting is appropriate if the failure investigation has determined that retesting is appropriate. Retesting is not appropriate if the error was process-related or for product failures. Retesting must be done on the same sample that produced the original, failing test result. It can substitute for the original result if the error was due to an analytical mistake, and it can supplement the original result if the investigation is inconclusive. There should be a predetermined testing procedure defining when retesting ends and results should be considered in terms of overall batch and product history (36).

Each type of laboratory test has its own specific retest procedure and the bacterial endotoxin test is no exception. The FDA Guideline on Validation details the retest requirements as follows from the routine testing section; one can see the similarities to the sterility retest requirements:

> The sampling technique selected and the number of units to be tested should be based on the manufacturing procedures and the batch size. A minimum of three units, representing the beginning, middle, and end, should be tested from a lot. These units can be run individually or pooled. If the units are pooled and any endotoxin is detected, repeat testing can be performed. The LAL test may be repeated no more than twice. The first repeat consists of twice the initial number of replicates of the sample in question to examine the possibility that extrinsic contamination occurred in the initial assay procedure. On pooled samples, if any endotoxin is detected in the first repeat, proceed to second repeat. The second repeat consists of an additional 10 units tested individually. None of the 10 units tested in the second repeat may contain endotoxin in excess of the limit concentration for the drug product (24).

A point easily overlooked is that "if the units are pooled and any endotoxin is detected, repeat testing can be performed." The implication is, conversely, that if the units are tested individually and endotoxin is detected (at the limit concentration), repeat testing may not be performed if a laboratory error cannot be demonstrated by a detailed investigation. This situation presents manufacturers with another incentive to pool vials for testing (the first being reduced sample testing).

SAFEGUARDS FOR WATER USED IN PARENTERAL PHARMACEUTICAL MANUFACTURING

The predominate potential source of endotoxin in a pharmaceutical manufacturing environment is the purified water used as a raw material (also used in component sterile rinse depyrogenation processes). Many different grades of water are used and may be variously labeled according to their origin, the treatment they have undergone, quality, or use and different groups employ different nomenclature (37). The only water required to be tested for endotoxin content is "water for injection" (WFI) and purified water with endotoxin control and is prepared via a validated distillation or reverse osmosis process. Distillation is the preferred method and results in sterile, endotoxin-free condensate. However, any water may become contaminated via a number of subsequent distribution or storage mechanisms including: the cooling or heating system, storage container, or distribution method such as hoses.

Water used to manufacture WFI of necessity originates from a local water supply, such as a deep well or lake. Lake or surface water is known to contain higher levels of bacteria than deep well water sources. Prior to purification water contains a number of contaminants.

> Most raw or potable water used in pharmaceutical processes contains a wide variety of contaminating electrolytes, organic substances, gross particulate matter, dissolved gases, such as carbon dioxide, and microorganisms. Bacteria indigenous to fresh water are predominately gram-negative rods and include *Pseudomonas* sp., *Alcaligenes* sp., *Flavobacter* sp., *Chromobacter* sp., and *Serratia* sp. (37).

Drainage and decaying matter bring in *Bacillus, Klebsiella,* and *Enterobacter* species (37). Water susceptible to sewage drainage may include pathogens: fecal coliforms, *S. faecalis*, and *Clostridium* sp. Stored water may grow any of the above organisms and favors (endotoxin-containing) gram negatives. Water systems must employ stored water at some point and require microbiological monitoring to prevent the occurrence of contamination. Gaining an accurate perspective of the microbiological quality of water from any given system requires that the frequency, points of sampling, and test methods should be carefully chosen and performed in a timely manner. Bacteria can multiply rapidly after gaining entry into a water distribution system at one of several points such as outlets used as sampling ports, and may proliferate in "dead legs" of pipes, pumps, hoses, outlets, and meters. The *Federal Register* lists standards for potable water often used to feed pharmaceutical water manufacturing processes.

The USP specifies limits for both viable organisms and endotoxin levels that must be met for various purified water and WFI. The FDA has established relevant cGMPs for pharmaceutical manufacturing processes. Regulations governing the control of contamination of pharmaceutical manufacturing products and processes includes 21 CFR 211.22, describing the authority and role of quality control unit in approving or rejecting all drug products, containers, components closures, in-process materials, etc. and 21 CFR 211.113 requiring the designation of written procedures to prevent the occurrence of objectionable microorganisms in nonsterile drug products and all microorganisms in drug products purported to be sterile.

The above requirements, while only a limited referencing of existing requirements, illustrate the degree to which pharmaceutical manufacturers (are required to) ensure the identity, safety, purity, strength, and quality of the production of sterile water and maintenance of the suitable manufacturing control over the environment and materials used in parenteral manufacturing according to cGMP requirements. Manufacturing operations are required to produce a parenteral drug that are guaranteed to do no harm to the patient from a microbiological perspective. Furthermore, as we have seen, endotoxin due to its enduring nature and low contaminating levels, presents the industry with what may be thought of as a "worst case" microbiological indicator.

CONTAMINATED WATER CAN GET WORSE

Travenol Laboratories (38) monitored the pyrogenicity of increasing doses of gram-negative bacteria using the LAL assay and the rabbit pyrogen test. *Klebsiella pneumoneae, Pseudomonas putida, E. coli, Serratia marcescen*, and *P. aeruginosa* were suspended in sterile distilled water that contained no demonstrable endotoxin as measured by the LAL assay. All bacteria that were evaluated induced a rabbit test failure at approximately 10^5 bacteria per milliliter when tests were performed just after suspension was made. Representative data are presented in Table 2. When the same solutions were tested using rabbit and LAL assays one year later, rabbit test failures and LAL test failures showed significantly altered thresholds. For example, original test results on *S. marcescens* showed clear LAL and rabbit test failure at 1.0×10^5 organisms per milliliter, but one year later 1.8×10^3 bacteria/mL remained in the solution and produced significant LAL and rabbit test failures. These data demonstrate the striking ability of *S. marcescens* to survive in distilled water for protracted periods of time and the capacity of heavily contaminated solutions to become more pyrogenic over time, even though viable counts decrease.

It is interesting that although viable cell counts decreased by approximately two orders of magnitude over one year, the number of viable cells required to

TABLE 2 Pyrogenicity of Whole Gram-Negative Bacteria

Bacterial strain	Viable count $(? \times 10^5)$	Sum of temperature increase, three-rabbit test	LAL test (pg/mL)[a]
K. pneumoniae	2.0	3.10	>200
P. putida	1.7	2.35	>200
E. coli	3.6	3.20	106
S. marcescens	1.0	2.30	166
P. aeruginosa	1.0	2.75	114

[a]The threshold pyrogenic response level is about 1 ng (1000 pg) per kilogram for *E. coli* and *S. typhosa* (approximately 0.1–1.0) and 50 to 70 ng/kg for *Pseudomonas*.
Abbreviation: LAL, *Limulus* amebocyte lysate.

induce a pyrogenic response and an LAL failure also decreased by two orders of magnitude. These results clearly indicate the continuous release of endotoxin by cells undergoing autolysis and suggest the biosynthesis of new endotoxin during the hold time. The results of a typical experiment using *P. putida* can be seen in Table 3. The LAL test produced failures one order of magnitude earlier than the rabbit pyrogen test did when 50 pg endotoxin per milliliter (referenced to *E. coli* 055:B5) was used as a pass–fail limit.

CELL CULTURE SUSCEPTIBILITY TO ENDOTOXIN CONTAMINATION

Endotoxin contamination is a critical concern in vertebrate tissue culture media and growth additives. The introduction of the LAL test brought about the revelation that most tissue culture media and additives contained high levels of endotoxin (39,40). Though establishing that cell cultures were routinely contaminated, these researchers did not quantify the levels or establish that the contamination had a deleterious effect on the culture or resultant by-products. Animal serum can be a significant source of endotoxin in tissue culture media. Gould (41) tested the fetal bovine serum (FBS) from ten different manufacturers and found endotoixin concentrations from 6 pg/mL to 0.8 µg/mL. Gould relates that early findings of contamination led many serum manufacturers to take extra care in the collection and

TABLE 3 Pyrogenicity of Whole *Pseudomonas putida* ATCC 12633

	Test performed just after suspension is made			Test performed 1 yr later		
Counts/mL	LAL estimate (pg/mL)	Sum of temperature increases (three-rabbit test)	Counts/mL	LAL estimate (pg/mL)	Sum of temperature increases (three-rabbit test)
0 (Negative control)	0.5	0.30	0	7	0.3
20	4	0.35	15	9	0.15
2×10^2	16.5	0.35	0	18	0.60
3×10^3	50	0.30	0	28	0.25
2.3×10^4	134	1.25	1.1×10^3	59	1.70
1.7×10^5	>200	2.35	4.0×10^3	102	1.90
1.6×10^6	>200	4.15	2.5×10^4	135	4.45

LAL test produced failures one order of magnitude earlier than the rabbit pyrogen test did when 50 pg endotoxin per milliliter (referenced to *E. coli* 055:B5) was used as a pass-fail limit.
Abbreviation: LAL, *Limulus* amebocyte lysate.

handling of blood used to make serum to ensure that their sera contain low levels of endotoxin. Being a blood product, serum is highly prone to gram-negative bacterial overgrowth subsequent to slaughterhouse collection, transport, and (like a food product) temperature abuse and contain high levels of gram-negative organisms in its raw, collected state.

The use of the LAL test allowed the detection of contamination in serum, but the use of LAL to quantify endotoxin in serum has demonstrated significant variability of results. Gould and others (41,42) suggest that the serum serves as a lipid detoxifying agent in which LPS is reversibly disaggregated to such an extent that it does not react well with LAL and that the lipid concentration may vary between batches of serum. A method that has been used to inactivate some of the capacity of serum samples to interfere with the LAL method is to heat the sample at 70°C in a water bath for 10 minutes prior to dilution and subsequent LAL testing.

Some manufactured biotechnology products today are cytokines (interferons, interleukins, growth factors, etc.) and the effects of the presence of minute amounts of endotoxin in such products may be the source of clinical and/or analytical confusion. According to Gould (41):

> Only after the effects of endotoxin have been measured under controlled conditions can investigators determine the extent of variability introduced by subnanogram amounts of endotoxin. They may then make realistic decisions regarding acceptable concentrations of endotoxin in cell culture media and additives.

Dawson (43) lists a number of products (other than cytokines) whose synthesis in cell culture is either enhanced or inhibited by endotoxin. Those he lists as being enhanced include: prostaglandin, acid phosphatase, fibrinolytic inhibitor, collagenase production, nerve growth factor, secretion of factor B, polypeptides, platelet activating factor, adhesion inhibitor, adhesion molecule-1, and procoagulant. Those listed as being inhibited include: angiotensin converting enzyme activity and synthesis of proteoglycan and alpha 2 macroglobulin. Both the amount and bacterial type of endotoxin contamination may affect the production of products from cell culture processes. Drug developers will do well to ensure that their cell culture media are as endotoxin-free as possible to avoid potential study variation as variable endotoxin content may confound a number of study criteria. Drugs designed to have immunostimulatory, mitogenic, or tumoricidal activity may be affected by the presence of endotoxin and the effect may vary with differing amounts of (very low) contamination present from batch to batch. Note that if the levels vary but remain below the limit of detection or at least below the specification assigned to it, then the endotoxin effects (not content as this is an expression system and not yet a product) will be most likely not even be a consideration in any investigation into the cause of lot-to-lot variability in either clinical efficacy or manufacturing efficiency.

INSTANCES OF PHARMACEUTICAL CONTAMINATION IN THE LAL ERA

In contrast to the occurrence of fever that has plagued man for centuries and has been associated with many of the most devastating diseases including plague, cholera, typhus, polio, etc. (Chapter 1), the occurrence of contamination in parenteral drugs, devices, and infusion and transfusion solutions has been relatively rare since the introduction of the LAL test. This is a testimony to both industry and

---

Case 1

October 1996: 35 newborns died in a small hospital in Roraima, Brazil (44). The deaths were >3X the normal death rate for the hospital nursery. The Brazilian Ministry of Health requested the CDC's assistance in an investigation which revealed that locally manufactured intravenous solutions were contaminated with endotoxin. Sampling of parenteral fluids was tested by the LAL method with the following results.

All cultures of these solutions were negative for bacterial growth. However, 6 of 13 unopened vials of bidistilled WFI and 12 of 15 unopened vials of 25% glucosehad elevated levels of 0.8 to 5.8 endotoxin units (EU)/mL (mean: 3.8 EU/mL) and 0.8 to 1.9 EU/mL (mean: 1.2 EU/mL), respectively. The USP endotoxin limit on WFI is 0.25 EU/mL and for glucose (5–7%) is 0.5 EU/mL. Caked amorphous-like material and bacterial cells were observed by scanning electron microscopy in samples of bidistilled water containing elevated levels of endotoxin.[d,e]

November 1996: 33 infant deaths were attributed to unopened vials of distilled water used to dilute IV medications (also) in Brazil in a single hospital. Though not tabulated in this reference, the outbreak was reported to have occurred nationally (45).

Red blood cell (RBC) transfusion is rarely associated with bacteremia and sepsis with gram negative, endotoxin containing, bacteria. MMWR (46) reported 10 cases of sepsis from RBC's specifically contaminated with *Yersinia enterocolitica* during the March 1991 to November 1996 period and cites 11 cases as having occurred during the November 1985 to February 1991 period. The transfusions were associated with "fever, chills, or respiratory distress." Five of the 10 more recent cases resulted in death within at least six days of the transfusion.

In Maine (1990) two patients developed fever and hypertension within two hours postsurgery (47). An investigation revealed that the likely cause was an intravenous anesthetic (propofol) contaminated by an infusion pump. *Moraxella osloensis* was cultured from the pump and LAL assays revealed 3900 to 5000 ng/mL of endotoxin. Implicating the pump as well was the fact that "cultures and endotoxin assays of unopened ampules of propofol from the same lot being used at the hospital were negative." The other cases of extrinsic contamination of the same drug, propofol, involved a gram-positive organism (*S. aureus*) and a yeast (*C. albicans*).

---

regulatory participants as well as a testimony to the LAL assay itself. Though scattered and usually limited in severity, there have been numerous events involving contaminated fluids introduced into unsuspecting patients. Examples are shown

---

[d]*MMWR Editorial Note*: Such reactions are highly dependent on the body mass of the patient. Because the minimal pyrogenic dose of endotoxin is 5 EU/kg, 2 to 3 mL of the contaminated bidistilled water (mean level of contamination: 3.8 EU/mL) would have been sufficient to evoke a pyrogenic reaction in an average 4 lbs, 8 oz (2000 g) infant. As a result, IV administration of these endotoxin-contaminated fluids explained the increased number of febrile reactions detected during this outbreak. All infants receiving parenteral medications were receiving bidistilled water and glucose. Attack rates of 70% among these infants suggest that not all lots of bidistilled water and glucose were contaminated.

[e]*MMWR Editorial Note*: Unopened vials of contaminated medication were undamaged and had no evidence of tampering, suggesting that contamination most likely occurred during the manufacturing process. Without appropriate manufacturing processes, endotoxin can contaminate solutions and reagents. Many gram-negative organisms, which can release endotoxin, require few nutrients and can grow in distilled water at 39.2°F (4°C). In addition, endotoxins can survive exposure to steam autoclaving, organic solvents, acids, ethanol, and sterilizing liquids. Only dry heat [greater than or equal to 482°F (greater than or equal to 250°C) for 30 minutes or greater than or equal to 356°F (greater than or equal to 180°C) for 3 hours] can assure the elimination of endotoxin.

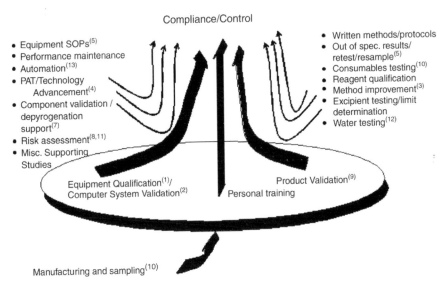

Compliance/Control

- Equipment SOPs[5]
- Performance maintenance
- Automation[13]
- PAT/Technology Advancement[4]
- Component validation / depyrogenation support[7]
- Risk assessment[8,11]
- Misc. Supporting Studies

- Written methods/protocols
- Out of spec. results/ retest/resample[5]
- Consumables testing[10]
- Reagent qualification
- Method improvement[3]
- Excipient testing/limit determination
- Water testing[12]

Equipment Qualification[1]/ Computer System Validation[2]

Personal training

Product Validation[9]

Manufacturing and sampling[10]

Selected References:

(1) Hubber, L., Validation of computerized analytical and networked systems, interpharm Press, Englewood, CO, 2002.
(2) 21 CFR Part 11: http://www.fda.gov/cder/guidance/5667fnl.htm
(3) Cooper, J.F., Resolving LAL Test Interferences, Journ. Science & Technology, vol. 44 (1). Jan./Feb. 1990, pp. 13–15.
(4) http://www.fda.gov/cder/guidance/6419fnl.htm
(5) United States District Court For the District of New Jersey, USA, Plaintiff, v. Barr Laboratories Inc., Civil Action No. 92-1744.
(6) USP-29 NF-24 Chapter <85>
(7) 21 CFR 211.80 Subpart E- Control of Components and Drug Product Containers and Colsures
(8) http://www.fda.gov/cder/guidance/index.htm
(9) FDA Guideline on Validation of the Limulus Amebocyte Lysate Test as an End-Product Test for Human and Animal Parenteral Drugs, Biological Products, and Medical Devices, Dec. 1987: http://www.fda.gov/cder/gdlns/lal.pdf
(10) http://www.fda.gov/cder/guidance/5882fnl.htm
(11) http://www.fda.gov/oc/guidance/gmp.htm
(12) USP-29 NF-24 Chapter <1231>
(12) USP-29 NF-24 Chapter <16>

FIGURE 3 Compliance and control references. *Abbreviation*: SOP, standard operating procedure; PAT, process analytical technology.

in Case 1. The instances are anecdotal and many other instances likely occur and go unreported due to their transitory nature and the fact that parenteral drug and medical device use occurs concurrent with disease.

Endotoxin-like reactions were associated with a contaminated batch of gentamicin traced back to the bulk drug used that was manufactured in China (48). The reactions were discovered in seven states. Of the 222 patients documented (some were excluded for various reasons) to have received the antibiotic, 24 had a definite adverse reaction. The off-label, once daily dose being used for pharmacological reasons (lower kidney toxicity, etc.) put the patients at risk due to the endotoxin content at that greater dose around the TPR. This episode is discussed as a case study in Chapter 12.

COMPLIANCE AND CONTROL REFERENCES

There are a myriad of control points to control endotoxin in the manufacture of parenteral drugs with quality control oversight being one. More and more such oversight is not layered onto the end product via an end product test, but is built in to the entire process of manufacturing parenteral drugs from the first acquisition of a raw material to the final filling of the final vial of a batch. Figure 3 highlights from a quality control vantage three "silos" of compliance and associates relevant references with each.

REFERENCES

1. Mayer H, Weckesser J. The Protein component of bacterial endotoxin. In: Rietschel ET, ed. Handbook of Endotoxin. Elsevier Science Publishers, 1984:339.
2. Dinarello CA. Production of endogenous Pyrogen. FASEB 1979; 38:52–56.
3. Hochstein HD. The LAL test versus the rabbit Pyrogen test for endotoxin detection. Pharm Technol 1987; 1:124–129.
4. Raetz C et al. Gram negative endotoxin: an extraordinary lipid with profound effects on eukaryotic signal transduction. FASEB 1991; 5(12):2652–2660.
5. Rietschel et al. Bacterial endotoxins: molecular relationship of structure to activity and function. FASEB 1994; 18(Feb):217–225.
6. Bowman JP et al. Diversity and association of psychrophilic bacteria in antarctic sea ice. Appl Environ Micro 1997; 63(8):3068–3078.
7. Stanley JT, Gosink JJ. Poles apart: biodiversity and biogeography of sea ice bacteria. Annu Rev Microbiol 1999; 53(1):189–215.
8. Novitsky TJ. Discovery to commercilization: the blood of the horseshoe crab. Oceanus 1991; 27(1):13–18.
9. Dinarello CA et al. New concepts in the pathogenisis of fever. Rev Infect Dis 1988; 10(1):168–189.
10. Dinarello CA, Wolff SM. Molecular basis of fever in humans. Am J Med 1982; 72(May):799–819.
11. Kluger MJ et al. The adaptive value of fever. In: Infectious Disease Clinics of North America. W. B. Saunders: Philadelphia, 1996:1–20.
12. Kluger MJ. Fever: role of pyrogens and cryogens. Physiol Rev 1991; 71(1):93–127.
13. Beveridge TJ. Structures of gram-negative cell walls and their derived membrane vesicles. J Bacteriol 1999; 181(16):4725–4733.
14. Swarbrick E, Boyan JC, eds. Pyrogen and depyrogenation. In: Encyclopedia of Pharmaceutical Technology. New York: Marcel Dekker, 1988:467.
15. Alberts B et al. Membrane Structure. Molecular Biology of the Cell. 3rd ed., ch. 10. New York: 9–13. Garland Publishing, 1994.
16. Horn DL, Opal SM, Lomastro E. Antibiotics, cytokines, and endotoxin: a complex and evolving relationship in gram-negative sepsis. Scand J Infect Dis 1996; 101:9–13.
17. Greisman S. Hornick RB. Comparative pyrogenic reactivity of rabbit and man to bacterial endotoxin. Proc Soc Exp Biol Med 1969.
18. Weary ME. Pyrogens and pyrogen testing. In: Swarbrick E, Boyan JC, eds. Encyclopedia of Pharmaceutical Technology. New York: Marcel Dekker, 1988:179–205.
19. Braude et al. Fever from pathogenic fungi. J Clin Invest 1960; 39:1266–1276.
20. Wolff SM. Biological effects of bacterial endotoxin in man. J Infect Dis 1973; 128(suppl):S259–S264.
21. Pearson F. A comparison of the pyrogenicity of environmental endotoxins and lipopolysaccharides. LAL Rev 1984; Summer:2–3.
22. Dinarello CA et al. Human leucocyte pyrogen test for detection of pyrogenic material in growth hormone produced by recombinant *Escherichia coli*. J Clin Micro 1984; 20(3): 323–329.
23. FDA. FDA Biological Inspection Guide Reference Materials and Training Aids. U.S. Department of Health and Human Services, Division of Field Investigations, 1991.
24. U.S. Dept. of Health and Human Services, FDA Guideline on Validation of the *Limulus* Amebocyte Lysate Test as an End-Product Endotoxin Test for Human and Animal Parenteral Drugs, Biological Products, and Medical Devices. Dec 1987.

25. Kopp-Kubel S. Compendial issues: WHO. J Parenter Sci Technol 1992; 46(6):201–205.
26. Wade A, Weller PJ, eds. Handbook of Pharmaceutical Excipients. Washington and London: American Pharmaceutical Association and the Pharmaceutical Press, 1994.
27. USP. Sterilization and Sterility Assurance of Compendial Articles, ch. 1211. USP, 2000. Rockville, Maryland.
28. Akers J, Agalloco J. Sterility and sterility assurance. J Parenter Sci Technol 1997; 51(2): 72–77.
29. Bruch CW. Quality assurance for medical devices. In: Avis KE, Lieberman HA, Lachman L, eds. Pharmaceutical Dosage Forms: Parenteral Medications. New York: Marcel Dekker, 1993:487–526.
30. FDA. Guideline on General Principles of Process Validation. Rockville, Maryland: FDA, 1987.
31. Sharp J. Validation—how much is required? PDA J Pharm Sci Technol 1995; 49(3): 111–118.
32. Munson TE et al. Federal regulation of parenterals. In: Avis KE, Lieberman HA, Lachman L, eds. Phamaceutical Dosage Forms: Parenteral Medications. New York: Marcel Dekker, 1993:289–361.
33. Avallone HL. Sterility retesting. PDA J Sci Technol 1986; 40(2):56–57.
34. Russell E, Madsen J. U.S. vs. Barr laboratories: a technical perspective. PDA J Pharm Sci Technol 1994; 48(4):176–179.
35. Rothschild A. FDA regulations and guidelines. PDA J Sci Technol 1990; 44(1):26–29.
36. Madsen RE. U.S. vs. Barr laboratories: a technical perspective. PDA J Sci Technol 1994; 48(4):176–179.
37. Artiss DH. Water systems validation. In: Carlton FJ, Agalloco J, eds. Valid. Aseptic Pharm Processes. New York: Marcel Dekker, 1998:207–251.
38. Pearson F. Pyrogens, Endotoxins, LAL Testing, and Depyrogenation. New York: Marcel Dekker, Inc., 1985.
39. Bito LZ. Inflammatory effects of endotoxin-like contaminants in commonly used protein preparations. Science 1977; 196:83–85.
40. Fumarola D, Jirillo E. Endotoxin contamination of some commercial preparations used in experimental research. In: Cohen E, ed. Biomedical applications of the horseshoe crab (Limulidae). New York: Alan R. Liss, Inc.,1979:379–385.
41. Gould MC. Endotoxin in Vertebrate Cell Culture: Its Measurement and Significance, Uses and Standardization of Vertebrate Cell Cultures. Monograph 5, 1984.
42. Berger D et al. Correlation between endotoxin-neutralizing capacity of human plasma as tested by the limulus-amebocyte-lysate-test and plasma protein levels. FESB letters 1990; 277(1,2):33–36.
43. Dawson ME. LAL Update, Associates of Cape Cod, 1988; 16(1). Newletter published by the LAL manufacturer ACC at Falmouth, Mass http://www.acciusa.com.
44. Clinical sepsis and death in a newborn nursery associated with contaminated parenteral medications—Brazil, 1996. Morb Mortal Wkly Rep 1998; 47(29):610–612.
45. HIP investigates infant deaths in Brazil. In: National Center for Infectious Diseases. CDC 1997; 1.
46. Red blood cell transfusions contaminated with *Yersinia enterocolitica*—United States, 1991–1996, and Initiation of a national study to detect bacterial-associated transfusion reactions. Morb Mortal Wkly Rep 1997; 46(24):553–555.
47. Postsurgical infections associated with an extrinsically contaminated intravenous anesthetic agent—California, Illinois, Maine, and Michigan. Morb Mortal Wkly Rep 1999; 39(25):426–427, 433.
48. Endotoxin-like reactions associated with intravenous Gentamicin—California. CDC Morb Mortal Wkly Rep, www.cdc.gov/mmwrhtml/00055322.htm.

3

Fever and the Host Response

Kevin L. Williams

Eli Lilly & Company, Indianapolis, Indiana, U.S.A.

Metazoans are born with the genetically encoded knowledge of the artifacts and signatures that arise from the "bad guys" of the microbial world. . . .

FEVER AND THE HOST RESPONSE TO ENDOTOXIN

From an early date, investigators realized that there was more to the febrile (fever) response than a simple reaction of the body to bacterial infection. Burdon-Sanderson in 1896 (1) described an additional fever mechanism commonly observed (other than that caused by infection). In cases of sever trauma or fractures in which the skin was not broken and, therefore, in which no bacterial infection could have occurred, fever was commonly observed. Albert Charrin claimed that cells contained "thermogenic substances" (1) and substances from which thermogenic substances could be generated. These concepts were forerunners of today's modern understanding of a complex host response (of which fever is a component) to a variety of exogenous triggers (of which endotoxin is considered the most potent) via endogenous mediators known as cytokines. Lewis Thomas, in *Lives of a Cell* (2) vividly described the host response to endotoxin as follows:

> The gram-negative bacteria . . . display lipopolysaccharide (LPS) endotoxin in their walls, and these macromolocules are read by our tissues as the very worst of bad news. When we sense lipopolysaccharide, we are likely to turn on every defense at our disposal; we will bomb, defoliate, blockade, seal off, and destroy all the tissues in the area. Leukocytes become more actively phagocytic, release lysosomal enzymes, turn sticky, and aggregate together in dense masses, occluding capillaries and shutting off the blood supply. Complement is switched on at the right point in its sequence to release chemotactic signals, calling in leukocytes from everywhere. Vessels become hyper-reactive to epinephrine so that physiologic concentrations suddenly possess necrotizing properties. Pyrogen is released from leukocytes, adding fever to hemorrhage, necrosis, and shock. It is a shambles. All of this seems unnecessary, panic-driven. There is nothing intrinsically poisonous about endotoxin, but it must look awful, or feel awful, when sensed by cells. Cells believe that it signifies the presence of gram-negative bacteria, and they will stop at nothing to avoid this threat. . . It is, basically, a response to propaganda. . . .

Fever is historically the most studied of host responses to exogenous pyrogen. Fever serves a purpose as a host survival mechanism in all vertebrates. Dinarello et al., cited evidence of this, including leukocyte migration into infected dermal sites in lizards (3), reduction of microbial reproduction at elevated host temperatures (4), and augmentation of mammalian lymphocyte function (5–7). Skarnes et al. (11) cite several studies that correlate increased body temperature with improved survival from bacterial infections. In one such study, Vaughn et al. (8) administered an antipyretic drug concomitantly with introduction of bacterial infection into the preoptic-anterior hypothalamus of rabbits. The antipyretic reduced fevers by about 50% and this group of rabbits had significantly increased mortality compared to the control group.

In the bloodstream, two early or acute phase events occur in response to bacterial infection: attack by serum proteins called complement and attachment (opsonization) or engulfment (phagocytosis) by tissue-resident or circulating host cells, called monocytes and macrophages. In the presence of LPS or bacterial microbial pyrogens, monocytes/macrophages become "activated." The activation of macrophages can be seen microscopically as host monocyte/macrophage cells change from their normally rounded shape to an extremely elongated form as shown in Figure 1 (9).

Upon activation, these host cells release cytokines, a family of small molecular weight soluble protein or glycoprotein molecules, which exercise powerful effects on surrounding tissues and distant organs. Some of these cytokines travel through the blood to the hypothalamus (notably Interleukin-1 and TNF-α), the body's thermoregulatory center in the brain. The temperature of the body is regulated via the (preoptic/anterior) hypothalamus, a part of the brain responsible for regulating involuntary (so-called vegetative) functions such as hunger and sleep, by secreting several neurocrine-releasing factors (brain prostaglandins) (10).

Once in the brain, cytokines stimulate cells to produce arachidonic acid metabolites (including cyclooxygenase-derived prostaglandins, prostacyclins, and thromboxanes). Prostaglandin E_2 (PGE$_2$) is believed to be the major arachidonic acid metabolite associated with adjusting the hypothalamic setting to a febrile level (11,12). Evidence of this includes elevated cerebral spinal fluid PGE$_2$ levels and antipyretic blockage of the cyclooxygenase pathway (13), cytokine stimulation of PGE$_2$ production in vitro in hypothalamic tissue, and fever induction only minutes after the injection of PGE$_2$ directly into the hypothalamus (12) (Fig. 2)

All vertebrates, even reptiles considered to be cold-blooded, have the ability to regulate their body temperature, either biochemically or through their behavior. The hypothalamus contains thermosensitive neurons that discharge to adjust for

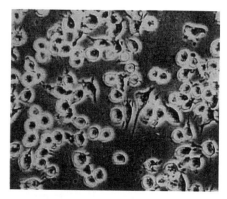
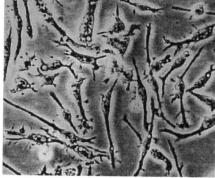

FIGURE 1 Macrophages (*left*) spread and enlarge (*right*) when they are exposed to lipopolysaccharides, indicating that they have become activated. The cells, which play a central role in inflammation and immunity and can kill cancer cells, secrete dozens of factors, including tumor necrosis factor, that carry out many of their activities. *Abbreviation*: LPS, lipopolysaccharide. *Source*: From Ref. 9.

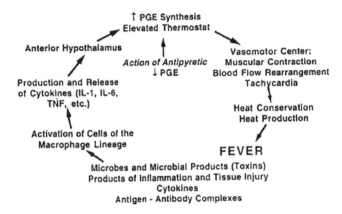

FIGURE 2 The sequential events that produce fever in humans and animals. *Abbreviations*: IL, interleukin; PGE, prostaglandin E_2; TNF, tumor necrosis factor. *Source*: From Ref. 76.

the temperature of the blood supply and in response to nerve stimuli from heat receptors in the skin and muscle tissues (10). Hypothalamic control has been likened to a home thermostat (10,14). Normally, in healthy people, it is set and performs within a narrow range ($\pm 10°C$), but during infection is reset to a higher level. Fever is, therefore, a controlled rise in the body's temperature beyond the normal range resulting from a change in the hypothalamic set point. Hyperthermia is different in that it occurs when the body's temperature rises above the hypothalamic set point due to either impairment of the body's heat-dissipating ability by drugs, through disease, or via extreme environmental effects (excessive heat).

The fundamental requirement for any substance to be considered a pyrogen is its ability to raise the hypothalamic set point by bringing about the manufacture of arachidonic metabolites. To accomplish this feat, two conditions must be met: (*i*) actual resetting of the set point and (*ii*) retention of the body's routine ability to regulate heat production or loss. Therefore, for fever to occur the normal operation of the central nervous system (CNS) is required. Drugs that affect neural transmission can short-circuit thermo-regulation resulting in fever or its suppression (10). The underlying principal of fever production is that exogenous pyrogens (LPS, bacteria, toxins, etc.) cause fever by inducing the host's cells (macrophages/ monocytes) to produce cytokines and other mediators, which in turn increase the production of arachidonate metabolites (10). As can be seen in Figure 2, the step of activation via exogenous pyrogen may be bypassed entirely upon injection with endogenous pyrogen to produce identical results. Additionally, endogenous pyrogens may induce the production of more of their kind (10) including: antigen-antibody complexes, androgenic steroid metabolites, inflammatory bile acids, complement components, and additional cytokines.

A difference in the pattern of fever response can be observed in the administration of endogenous versus exogenous pyrogens (11). Endogenous pyrogen injection induces a rapid, monophasic fever curve whereas the curve associated with large doses of exogenous pyrogen (including endotoxin) is biphasic, in that it rises rapidly but falls off and rises again before subsiding. The delayed effect of the second rise is presumably due to the production of additional endogenous pyrogen(s). The injection of low levels of endotoxin is monophasic, but of a slower onset than endogenous pyrogen. The slower onset time for endotoxin is, again, due to the time needed to produce the mediators that affect the hypothalamic set point (10).

Endogenous pyrogens (whether injected or induced via exogenous pyrogen) affect the production of arachidonic acid metabolites, mostly prostaglandin, derived from cyclooxygenase with resultant fever. Aspirin, acetaminophen, ibuprofen, and other antipyretics block cyclooxygenase production and not endogenous pyrogen production (15). The body's thermostat can be "turned down" to normal again if the concentration of endogenous pyrogen falls, if prostaglandin synthesis is blocked by antipyretics, or if endogenous antipyretics are introduced, such as inhibitors of protein synthesis that act to halt the synthesis of enzymes involved in producing PGE_2 (16,17).

Fever is, of course, only the most obvious portion of the underlying host response to invasion by microbes and microbial by-products such as endotoxin. The onset of fever has historically served as the only standard for gauging the allowable levels of such contaminants in parenteral drugs. However, given the advancements in knowledge surrounding the adverse host induction capacity of cytokines at sub-threshold pyrogenic response levels (Gentamicin Case Study in Chapter 13), some have suggested that the industry "must also consider that inflammatory reactions occur in the absence of fever" (18) and have suggested that the conformation of such currently unmonitored deleterious effects "would require the introduction of new testing procedures and a reevaluation of pyrogenicity standards."

ROUTES OF HOST INVASION AND TYPES OF ORGANISMS IMPLICATED

Sepsis is a modern epidemic created by the success of medical technology (19). The use of antibiotic therapy, invasive medical procedures and devices, immunosuppressive therapy for transplant patients, radiation and chemotherapy in cancer patients, an increased elderly population and those with serious underlying diseases, as well as the gathering of patients into critical care units and nursing homes have all contributed to increasing the pool of potential sepsis victims (20). The use of antibiotics has paralleled the rise in the number of fatal infections due to gram-negative bacteria as a result of (*i*) the fact that antibiotics "select" for gram-negative organisms (due in part to LPS provided protection from antibiotic efficacy) and (*ii*) the rise of increased bacterial antibiotic resistance (21).

Studies have implicated various organisms including *Klebsiella* (*K. pneumoniae*), *Enterobacter*, *Serratia*, and *Escherichia coli* as frequently implicated gram-negative organisms (bacteremia) in the hospital (nosocomial) environment in which sepsis predominates (22). However, according to Bone, more recently 55% of such infections were caused by gram-positive organisms, particularly *Staphylococcus epidermidis* ("associated with long-term indwelling catheters") (23). A notable study (SENTRY Antimicrobial Surveillance Program) was undertaken in 1997 to determine the predominant pathogens and antimicrobial resistance patterns of nosocomial and community-acquired infections in a wide group of Sentinel hospitals in the United States, Canada, South America, and Europe (72 sites total)(24). The program is intended to span a—five to ten years period, but the current report only includes the first six months of the study, which monitored a total of 5,058 bloodstream infections (BSI). The two most frequent isolates were *S. aureus* and *E. coli*, after which coagulase-negative staphylococci and enterococci predominated. Notable among the top ten offenders were *Klebsiella* spp., *Enterobacter* spp., *Pseudomonas aeruginosa*, *S. pneumoniae*, and β-hemolytic streptococci (24). The preliminary results among 4119 U.S. BSI cases, 20% were of nosocomial origin (acquired after 72 hours of hospitalization), 36% were non-nosocomial or community acquired, and 44% could not be determined one way or the other. According to Reimer et al. (25) "many septic episodes are nosocomial and in some hospitals represent a majority; such episodes may be due to microorganisms with increased antimicrobial resistance and are associated with greater mortality than are community-acquired episodes." Results of a 2006 update of that continuing study (26) revealed that *S. aureus* (∼19% vs. ∼ 17% *E. coli*) and *E. coli* (∼39% vs. ∼15% *S. aureus*) are the two most frequent isolates from inpatient and outpatient respectively, given the ongoing survey from 1998 to March 2005, and based on a total of 3,209,413 bacterial isolates.

Bodily routes of invasion include: genitourinary tract, gastrointestinal tract, biliary tract, and respiratory tract. Invasion more typically occurs as a result of drainage from a primary locus of infection (i.e., from the lymphatic to vascular system) or direct medical intervention such as from devices, needles, catheters, or graft material (25). Transfusion of bacterially contaminated blood has also been implicated as a significant source of bacterial sepsis (27). Beebe and Koneman (28) have described the recovery of uncommon bacteria as well as a greater prevalence of polymicrobic bacteremia from the blood as a routine occurrence in cancer patients, presumably due to the breakdown of the host's defense mechanisms and the resultant susceptibility to microbial invasion and proliferation. They list cancer chemotherapy and intravenous catheterization as allowing a host–barrier break for microbes while associated liver disease renders the host less able to rid the circulatory system of invaders (Table 1).

INNATE IMMUNITY AND THE ACUTE HOST RESPONSE

The understanding of the mechanisms of innate immunity[a] has increased in the past few years, since Charles Janeway first theorized the broad mechanism of their action in the late 1980s. Endotoxin has served as a prototype for understanding the mode of operation of pathogen associated microbial patterns (PAMPs) and has led to the knowledge of host pattern recognition receptors (PRRs), the most relevant of which are known specifically as Toll-like receptors (TLR). These "innate" receptors are coded in the genome and have been conserved across all multicellular life forms, presumably from primordial times. Metazoans are born with the genetically encoded knowledge of the artifacts and signatures that arise from the "bad guys" of the microbial world including endotoxin (the residue of gram-negative cells), peptidoglycan (the residue of gram-positive cells), single and double-stranded RNA (from viral particles), flagellin (present in an assortment of bacteria), and β-glucans (from mold and yeast). TLRs straddle the outer membrane of host cells with the receptor acting as a sentinel outside the cell and communicating contact with PAMPs inside the cell upon contact. See Table 2 for list of TLRs and associated PAMPs.

---

[a]Innate immunity—the paramount antimicrobial response of metazoans—depends on germline encoded receptors that recognize repeated patterns of molecular structures on the surface of microorganisms; these patterns are absent from eukaryotic cells (78).

TABLE 1   Selected Toll-Like Receptors and Associated Pathogen Associated Microbial Patterns

Toll/TLR	PAMP(s) Recognized	Comments
TLR1/IL-1 (cytoplasmic[a])	Activated by end product of proteolytic cascade (Spätzle)	Toll discovered in *Drosophila* and subsequently IL-1 as a mammalian homolog
TLR4	LPS, LTA	Prototypical pattern recognition receptor for endotoxin
TLR2	Peptidoglycan, LTA, atypical LPS[b], mycobacterial cell walls (glycosylphospha-tidylinositol lipid from *T. cruzi*[c]), a *S. epidermidis* modulin of yeast cell walls	The range of PAMPs recognized is explained by TLR2 associating with TLR1 and TLR6
TLR3	dsRNA	Present in virions
TLR5	Flagellin - protein that comprises bacterial flagella	Unique among TLR in that it recognizes a protein
TLR9	Unmethylated CpG motifs in bacterial DNA	Theorized to be an indicator of bacterial infection

[a]Noted in 1991 that cytoplasmic domain of IL-1 was homologous to Toll (TLR1).
[b]Associated with *Leptospira interrogans* and *Porphyromonas gingivitis*.
[c]*Trypanosoma* is a protozoan parasite.
Abbreviations: IL, Interleukin; LPS, lipopolysaccharides; LTA, lipoteichoic acid; PAMP, Pathogen Associated Microbial Patterns; TLR, Toll-like receptors.

   TLR4, which is generally associated with endotoxin host detection, was discovered in Drosophila (and subsequently in mammals), but was not associated with a specific function in innate immunity until many years later when mutant mice deficient in the receptor were shown to be insensitive to endotoxin. The discovery "indicated immediately how mammalian innate immune sensing might operate in relation to other microbes and other inducing molecules" (25). Numerous TLRs have since been discovered and the identified number of PAMPs (though pathogen-associated is surely a misnomer as the given molecular patterns are associated with all the organisms of a class, pathogen or not; such as LPS which is associated with all gram-negatives) has increased even more. Indeed, the conserved nature of the PAMP is the reason for its use as a marker in multicellular hosts. Any mutation in necessary microbial organisms would render them nonviable (again, as in the case of LPS in gram-negatives), as contrasted with the ever-changing structure of various virulence factors. Interestingly, the list of PAMPs has grown to include a plethora of microbial artifacts, reading as a "who's who" of originating microbial culprits.

TABLE 2   The Six Cytokine Families

Family	Example(s)
Interleukins	IL-1 to IL-16
Cytotoxic cytokines	TNF-α, TNF-β
Colony-stimulating factors	IL-3, G-CSF, M-CSF
Interferons	IFN-α, IFN-β, IFN-γ
Growth factors	Platelet-derived growth factor (PDGF)
Chemokines	IL-8, Rantes

Abbreviations: CSF, colony-stimulating factors; IL, Interleukin; TNF, tumor necrosis factor.
Source: From Ref. 16.

The basic pattern of innate response, therefore, can be characterized as (*i*) microbial intrusion (invasion), (*ii*) host recognition by either a soluble PRR (Lipopolysaccharide Binding Protein, LBP) or cell-embedded PRR (CD14) or both (as in binding by LBP and presentation to CD14), and sometimes an intracellular PRR, (*iii*) host cell transcription (via NF-κB) of response factors (cytokines, etc.) and antimicrobial peptides[b], (*iv*) macrophage activation/phagocytation, and (*v*), (eventual[c]) activation of an adaptive immune response via TLR expressed on antigen presenting cells (APCs) contributed by the activation of intruder-specific (differentiated) T cells (30). Innate immunity involving TLRs is described in Chapter 5. The mechanism of specific response of Limulus infection with gram-negative organisms bearings endotoxin will be described in Chapter 10 in great detail, as it is well characterized. In this regard innate immunity is highly pertinent to a discussion of endotoxin whereas adaptive immunity is much less relevant as a delayed means of immunity. The latter is an ineffective mechanism in regard to host defense against endotoxin.

Organisms may gain access to the bloodstream by overrunning the boundaries put in place by the host's initial defense mechanisms by any of several artificial medical procedures mentioned earlier, or, from the parenteral manufacturing perspective, very rarely from parenteral drug or nutrition contamination. There are two major nonspecific, so-called "cell mediated immunity"[d] or acute responses elicited by endotoxin of gram-negative bacteria that occur before specific B-cell and T-cell immunity can begin[e], including:

1. Cytokine production (TNF and IL-1) and release from macrophages in turn increases the microbicidal potential and chemotaxis[f] of phagocytes and increases adherence of blood cells to endothelial cells, accompanied by characteristic intravascular coagulation. It was the phenomenon of disseminated intravascular coagulation that alerted Fredrick Bank to the effect of bacterial infection on horseshoe crabs. Cytokine production and release from macrophages and monocytes have multiple, various, potentially redundant, additive, and in some cases contradictory effects on different organ systems. The interactions vary from synergistic, to a cascade or sequential synergy, to antagonistic effect. Pro-inflammatory cytokines are counterbalanced by anti-inflammatory cytokines that include IL-10, IL-4, and IL-13 (31). Cytokines travel to the hypothalamus to trigger an increase in the body's set point, thus bringing about fever.

---

[b]Cationic host defense peptides ... that fold into ampiphilic structures with hydrophobic and hydrophilic (charged) faces.

[c]Adaptive immune response (as opposed to innate immune response) is said to occur four to seven days subsequent to infection.

[d]The term "cell mediated immunity" (CMI) was originally coined to describe the localized reactions to organisms, usually intracellular pathogens, mediated by lymphocytes and phagocytes rather than by antibody (humoral immunity). It is now often used in a more general sense for any response against organisms or tumors in which antibody plays a subordinate role (34).

[e]Cell-mediated immunity is the only response in lower organisms (such as Limulus) that have only phagocytes (i.e., no T- or B-cells) and complement-like proteins.

[f]Movement of phagocytes toward invading microorganisms.

2. The complement activated response is an initial nonspecific host reaction to gram-negative invasion that acts to coat the intruder with any number of a group of about 20 serum proteins (complement) that act sequentially. Low doses of injected LPS (2 to 4 ng/kg) do not activate the complement system, indicating a high relative pathway cascade threshold (31). However, increasing levels of LPS generate a dose-dependent activation of complement, which leads to the generation of anaphylatoxins. Genetic deficiencies have been described, which involve the lack of virtually each of the approximately 20 serum complement proteins and are demonstrated in a wide range of resulting impairments culminating usually in increased susceptibility to infection (32). For example, those genetically deficient in late complement components are prone to Neisserial (meningococcemia) infection but experience an attenuated form of disease progression (33). Complement activation (physical attachment to the invader) leads to recognition by phagocytes. Complement can also be activated by antigen present on pathogens to induce a specific or immunological response. Complement activation, whether it is begun as a result of nonspecific (called the alternate pathway) or immunological response (called the classical pathway) that produces an antibody–antigen complex, brings about the following cascade of events designed to mediate bacterial opsonization (lysis) and promote the inflammatory response (34):

A. generate complement peptides (predominately in the liver but also by macrophages) to opsonize the microbes for phagocyte uptake and intercellular death
B. draw phagocytes to the infection site by means of chemotaxis
C. increase blood flow to the site
D. damage plasma membranes to lysis bacterial cells or enveloped viruses to reduce infection
E. release inflammatory mediators from mast cells to increase capillary permeability to allow more soluble mediators to reach the site

The *Limulus* amebocyte assay used to detect endotoxin is based upon a complement type of pathway that forms fibrin to seal off the advance of endotoxin bearing organisms in *Limulus polyphemus* blood. Brandtzaeg (31) notes that such a "walling off" of intruders in local tissues is an appropriate host reaction, but that "the response is highly inappropriate when it causes generalized intravascular fibrin formation, plugging of the microvasculature, and bleeding."

THE CLINICAL RESPONSE TO ENDOTOXIN ADMINISTRATION IN HUMANS

Endotoxin that is administered intravenously produces effects similar to the onset of sepsis and for this reason has been used widely as a model in humans and animals to study the mechanism of sepsis (35). The important effects of endotoxin upon the host have been an intense area of modern clinical research and the literature contains an overwhelming array of related information. The focus on sepsis in current research efforts is due to the predominance of its occurrence and the associated mortality. Estimates are upwards of 500,000 cases per year in the United States alone of which approximately 35% of those patients do not recover (36). In terms of mortality, sepsis ranked twelfth in 1997 (1% of 2,314,245 deaths in the United States) ahead of homicide, AIDS, and atherosclerosis (37). The host response is of interest to pharmaceutical and device manufacturers because it creates the concern for endo-toxin contamination control in the first place. While this overview cannot do justice to such a complex field, an appreciation can be gained for current research and for the importance of contamination control in parenteral manufacturing.

Many controlled studies have been done involving bolus injections of endotoxin into human subjects (38–45). Typically, such studies involve administering an injection of between 2 and 4 ng/kg of *E. coli* derived purified LPS. Within about an hour to an hour and a half most injection subjects commonly complain of influenza-like symptoms, including myalgia, headache, and nausea. Some two-thirds of a typical group develop chills and all develop fever of 1°C or 2°C above baseline accompanied by an increased heart rate. Leukocyte count initially decreases for the first hour, then abruptly begins to rise rapidly and is accompanied by neutrophilia. At about two hours post injection a lowering of the blood pressure occurs. Whereas peak endotoxin concentrations in the blood are reached within five minutes, peak body temperature is not reached until 60–90 minutes and correlates well with peak TNF and IL-6 cytokine levels. The initial and peak levels of IL-6 typically occur 15 minutes after the initial and peak TNF levels. The peak of fever occurs at three hours post injection after which the patient begins to show symptomatic improvement (42). The low doses (2 to 4 ng/kg) used in such studies do not activate the complement system and therefore differ in this respect from what occurs in septic shock patients (31).

The latency period prior to the detection of TNF is considered to be due to the time required by macrophages to produce and release it. The delay of IL-1 and IL-6 production supports the belief that TNF stimulates the release of these cytokines from macrophages and endothelial cells. In one study, cyclooxygenase inhibition in the form of ibuprofen pretreatment did not affect the circulating concentration of TNF but did affect the fever and endocrine responses, suggesting that cyto-kine-induced pyrogenic responses are accomplished via the cyclooxygenase pathway (38). Among the many factors found to be elicited by endotoxin are: serum-derived anaphylatoxins (complement factors), prostaglandins (PG), interlu-kins (IL), interferons (INF), colony-stimulating factors (CSF), hemopoietins, tumor necrosis factor (TNF-α also called Cachectin and TNF-β), platelet activating factor (PAF), and endorphins.

CYTOKINES

Cytokines are involved in all the body's major biological processes including cell growth and activation, hemopoeisis, inflammation, immunity, tissue repair, fibro-sis, and morphogenesis. These mediators are a "family" only in the sense of their functionality, not their structure; although, many of them are structurally similar, such as IL1-α, IL-1β, TNF-α. Initially, this class of compounds was believed to be a single substance and was called "endogenous pyrogen." Morrison expresses the unique relationship of endotoxin to cytokines:

> Probably the most unique feature of endotoxin, therefore, is its almost ubiquitous capacity to elicit the entire spectrum of host effector molecules. In fact, the diversity of such molecules that can be mobilized by endotoxin is primarily what has con-founded as efforts to define a singular unifying concept of endotoxin action. This in turn suggests that while appropriate regulation of any single mediator may modify and, at least partially, abrogate the deleterious effects of endotoxin, it is highly unlikely that any single modulatory regimen will be totally successful either in an experimental model of endotoxemia or in a clinical setting of infectious disease (46).

A modern study of the host response to endotoxin (or any pyrogen) quickly becomes a study of cytokines. Once an exogenous agent (or event) has triggered the inflammatory response, the host's response is believed to no longer depend upon the agent activating the cascade but rather becomes self perpetuating. The symptoms and progressive effects may continue on the given course, and even intensify after the agent has been cleared from the system and/or after the event (burn, wound, etc.) has passed. The study of cytokines and their effects has been a field of explosive and fertile growth during the biotechnology revolution. Many genes encoding these substances have been cloned and expressed, and several have been commercialized as treatments for a variety of diseases including viral infections, multiple sclerosis, and certain cancers.

These mediators were initially identified from lymphocytes and were called lymphokines(47). Cytokines are now known to be mainly the product of macrophages[g] (but are also produced by T-cells, and endothelial cells), which are the predominant long-lived blood monocytes. As phagocytes, macrophages internalize antigens and pathogens in order to degrade them. There are resident (noncirculating) macrophages, or phagocytic cells from the monocyte lineage, in many tissues including alveolar (lung), liver (Kuffer cells), splenic, blood, lymph node, recirculating, and kidney mesangial(34). Six families of cytokines have been described and are shown in Table 2 (52).

In response to gram-negative bacterial or LPS stimulation, TNF-α, IL-1, and IL-6 have been indicated as the major cytokines induced. See Table 3 for a list of biological actions associated with each cytokine. Cytokines are included in a class of intercellular signaling molecules, which includes neurotransmitters, endocrine hormones, and autocoids (47). Cytokines have been defined in detail to be "soluble (glyco) proteins, nonimmunoglobulin in nature, released by living cells of the host, which act nonenzymatically in picomolar to nanomolar concentrations to regulate host cell function"(47).

SEPSIS, BACTEREMIA, ENDOTOXEMIA, AND THE SYSTEMATIC INFLAMMATORY RESPONSE

Sepsis has been defined as the "systemic response to infection"(48), whereas bacteremia, endotoxemia, fungemia, and viremia more specifically represent the presence of viable bacteria, endotoxin, fungi, and virus respectively in the blood. Definitions often overlap, as determined by the severity of the response or by the type of offender isolated from the blood. The more general phrase "systematic inflammatory response" is often used to describe a generalized host response to microbial or traumatic insult (49). Septic shock is the end result of sepsis and has been defined as "a state of inadequate tissue perfusion induced by microbial products and characterized by low blood pressure and biochemical signs of oxygen deficit"(23). The reduced oxygen and nutrient-transport capability to vital organs is caused by a generalized intravascular inflammatory response resulting in vasodilation. The associated occurrence and mortality of sepsis has proven difficult to accurately estimate. Some

---

[g]Cells of the monocyte/macrophage lineage derive from myelomonocytic stem cells in one marrow. These cells give rise to monoblasts, which then develop into monocytes. Monocytes go into the blood where they circulate with a half life of one to three days. They then go into the various tissues and here they are collectively called macrophages (79).

TABLE 3 Biological Actions of IL-1, IL-6, and TNF

Biological action	Action displayed by		
	IL-1	IL-6	TNF
Endogenous pyrogen	+	+	+
Induction of acute-phase proteins	+	+	+
Activation of T- and B-lymphocytes	+	+	+
Stimulation of immunoglobulin sythesis	–	+	–
Stimulation of fibroblast proliferation	+	+	+
Stimulation of cyclooxygenase II induction	+	–	+
Stimulation of cartilage breakdown	+	–	+
Stimulation of endothelial cells	+	–	+
Stimulation of murine bone breakdown	+	+	+
Induction of endothelial adhesion molecules	+	–	+
Induction of septic shock-like syndrome	+	–	+
Induction of IL-1, TNF, and IL-8	+	–	+
Induction of IL-6	+	–	+
Induction of hyperalgesia	+	–	+

Abbreviations: IL Interleukin; TNF, tumor necrosis factor.
Source: From Ref. 52.

estimates range up to 60% and the overall occurrence at a rate of about 1% of all hospitalized patients and 20% to 30% of ICU patients in the United States per year (50). Mortality has been shown to depend upon the bacterial type, seriousness of the underlying disease, use and type of antibiotic therapy, use of invasive devices, and even the use of parenteral nutrition shown to result in increased TNF production (51).

Although LPS is the most potent inducer of cytokine production in septic shock, sepsis is not entirely specific or unique to either infection or infection with LPS-bearing bacteria (such as *E. coli*, *Salmonnela*, *Klebsiella*, *Pseudomonas*.). The inflammatory cascade may be initiated by trauma, ischemia-reperfusion injury, transplant rejection, antigenic-immune responses, and inflammatory states including hepatitis and pancreatitis (52,53). In a clinical setting, many microbial pathogens and by-products arising from infection other than gram-negative bacteria have been found to be deadly. The list includes gram-positive bacteria, which produce peptidoglycan, teichoic acid, and exotoxins (*Staphylococcus aureus* and *Streptococcus pyogenes*)(54), though the levels needed to arrive at such a state are believed to be higher with gram-positive organisms and their by-products than with either gram-negative organisms or LPS. Gram-negative organisms have been found to be responsible for in excess of 50% of sepsis cases and are associated with greater mortality (36). Levels of lethal endotoxin may vary greatly and even low circulating mediator (cytokine) concentrations may prove harmful if the host is in a hyperreactive state, which may be caused by exotoxins, chronic infection, tumors, or interferon.

In septic shock, septicemia, and endotoxiemia, not only are systemic changes such as fever and intravascular coagulation elicited, but also specific and multiple organ changes, which can include renal failure and adult respiratory distress syndrome (55). When the body's counter-reaction to endotoxin recognition remains localized the infected tissue, it forms an effective barrier to invasion, localizing the infection and disabling the invader. However, when the infection spreads into the blood, systemically, then the macrophages of the entire body produce an overwhelming response with the release of cytokines that cause fever, circulatory collapse, hemorrhagic fever, shock, multiple organ failure, and eventually death. Unlike hormones, the apparent purpose of cytokine action is limited to their local effects amongst a small number of individual cells (i.e., "within a few cell diameters") (19).

That cytokines are, in fact, the cause of the host response to endotoxin exposure is generally accepted as a fact that explains a plethora of modern data. Proof of this includes the purification and subsequent cloning and recombinant production of TNF-α and its injection into healthy hosts (48). The effects elicited are virtually identical to those obtained upon injection of purified LPS and endotoxin via gram-negative infection. The converse situation has also been shown in that the adverse effects of LPS have been prevented by the use of anti-TNF monoclonal antibodies (56). The effects caused by some bacterial diseases are almost wholly caused by the release of endotoxin and include plague (*Yersinia pestis*) and typhoid fever (*Salmonella typhimurium*) as well as other "classical" gram-negative pathogens (43).

LIPOPOLYSACCHARIDES INTERACTION WITH CELL MEMBRANES

At least three types of LPS interactions with cellular membranes have been described: (*i*) binding via a cell bound receptor that recognizes a soluble protein complexed with LPS, (*ii*) binding via membrane bound receptors, and (*iii*) direct LPS membrane interaction.

1. Perhaps the best characterized of several known LPS host macrophage receptors is a 55 kD surface glycoprotein called CD14 (57). This glycoprotein is also found in soluble form (sCD14) and acts as a receptor for host cells that do not express CD14 on their surface (58). In an unusual mechanism, LPS is not mediated directly by the membrane bound protein, but first by a soluble 60 kDa protein synthesized in hepatacytes called lipopolysaccharide binding protein (LBP). The soluble protein opsonizes (free or gram-negative bacterial associated) LPS forming a soluble complex, and, through an affinity for a macrophage bound receptor, CD14, facilitates LPS adhesion to macrophage for internalization. The adhesion of the LPS–LBP complex induces the synthesis of TNF-α at the mRNA level. The genes for both human and murine CD14 have been cloned, sequenced, and shown to share in homology with one another and with another endotoxin binding protein called bacterial permeability increasing protein (BPI). Besides LPS, CD14 has been found to bind other microbial by-products including lipoarabinomannan (LAM), peptidoglycan and other *Streptococcus* and *Staphylococcus* cell wall glucose polymers, and yeast W-1 antigen (58).
2. The 95 kdDa CD18 receptor directly recognizes LPS on whole *E. coli* and results in adhesion, phagocytic uptake, and transport to a degradative host-cell compartment (57). Whereas binding of the soluble LPS–LBP complex induces the synthesis of TNF, binding of LPS by CD18 results in the clearance of bacteria from the bloodstream without resulting in cytokine release (57).
3. Electronmicroscopic studies have shown that LPS binds monocyte membranes directly in perpendicular and parallel orientations leading to their being "solubilized" into the plasma membrane (59). Such insertion of lipid A into the phospholipid bilayer causes membrane disruption. In vitro studies have shown that

disruption facilitates migration of LPS bilayers into the cytoplasm of monocytes by passive diffusion. Such ingestion of LPS and associated membrane destruction can cause cell death. Once inside, LPS disrupts the cell machinery (mitochondria, rough endoplasmic reticulum, and golgi apparatus) and causes cellular disruption. Hepatic Kupffer cells and hepatacytes as well as lung macrophages play a role in clearing and detoxifying LPS by converting lipid A to less toxic precursor-like molecules. The ultra-structural localization of LPS in the cell nucleus indicates that LPS may gain access to DNA in the nucleus (59).

Binding of LPS to the plasma membrane causes dramatic changes in host macrophage cell shape, behavior, and enzyme activities. The reversibility of the changes suggests alterations in the cell "membrane fluidity and microfilament cytoskeleton"(59). LPS extracted from rough strains (r-LPS) are deficient in O-antigen and therefore contain more lipids on a weight basis and may, therefore, be more membrane reactive. LPS in physiological conditions are released in "blebs." The released blebs contain LPS, protein, and phospholipids. In vitro bleb release is related to peptidoglycan breakdown in the cell wall, proliferitive activity, and quantity of capsular polysaccharide. In vitro and in vivo endotoxin release from host cells is enhanced by antibiotic use.

Ultimately, it has been theorized that the fate of endotoxin in the body depends on the competition of receptors for LPS attachment. Therefore, factors affecting the availability of various receptors may determine the course of the body's response to LPS (60), given the requisite presentation of the endotoxic lipid A structure. Multiple LPS binding proteins (LBP, sCD14, BPI), multiple receptors (CD14, CD18, scavenger receptor), multiple soluble mediators and classes (cytokine, complement, etc.), synergistic as well as antagonistic effects of specific elicited mediators (TNF, IL-1, IL-6), as well as the ability of LPS to directly bind membranes have served to, if not completely clarify, then at least to illuminate the complexity of LPS-host cell interactions.

TUMOR NECROSIS FACTOR ALPHA

The cytokine that has been implicated as the most direct result of endotoxin administration and of the systematic proinflammatory response is TNF$-\alpha$. Along with IL-1 and IL-6, TNF is believed to be the major endogenous mediator of LPS. TNF was discovered in the mid-1970s by a group lead by Old, but was not isolated and purified until the mid-1980s. Its purification allowed the cloning of its encoding gene and subsequently allowed its production in sufficient quantities to allow extensive study(9). Initially, two seemingly different compounds were isolated, Cachectin isolated due to its role in wasting disease and TNF due to its antitumor activity(61). Later both were shown to be one and the same molecule(62). TNF$-\alpha$ is a 17 kilodalton polypeptide proposed to be a primary mediator associated with gram-negative (LPS induced) bacterial sepsis and endotoxiemia as well as a number of beneficial host effects including that associated with its namesake (9,63,64). Although some casual relationships have been described that appear to underscore the importance of TNF as at least one of several key mediators in endotoxemia and septicemia, attempts to attenuate the deleterious host response to TNF$-\alpha$ have been notably unsuccessful. Michie et al. (38) list four primary findings supporting the importance of TNF in endotoxemia and sepsis:

> First, tumor necrosis factor has been detected in the circulation of laboratory animals after the administration of a lethal injection of endotoxin. Second, infusion of tumor necrosis factor in laboratory animals caused physiological changes similar to those observed in animals with gram-negative septicemia. Third, C3H HeJ mice, which are unable to elaborate tumor necrosis factor because of a genetic defect, are resistant to otherwise lethal doses of endotoxin. Finally, passive immunization of endotoxin-sensitive mice with antiserum to tumor necrosis factor substantially reduced the lethal effects of endotoxin and pretreatment of baboons with a monoclonal antibody to tumor necrosis factor prevented their deaths after injection with a lethal dose (LD_{100}) of live *E. coli* organisms.

Because the half life associated with a given molecule of TNF is very short (a few minutes), and it may disappear before symptoms are observed, studies designed to correlate the levels of TNF with the degree of severity of sepsis have been variable (60). Attempts to attenuate the effects of septicemia by preventing TNF production would have to be undertaken before it can become apparent that such an effort would even be needed (i.e., when a patient is asymptomatic). Studies have also shown similar sepsis-associated increases in IL-1 and IL-6. While the septic studies implicate TNF in a systemic role, other studies have also implicated TNFs role in specific organ responses such as ARDS, inflammatory bowel disease, Crohn's disease, and rheumatoid arthritis. Modern monoclonal antibodies have been successful in attenuating the TNF role in the latter two diseases[h].

Although TNF can induce systemic inflammatory response similar to endotoxemia and septic shock, it is the state of the host rather than the dose ("seed versus soil") that is believed by many to determine the final outcome of endotoxin exposure (60). Suffice it to say that TNF is an important letter of a cytokine network, which forms the language of inflammatory response, the exact combination and sequence and amounts of which have not been deciphered in spelling out the fatal septic epithet.

Even with overwhelming evidence of a major TNF role in the endotoxin inflammatory response, the exact interplay of the various cytokines has been called into question by other findings. Brouckaert and Fiers (60) provide several points that suggest a more moderate role of TNF in the host response to LPS:

1. TNF levels do not discriminate between survivors and nonsurvivors
2. patients treated with TNF have higher levels of TNF than septic shock patients but the toxicity does not mimic septic shock and is reversible
3. Offner et al. (53) (1990) suggest that sustained low doses of TNF are correlated with fatal septic shock outcome (such as those potentially present in parenteral nutrition and other chronic states of medical intervention)
4. in bacterial peritonitis TNF proves to be protective rather than detrimental
5. hampering anticytokine strategies is the observation that low levels of some cytokines may be necessary for protection from excessive inflammatory responses

---

[h]REMICADE™ (infliximab) for the treatment of Crohn's disease and rheumatoid arthritis (anti-TNFα chimeric monoclonal antibody) launched in 2002 by Centocor in the U.S.

The types of (endotoxin) "bad seeds" are described in Chapter 3 and none-ndotoxin modulators in Chapter 5. The "seeds" refer to either the specific endo-toxic conformation of LPS, the presence of additional microbes and/or microbial by-products, or a combination of both. Types of "bad soil" may include a number of contributing host states such as blood factors (e.g., lipid content, comp-lement, LPS receptor availability, etc.), additional disease states, and even genetic predispositions of the host. Westendorp et al. (66) studied the inheritability of cytokine production ("the proportion of the population variation attributable to genetic variation") using statistical methods involving 190 first-degree relatives of 61 patients of meningococcal disease as well as 26 monozygotic twins. Cytokine production was stimulated and measured in whole-blood by an ex vivo method. According to the authors, families with low TNF production had a 10 times greater risk of fatal outcome, while a 20 times increased risk of fatality was (retro-spectively) associated with high IL-10 production. Families with both low TNF and high IL-10 production had the greatest risk. Therefore, pro-inflammatory TNF was seen to act as a protector against fatal meningococcal disease progression while the anti-inflammatory IL-10 cytokine was viewed as a hindrance to the body's efforts against the bacterial infection. The authors state, "taken together the data suggest that innate capacity to produce cytokines contributes to familial susceptibility for fatal meningococcal disease." However, the authors also indicate that it is premature to generalize these findings with regard to other types of infections.

In another study implying that the susceptibility to endotoxic shock may reside to some degree in a patient's genome, a multicenter study found that specific sequences of the TNF-α gene (TNF2 as opposed to the TNF1 allele) were statistically associated with a higher number of cases of septic shock and death (3.7 fold increased risk) due to septic shock (67). The later two findings can now be under-stood in terms of TLR polymorphisms, which are heritable differences in the ulti-mate endotoxin signaling receptors to be discussed in some detail in Chapter 4 and in regard to sepsis in Chapter 17. The "right" types and amounts of both pro-inflammatory and anti-inflammatory cytokines desired for survival are far from clear, though the body knows and is very sensitive to changes instigated by outsiders including both man-made concoctions and infecting invaders. Quakyi et al. (68) maintain that because endotoxin-associated preparations are generally heterogeneous, associated non-LPS cellular components may provide crosscurrents in the cytokine mix resulting in beneficial effects that could possibly modulate some of the toxic effects of TNF.

ANTIBIOTIC RELEASE

Endotoxin liberation via antibiotic usage has been well documented and was actu-ally proposed over a century ago (1895) when Jarisch Herxheimer described the reactions occurring when mercurials were used to treat syphilis (69). The advent of antibiotic therapy brought with it the realization that certain ailments were aggravated by antibiotic treatment including typhoid, other classical gram-negative infections, and malaria. It has been widely recognized that the rise of sepsis has stat-istically paralleled the rise in antibiotic usage. Considering that many antibiotics are designed to destroy bacterial cell walls, it is not too surprising that their use could provoke the freeing of endotoxin in human hosts. Factors affecting such release include bacterial strain, antibiotic type, and time of exposure (70).

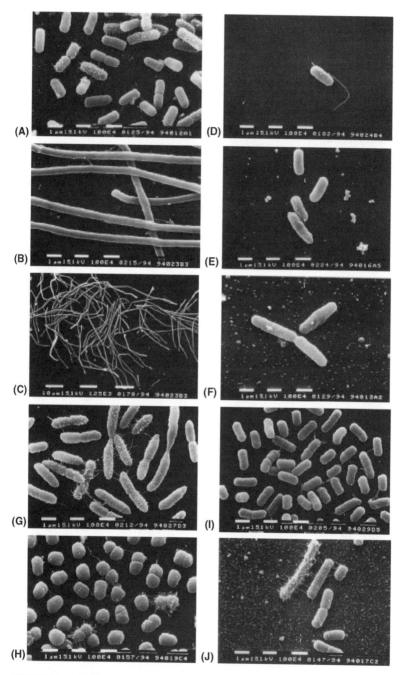

FIGURE 3 Scanning electronmicrographs (magnification X 7,000) of *E. coli* O4:K2 after 4 hours of incubation without antibiotics (**A**), with ceftazidime at magnifications of X7,000 (**B**) and X875 (**C**) imipenem (**D**), gentamicin (**E**), or ciprofloxacin (**F**), all in a concentration of 50 times the MIC; or with ceftazidime (**G**), imipenem (**H**), gentamicin (**I**), or ciprofloxacin (**J**) in a concentration of 0.5 times the MIC. *Source*: From Ref. 77.

Antibiotic therapy is used to eliminate bacteria from the host and, therefore, the source of endotoxin as well. However, the endotoxin liberating ability of antibiotics is tied to their antimicrobial properties, particularly those such as the beta lactam antibiotics that act by attacking the bacterial cell wall. Mock et al. summarized the totality of recent evidence for the relevance of antibiotic induced endotoxin in the clinical setting (70). They conclude that three broad assumptions can be drawn but that the evidence is not sufficient to "advocate changes in current antibiotic prescribing or dosing decisions." They found that (*i*) different types of antibiotics induce different amounts of endotoxin release in human antibiotic treatment, (*ii*) endotoxin release probably has biological consequences, and (*iii*) the biological result is possibly clinically relevant (70).

While β-lactam antibiotics have been most associated with the release of endotoxin during treatment, Jackson and Kropp have found differences in the ability of subclasses to free endotoxin in vivo with the traditional cephalosporin, monobactam, and penicillin antibiotics liberating more endotoxin than the carbapenems (and also the non β-lactam aminoglycosides) (71) using hypersensitive mouse models infected with *P. aeruginosa*. Interestingly, they determined from electronmicrographs that treatment with specific antibiotics such as ceftazidime and aztreonam induces filament formation (elongation) bringing about increased microbial biomass without a resultant increase in cell counts (i.e., bacteria stop proliferating but continue to grow). Filament formation allows for the continual biosynthesis of endotoxin and the antibiotic dosing schedule may have an effect on filament formation.

Prins et al. give three mechanisms to account for the increased endotoxin concentration observed following antibiotic treatment including: (*i*) increased bacterial biomass such as filament formation (*ii*) increased accessibility of cell bound endotoxin, and (*iii*) the release of free endotoxin (72). The use of ciprofloxacin and ceftazidime produced extraordinary elongation of *E. coli* cells in the Prins study as compared to the use of Imipenem (which produced rounded cells) and gentamicin, which had little visible effect (Fig. 3). The filaments produced by Ciprofloxacin and ceftazidime corresponded with an increase in endotoxin, TNF-α, and IL-6 levels as compared to the imipenem and gentamicin treatments

Kirckae et al. studied the phenomenon of antibiotic facilitated LPS release by culturing *P. aeruginosa* in the presence of ceftazadime, removing the whole cells by filtration (0.22 micrometer filter) and characterizing the bioactivity of the filtrate (73). The resulting LPS solution was shown to be comparable to phenol water extracted LPS in bioactivity. They also demonstrated that excess endotoxin liberated by cell wall–active antibiotic treaments (such as β-lactams) are highly associated with cellular proteins. They subsequently neutralized the LPS activity by binding the lipid A portion of the complex with polymyxin B to demonstrate that the lipid A portion is the active molecule released by ceftazidime treatment. Though the associated protein is not endotoxic it has been shown to be a potent mitogen for C3H/HeJ mouse cells and human lymphocytes [hyporesponsive to LPS (74)].

REFERENCES

1. Westphal O, Westphal U, Sommer T. History of pyrogen research. In: Schlessinger D, ed. Microbiology. Washington: American Society for Microbiology, 1977:221–238.
2. Thomas L. Lives of a Cell. Penguin, 1975:153.

3. Bernheim HA, D. C. A. Effect of protein synthesis inhibitors on leukocytic pyrogen-induced in vitro hypothalamic prostaglandin production. Yale J Biol Med 1985; 58:179–187.
4. Mackowiak PA. Direct effects of hypothermia on pathogenic microorganisms: teleologic implications with regard to fever. Rev Infect Dis 1981; (3):508–520.
5. Roberts NJJ. Temperature and host defense. Microbiol Rev 1979; 43:241–259.
6. Duff, Durum. Fever and immunoregulation: hyperthermia, interleukins 1 and 2, and T-cell proliferation. Yale J Biol Med 1982; 55:437–442.
7. Hanson DF, et al. The effect of temperature on the activation of thymocytes by interleukins I and II. J Immunol 1983; 130:216–221.
8. Vaughn LK, et al. Antipyresis: its effect on mortality rate of bacterially infected rabbits. Brain Res Bull 1980; 5:69–73.
9. Old LJ. Tumor necrosis factor. Sci Am 1988; 258(May):59–75.
10. Dinarello CA, et al. New concepts in the pathogenesis of fever. Rev Infect Dis 1988; 10(1):168–189.
11. Skarnes RC, et al. Role of prostaglandin E in the biphasic fever response to endotoxin. J Exp Med 1981; 154:1212–1224.
12. Ashman RB. Fever. In: Roitt IM, Delves PJ. eds. Encyclopedia of Immunology. London: Academic Press Limited, 1992:559–561.
13. Weary M. Pyrogens and pyrogen testing. In: Swarbrick E, Boyan JC, eds. Encyclopedia of Pharmaceutical Technology. New York: Marcel Dekker, 1988:185.
14. Dinarello CA, Wolff SM. Molecular basis of fever in humans. Am J Med 1982; 72: 799–819.
15. Arend WP. Effects of immune complexes on production by human monocytes of interleukin 1 or an interleukin 1 inhibitor. J Immunol 1985;134:3868–3875.
16. Bernheim HA, Dinarello CA. Effect of protein synthesis inhibitors on leukocyte pyrogen-induced in vitro hypothalamic prostaglandin production. Yale J Biol Med 1985; 58: 179–187.
17. Townsend Y, et al. Inhibition of brain protein synthesis suppresses the release of prostaglandin E2 in febrile rabbits. Brain Res Bull 1984; 13:335–338.
18. Grandics P. Pyrogens in parenteral pharmaceuticals. Pharm Technol 2000; (April):26–34.
19. Bone RC. Gram-negative sepsis: a dilema of modern medicine. Clin Microbiol Rev 1993; 6(1):57–68.
20. Martin MA. Epidemiology and clinical impact of gram-negative sepsis. In: Young LS, Glauser MP. eds. Gram-Negative Septicemia and Septic Shock. Infect Dis Clin North Am. 1991:739.
21. Burd RS, Cody CS, Dunn DL. Immnothertherapy of gram negative bacterial sepsis. In: The Clinical Problem. ch. 2. Austin: R.G. Landes Company, 1992.
22. Maki DC. Nosocomial bacteremia: an epidemiologic overview. Am J Med 1981; 70(March):719–732.
23. Bone RC. The Sepsis syndrome. In: Dorinsky PM, ed. Clin Chest Med 1996; 175–181.
24. Pfaller MA, et al. Bacterial pathogens isolated from patients with bloodstream infection: frequencies of occurrence and antimicrobial susceptibility patterns from the SENTRY antimicrobial surveilance program (United States and Canada, 1997). Antimicrob Agents Chemother 1998; 42(7):1762–1770.
25. Reimer LG, Wilson ML, Weinstein MP. Update on detection of bacteremia and fungemia. Clin Microbiol Rev 1997; 10(3):444–465.
26. Styers D, et al. Laboratory-based surveillance of current antimicrobial resistance patterns and trends among *Staphylococcus aureus*: 2005 status in the United States. Ann Clin Microbiol Antimicrob Res 2006; 5:2, doi:10.1186/1476-0711-5-2, http://www.ann-clinmicrob.com/content/5/1/2.
27. Wagner SJ, Friedman LI, Dodd RY. Transfusion-associated bacterial sepsis. Clin Microb Rev 1994; 7(3):290–302.
28. Beebe JL, Koneman EW. Recovery of uncommon bacteria from blood: association with neoplastic disease. Clin Microb Rev 1995; 8(3):336–356.
29. Beutler B, Ernst Th, Rietschel. Innate immune sensing and its roots: the story of endotoxin. Nat Rev Immunol 2003; 3:169–176.

30. Janeway CA Jr. Approaching the asymptote? Evolution and revolution in immunology. Cold Spring Harbor Symposium. Quant Biol 1989; 1:1–13.
31. Brandtzaeg P. Significance and pathogenesis of septic shock. In: Rietschel ET, Wagner H, eds. Pathology of Septic Shock, Current Topics in Microbiology and Immunology (CTIMI). Berlin: Springer, 1996:15–37.
32. Colten HR, Rosen FS. Complement deficiencies. Annu Rev Immunol 1992; 10:809–834.
33. Barton PA, Warren JS. Complement component C5 modulates the systemic tumor necrosis factor response in murine endotoxic shock. Infect Immun 1993; 61(4):1474–1481.
34. Roitt I, Brostoff J, Male D. Immunology. London: Mosby, 1996,28:15.
35. Bone RC. A critical evaluation of new agents for the treatment of sepsis. JAMA 1991; 266(12):1686–1691.
36. Rangel-Frausto MS. The epidemiology of bacterial sepsis.In: Opal SM, Cross AS, eds. Infect Dis Clin North Am 1999; 299–312.
37. National Vital Statistics Reports. June 30 1999, 47.
38. Michie HR, et al. Detection of circulating tumor necrosis factor after endotoxin administration. NEJM 1988; 318(23):1481–1486.
39. Wolff SM. Biological effects of bacterial endotoxins in man. J Infect Dis 1973; 128(Suppl):S259–S264.
40. Engelhardt R, et al. Biological response to intravenously administered endotxoin in patients with advanced cancer. J Biol Response Modif 1990; 9:480–491.
41. Deventer SJV, et al, Experimental endotoxemia in humans: analysis of cytokine release and coagulation, fibrinolytic, and complement pathways. Blood 1990; 76(12):2520–2526.
42. Martich GD, Boujoukos AJ, Suffredini AF. Response of man to endotoxin. Immunobiology 1993; 187:403–416.
43. Glauser MP, et al. Septic shock: pathogenesis. Lancet 1991; 338(September): 732–736.
44. Suffredini AF, et al, The cardiovascular response of normal humans to the adminstration of endotoxin. NEJM 1989; 321:280–287.
45. Taveira D, et al, Brief report: shock and multiple organ dysfunction after self-administration of *Salmonella* endotoxin. NEJM 1993; 328:1457–1460.
46. Morrison DC, Ryan JL. Endotoxins and disease mechanisms. Annu Rev Med 1987; 38:417–432.
47. Nathan C, Sporn M. Cytokines in context. J Cell Biol 1991; 113(5):981–986.
48. Marsh CB, Wewers MD. The pathogenesis of sepsis, The sepsis syndrome. Clin Chest Med 1996; 17(2):83–197.
49. Bone RC. Sepsis syndrome-new insights into its pathogenesis and treatment. Infect Dis Clin North Am 1991; 793–805.
50. Vincent JL. Definition and pathogenesis of septic shock. In: Rietschel ET, Wagner H, eds. Pathology of Septic Shock, Current Topics in Microbiology and Immunology (CTIMI). New York: Springer Publishing, 1996.
51. Fong Y, et al. Total parenteral nutrition and bowel rest modify the metabolic response to endotoxin in humans. Ann Surg 1989; 210(Oct.):449–457.
52. Henderson B, Poole S, Wilson M. Bacterial modulins: a novel class of virulence factors which cause host tissue pathology by inducing cytokine synthesis. Microbiol Rev 1996; 60(June):316–341.
53. Bone RC. Systemic inflammatory response syndrome, sepsis and multiorgan failure. In: Fein AM, et al. ch. 1. Williams & Wilkins, 1997.
54. Trenholme GM. Microbiology of sepsis.In: Fein AM, et al. ch. 3. Williams & Wilkins, 1997.
55. Maier RV. Endotoxin Requirements for Alveolar Macrophage Stimulation. Ad. In Understanding Trauma and Burn Injury. 1991; 30(12): S49–S57.
56. Tracey KJ, et al. Anti-cachectin/TNF monoclonal antibodies prevent septic shock during lethal bacteraemia. Nature 1987; 330:662–664.
57. Wright SD. Multiple receptors for endotoxin. Curr Opin Immunol 1991; 3:83–90.
58. Ingalls RR, et al. Lipopolysaccharide recognition, CD14, and lipopolysaccharide receptors. In: Opal SM, Cross AS, eds. Bacterial Sepsis and Septic Shock. Philadelphia: W. B. Saunders Company, 1999:341–353.

59. Kang Y-H, et al, Uptake, distribution and fate of bacterial lipopolysaccharides in monocytes and macrophages: an ultrastructural and functional correlation. Electron Microsc Rev 1992; 5:381–419.

60. Brouckaert P, Fiers W. Tumor necrosis factor and the systemic inflammatory response syndrome. In: Rietschel ET, Wagner H, eds. Pathology of Septic Shock. Berlin: Springer,1996:167–187.

61. BeutlerB, Cerami A. The biology of cachectin/TNF- a primary mediator of the host response. Annu Rev Immunol 1989; 7:625–655.

62. Beutler B, Cerami A. Cachectin and tumor necrosis factor as two sides of the same biological coin. Nature 1986; 320:584–588.

63. Mannel DN, et al. Tumor necrosis factor: a cytokine involved in toxic effects of endotoxin. Rev Infect Dis 1987; 9(Suppl 5):S602.

64. Urbaschek R, Urbaschek B. Tumor necrosis factor and interleukin 1 as mediators of endotoxin-induced beneficial effects. Rev Infect Dis 1987; 9(Suppl 5):S607.

65. Offner F, Philippe J, Vogelaers D, et al. Serum tumor necrosis factor levels in patients with infectious disease and septic shock. J Lab Clin Med 1990; 116:100–105.

66. Westendorp R, et al. Genetic influence on cytokine production and fatal meningococcal disease. Lancet 1997; 349(18):170–173.

67. Mira J P, et al. Association of TNF2, a TNF-a promoter polymorphism, with septic shock susceptibility and mortality. JAMA 1999; 282(6):561–568.

68. Quakyi EK, Hochstein HD, Tsai CM. Modulation of the biological activities of meningococcal endotoxins by association with outer membrane proteins is not inevitably linked to toxicity. Infect Immun 1997; 65:1972–1979.

69. Arditi, et al. Antibiotic induced bacterial killing activates vascular endothelial cells and whole blood cells: role of free lipopolysaccharide and soluble CD14. J Endotoxin Res 1996. 3(3): p. 179–185.

70. Mock CN, et al. The clinical significance of endotoxin released by antibiotics: what is the evidence? J Endotoxin Res 1990; 3(3): 253–259.

71. Jackson JJ, Kropp H. Differences in mode of action of β-lactam antibiotics influence morphology, LPS release and in vivo antibiotic efficacy. J Endotoxin Res 1996; 3(3):201–218.

72. Prins JM, et al. Cytokine production during killing of E. Coli. Infect Immun 1995; June: 2236–2242.

73. Kirikae, et al. Biological characterization of endotoxins released from antibiotic-treated Pseudomonas aeruginosa and Escherichia coli. Antimicrob Agents Chemother 1998; 42(5):1015–1021.

74. Mangan D, et al. Stimulation of human monocytes by endotoxin-associated protein: inhibition of programmmed cell death. Infect Immun 1992; 60:1684–1686.

75. Dofferhoff ASM, Buys J. The influence of antibiotic-induced filament formation on the release of endotoxin from gram-negative bacteria. J Endotoxin Res 1996; 3(3):187–194.

76. Weary M. Pyrogens and pyrogen testing. In: Swarbrick E, Boyan JC, eds. Encyclopedia of Pharmaceutical Technology. New York: Marcel Dekker, 1988:185.

77. Dofferhoff ASM, Buys J. The influence of antibiotic-induced filament formation on the release of endotoxin from gram-negative bacteria. J Endotoxin Res 1996; 3(3):187–194.

78. Hoffmann JA, Reichhart JM. Drosophila innate immunity: an evolutionary perspective. Nat Immunol 2002; 3(2):121–126.

79. Ziegler-Heitbrock HWL. Definiiton of human blood monocytes. J Leukoc Biol 2000; 67:603–606

4

Endotoxin Structure, Function, and Activity

Kevin L. Williams

Eli Lilly & Company, Indianapolis, Indiana, U.S.A.

Endotoxin molecules are often thought of simplistically as singular, static structures; however, the endotoxin molecule is a chimera, able to change form depending not only upon intrinsic factors ultimately determined in the genetic code for a given bacterium, but also upon extrinsic factors.

STRUCTURE OVERVIEW

The outer membrane of the gram-negative bacterial cell wall is an asymmetrical distribution of various lipids interspersed with proteins. The membrane is "asymmetrical" in that the outer layer has an inner and outer leaf made up of different constituents. The outer layer contains almost all of the lipopolysaccharide (LPS) and the inner leaf contains phospholipids (PL) and no LPS. The outer face is highly charged and interactive with cations; so much so that the anionic groups can bind the fine-grained minerals in natural environments (1). LPS contains more charge per unit of surface area than any other phospholipid and is anionic at neutral physiological pH due to exposed ionizable phosphoryl and carboxyl groups (1). The biochemical pathways for the biosynthesis of each part of the LPS molecule have been deciphered (2). The biosynthesis of O-antigen, lipid A, and the core polysaccharide region are independent, arising from different genes and transported to the outer-membrane separately by a partially characterized mechanism (2,3).

The basic architecture of endotoxin (LPS) is that of a polysaccharide covalently bound to a lipid component, called lipid A (4). Lipid A is embedded in the outer membrane of the bacterial cell whereas the highly variable polysaccharide extends into the cell's environment. The long hair-like, protruding polysaccharide chain is responsible for the gram-negative cell's immunological activity and is known as "O-specific side chain" [Oligosaccharide(O)] or "O-antigen" or "somatic-antigen chain" and has been used for years as a means of distinguishing strains of *Escherichia coli*, *Salmonella*, and other gram-negative pathogens. Endogenous endotoxin contains cell membrane–associated PL and proteins, as well as nucleic acids and glucans (4). Figure 1 shows LPS of a gram-negative bacteria contrasted with the outer shell of a gram-positive bacteria. Rietschel and Brade (5) have likened the structure of LPS to that of a set of wind chimes. The fatty acids resemble the musical pipes and are embedded in the outer membrane parallel to one another and perpendicular to the cellular wall and to the pair of phosphorylated glucosamine sugars, which form the plate from which they dangle. The "plate" is somewhat skewed at a 45-degree angle relative to the membrane[a]. This can be seen clearly in Figure 2 (6,7). Connected to the plate is the O-specific chain, which, in

---

[a]For *E. coli*; much will be made of this angle later.

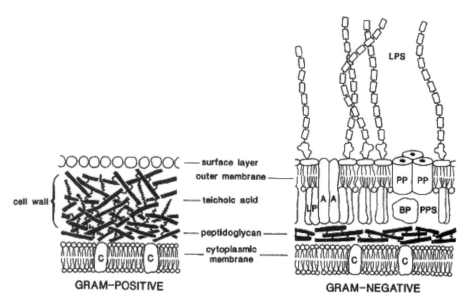

FIGURE 1 Schematic diagram of gram-positive and gram-negative cell envelopes. *Abbreviations*:
A, outer membrane protein; BP, binding protein; C, cytoplasmic membrane-embedded protein; LPS,
lipopolysaccharide; PP, porin; PPS, periplasmic space. *Source*: From Ref. 56.

this analogy, is the long filament from which the wind chime hangs (if in fact it did
hang rather protrude from the lipid A "plate" backbone and fatty acid "pipes"
embedded in the outer cell layer).

ENDOTOXIN NOMENCLATURE AND EXTRACTION

Although used interchangeably, Hitchcock and others have proposed reserving the
term "lipopolysaccharide" for "purified bacterial extracts, which are reasonably
free of detectable contaminants, particularly protein" (8) and the term "endotoxin"
for "products of extraction procedures, which result in macromolecular complexes
of LPS, protein, and phospholipid." Trichloroacetic acid (Boivin-TCA), butanol, and
EDTA methods of extractions (8) yield associated outer membrane proteins (OMP)
also known as lipid associated proteins (LAP). LAPs, in some cases, have been
shown to have potent host effects of their own and act synergistically in association
with LPS. Mangan et al. (10) demonstrated that LAP from *S. typhimurium* is three to
four times more active in inducing IL-1 from monocytes than protein-free LPS.
Since so many additional components of the bacterial cell wall have recently
been implicated in inducing the production of cytokines, this distinction is becoming more widely appreciated. Furthermore, in discussing the endotoxin of the
family *Enterobactereacea*, the use of the term "endotoxin" implies a known configuration of LPS because the molecules are similar enough to speak of as multiples of
the single type, whereas the same term (endotoxin) used to describe LPS derived
from other families cannot be said to necessarily consist of the same prototypical
structure (see Chapter 6 for a discussion of atypical structures).

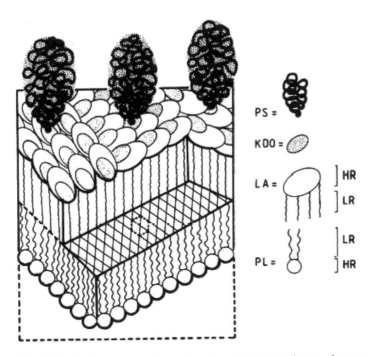

FIGURE 2 Tentative view of a section of the outer membrane of gram-negative bacteria. To emphasize the packing of lipopolysaccharide molecules, only a small section of the outer membrane from which proteins and other membrane constituents are omitted is depicted. Lipid A (LA) [HR, hydrophilic region = bisphosphorylated glucosamine disaccharide; LR, lipophilic region (fatty acid chains)] tends to form oriented domains, resulting in the shed roof-like appearance of areas of the external leaflet of the outer membrane. Compared with phospholipids (PL) the fatty acid chain conformation of lipid A is remarkably well ordered; the hexagonal packing of the schematically drawn acyl residues is indicated. The polysaccharide portion (PS), which is drawn schematically, can adopt a heavily coiled conformation and may or may not be intermingled. For better clarity only some of the polysaccharide chains are shown. *Abbreviation*: KDO, 2-Reto 3-deoxy D-manno Octulosonic OH acid. *Source*: Ref. 6, 7, 22.

The term "lipid" refers to biologically derived molecules that dissolve in organic solvents but are poorly soluble in water. Purified LPS is derived from the organic extraction of dried, dense cultures of gram-negative bacteria. Various organic solvents have been employed throughout the years to yield LPS preparations of varying degrees of purity beginning with Trichloroacetic acid (Boivin and Mesrobeanu in 1935). The most commonly used modern methods of extraction are derived from the phenol-water method originally developed by Palmer and Gerlough and later modified by Westphal et al. (1952) (10). Henderson and Wilson (11) maintain that preparations obtained via Westphal extraction are considered the "starting point" for LPS, from a nomenclature vantage. The current international reference standard (EC-6, IS-2) derived from the EC line is extracted in this way. The process involves treatment of a dried bacterial mass with a 45:55 (v/v) mix of phenol and water at 68°C for 30 minutes. Upon cooling, the solution separates into an upper water phase and a lower phenol phase. The endotoxin in this mixture ends up in the water phase with cellular nucleic acids. The water phase is centrifuged at 105,000 × g and the endotoxin forms a nearly nucleic acid-free sediment. The sediment is lyophilized to yield 1% to 4% of the original dry bacterial weight (10).

STRUCTURE AND FUNCTION

The function of each of the three moieties of the LPS molecule as seen in Figures 1 and 2 can be summarized in terms of how each affects biological systems: the O-antigen act "antigenically," providing the basis for an immunogenic response; the core region provides the molecule with its overall negative charge thus affecting many of the biological properties of the molecule, and the lipid A portion contains the endotoxic principle with its well-known deleterious host effects. A brief discussion of each moiety is given below.

Oligosaccharide-Specific Side Chains

The O-specific side chain consists of a polymer of repeating sugars and determines the O-specificity of the parent bacterial strain (4). The O-chain can be highly variable, even within a given gram-negative bacterial species, and is responsible for the LPS molecule's ability to escape an effective mammalian antigenic response due to the number of different sugars and combinations of sugars that are presented by different strains. Serological identification of members of the family *Enterobacteriaceae* utilizes the variation inherent in this region of LPS and is the only means of identifying certain pathogenic strains of *E. coli* (12) such as *E. coli* O157, which has been implicated in recent outbreaks of food-borne illness (13). The O-chain generally (for the most highly studied family, *Enterobactereaceae*) contains from twenty to forty repeating saccharide units that may include up to eight different six-carbon sugars per repeating unit and may occur in rings and other structures. Some organisms lack O-chain entirely [*Chlamydia trachomatis* consits of only KDO[b] and lipid A (3)]. At the other end of the O-chain variability spectrum lies the *Legionella pneumophilia* (serogroup 1), which contains up to 75 residues of a single sugar (a homopolymer) (14). Whereas there are in excess of 2000 O-chain variants in *Salmonella* and 100 in *E. coli*, there are only two closely related core types in the former (15) and five in the latter (14). Strains with identical sugar assembly patterns may be antigenically different due to different polysaccharide linkages (3). For this reason, an immune response evoked for one variant of *Salmonella* will produce antibodies that may be oblivious to 2000 other *Salmonnella* invaders. A great many studies have been performed and show that the O-antigen induces (either by infection or vaccination) immunity to subsequent LPS exposure, however, such immunity is limited in duration and is not cross-protective between serotypes (15).

Historically, studies of mutant bacteria unable to produce the O-specific side chain, or producing only partial side chain with whole or partial core region, have been extensively studied for their ability to retain their endotoxic properties (16). Most gram-negative bacteria have complete LPS and are referred to as "smooth" (s-LPS), given their unwrinkled visible colony morphology. Mutant isolates have been obtained that lack various polysaccharides, including O-specific side chain and core components. These isolates, called *Chemotypes*, have been labeled

---

[b]2-Keto 3-deoxy-D-manno octulosonic acid, an unusual eight carbon sugar that is a highly conserved structure in the LPS outer core.

"rough" (r-LPS) mutants due to their distinctive wrinkled colony morphology. Various mutants, ranging from Ra (most complete core) to Re (most deficient containing only KDO), have aided researchers in determining the chemical structure of LPS and its related endotoxic properties (16–18). (See Fig. 8 in Chapter 18 which shows various chemotypes.) Galanos et al. (19) modified the Westphal method in 1969 to extract the LPS of rough (r) mutants by using phenol/chloroform/petroleum ether at room temperature to yield incomplete, purified LPSs.

While the O-antigen side chain is not necessary for in vitro survival, it has been shown to be necessary to provide in vivo protection from phagocytosis and serum (complement) mediated lysis for some gram-negative pathogens (5,20). The O-specific chain in *S. enterica, Vibrio Cholerae, Shigella, E. Coil,* and *P. aerugenosa* is encoded by a cluster of genes termed *rfb* (21). A defect in the *rfb* gene cluster forms LPS without O-specific side chains (r-form LPS or r-LPS). These r-forms can grow only in vitro. According to the molecular modeling of LPS structure by Kastowsky et al. (22), the O-specific chain is flexible and may be stretched out significantly into the bacterial environment. The repeating saccharride units (folded on the cellular surface) are slightly greater than 1 nm in length per unit compared to approximately 2.4 nm for the entire length of lipid A. Of course, the number of repeating units in the given bacterial serotype will determine the length of the O-antigenic chain and the molecular weight for a given LPS monomer. Given the large number of O-antigen chains on a given cell, they produce a "felt-like network" and form an effective barrier or filter for unwanted substances (22).

Inner and Outer Core

The O-antigen side chain connects to the core oligosaccharide, which is made up of an outer (proximal to the O-chain) and inner (proximal to lipid A) core. The outer core contains common sugars: D-glucose, D-galactose, N-acetyl-D-glucosamine, and N-acetyl-D-galactosamine (in *E. coli* and *Salmonella).* The inner core contains two uncommon sugars: a seven-carbon heptose and 2-keto 3-deoxy-D-manno-octulosonic acid (KDO, systematically called 3-deoxy-D-manno-2-octulosonic acid) (22). These residues are usually substituted by charged groups such as phosphate and pyrophosphate, giving the LPS complex an overall negative charge that binds bivalent cations such as Ca^{2+} and Mg^{2+}. The minimal bacterial LPS structure capable of retaining bacterial reproductive capability consists of one KDO residue linked to lipid A (22). KDO contains an unusual eight-carbon atom structure and is a more conserved structure than the O-specific side chain or the outer core region but not as conserved in structure as lipid A. KDO very rarely occurs in nature outside of the LPS molecule. KDO as a polysaccharide acts to solubilize the lipid portion of LPS in aqueous systems (as does O-antigen when it remains attached).

The prototypical structure of LPS is contained in the family *Enterobacteriaceae,* which have caused many historically devastating diseases, including plague, cholera, and typhoid fever. The search for vaccines against such diseases has included LPS and the conserved core region. Vaccines against the O-antigenic region have been found to provide immunity; however, the region is too hypervariable and diverse to be of practical use as there are in excess of 2000 *Salmonella* O-antigen variants, whereas there are only two closely related core types (15). Nine such "epitopes" studied for immunological induction studies are shown in Figure 3. The vertical lines represent truncated chemotypes and are denoted as "R" types with the exception of SL5007.

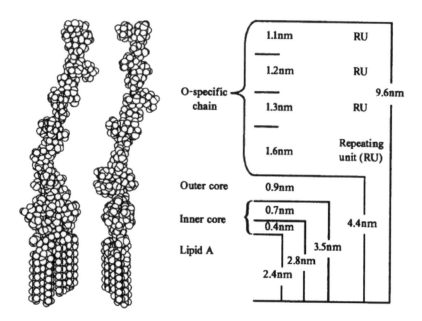

FIGURE 3 Dimensions of the calculated lipopolysaccharide (LPS) model and of partial structures. The conformer depicted shows the O-antigenic chain as an upper limit, whereas dimensions for other molecular portions are typical values. The dimensions of partial LPS structures up to the Ra-LPS structure (including the outer core) fit quite well with experimental data. *Source*: From Ref. 22.

In Figure 3 one can gain an appreciation for the relative sizes of each moiety in the LPS molecule with the core region roughly equal to the Lipid A group. The O-antigenic chain, of course, shows great variability in the length of the sugars added in various organisms. Also, the lipid A acyl groups contain elongated carbon chains in some bacterial species.

Lipid A

Westphal and Luderitz first precipitated the lipid-rich hydrolytic fragment of LPS and named it "lipid A" (16) (and the other more easily separated portion: Lipid B) (23). Lipid A is a disaccharide of glucosamine, which is highly substituted with amide and ester-linked long-chain fatty acids. Lipid A is highly conserved across gram-negative bacterial LPS and varies mainly in the fatty acid types (acyl groups) and numbers attached to the glucosamine backbone. The molecular weight of lipid A has been determined to be approximately 2000 daltons (18) as a monomer, but largely exists in aggregates of 300,000 to 1,000,000 daltons in aqueous (physiological) solutions (24).

The structure of lipid A included in Figure 4A demonstrates the general form of lipid A as seen in the *E. coli* structure and natural variants that occur in the fatty acid part of the molecule. Bacterial LPS inside the family Enterobactereaceae share the prototypical asymmetrical structure with *E. coli* and *Salmonella*, but other gram-negative organisms may or may not share the structure. The fatty acid groups (acyl groups) may be in either an asymmetrical or symmetrical repeating series and occur

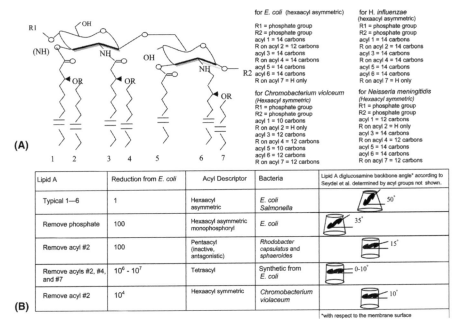

(A)

for *E. coli* (hexaacyl asymmetric)
R1 = phosphate group
R2 = phosphate group
acyl 1 = 14 carbons
R on acyl 2 = 12 carbons
acyl 3 = 14 carbons
R on acyl 4 = 14 carbons
acyl 5 = 14 carbons
acyl 6 = 14 carbons
R on acyl 7 = H only

for *H. influenzae*
(hexaacyl asymmetric)
R1 = phosphate group
R2 = phosphate group
acyl 1 = 14 carbons
R on acyl 2 = 14 carbons
acyl 3 = 14 carbons
R on acyl 4 = 14 carbons
acyl 5 = 14 carbons
acyl 6 = 14 carbons
R on acyl 7 = H only

for *Chromobacterium violceum*
(Hexaacyl symmetric)
R1 = phosphate group
R2 = phosphate group
acyl 1 = 10 carbons
R on acyl 2 = H only
acyl 3 = 14 carbons
R on acyl 4 = 12 carbons
acyl 5 = 10 carbons
acyl 6 = 12 carbons
R on acyl 7 = 12 carbons

for *Neisseria meningitidis*
(Hexaacyl symmetric)
R1 = phosphate group
R2 = phosphate group
acyl 1 = 12 carbons
R on acyl 2 = H only
acyl 3 = 14 carbons
R on acyl 4 = 12 carbons
acyl 5 = 14 carbons
acyl 6 = 14 carbons
R on acyl 7 = 12 carbons

Lipid A	Reduction from *E. coli*	Acyl Descriptor	Bacteria	Lipid A diglucosamine backbone angle* according to Seydel et al. determined by acyl groups not shown.
Typical 1—6	1	Hexaacyl asymmetric	*E. coli Salmonella*	50°
Remove phosphate	100	Hexaacyl asymmetric monophosphoryl	*E. coli*	35°
Remove acyl #2	100	Pentaacyl (inactive, antagonistic)	*Rhodobacter capsulatus and sphaeroides*	15°
Remove acyls #2, #4, and #7	10^6 - 10^7	Tetraacyl	Synthetic from *E. coli*	0-10°
Remove acyl #2	10^4	Hexaacyl symmetric	*Chromobacterium violaceum*	10°

(B)

*with respect to the membrane surface

FIGURE 4 (**A**) Chemical structure of the lipid A component of various gram-negative bacteria. (**B**) Shows lipid A diglucosamine backbone angle relative to the membrane according to Seydel et al. as determined by the underlying acyl groups of various representative organisms. *Source*: From Refs. 20, 65, 66.

almost exclusively with even-numbered carbon chains. Nontoxic lipid A analogs are being studied as a way of foiling the endotoxic reaction by competing with natural lipid A for receptor binding sites on host cells to prevent the release of endogenous pyrogens. Optimally, endotoxic lipid A structures are invariably asymmetrical (23).

The structure of the lipid A found in *E. coli* and *Salmonella* consists of a $\beta(1-6)$-linked D-glucosamine disaccharide with phosphoryl groups at position 4′ of the nonreducing glucosamine residue (GlcN II), and position 1 of the reducing glucosamine residue (GlcN II) (12). Long-chain fatty acids occupy positions 2, 3, 2′, and 3′. GlcN I contains nonacylated (R)-3-hydroxytetradecanoic acid, amide and ester-linked at positions 2 and 3 respectively. GlcN II is substituted at position 2′ with amide-linked (R)-3-dodecanoyloxytetradecanoic acid and at 3′ with ester-linked (R)-3-tetradecanoyloxytetradecanoic acid (14 carbons). The KDO disaccharide at position 6′ connects lipid A to the core polysaccharide region (20).

Galanos et al. (19) used synthetic lipid A (complexed with serum albumin) injected into laboratory animals to bring about endotoxic reactions nearly identical to those of native LPS, including lethal toxicity, pyrogenicity, local Shwartzman reactivity, *Limulus* amoebocyte lysate gelation capacity, tumor necrotizing activity, B-cell mitogenicity, induction of prostaglandin synthesis in macrophages, and antigenic specificity. This provided conclusive proof that the endotoxic principle resided in the lipid A structure. In addition to chemotypes, lipid A partial structures and precursors have been extensively studied to reveal the specific and various toxicities associated with individual Lipid A and Lipid A-like substructures

(25–29). Much of the accumulated knowledge of structure to function studies is shown graphically in Figure 4A and B. Each Lipid A substructure denoted has been found in natural organisms, synthetically produced, or created via mutation to allow researchers to define the exact structure believed to be necessary for endotoxicity. As a general rule, as lipid A structures drift away from the enteric (*E. coli*, *Salmonnella*, etc.) structure they become less endotoxic. Studies have centered around the concept of determining the resulting biological effects caused by specific changes in the geometry of the lipid A glucosamine backbone (Fig. 4B) as brought about by the specific attached fatty acid (acyl) groups.

EXTRINSIC FACTORS AFFECTING ENDOTOXIN ACTIVITY

Endotoxin molecules are often thought of simplistically as singular, static structures, however, the endotoxin molecule is a chimera, able to change forms depending not only upon intrinsic factors ultimately determined in the genetic code for a given bacterium, but also upon extrinsic factors. Much of the physical and chemical characterization of endotoxin have been carried out using purified LPS. The use of a purified LPS in research and quality control testing involves the use of a standardized material chosen to meet certain criteria that were agreed upon and does not represent many of the specific properties of a broader population of natural endotoxin molecules. The resulting standard is an artifact of the endotoxin complex not present in nature (even in the specific bacterial species from which it was derived), but refined to allow different users to enjoy a uniform testing experience and reproduce the detection, quantification, and characterization of an otherwise overly complex material. Real-world endotoxin has attributes that differ from purified LPS. Some recent discoveries shed some light on endotoxin as a living and changing part of the organism from which it is derived including the various effects of antibiotic treatment on bacterial endotoxin in host systems, the phenomenon of biofilms, and the phenomenon of gram-negative membrane vesicle (MV) production.

Extrinsic factors affecting the heterogeneity of LPS include:

1. The environment in which the bacterial culture is grown can cause slight structural variations in lipid A due primarily to changes in the attached amide-linked fatty acid chain lengths as well as variable O-antigenic side chain length and sugar constituents (30,31). Therefore, an exact structure of endotoxin cannot be absolutely defined for a population of bacteria without carefully controlling extrinsic factors such as cultural conditions.
2. The method of extraction used to obtain LPS from whole cells results in endotoxin or lipid A structures that differ both chemically and in their biological activity in host systems (32). Large macromolecular structures such as endotoxin can be expected to result in hybrid preparations with most extraction procedures resulting in a population of various chemical constituents with accompanying varying attributes.
3. The toxic properties of endotoxin and specifically, lipid A, have been determined to be dependant upon the non-LPS cellular constituents to which it is attached (33,34). Free lipid A is all but biologically inactive unless solubilized in human or bovine serum albumin or other carriers (35,36). Even though the lipid A portion clearly contains the endotoxic principle, it must be solubilized to make it available to interact with host cells. Non-LPS constituents serve to

help solubilize lipid A. In commercial LPS preparations (Reference standard endotoxin and control standard endotoxin), fillers are used to stabilize LPS and to aid the filling of vials during manufacture. Common fillers such as human serum albumin, PEG, and lactose can cause *Limulus* amebocyte lysate (LAL) reactivity differences in different product testing matrices (37). The relative biological activity or exposure of various "real-world" bacterial endotoxins in a host are also affected by the degree of association of endotoxin with cellular wall material including (*i*) the presence of non-LPS cellular fragments (i.e., polysaccharides, K antigen, protein content) and (*ii*) the disassociation of free endotoxin from whole cells. A basic tenant of endotoxin knowledge is that LPS is the biologically toxic portion of the endotoxin complex and, more specifically, the endotoxic principle resides in the Lipid A moiety[c]. However, it is also a given that rarely, if ever, is LPS in host systems disassociated from other cellular components, such as cellular membrane proteins (38). Mutants without O-antigen polysaccharide (rough types) have been shown to be more endotoxic and shed 10 times more free endotoxin into the environment than s-forms (39). Morrison and coworkers reported that as the length of the LPS polysaccharide chain is shortened, the resulting LAL activation capability increases. Interestingly, LPS molecules with longer (polysaccharide) chains have also been shown to differ in fatty acid content from the shorter, r-LPS types (40).

Another major but variable component of bacteria, including *E. coli* strains, is the capsular polysaccharide outermost coating produced by so-called K strains capsule producers) Mattsby-Baltzer et al. (37) studied the effect of K antigen in *Limulus* assays and found that K(+) and K(−) strains did not differ appreciably in activity. This surprised the researchers who speculated that the polysaccharide capsule may have been removed by washings of the bacterial cells prior to analysis as well as the fact that K antigens usually cover only part of the cell wall. Apparently of greater importance is the absence of associated O-antigen, which may allow greater interaction between cell-bound lipid A and *Limulus* proclotting enzyme in the LAL assay and soluble receptors in host systems (such as sCD14). A notable exception to the muted activity of endotoxin with associated cellular residues is the potent cytokine inducing capability attributed to several bacterial OMP. Henderson, Poole, and Wilson (40) identify three types of OMPs: (*i*) porins (permeable to <600 Da molecules), (*ii*) lipid-A-associated proteins (LAP) or endotoxin-associated proteins, and (*iii*) other OMPs. The lowest associated concentration inducing cytokine synthesis (in ng/ml) is reported by Henderson to be in a range of activity similar to LPS (0.01 ng/ml) although via a different mechanism.

Wahl et al. (41) demonstrated the contribution of proteins in some LPS preparations by comparing protein-free LPS by phenol extraction and LAP-containing LPS by butanol extraction. Using "endotoxin-unresponsive" C3H/HeJ mice, they showed that only the protein-containing preparation produced a lethal effect. Doses of purified, protein-free LPS five times that of LPS–LAP were completely nontoxic to the mice even though the phenol extracted LPS was twice as potent in normal mice. A question evoked by the contrast of environmental and standard or purified LPS concerns the relative biological activity of free (soluble)

---

[c]Part of a molecule, often with a specific function.

versus bound (cell-embedded) endotoxin. Morrison et al. (23) showed free endo-toxin to be 20 to 50 times more biologically active than bacterial cell-bound endo-toxin. Their study used TNF-α secretion and tissue factor procoagulant activity of human monocytes in vitro to quantitate the relative endotoxicity of bacterial bound versus free endotoxin. Morrison acknowledges that the choice of the system used to measure "pro-inflammatory" biological activity may explain the conflicting results obtained in his group's study versus some other studies. His group used nonreplicating *E. coli* minicells and LPS adsorbed to latex particles to approximate the size of the microbe as a particulate. However, Katz et al. (42) found that whole *E. coli* cells were fully capable of potent CD14-mediated signaling of human leukocytes, and were absent in the existence of free (released) endotoxin.

4.   Means of (assay) measurement affect the potency and determination of biologi-cal activity. Table 1 shows the reactivity of a constant dose of various gram-negative bacteria and endotoxin as a ratio, where the rabbit pyrogen test results are comparable to the LAL assay results. At the extreme, in the studies cited, the dose varies by a thousand-fold in the case of *Legionella pneu-mophilia* and 10 to 50 times for some members of the same family (*Salmonella, Serratia, Klebsiella*) to that of the commonly used standard, *E. coli*. Table 1

TABLE 1   Comparative Reactivity to a Dose of Various Gram-Negative Organisms as a Ratio where the Rabbit Pyrogen Test Result Is Comparable to the *Limulus* Amebocyte Lysate Assay Result

Reference	Gram-negative organism	Ratio of reactivity in rabbit pyrogen test to that of LAL assay[a]
Wachtel and Tsuji (66)	*E. coli*	35–52
	S. typhi	"
	P. mirabilis	"
	Pseudomonas spp.	"
Sween et al. (67)	*S. enteritidis*	4.3
	Veillonella spp. *(2 strains)*	84–896
	Fusobacterium spp. *(2 strains)*	"
	Bacteroides spp. *(3 strains)*	"
Wong et al. (68)	*Legionella pneumophilia*	1000
Weary et al. (69)	*Y. enterocolitica*	2–6
Group 1	*A. calcoaceticus*	"
	S. abortus-equi	"
	S. dysenteriae	"
	E. coli (3 strains)	"
Group 2	*V. cholerae*	26–75
	S. marcescens	"
	P. aeruginosa (2 strains)	"
Devleeschouwer et al. (70)	*E. coli*	1
	K. pneumoniae	9–12
	S. marcescens	10–11
	P. aeruginosa	1–15
	P. putida	15–500

[a]Ratio of dose of endotoxin (7,67,68) or bacteria (69,71) required for reactivity with the rabbit pyrogen assay to dose for reactivity with the LAL assay.
Source: From Ref. 6.

demonstrates not only that the relative pyrogenicity/endotoxicity differs by bacterial type but also by the method of measurement. In each case, according to the table, the rabbit pyrogen assay underestimates (or is at most equal to) the activity of endotoxin from environmental isolates as determined by the LAL assay. Gram-negative bacteria are noted for their ability to shed endotoxin during normal growth (43). Shed endotoxin is believed to resemble the endotoxin released during gram-negative infection in that the endotoxin may contain even less phospholipid and protein than extracted LPS (37). Mattsby-Baltzer et al. (37) compared the activity of several enteric bacteria (*E. coli*, *Salmonella*) by various methods including chromogenic LAL (cLAL) and GC detection of the β-hydroxymyristic acid (β-OHC$_{14:0}$) marker indicative of the presence of lipid A. By comparing the activity of whole cell cultures and supernatants (filtered through a whole cell excluding 0.22 micrometer filter), they showed the cLAL activity of the supernatants to be up to 20 times greater. The β-OHC$_{14:0}$ measured contents in the supernatants were approximately half to one-fourth that of the whole cell cultures. Their study indicates that the method of presentation of LPS is an important factor in cLAL reactivity. Morrison et al. (36) relate that the biological activity of lipid A may vary with the relative types of lipid A subfractions generated by various methods of cellular release. Johnson et al. (44) speculate that the cellular attached versus free endotoxin differential may be a "virulence characteristic" observed in "shedders" versus "nonshedders," at least in some species such as *Neisseria*.

Hurley and Tosolini (45) related the increase in endotoxin content as determined by a modified kinetic LAL assay in infected urine. Given a constant CFU count, the group determined that the endotoxin counts from members of the family Enterobacteriaceae were two to three times higher than those infected with *Pseudomonas*, indicating that the type of bacterial infection determines the toxicity of the endotoxin released. Bacteria considered to emit relatively greater amount of endotoxin include those with rough phenotypes and certain pathogens. Gram-negatives with rough LPS were found by Mattsby-Baltzer et al. (37) to shed up to ten times more endotoxin than their smooth counterparts. Virulent pathogens associated with meningitis and gonorrhea have been implicated as shedding more endotoxin than less virulent variants (44).

While the range of relative reactivity between the pyrogen and LAL assays is great in some instances, in general the LAL assay results parallel other measures of adverse host reactivity such as mitogenicity as well as mice and chick embryo lethality, at least for the smaller group of most studied enteric organisms (6).

5. The mechanism of LPS release from bacterial cells affects the biological activity of the resulting endotoxin. Given that the release of LPS from microbes (as well as the attachment or lack thereof of specific non-LPS components) affects the biological activity, the method of release may also be important in determining the resultant structures formed. Endotoxin release from whole gram-negative bacteria has been characterized as arising via several mechanisms:

- natural cell death and bacteriolysis
- LPS shedding via bleb or MV release
- serum protein and complement-mediated release
- host phagocyte ingestion with subsequent exocytosis of LPS
- antibiotic-mediated release

Bacterial cell death and lysis occur as a normal part of the growth curve of populations of bacteria and contribute predominately to the existence of free endotoxin complex in aqueous solutions in which they grow. Shedding (46) has been studied in meningococcus, where blebbing of outer membranes results in large amounts of free endotoxin. The resulting endotoxic effects are notably severe in meningitis due to the potency of the endotoxin released and given the access to the hypothalamus via the cerebral spinal fluid route.

Beveridge (47) has described a phenomenon common to gram–negative organisms in which MV are formed. MVs have been characterized as 50–250 nm-diameter bilayered spheres released from the surface of virtually all gram-negative bacteria. MVs resemble the buds on a microscopic yeast cell (Fig. 5). Cells can become covered by MVs, as seen in Figure 6, which consist of the gram-negative membrane enclosing cellular protoplasm (1). Prior to release, the normal curvature of the outer cell membrane is changed to a high curvature structure that, curiously, only contains one of the two different kinds of LPS characterized in *Pseudomonas aerugiona* (1). MVs have been found to attach to (gram-negative and positive) bacterial cells by inserting themselves into the bacterial cellular membrane (47). For this reason, they are being studied as potential delivery vehicles for antibiotics, vaccines, and virulence factors. However, if the endotoxicity associated with MVs cannot be attenuated, the delivery method would be reserved for oral delivery.

Gram-negative bacteria are phagocytized by macrophages and neutrophils in vitro and in vivo (17,18). LPS may be subsequently released after being engulfed. This process has been termed exocytosis. Shnyra et al. (48) demonstrated an increase in biological activity with increased aggregation (other factors such as solubility being equal). Phagocytic cellular uptake of invading particles has been described as occurring when the particle encountered is of a sufficient aggregate size and when its hydrophobicity exceeds that of the phagocyte (48). LPS

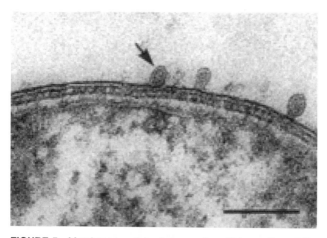

FIGURE 5   Membrane vesicle close up view: Thin section of *P. aeruginosa* PAO1 showing the development of n-membrane vesicles before they are liberated from the cell. The arrow points to one vesicle in which the membrane bilayer and the periplasm within its lumen (i.e., electrondense area inside the vesicle) can be seen. Bar = 250 nm. *Source*: From Ref. 1.

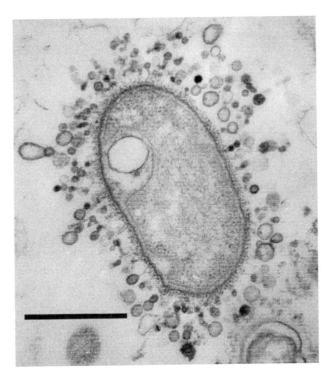

FIGURE 6 Membrane vesicles covering an entire gram-negative bacterial cell: Thin section of an unidentified gram-negative bacterium found in a freshwater biofilm in a river near laboratory. This bacterium possesses a microcapsule and is liberating a prodigious amount of membrane vesicles. Bar = 1 μm. *Source*: From Ref. 1.

aggregates satisfying the hydrophobic criteria are actively taken up by monocytes/macrophages with the resultant production and release of cytokines.

Complement-mediated killing is another method by which endotoxin is liberated from invading cells and occurs upon bacterial entry into host blood systems. Tesh et al. (49) have studied complement-mediated endotoxin release extensively by treating *E. coli* in vitro with human serum. They found that approximately 50% of the cellular endotoxin is able to be freed by the insertion of complement complexes into the cellular outer membrane by both alternative and classical complement pathways, and that the released LPS is rapidly bound by multiple serum constituents and rendered reversibly biologically inactive (50).

In addition to complement proteins active in attaching and facilitating the uptake of LPS, various lipoproteins present in blood plasma bind and neutralize free LPS and release LPS that has already been bound to leukocytes (monocytes). The predominant lipoprotein in plasma is high-density lipoprotein (HDL). Kitchens et al. (51) studied the binding of monocytes in plasma with radiolabeled LPS [(^{3}H)LPS] with and without HDL [with added plasma lipid transfer proteins LPS-binding protein (LBP) and phospholipid transfer protein (PLTP) needed to facilitate binding to the LPS receptor CD14 on membranes (mCD14) and in solution (sCD14)]. They showed that in plasma containing monocyte bound (^{3}H)LPS and either native or reconstituted HDL, 70% of the cell-associated labeled LPS was

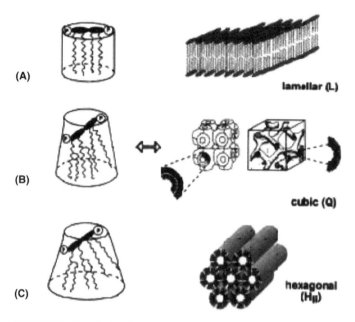

(A)

lamellar (L)

(B)

cubic (Q)

(C)

hexagonal (H$_{II}$)

FIGURE 7 Correlation between the molecular shape of lipid A and the three-dimensional supramolecular structure formed. Figure shows the interrelationship between Lipid A type, supramolecular structure formed (lamellar versus inverted (conical)), biological activity (endotoxicity) and blood reactivity (anti-complement activity). *Abbreviations*: H$_{II}$, hexagonal; L, Lamellar; Q, cubic. *Source*: From Ref. 54.

released whereas (^{3}H)LPS in the control sample (serum-free medium) remained bound to the cells. Specific cellular responses were also reduced indicating that the migration of cellular bound LPS to lipoprotein-associated LPS serves to attenuate the host response to LPS in host systems.

LIFE AS AN AMPHIPHILE: SOLUBILITY, IONIC CHARGE/PH, AND AGGREGATE SIZE

In solution, endotoxin molecules stick to each other or aggregate to form supramolecular structures ranging in molecular weight from 300,000 to 1,000,000 daltons (24). It has been known for some time that LPS is an ampiphilic (amphipathic) molecule consisting of a hydrophilic polysaccharide end and a hydrophobic lipid (A) end (with a negative net charge). In aqueous solution (physiological solutions), the molecules form spheres or ribbons consisting of bilayers (52,53). The bilayers hydrophobic fatty acid tails are sandwiched in the center of the resulting bilayer of hydrophilic polysaccharides (24). Adding detergent or bile salts to yield molecular weights of between 10,000 to 20,000 daltons can reduce the micelle aggregation size. If the detergent is then dialyzed out, the larger structures reversibly reassemble. Such aggregates have been shown to occur in micellar, hexagonal, lamellar, and nonlamellar cubic and inverted hexagonal form (54) as shown in Figure 8. The adoption of different three-dimensional, supramolecular structures occurs once the crital micellar concentration of LPS in a given solution has been reached. The structures formed depend upon the underlying chemical structure of the specific LPS as well as factors present in the environment in which LPS molecule finds itself, such as temperature, pH, and divalent cation concentration, mainly Ca^{2+} and Mg^{2+}, which are important in stabilizing the three-dimensional structure of the molecule and in forming the endotoxic three-dimensional conformation (20).

Aggregation (which will be discussed in the next section) as measured in molecular weight of the aggregate is related to solubility and is the tendency of amphiphiles to gather with like hydrophobic molecular moieties attaching to like hydrophobic moieties of other like molecules. Hartley called ionic or polar derivatives of hydrocarbons "amphipathic" in 1936 to describe them as one part "sympathy" and one part "antipathy" for water (55). As the hydrophobic tail lengthens, the amphiphile becomes more and more water insoluble. Many such combined molecules are generally called micelles, although the term is also used specifically by some to describe various forms of aggregates.

Micelle formation has been described as the segregation of amphiphilic molecular portions from aqueous solvents by self-aggregation (55). If the hydrophobic portion is a hydrocarbon chain, as in the case of LPS fatty acids, then the core consists entirely of hydrocarbons while the polar head groups (core polysaccharides) serve to solubilize the material in its aqueous environment. The forms such amphiphiles take include: spheres or disks, oblate or prolate ellipsoids (long cylinders), or bilayers (parallel layers with polar groups facing out). The hydrocarbon center is considered to be disorderly. In effect, according to Tanford (55), the hydrophobic core is a small volume of liquid hydrocarbon. Other hydrophobic substances may become dissolved within the hydrophobic core (56). It is interesting to view some general hydrocarbon micelle postulates as described by Tanford to LPS aggregation theory to see that they are governed by common laws of hydrocarbon interaction:

1. The number of monomers that may aggregate is a function of the number of hydrocarbon chains attached to each amphiphile
2. the dimension of the micelle is limited by the maximum extension of hydrocarbon chain (the smaller the acyl chains, the smaller the micelles that may

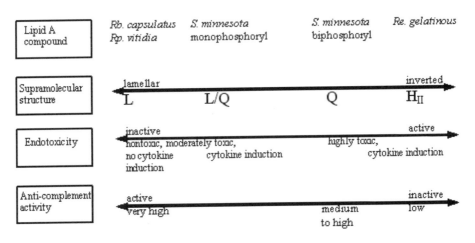

FIGURE 8

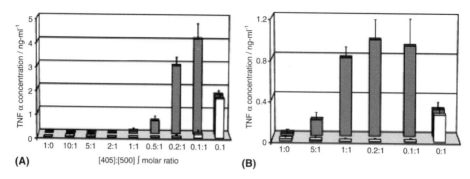

FIGURE 9 The molecular composition of aggregates critically determines their biological activities. TNF production from human MNCs after stimulation under serum-free conditions with aggregate mixtures (aggr.(506+406), *light boxes*) and mixed aggregates (aggr.(506) plus aggr.(406), *dark boxes*) of compound 506 and compound 406 (A) and aggregate mixtures (aggr.(506+CL), *light boxes*) and mixed aggregates (aggr.(506) plus aggr.(CL), *dark boxes*) of compound 506 and diphosphatidylglycerol (*CL*) (**B**), in varying molar ratios. Data represent one out of three independent experiments, and data given are mean of triplicates ± S.D. *Source*: From Ref. 62.

be formed). Note that the proposed endotoxic conformation requires fatty acid chains of 10 to 16 carbons.

3. for enclosed volumes of hydrocarbons, the surface/volume ratio decreases with increasing volume
4. given the fluid nature of the micelle interior, the surface can be viewed as "rough" with spikes and troughs correlating to the state of flux of the interior.
5. the presence of odd or even acyl chains affects the internal packing structure (note that endotoxic LPS consists of even carbon fatty acid chains in an asymmetrical pattern)

These axioms are interesting given that the aggregation-state (molecular weight) of endotoxin is a critical determinant of biological activity. Luderitz et al. (38) demonstrated this principle by using various salt forms of a highly purified LPS from *Salmonella abortus equi*. The aggregation of endotoxin is not only a function of its hydrophobic lipid A moiety's ability to interact (thereby forming higher molecular weight aggregates), but also the electrostatic nature of cationic components associated with the acidic phosphate and carboxyl groups of the molecule. LPS is acidic due to the presence of negatively charged carboxyl and phosphate groups (4). Neutralization of (acidic) LPS by electrodialysis in base yields a corresponding uniform salt. Salts formed from various LPS molecules have different solubility characteristics in water. Luderitz et al. demonstrated that, when a highly purified LPS was converted to the triethylamine, sodium, or putrescine salt the molecular weight increased and the water solubility decreased (26). As the molecular weight increased, toxicity in rats, rate of clearance from blood, interaction with complement, and affinity for cells also increased, but lethality decreased in mice (but increased in rats), as did pyrogenicity in rabbits. The latter two phenomena increased with decreasing molecular weight (sedimentation coefficient) or increasing water solubility. The relationship between molecular weight and biological activity can be seen in Table 2. Since the molecular weight of an endotoxin preparation is a critical determinant of its biological activity substances that either reduce surface tension (such as Tween-20) or sequester divalent cations (such as ethylenediaminetetraacetic acid, EDTA) will decrease molecular aggregation as measured by (increased) LAL activity.

In the presence of magnesium and calcium, LPS forms bilayer sheets or vesicles with a diameter of approximately 0.1 μm. When endotoxin preparations are reduced by a chelating agent or surfactant, rod-shaped subunits appear, which have a molecular weight of approximately 20,000 daltons, a diameter of 8 to 12 Angstroms, and a length of 200 to 700 Angstroms. These structures are interconvertible, as has been demonstrated using molecular filtration (18). Sweadner's studies showed that vesicles and bilayer sheets pass through a 0.22 μm membrane filter, but are retained by a 0.025 μm pore size and that the small micellar forms pass through a 0.025 μm filter but are retained by a 1,000,000 nominal molecular weight limit (NMWL) molecular filter. When LPS is reduced to its smallest subunit by a surface-active agent, such as sodium deoxycholate, it will pass through a molecular filter with a NMWL of 1,000,000, but will be retained by a molecular weight filter with a NMWL of 10,000. However, from a practical point of view, endotoxin can be considered to have a molecular weight of 10^6 daltons in an aqueous environment in the absence of significant levels of divalent cations and surface-active agents. This is the approximate molecular aggregate most frequently encountered in large-volume parenteral and medical device rinse solutions.

In another series of classical studies, Sweadner et al. (24) demonstrated the effect of the state of aggregation on the filtration of endotoxin solutions. These studies may be summarized as defining a gradient after manipulation of a given LPS solution to yield a characteristic resultant LPS type as shown in Table 2.

Impurities (considering non-LPS cellular components as impurities) and cations present in a given (parenteral) solution affect the solubility of the resulting endotoxin suspension. In general, the solubility of a given endotoxin preparation will increase in proportion to the increase in the polysaccharide to lipid ratio (4). The richer the polysaccharide content, the more soluble the preparation will be. For extracted endotoxin, the general rule is that s-LPS is more soluble than r-LPS and Ra mutants are more soluble than Re mutants (20). This is not always the case, however, and some PCP prepared r-LPS may be more soluble than the same prepared in phenol-water and even, rarely, more soluble than phenol-water extracted s-LPS (4).

The negatively charged carboxyl and phosphate groups also help to determine the solubility of the LPS molecule (4). Low phosphate and/or phosphate content is associated with poor solubility. The presence of environmental charged groups helps to determine the solubility of LPS in a given solution. The presence of divalent cations Ca^{2+} and Mg^{2+} neutralize the anionic phosphate and carboxyl groups. These

TABLE 2

Solution	LPS form present	Mol. weight in Daltons
Aqueous solution	bilayer	>1,000,000
Removal of Ca^{2+} and Mg^{2+}	micelles (diameters 3–7 nm)	300,000 – 1,000,000
Detergent or bile salt treatment	decreased diameters (0.8–1.2 nm)	10,000 – 20,000[a]

[a]Invisible in electron microscope.

internal anionic (−) groups help solubilize the LPS molecule, but also depend on the presence of external cations to be available to neutralize them. If enough divalent cations are added to a given solution, LPS may precipitate from solution altogether. Even in its purified salt forms, LPS has not been found to be present as a monomer. Galanos and Luderitz demonstrated that the lowest sedimentation coefficient obtained corresponded to molecular weights of 30,000 daltons, which equates to the smallest aggregation size of 15 to 20 molecules for the common s-form (4).

In continuing the analogy of LPS to hydrocarbon activity, the dispersion of LPS in solution is achieved by several means (56); each is used in some manner to facilitate the recovery of (standard) endotoxin from pharmaceutical products, for LAL testing. They include: (*i*) increasing the surface area of the hydrocarbon relative to the solvent (water in physiological environments) by the addition of mechanical energy such as shaking, stirring, vortexing, sonication and so on, and so on, (*ii*) chemical dispersions, such as with deoxycholate (57), (*iii*) emulsification via surface-active compounds such as polysorbate or Pyrosperse™. Liquid–liquid extraction (*iv*) may also serve as a means of coaxing the fatty acid dominated LPS into aqueous phase from which it may be quantified. High salt concentrations and extreme pH values (56) bring about the opposite effect of lowered dissolution (solubility). Not surprisingly, the LPS–LAL reaction is optimum under physiological conditions that mimic those occurring in biological systems.

The fluidity state of a hydrocarbon structure is a description of the state of order of its carbon constituents. Luhm et al. (58) examined the effect of LPS fluidity on biological activity as measured by resultant cytokine production at various temperatures. They found that cytokine production in serum as initiated by heat-killed *E. coli* as well as various chemotypes of LPS was significantly higher at 30°C compared to 37°C. Thus, they established an inverse relationship between cytokine production and fluidity. Cytokine secretion increased with decreasing fluidity. The authors speculate that the binding of LBP (or low density lipoproteins-LDL) to lipid A is facilitated by low fluidity (i.e., lower temperature) accompanied (in the case of LBP) by the enhanced ability of the LPS–LBP complex to activate the CD14 LPS cellular receptor due to the increase in order of its hydrocarbon residues (i.e., increasing geometric specificity).

ARE AGGREGATES OR MONOMERS MORE BIOLOGICALLY ACTIVE?

In water-based environments endotoxin aggregates and the type of aggregates that form are based upon the chemical structure of the underlying LPS molecules. Many interrelated physical factors affect the pyrogenicity/endotoxicity of endotoxins in solution by affecting the ability to form aggregates as well as the underlying conformation (geometrical arrangement) of those aggregates. The resulting changes affect the availability of the endotoxic lipid A portion of the LPS molecule to interact with host cell membranes and, therefore, its biological activity.

Recent studies have focused on the so-called "endotoxic conformation" and upon the complex interaction of LPS with serum proteins in host systems (59). Din et al. express the aggregate versus monomeric biological activity dilemma:

> Is it an aggregate with a defined surface topography or a monomeric LPS exhibiting specific structural features in the lipid A region that are recognized by the biological system? If monomer, what are its solubility properties? Is the available monomer concentration adequate for activating the biological systems?

The answers to these questions are basic to how we interpret the results of studies on the ... structure-to-function relationship of LPS or lipid A in the activation of responding cells (macrophages, B cells, neutrophils, monocytes, and endothelial cells). These questions have not been adequately resolved (60).

Din et al. favor the view that LPS monomers are the more biologically active units. Their reasoning is as follows: diphosphoryl lipid A derived from nontoxic LPS of *Rhodobacter sphaeroides* is inactive, whereas the lipid A from *E. coli* is active; the structural differences between the two consist of the number of fatty acid chains (five vs. six) and the chain length of the hydroxyl fatty acids (10 vs. 14). From such chain-length variations, "it is difficult to rationalize how such a structural specificity can be achieved with aggregated LPS." Although, according to Tanford (55) such fine structure changes profoundly affect the resulting supramolecular aggregation geometry. Din et al. prepared a Re-LPS-bovine serum albumin complex containing Re-LPS in a highly disaggregated state. This complex was shown to activate pre-B cells. Furthermore, the degree of solubilization of Re-LPS was not affected by temperature or ionic concentration as one would predict, if the micellar model were active in this case (60). Takayama et al. (61) successfully prepared LPS monomers and demonstrated that such solutions displayed significantly greater in vitro biological activity as compared to aggregated solutions. An opposing camp is aligned for aggregation as a prerequisite for significant endotoxicity. Shnyra et al. (48) found that *Salmonella* LPS could be detoxified reversibly by changing its physical state toward disaggregation. In the application of LAL testing, increased aggregation correlates to inhibition of control standard endotoxin recovery. For this reason, dispersing solutions and vortexing are routinely used to aid in disaggregating control standard endotoxin spike solutions used in validating parenteral product tests. In this setting, aggregation clearly favors an inhibition of endotoxicity as measured by LAL testing, albeit this is an artificial environment compared to the interaction of physiological systems and endogenous endotoxin.

Mueller et al. (62) more recently (2004) studied this question using lipid A compounds 506 (synthetic *E. coli*-like hexaacylated) and 406 (tetraacylated precursor IVa) mixed at different ratios and also mixed together in various aggregates. They found that a mixture up to 20% of 406 and 80% of 506 was more endotoxic than 506 alone. The researchers surmise: "These observations can only be understood by assuming that the active unit of endotoxin is the aggregate." The data are summarized in Figures 10A and B. The group further confirmed the active aggregate versus inert monomer findings using 506 and 406 prepared monomeric lipid A preparations via dialysis membrane separation of the solution[d]. They used solutions from each side of the dialysis chamber and exposed them to human mononuclear cells with detection via TNF-α production as well as testing the solutions using LAL. The results for both clearly show that only the aggregate solutions are biologically active. LAL results are shown in Figure 11.

ENDOTOXIC CONFORMATION SUMMARY

There is a prerequisite molecular lipid A structure that forms the prerequisite supramolecular aggregate structure that in turn interacts biologically with host

---

[d]Monomeric lipid A is 1797 Da and thus monomers and not dimmers could pass the membrane (62). The authors also quote the critical micillar concentration of lipid A as $\sim 10^8$ M.

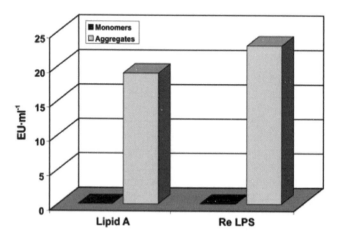

FIGURE 10   Endotoxin aggregates are more active in the *Limulus* amebocyte lysate (LAL) assay than monomers. Endotoxic activity of Lipid A and Re LPS aggregates (*light boxes*) and monomers (*dark boxes*) in same concentrations (10^{-9} M) in the LAL assay. Data shown are mean of duplicates. *Source*: From Ref. 62.

systems via pattern recognition receptors to bring about the host response. The characteristics of the unique lipid A endotoxic conformation have been refined from many studies correlating the three-dimensional structure of supramolecular aggregates of different bacterial species with the resulting differences in biological activity. *E. coli* and *Salmonella* have generally been used as the reference LPS structures as a means of relating the degree of similarity. The prerequisite chemical structure of endotoxic lipid A has been found to consist of: the lipid A backbone composed of a β 1,6-linked D-glucosamine disaccharide substituted with two phosphate groups in positions 1 and 4' and six fatty acid residues of specific length, from 10 to 16 carbon atoms (54,63). This is the lipid A structure present in *E. coli* and *S. minnesota* and *S. typhimurum* and other *Enterobactereaceae* [and some nonenterics as well such as *Hemophilus* and *Providencia* (64)]. This is not the form seen in nonendotoxic structures represented in such gram-negative organisms as *Bacteroides fragilis*, *R. capsulatum*, and *R. sphaeroides* (29). Other investigators have found that the glucosamine backbone as substituted glucosamine with short peptide chains as well as the phosphate groups are not significant to the endotoxicity of lipid A (if replaced by synthetic, mimicking groups), but have confirmed the importance of the acyl group conformation (26). Given the fact that the lipid A region contains the endotoxic portion of the molecule and the preference for aggregates to form in solution that hide lipid A from the environment, the question remains: How does Lipid A in such an arrangement interact with cellular membranes to trigger the host response?

Many studies have been undertaken to answer this question and to determine the precise characteristics that endow the lipid A portion of LPS with its endotoxic properties. Puzzling as well is the contrast of gram-negative organisms of low (or no) biologically active endotoxin (such as *Rhodobacter* and *Rhodo-pseudomonas*) to those of highly active endotoxin, such as those of the *Enterobacteriaceae* family. Rietschel et al. (20) at the Borstel Center for Medicine and Biosciences in Germany have postulated that specific chemical, three dimensional, structural variations (conformations) in LPS correlate with the relative endotoxin biological activity. For enterobacterial-free lipid A, the tendency is to adopt, at physiological conditions, a nonlamellar cubic structure. The inference from such studies has been that a prerequisite for biological activity is the inverted conical shape (as opposed to cylindrical) of the individual endotoxin molecule that leads to nonlamellar inverted aggregate structures. What appears to be important is the higher surface area of the hydrophobic (lipid) versus hydrophilic regions of such nonlamellar inverted structures, thus exposing the Lipid A acyl group structures. This appears to indicate that the flipping of the Lipid A acyl groups from inside (lamellar) to outside (cubic < hexagonal) of the aggregated molecules brings about the ability to interact with host cell receptors.

The toxicity of lipid A has been theorized to be dependent on the tendency of a given species' LPS to adopt nonlamellar (cubit or hexagonal) structures as determined by its prerequisite chemical structure (14). LPS (free lipid A or the entire LPS complex) that prefers a lamellar structure exhibits little or no biological activity. Seemingly, this would explain preliminarily, if not conclusively, how the Lipid A portion determines the endotoxicity of LPS. That is, when the hydrophobic lipids are in an outwardly presented conformation (not an inward aggregate as are lamellar structures) and consists of at least the minimum required chemical structure, it presumably fits a host cell receptor or family of receptors and triggers a transmembrane signaling event and subsequent cytokine gene transcription, manufacture, and release. Brandenburg et al. have theorized that it is specifically the conical molecular geometry that causes the disturbance in the target cell membrane and provides the trigger that signals a specific membrane protein (receptor) to actively manufacture and subsequently release endotoxic mediators. Structural analogs and precursors of lipid A that act as competitive antagonists of LPS to reduce or eliminate LPS biological activities provide further evidence that the effects of LPS are indeed mediated by specific receptors on host cells (6,25–29).

Seydel et al. (65) have summarized the hypothesized "general endotoxic principle" as follows:

> . . . prerequisites for agonistic (endotoxic) action are amphiphilic molecules with clearly separated polar and apolar moieties and a conical conformation of the molecules with a larger conical conformation of the molecules with a larger cross-section of the hydrophobic than of the hydrophobic moiety. For antagonistic action, a cylindrical rather than a conical conformation of the molecules is required, usually guaranteed by a less acylated apolar moiety. For both, agonism as well as antagonism, the presence of at least two negative charges in the polar headgroup is an important prerequisite, no matter whether these are provided by phosphate or carboxylate groups.

These principles have been depicted graphically and shown as a function of the degree (angle) of divergence from perpendicular to the attached acyl chains in Figure 4B.

REFERENCES

1. Beveridge TJ. Structures of gram-negative cell walls and their derived membrane vesicles. J Bacteriol 1999; 181(16):4725–4733.
2. Raetz C et al. Gram negative endotoxin: an extraordinary lipid with profound effects on eukaryotic signal transduction. FASEB 1991; 5(12):2652–2660.
3. Raetz C. Biochemistry of endotoxins. Annu Rev Biochem 1990; 59:129–170.

4. Galanos C, Luderitz O. Lipopolysaccharide: properties of an amphipathic molecule. In: Rietschel ET, ed. Handbook of Endotoxin, Chemistry of Endotoxin. Vol. 1. Elsevier Science Publishers, 1984.

5. Rietschel, Brade. Bacterial endotoxins. Sci Am 1992; Aug:54–61.

6. Hurley J. Endotoxemia: methods of detection and clinical correlates. Clin Micro Rev 1995; April:268–292.

7. Barnickel G, Bradaczek H, Naumann D, Rietschel ET, Giesbrecnt P, Labischinski IH. High state of order of isolated bacterial lipopolysaccharide and its possible contribution to the permeation barrier property of the outer membrane. J Bacteriol 1985; 162(1):9–20.

8. Hitchcock PJ et al. Lipopolysaccharide nomenclature-past, present, and future. J Bacteriol 1986; 166:699–701.

9. Mangan DF et al. Stimulation of human monocdytes by endotoxin-associated protein: inhibition of programmed cell death (apoptosis) and potential significance in adjuvanticity. Infect Immun 1992; 60:1684–1686.

10. Kabir ST, et al. Bacterial toxins and cell membranes. In: Jeljaszewicz T, Wadstrom, eds. New York: Academic Press New York, 1978.

11. Henderson B, Wilson M. Cytokine induction by bacteria: beyond lipopolysaccharide. Cytokine 1996; 8(4):269–282.

12. Kelly MT, Brenner DJ, JJ Farmer III. Enterobacteriaceae. In: Lennette EH, ed. Manual of Clinical Microbiology. Washington: American Society for Microbiology, 1985:263–277.

13. Dundas S, Todd WTA. *Escherichia coli* O157 and human disease. Curr Opin Infect Dis 1998; 11:171–175.

14. Rietschel et al. Bacterial endotoxins: molecular relationship of structure to activity and function. FASEB 1994; 18:217–225.

15. Nnalue AN. All accessible epitopes in the *Salmonella* lipopolysaccharide core are associated with branch residues. Infect Immun 1999; 67(2):998–1003.

16. Luderitz OH. Endotoxins and other cell wall components of gram negative bacteria and their biological activities, p. 234–246. In: Schiessinger D (ed)., Microbiology-1977, American Society Microbiology, Washington, D.C. Annu Rev Microbiol 1977; 239–246.

17. Nowotny A. Relation of structure to function in bacterial endotoxin. Annu Rev Microbiol 1977:247–252.

18. Rietschel et al. Chemical structure of lipid A. Microbiology 1977; 262.

19. Galanos C et al. Synthetic and Natural *E. coli* free lipid A express identical endotoxic activities. Eur J Biochem 1985; 148:1–5.

20. Rietschel, E. Th., et al., Bacterial endotoxin: molecular releationships of structure to activity and function, FASEB J. 1994; 8:217–225.

21. Schnaitman CA, Klena JD. Genetics of lipopolysaccharide biosynthesis in enteric bacteria. Microbiol Rev 1993 September; 57:655–682.

22. Kastowsky et al. Molecular modeling of the three-dimensional structure and conformational flexibility of bacterial lipopolysaccharide. J Bacteriol 1992; July: 4798–4806.

23. Morrison DC et al. Structure-function relationships of bacterial endotoxins, contribution to microbial sepsis. In: Opal SM, Cross AS, eds. *Infect Dis Clin North Am*, Philadelphia: Harcourt Brace & Co 1999; 13(2):313–340.

24. Sweadner et al. Filtration removal of endotoxin (pyrogens) in solution in different states of aggregation. Appl Environ Micro 1977; 34(4):382–285.

25. Pedron T et al. New synthetic analogs of Lipid A as lipopolysaccharide agonists or antagonists of B lymphocyte activation. Int Immunol 1992; 4(4):533–540.

26. Loppnow H et al. IL-1 Induction-capacity of defined lipopolysaccharide partical structures. J Immunol 1989; 142(9):3229–3238.

27. Nowotny A. Review of the molecular requirements of endotoxic actions. Rev Infect Dis 1987; 9(suppl 5):S503–S511.

28. Lynn WA, Golenbock DT. Lipopolysaccharide antagonists. Immunol Today 1992.

29. Johnson AG et al. Characterization of a nontoxic monophosphoryl lipid A. Rev Infect Dis 1987; 9(suppl 5):S512–S516.

30. Morrison D, Ulevitch R. The effects of bacterial endotoxins on host mediation systems. Am J Pathol 1978; 93(527).

31. Galanos C et al. Immunogenic properties of lipid A. Rev Infect Dis 1984; 6:546–552.

32. Brade L et al. The immunogenicity and antigenicity of lipid A are influenced by its physicochemical state and environment. Infect Immun 1987; 55:2636.
33. Galanos C et al. Biological activities of lipid A complexed with bovine serum albumin or human serum albumin. Infect Immun 1972; 31:230.
34. Rietschel E et al. Pyrogenicity and immunogenicity of lipid A complexed with bovine serum albumin or human serum albumin. Infect Immun 1973; 8:173.
35. Novitsky TJ. Factors affecting the recovery of endotoxin. 1992; 10(1):1–2.
36. Morrison DC et al. Structural requirements for gelation of the Limulus amoebocyte lysate by endotoxin. Prog Clin Biol Res 1987; 231:55–73.
37. Mattsby-Baltzer et al. Endotoxin shedding by enterobacteria free and cell-bound endotoxin differ in Limulus activity. Prog clin Biol Res 1991; 59:689–695.
38. Luderitz O, Galanos C. Lipid A: chemical structure and biological activity. J Infect Dis 1973; 128(17).
39. Jiao B, Freudenberg M, Galanos C. Characterization of the lipid A component of genuine smooth-form lipopolysaccharide. Eur J Biochem 1989; 180:515–518.
40. Henderson BS, Poole S, Wilson M. Bacterial modulins: a novel class of virulence factors which cause host tissue pathology by inducing cytokine synthesis. Microbiol Rev 1996; 60:316–341.
41. Reitschel ET, Wahl. In: Rietschel, ed. Handbook of Endotoxin. Elsevier Science Publishers, 1984.
42. Katz et al. Potent CD14-mediated signalling of human leukocytes by *E. coli* can be mediated by interaction of whole bacteria and host cells without excessive prior release of endotoxin. Infect Immun 1996; 64:3592.
43. Cadieux JE et al. Spontaneous release of lipopolysaccharide by Pseudomonas aeruginosa. J Bacteriol 1983; 155:817–825.
44. Johnson KG et al. Cellular and free lipopolysaccharides of some species of Neisseria. Can J Microbiol 1975; 21:1969–1980.
45. Hurley JC, Tosolini FA. A Quantitative micro-assay for endotoxin and correlation with bacterial density in urine. J Microbiol Methods 1992; 15:91–99.
46. van Deuren M, Brandtzaeg P, Meer JWMVD. Update on meningococcal disease with emphasis on pathogenesis and clinical management. Clin Microbiol Rev 2000; 13:144–166.
47. Li Z, Clarke A, Beveridge T. Gram-negative bacteria produce membrane vesicles which are capable of killing other bacteria. J Bacteriol 1998; 180(20):5478–5483.
48. Shnyra A et al. Role of the physical state of *Salmonella* lipopolysaccharide in expression of biological and endotoxin properties. Infect Immun 1993; 61(12):5351–5360.
49. Tesh TL, Morrison DC. The interaction of *E. coli* with normal human serum: factors affecting the capacity of serum to mediate lipopolysacharide release. Microb Pathog 1988; 4(175).
50. Tesh TL, Morrison DC. The physical chemical characterization and biological activity of serum-released lipopolysacharides. J Immunol 1988; 141:3523.
51. Kitchens RL et al. Plasma lipoproteins promote the release of bacterial lipopolysaccharide from the monocyte cell surface. J Biol Chem 1999; 274(48):34116–34122.
52. Shands JW. Affinity of endotoxin for membranes. J Infect Dis 1973; 128(suppl):197–201.
53. Shands JW. Morphological structures of isolated bacterial lipopolysaccharide. J Mol Biol 1967; 25:15–21.
54. Brandenburg K, Rietschel ET, Brade H. Conformation of lipid A-the endotoxic center of bacterial lipopolysaccharide. J Endotoxin Res 1996; 313:173–178.
55. Tanford C. The hydrophobic effect: formation of micelles and biological membranes. 2nd ed. New York: John Wiley & Sons, 1980.
56. Sikkema J, De Bont JAM, Poolman B. Mechanisms of membrane toxicity of hydrocarbons. Microbiol Rev 1995; 59(2):201–222.
57. Shands JW, Chun PW. The dispersion of gram-negative lipopolysaccharide by deoxycholate. J Biol Chem 1980; 255(3):1221–1226.
58. Luhm J et al. Hypothermia enhances the biological activity of lipopolysaccharide by altering its fluidity state. Eur J Biochem 1988; 256:325–333.

59. Falk MC et al. Aggregation of serum proteins with lipopolysaccharide (LPS): characterization of the precipitable LPS-protein complex. J Endotoxin Res 1996; 3(2):129–142.
60. Din ZZ et al. Effect of pH on solubility and ionic state of lipopolysaccharide obtained from the deep rough mutant of *Escherichia coli*. Biochemistry 32:4579–4586.
61. Takayama et al. Physiochemical properties of the lipopolysaccharide unit that activates B lymphocytes. J Biol Chem 1990; 265(23):14023–14029.
62. Mueller M, Linder B, Kusumoto S, Fukase K, Andra B Schromm, Ulrich Seydel. Aggregates are the biologically active units of endotoxin. J Biol Chem 2004; 279(25):26307–26313.
63. Brandenburg KJ, Rietschel ET, Mayer H, Koch MH, Weckesser J, Seydel U. Influence of the supramolecular structure of free lipid A on its biological activities. FEBS J Eur Biochem 1993; 218:555–563.
64. Kato H et al. Chemical structure of lipid A isolated from *Flavobacterium meningosepticum* lipopolysaccharide. J Bacteriol 1998; 180(15):3891–3899.
65. Seydel U et al. The generalized endotoxic principle. Eur J Immunol 2003; 33:1586–1592.
66. Schromm AB, Brandenburg K, Loppnow H, et al. Biological activities of lipopolysaccharides are determined by the shape of their lipid A portion. Eur J Biochem FEBS 2000; 267:2008–2013.
67. Wachtel RE, Tsuji K. Comparison of *Limulus* amebocyte lysates and correlation with the United States Pharmacopeial pyrogen test. Appl Environ Microbiol 1977; 33:1265–1269.
68. Sveen K, Hofstad T, Milner KC. Lethality for mice and chick embryos, pyrogenicity in rabbits and ability to gelate lysate from amoebocytes of *Limulus polyphemus* by lipopolysaccharides from *Bacteroides*, *Fusobacterium* and *Veillonella*. Acta Pathol Microbiol Scand B 1977; 85:388–396.
69. Wong KH, Moss CW, Hochstein DH, Arko RJ, Schalla WO. Endotoxicity of the Legionnaire's disease bacterium. Ann Intern Med 1979; 90:624–627.
70. Weary ME, Pearson FC, Bohon J, Donohue G. The activity of various endotoxins in the USP rabbit test and in three different LAL tests. Prog Clin Biol Res 1982; 93:365–379.
71. Devleeschouwer MJ, Cornil MF, Dony J. Studies on the sensitivity and specificity of the *Limulus* amebocyte lysate test and rabbit pyrogen assays. Appl Environ Microbiol 1985; 50:1509–1511.
72. Luderitz O, Staub A, Westphal O. Immunochemistry of O and R antigens of *Salmonella* and related enterobacteriaceae. Bacteriol Rev 1966; 30(192).
73. Bradley S. Cellular and molecular mechanisms of bacterial endotoxins. Annu Rev Microbiol 1979; 33(67).
74. Galanos C et al. Chemical, physical, and biological properties of bacterial lipopolysaccharides. In: Cohen E, ed. Biomedical Applications of the Horseshoe Crab (Limulidae). New York: Alan R. Liss, 1979:319.
75. Komuro T, Murai T, Kawasaki H. Effect of sonication on the dispersion state of lipopolysaccharide and its pyrogenicity in rabbits. Chem Pharm Bull 1987; 35(12):4946–4952.
76. Kotra LP et al. Visualizing bacteria at high resolution. ASM News 2000; 66(1):675–681.
77. Seydel U, Oikawa M, Fukase K, Kusumoto S, Brandenburg K. Intrinsic conformation of lipid A is responsible for agonistic and antagonistic activity. Eur J Biochem 2000; 267:3032–3039.

5 | Descent of *Limulus:* Arthropoda and the New Biology

Kevin L. Williams

Eli Lilly & Company, Indianapolis, Indiana, U.S.A.

It has long been known that the modeling of the reaction of endotoxin with the human blood system has been wonderfully achieved using Limulus but it has only recently become apparent as to WHY this should be the case.

INTRODUCTION TO THE "NEW BIOLOGY"

This chapter contains a review of recent knowledge that has come about from the research into the superphylum Arthropoda, which includes *Limulus* and *Drosophila*[a]. *Limulus* served early on as a significant tool for medical research in large part due to the simplicity of its blood system and to its obvious primitive status (i.e., living fossil) among nature's creatures. More recently, *Drosophila* has dominated phylogenetic studies for similar reasons, but also due to its small size, ease of culture, small number of chromosomes, and short mating cycle (1,2). It is the blood system of the horseshoe crab that has allowed the in vitro determination of endotoxin content in various substances relative to the manufacture of pharmaceuticals. The relevance of the blood of an arthropod has fostered the elucidation of the "endotoxic" principle. Therefore, a study of *Limulus* as an ancient metazoan defender against prokaryotic invasion is in order. Such a study, in fact, tells several stories about the interrelatedness of the immune systems preserved in the blood, from *Limulus* to man. This interrelatedness is not confined to the immune system, but overlaps, and can be seen preserved in the DNA from arthropoda to man. It has long been known that the modeling of the reaction of endotoxin with the human blood system has been wonderfully achieved using *Limulus*, but it has only recently become apparent as to why this should be the case. At least five critical areas of interest have been recently illuminated by research on *Limulus* and its arthropod relatives.

1. The view of life as a continuous lineage from simple to complex (including terrestrialization) with an accumulating, chronologically progressive genetic and phenotypic gradient, from the simplest to the most complex organisms, is perhaps best visible within the superphylum Arthropoda (given the fossil record and great time span of their existence).
2. The discovery of *Hox* genes as the determinants of metazoan body formation are necessary to place *Limulus* relative to other arthropods and lead to the discovery of Toll and Toll-like receptors (TLRs).

---

[a]The importance of both creatures can be seen in the fact that three Nobel Prizes have been awarded to two researchers using *Drosophila* and one using *Limulus* (study of visual system).

3. The use of arthropods as models for human diseases (at least 75% of human disease genes have an arthropod homolog).
4. Expanding knowledge of innate immunity via the Toll and TLR family of receptors [i.e., the ultimate mediators of the host response to lipopolysaccharide (LPS)] has elaborated the "endotoxic principle" as seen in TLR-4 and TLR polymorphisms that have been shown to be a cause of autoimmune and microbial susceptibility diseases.
5. Arthropods are a vector and evolutionary incubator for pathogenic viruses and bacteria, including many fever-causing, gram-negative bacteria.

Woese (3), the father of microbial phylogenetics; describes the chronological, forward flow of life as a river (see Chap. 6).

> If they are not machines, then what are organisms? A metaphor far more to my liking is this: Imagine a child playing in a woodland stream, poking a stick into an eddy in the flowing current, thereby disrupting it. But the eddy quickly reforms. The child disperses it again. Again it reforms, and the fascinating game goes on. There you have it! Organisms are resilient patterns in a turbulent flow-pattern in an energy flow. A simple flow metaphor, of course, fails to capture much of what the organism is. None of our representations of an organism captures it in its entirety. But the flow metaphor does begin to show us the organism's (and biology's) essence. And it is becoming increasingly clear that to understand living systems in any deep sense, we must come to see them not materialistically, as machines, but as stable, complex, dynamic organizations.

The "New Biology," especially as it directly impacts the modeling of host-prokaryote interfaces, reveals Arthropoda to be a bridge to understanding the overly complex organisms above and the simpler prokaryotes below. Ultimately, the waging war is one of man against microbe, and along the way we have enlisted *Limulus*, *Drosophila*, and others to help us wage it, while others (i.e., pathogen vectors) serve to harbor, and even deliver, the culprits to our proverbial doorstep.

LIMULUS WITHIN ARTHROPODA

Arthropoda has been the most successful of multicellular life forms, comprising three-fourths of all known living and extinct organisms, an estimated 1 million species. By some estimates, 10 times that amount remain undiscovered (4). Distinguishing features of Arthropoda include their modular body parts, including segmented bodies and jointed appendages (antennae, legs, feeding appendages, etc.), and chitinous exoskeleton. They also demonstrate a dizzying array of life cycle adaptations that can include pupae and larvae, molting, and sometimes an adult form that has its being for only a very short time relative to its immature stages (i.e., fireflies, cicadas). Arthropoda consists of four extant (remaining) groups:

1. Chelicerata (*Limulus*, scorpions, spiders),
2. Crustacea [lobsters, shrimp, true crabs and woodlice, (also called sowbugs or pillbugs, which, lest we think they are all aquatic, are terrestrial crustaceans)].
3. Hexapoda (insects),
4. Myriapoda (centipedes and millipedes).

The subphylum Chelicerata contains four orders (three extant and one extinct):

(a) Arachnida—spiders, mites, ticks, scorpions
(b) Eurypterida, though now extinct, contained sea scorpions, purported to have reached lengths of six feet and to be among the first creatures to have crawled onto land (5)
(c) Xiphosura—horseshoe crabs
(d) Pycnogonida or sea spiders (6), some which survive today.

Trilobites are extinct but well-preserved and represented in the fossil record and said to be the horseshoe crab's nearest "recent" relative; although, according to Scholtz and Edgecombe (7), the Trilobites are derived from more basal Chelicerates, as are the other arthropod groups. Since the 19th century, those who have studied horseshoe crabs have separated them from the crabs and aligned them with the spiders. Kingsley (8) in 1893 lists six features in which "*Limulus* agrees with the Crustacea and differs from the Arachnida..." but 28 features in which "*Limulus* and Arachnids agree in, and both differ from other 'Tracheates'" (Hexapoda, Crustacea, and Myriapoda). Today, most phylogenies separate out the Chelicerates from the three other extant Arthropoda groups based upon various genetic and morphological features, including the presence of chelicerate instead of mandibular, mouthparts (9). The Mandibulata include hexapoda, crustacea, and myriapoda versus the Chelicerata (10). There remain today only three genera and four species of Xiphosura [all of which are horseshoe crabs (11)[b]], some of which are endangered.

Thus horseshoe crabs are not true crabs, but more akin to scorpions and spiders. The arthropod groups diverged from an original ancestor some 540 million years ago (11)[c]. The Chelicerates started out as aquatic but today are mostly terrestrial and consist mainly of predators and parasites (mites and ticks), significantly, many of the very insects that arose from them, as they are "fluid eaters" and dissolve their victim's tissues prior to feeding on their juices (arachnids). Alternatively, some crush them to the same effect. *Limulus* is a benign member subsisting on crabs and other invertebrates on the sea bottom. Though now declining, one can gain an appreciation of their historical numerical success as a species from Figure 1.

Figure 2 shows Arthropod body plans and phylogeny. The four major groups of extant arthropods are illustrated with a tree based on several recent molecular phylogenies that group the insects with the crustacean. Tagmatic boundaries and names for tagmata of different groups are indicated. Some groups of arthropods (e.g., the crustaceans) include species with a variety of tagmatic plans not included in Figure 2.

TERRESTRIALIZATION

The move from sea to land is said to have occurred as an escape from a teeming, competitive environment[d] to one of unbounded opportunity. Some of the adaptations that accompanied the move are being studied at the molecular level in present day arthropods to discover the sequence of events and the specific participants involved (Fig. 2). It has been proposed that three different terrestrialization

---

[c]Before the suspected divergence of the continents themselves around 350 million years ago.
[d]A proverbial barrel of crabs.

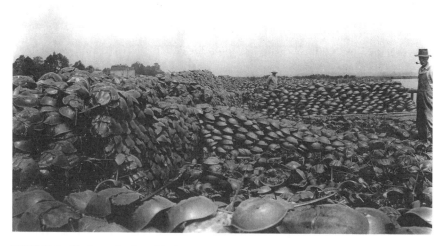

FIGURE 1 Photograph of stacks of tens of thousands of horseshoe crabs prior to being ground up for fertilizer in June of 1924 in Delaware. *Source*: From Ref. 67.

events occurred, one each by arachnids, myriapods, and insects. The fossil record points to gradations of each from land to sea. *Limulus* itself is semiterrestrial in that it crawls to shore to lay its eggs (Fig. 3). More recently, the underlying genes involved in morphological diversification are being explored (next section). The differences that have accrued are theorized to derive from common features as shown in Figure 4 with regard to a hypothetical arthropod ancestor to the aquatic chelicerates, including *Limulus*.

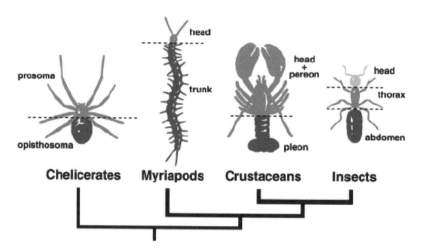

FIGURE 2 Arthropod body plans and phylogeny. The four major groups of extant arthropods are illustrated here with a tree based on several recent molecular phylogenies that groups the insects with the crustacean. Tagmatic boundaries are indicated by broken lines; names for tagmata of different groups are also indicated. Note that some groups of arthropods, for example, the crustaceans, include species with a variety of tagmatic plans not illustrated here. *Source*: From Ref. 42.

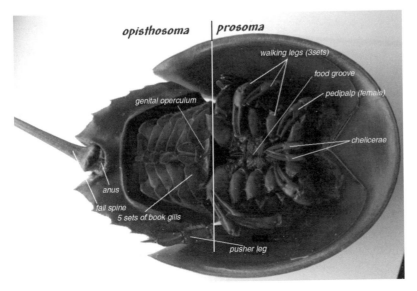

FIGURE 3   *Limulus* body parts relative to Figure 2 and as discussed in Table 1.

Damen et al. (12) provide a view of the current thinking on the common gen-etics (sequence homology) and structure (morphology) of various Chelicerates. These have been studied actively in a search for specialization related to both "terrestrialization," with Negrisolo et al. (13) maintaining four separate arthropod colonization events, one each by spiders, scorpions, millipedes, and centipedes, (14) and the morphological diversity of the arthropods, with arthropodal gills being proposed to have given rise to wings, book lungs, tracheal tubes, and spinnerets. According to Angelini and Kaufman (15), the book gills of the horseshoe crab "have been internalized into book lungs in the evolution of arachnids." The book gills have been retained by *Limulus* but have become epipods/gills in crustaceans and wings in insects; they are absent entirely in centipedes and millipedes and book lungs/tracheae, spinnerets in (terrestrial) spiders, and retained as book gills in some scorpions (12), but is not a feature homologous across the scorpions (16).

ADD *Hox*
Limulus has been critical in the understanding of innate immunity and endotoxicity. This beginning has recently been furthered by studying *Drosophila*, starting with the recognition that Toll had at least a dual function (17). Prior to its recognition as an innate immunity receptor, Toll was being studied for its regulatory function in the morphological development of the *Drosophila* embryo (Fig. 4) (18). The Homeobox or *Hox* gene discoveries (19) laid the groundwork for a new discipline: evolutionary development, the so-called evo-devo (20). The *Hox* genes have been found in virtually all multicellular organisms since their discovery: insects, crabs, spiders, *Limulus*, millipedes and centipedes, fish, frogs, mice, and humans (21), in another living fossil, the coelacanth (22), and even plants (23). The expression of specific *Hox* genes during embryotic development sets the stage for an organism's bilateral, symmetrical, anterior to posterior development and is associated with the

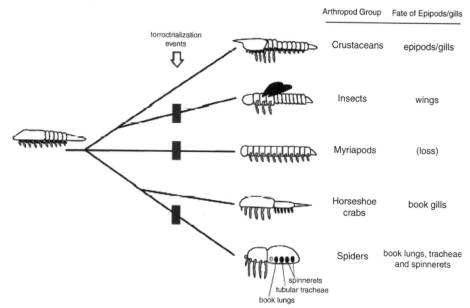

FIGURE 4 The evolutionary fate of gills in terrestrial arthropods. The last common ancestors of all arthropods were aquatic creatures with branched appendages. The ventral branches (in light gray) of these appendages were used mostly for locomotion (e.g., legs), whereas the dorsal branches, called epipods (in dark gray), were used mostly for respiration and osmoregulation (gills). Endopods/legs are preserved in most arthropods. Epipods/gills are preserved in aquatic arthropods but modified or lost in terrestrial groups, as indicated in the right of the figure. In terrestrial arachnids (spiders and scorpions), a series of related primordia arise in posterior segments of the body. In spiders, the first primordium fails to develop further, the second gives rise to book lungs, the third gives rise to book lungs or to the lateral tubes of the tubular tracheae (depending on the group of spiders), and the more posterior ones give rise to the spinnerets. For simplicity, some appendages or appendage parts are not shown (e.g., antennae, exopods). *Source*: From Ref. 12.

proper placement of body structures, such as segments and appendages in insects and other arthropods (24). As demonstrated in Table 1, it is increasingly difficult to assign relatedness of some creatures, such as *Limulus*, without a consideration of *Hox* gene alignment, therefore, a rudimentary discussion as a background is desirable (Fig. 5).

The expression of DNA transcription proteins via *Hox* occurs in a linear, sequential order, with those occurring first [DNA helix ($3' \rightarrow 5'$)] on a chromosome that it resides on expressed in cells in the anterior (i.e., head) region, and those occurring last on the helix expressed in cells of the posterior (i.e., rear), with the range of *Hox* between expressed in the trunk. The anterior (A) versus posterior (P) encoding and expression has been shown via antibody dye studies, in which the *Hox* genes from a certain embryonic stage are expressed in the embryo bearing the tale-tell dye color changes (25). The changes in *Hox* explain the myriad associated forms of arthropoda that have developed, including those with one (mites and ticks), two (*Limulus* and spiders), and three (insects) body regions or tagmata (27). Mutations in *Hox* are associated with drastic, though often survivable, body-type experimentation [i.e., the "hopeful monster" (21)].

TABLE 1 Summary of *Limulus* Scorpion and "Spiderlikeness"

Topic	Reference[a]	Comments (quotation marks indicate direct quotes)
Morphology		
Mouthparts	33	Arthropoda relatedness is by no means an area of universal agreement: "Our evidence [phylogenetic] analyses of concatenated (*Hox* gene protein) amino acid sequences from various arthropods...] that chelicerates are allied to myriapods argues against the idea of a clade of mandibulate arthropods (insects/crustaceans and myriapods). Rather, it supports the alternative notion that three taxa sharing a well-defined and complex character-the mandible-might not be monophyletic. This suggests that mandibles might have been present in the common arthropod ancestor and might subsequently have been lost in chelicerates. Alternatively, we must assume the convergent evolution of mandibles in myriapods and in the crustacean/insect clade." (i.e., which argues that myriapods are the most basal group and chelicerates, crustaceans, and hexapods are, respectively, more to most derived).
Head	34	Originally, it was thought, based upon morphological studies, that the lack of antennae for chelicerates as well as the lack of a true head segment that the chelicerates had "lost" the genetic machinery responsible for its formation, but this notion has been supplanted by the discovery of analogous *Hox* genes in chelicerates corresponding to the head sections of other arthropods (i.e., insects and crustacea)
Breathing	35	"The presence of five pairs of book-lungs in the East Kirkton scorpions, and the similarity of the respiratory lamellae with those of *Limulus*, may be regarded as primitive characteristics, and provide the strongest evidence yet that arachnid book-lungs were derived directly from book-gills in their aquatic ancestors."
Appendages	36	Horseshoe crabs have a small set of chelicerae, which resemble little legs above the mouth whereas in spiders, these are modified into fangs. The pedipalps (first set of legs posterior to the chelicerae) of both the male horseshoe crab and spiders are modified with a small hook for copulation purposes. In scorpions, the pedipalps are the large pincers. General observations support "... an increased degree of limb tagmosis among modern, as opposed to ancient, arthropods. This transition reflects both the relative decline of the weakly tagmatized marine arachnates and the increased dominance of derived, highly tagmatized mandibulates"
Terrestrialization	12	"In the horseshoe crab, a primitively aquatic chelicerate, pdm/nubbin is specifically expressed in opisthosomal appendages that give rise to respiratory organs called book gills. In spiders (terrestrial chelicerates), pdm/nubbin and apterous are expressed in... book lungs, lateral tubular tracheae, and spinnerets, novel structures that are used by spiders to breathe on land and to spin their webs. Combined with morphological and palaeontological evidence, these observations suggest that fundamentally different new organs (wings, air-breathing organs, and spinnerets) evolved from the same ancestral structure (gills) in parallel instances of terrestrialization"
Hemolymph		

(Continued)

TABLE 1 Summary of *Limulus* Scorpion and "Spiderlikeness" (*Continued*)

Topic	Reference[a]	Comments (quotation marks indicate direct quotes)
Phenoloxidase activity	37	"…in some chelicerates, a strong phenoloxidase activity has persisted in hemocyanins until the present. Tarantula hemocyanin from Eurypelma californicum is comparable to phenoloxidases based on activation mechanism, substratem specificity and inhibition…. The same holds for hemocyanins from the horseshoe crabs *L. polyphemus* and *Tachypleus tridentatus*… All three are ancient chelicerate species and unlike more modern crustaceans, myriapods and insects, no true phenoloxidases have been found in their hemolymphs to date"
Antimicrobials	38	"We have isolated, from the hemolymph of unchallenged scorpions of the species Androctonus australis, three distinct antimicrobial peptides…. (i) androctonin, a 25-residue peptide with two disulfide bridges, active against both bacteria (gram-positive and gram-negative) and fungi and showing marked sequence homology to tachyplesins and polyphemusins from horseshoe crabs…"
mtDNA/protein sequences combined with fossil record	39	The entire mtDNA sequence of *L. polyphemus* has been deciphered and compared in similarity to other Arthropoda including various insects *Drosophila*, spiders, scorpions, and crustacia. The differences in mtDNA of *Drosophila* and *L. polyphemus* consist of only a single tRNA (part of the mtDNA set) translocation and the *Limulus* sequence is identical to that of the tick, Ixodes, according to Boore.
	40	
	41	"…the failure of *Limulus* to share the same derived position for the mt-tRNA LeU(UUR) gene as insect and crustacean species supports the hypothesis that insects and crustaceans form a derived, monophyletic group from which chelicerates are excluded (see also Friedrich and Tautz 1995). The *Limulus* data indicate that the basic arrangement of genes in arthropod mtDNA was established prior to and has been relatively stable over at least 530 Myr. The chelicerate lineage to which *Limulus* belongs, Xiphosurida, was well established by the mid-Silurian, 420 MYA (Fisher 1984).), and the divergence of chelicerates and crustaceans had taken place prior to Middle Cambrian, 530 MYA, because a definitive chelicerate (Sunctucaris; Briggs and Collins 1988) and a representative crustacean (Cunaduspis; Briggs 1978.) are both present in the Burgess shale…"
Hox genes arrangement	42	"The chelicerates like spiders and mites have broadly overlapping expression of the *Hox* genes within the prosoma (lab, pb, Hox3, Dfd, Scr, and ftz) and within the opisthosoma (Antp, Ubx, abd-A, and Abd-B). The overlap of the chelicerate prosoma genes contrasts with the more subdivided pattern in the heads of insects and crustaceans…"
Note	43	"Pycnogonids (sea spiders) are most commonly placed as a sister taxon to the chelicerates or as a separate class, basal to all remaining extant arthropods"

[a]If applicable.

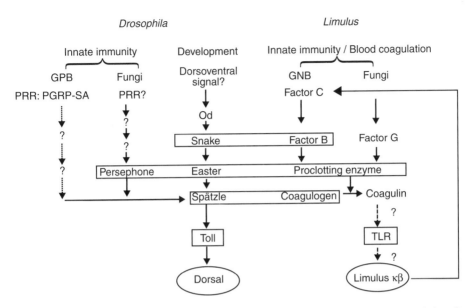

FIGURE 5 Serine protease cascades in development, innate immunity, and blood coagulation. On the left are the serine protease cascades in dorsoventral determination, immune response against gram-positive bacteria, and fungal infection in *Drosophila*. Dotted arrows with "?" indicate unidentified components in the cascades. On the right are the serine protease cascades in *Limulus* blood coagulation and innate immunity, which are activated by gram-negative bacteria and fungi, respectively. Factor G is the upstream serine protease in the alternate blood coagulation pathway that is triggered by β1,3-glucan. Discontinuous arrows annotate the putative LPS-mediated signaling pathway as proposed under "Discussion." Homologs in all the cascades are boxed. *Abbreviations*: Gd, gastrulation defective; GNB, gram-negative bacteria; GPB, gram-positive bacteria; PRR, pattern recognition receptors; TLR, toll-like receptors. *Source*: From Ref. 25.

The morphological orientation via *Hox* has been shown experimentally by rearranging *Hox* and producing *Drosophila* with extra body segments bearing wings or the notorious transposition of legs and antennae (28)[e].

> The body plan of *Drosophila* is encoded in part by the patterned expression of a set of transcription factors called the *Hox* proteins, which divide the embryo into a series of unique domains from anterior to posterior, and thereby assigns spatial identity to the segments. The *Hox* genes are now known to be crucial players in the development of nearly all animals, both protostomes and deuterostomes (Manak and Scott, 1994). Furthermore, because the *Hox* genes coordinate a large suite of downstream targets that work together to create segmental identity, a shift in the expression pattern of a *Hox* gene can cause major morphological change without necessarily being disastrous to the animal. Thus, changes in *Hox* gene expression may provide a mechanism of relatively rapid macroevolutionary change (29).

---

[e]It is interesting that some complex questions can be answered in regard to life's origins, but some of the most rudimentary questions remain enigmatic. For example, a specific set of 20 amino acids were "chosen" as the universal set of the building blocks to make proteins in living systems, but many more are available and, some that are used are not thought to have been available in the primordial environment. See Lu and Freeland. On the evolution of the standard amino-acid alphabet. *Genome Biology* 2006, 7:102.

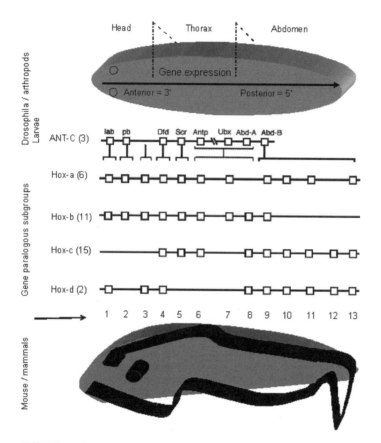

FIGURE 6 *Drosophila* larvae on the left and mouse embryo on the right. The common ancestor is assumed to be a worm-like prearthropod possessing the original *Hox* cluster. The mammals have four such sets of clusters (A, B, C, D) thought to have derived from two duplications of the original set. The relevant chromosome location for each *Hox* cluster is listed above each set. Some of the genes are so close that the mouse *HoxB6* gene has been inserted in *Drosophila* and substituted for Antennapedia to produce legs instead of antennae just as mutant *Antp* genes do. *Source*: From Refs. 29–31.

There are 10 *Hox* genes that have come to be known as the arthropod homeodomain; in 3′ → 5′/A-P order, they are: (*i*) labial, (*ii*) proboscipedia, (*iii*) Hox3/zen, (*iv*) deformed, (*v*) sex combs reduced, (*vi*) fushi tarazu, (*vii*) antennapedia, (*viii*) ultrabithorax, (*ix*) abdominal-A, and (*x*) abdominal-B (29). Nine core arthropoda *Hox* genes are seen as expressed in *Drosophila* with mammalian counterparts in Figure 6.

LIMULUS' SCORPION AND "SPIDERLIKENESS"

There is much historical and recent evidence of the relatedness of *Limulus* to spiders and scorpions (arachnids) as fellow Chelicerates. Lavrov et al. (32) describe the early efforts to categorize *Limulus*:

> *Limulus polyphemus* is one of the... extant species of Xiphosura (horseshoe crabs), one of the two extant major lineages of chelicerates (the other lineage, Arachnida...).

Originally thought to be crustaceans (hence the common name), xiphosurans[f] were recognized as aquatic chelicerates late in the 19th century (Lankester 1881). The fossil record of horseshoe crabs goes back to the Devonian, and modern-looking horseshoe crabs first appear in the mid-Mesozoic (Størmer 1952). Their apparently slow rate of morphological change since has led to their being dubbed "living fossils" (Fisher 1984) and regarded as a keystone group for studies of evolution and of arthropod phylogeny.

Some significant features supporting the current grouping of *Limulus* with spiders and scorpions rather than with true crabs are summarized in Table 1. Note that the table is a general overview, with many of the details debated among experts in various fields (Table 1).

Both the genetic similarity and the divergence displayed in *Hox* genes is striking among the broad group of Arthropoda, and, perhaps more surprising, is the conservation of structure and function in virtually all subsequent metazoans (Fig. 6). Due to its primitive status, *Limulus* has served as a genetic reference to which others are compared. Although the phylogeny of Arthropoda is still contested, much of the route of the lineage has been determined. The most noteworthy of gene functions shown to have diverged in an evolutionarily chronological gradient in the governing morphology of Arthropoda, can be used to place *Limulus* with the spiders and scorpions from a relationship standpoint, and this relatedness can be seen both phylogenetically and morphologically, albeit anecdotally, in Table 1.

The question: "How is *Limulus* like the spiders and scorpions?" has been answered in some detail, and along the way additional similarities have come to light between *Drosophila* and *Limulus* and Arthropoda and man. Perhaps the most surprising thing to come from the study of Arthropoda is a knowledge of the genetic features that have been conserved in modern vertebrates from the primordial divergence of the two groups. Some noteworthy gene functions conserved (studies with mice predominate), include:

1. The genetic sequence of "five Toll-like receptors-named TLRs1–5 are probably the direct homologs of the fly molecule..." (44).
2. The cytoplasmic part of the receptor is nearly identical in fly and man and utilized across the TLRs (45). (See section Toll and Toll-Like Receptors).
3. *Hox* gene homology; the Hox gene transcription factors regulate the orientation of the body segments and spatial arrangement in embryotic development, including bilateralism (29) from Arthropoda to mice to man.
4. Conservation of some blood constituents: Kairies et al. (46) report "...the crystal structure of tachylectin 5A (TL5A), a nonself-recognizing lectin from the hemolymph plasma of *T. tridentatus*. TL5A shares not only a common fold but also related functional sites with the γ fragment of mammalian fibrinogen. Our observations provide the first structural evidence of a common ancestor for the innate immunity and the blood coagulation systems."
5. A precomplement protease molecule: alpha2-Macroglobulin in *Limulus* is a homolog of a mammalian version that mediates the clearance of proteases from the plasma [(alpha2)(47)]

---

[f]Even with this knowledge "horseshoe xiphosuran" does not have the same ring as "horseshoe crab."

ARTHROPODA: MODELS FOR HUMAN DISEASE

Bier and McGinnis (30) make much of the presence of a complex system of Hox genes in the ancestor of both arthropods and mammals, and the criticality of this genetic conservation becomes apparent upon a closer examination.

> ...developmentally important genes have been phylogenetically conserved and ... disorders in humans (will) often involve genes controlling similar morphogenetic processes in vertebrates and invertebrates. A systematic analysis of human disease gene homologs in *Drosophila* supports this view since 75% of human disease genes are structurally related to genes present in *Drosophila* and more than a third of these human genes are highly related to their fruit fly counterparts.

The authors present several cases of genes present in *Drosophila* that are representative of human disease-causing genes, including polyglutamine repeat neurodegenerative disorders. In this instance, the size of the polyglutamine repeats can be related to the onset time and severity of the resultant neurological disorders in both flies and man. Indeed, the authors cite a broad spectrum of shared mechanisms including CNS, cardiac, cancer, immune dysfunction, and metabolic disorders that relate *Drosophila* genes to their human counterparts "in virtually every known biochemical capacity ranging from transcription factors to signaling components to cytoskeletal elements to metabolic enzymes." Specific examples (that are beyond the scope of this discussion) include (*i*) primary congenital glaucoma, (*ii*) Angelman syndrome, and (*iii*) Alzheimer disease.

In summary, Bier and McGinnis bring home the relevance of Arthropoda, including *Limulus*, to modern biology:

> An important practical consequence of the fact that vertebrates and invertebrates derived from a shared, highly structured, bilateral ancestor is that many types of complex molecular machine which were present in this creature have remained virtually unchanged in both lineages... These deep homologies between genetic networks can be exploited to understand the function of genes which can cause disease in humans when altered and should be very useful for identifying new genes in humans involved in disease states.

TOLL AND TOLL-LIKE RECEPTORS

The fact that virtually all organisms are born "knowing" that endotoxin from gram-negative bacteria is the "enemy" speaks to both the power of endotoxin as a host defense activator and to the universality (and thus the necessity of conservation) of the host's solution to endotoxin detection and elimination. It seems strange, at least to me, that an outside prokaryotic contaminant should have gene-encoded triggers to its presence in metazoans, but this is exactly what has happened and remains, in all multicellular life forms from plants to fungi to us. It is as if the metazoans have said "We are so concerned by these little monsters that we will include traps for them in our genetic code and when the traps are triggered a cascade of weapons will be unleashed to destroy them." The elucidation of the various, but analogous[g], mechanisms of immunity has exploded in the past few

---

[g]Arthropoda appears to contain the seeds of all three systems.

years and include: precomplement-[h], prophenoloxidase (PPo/melanin)-based[i], complement and adaptive immune[j] systems in various organisms (48).

The *Limulus* system long served as a prototype as it was characterized early on in terms of innate immunity mechanisms. By the early 1980s, researchers in the United States and Japan had characterized the process of degranulation and deciphered the resulting cascade beginning with factor C's autocatalization via endotoxin[k]. Subsequent to the quest to elucidate the reaction of the *Limulus* hemolymph with gram-negative endotoxin, other organisms have become more instrumental in clarifying the mechanisms of innate immunity. The endotoxin-*Limulus* pair thus has served as a prototype for understanding the mode of operation of both host innate immunity and corresponding pathogen-associated microbial patterns (PAMPs), prior to their being labeled as such. These advances in understanding predated the great strides made using *Drosophila* as a model, and in effect began the search for more specific and detailed knowledge of the host response to microbial invasion. Pattern recognition receptors (PRRs) became a relevant area of pursuit in the search for the functional facilitators of innate immunity. It is perhaps not too surprising that members of Arthropoda have developed extensive innate immunity mechanisms to ward off microbes because they spend their days in the trenches with the microbes—*Limulus* in the gram-negative–festering sandy shores and *Drosophila* in decaying fruit.

The Toll receptor family was found initially in *Drosophila* and subsequently in mammals and virtually all metazoans and called TLRs (49). Hence we are born with genetically encoded knowledge of the artifacts and signatures that arise from the "bad guys" of the microbial world, including endotoxin (the residue of gram-negative cells), peptidoglycan (the residue of gram-positive cells), single and double-stranded RNA (from viral particles), flagellin (present in an assortment of bacteria), and β-glucans (from mold and yeast) and more that are currently under investigation. TLRs straddle the outer membrane of host cells, with the receptor acting as a sentinel outside the cell and communicating, upon PAMP contact, to the cytoplasmic part of the receptor inside of cell.

In *Drosophila*, antimicrobial responses rely on two signaling pathways: the Toll pathway and the IMD pathway. In mammals, there are at least 10 members of the TLR family that recognize specific components conserved among microorganisms. Activation of the TLRs leads not only to the induction of inflammatory responses but also to the development of antigen-specific adaptive immunity. The signaling pathway of *Drosophila* Toll shows remarkable similarity to the mammalian IL-1 pathway, which leads to activation of NF-kB, a transcription factor responsible for many aspects of inflammatory and immune responses. Indeed, the cytoplasmic domains of *Drosophila* Toll and the mammalian IL-1 receptor are highly conserved and are referred to as the Toll/IL-1 receptor (TIR) domain (45).

---

[h]As in some arthropods, such as *Limulus, Carcinoscorpius,* and even pre-arthropods like the sea urchin and a coral (*Swiftia exserta*).

[j]In vertebrates, such as in mice and humans.

[k]"... the autoactivation of factor C, a serine protease that shares structural features with the initiating enzymes of the complement system (C1r, C1s, and MASP). The clotting enzyme cleaves coagulogen to coagulin, which polymerizes to cause a clot; although analogous in function, coagulogen is structurally unrelated to mammalian fibrinogen." (48).

The Toll receptor was initially discovered as a gene controlling some aspects of fly developmental morphology (50) and was subsequently observed by Gay and Keith (51) to share sequence similarity to the human IL-1 intracellular receptor domain (1991). But it was not associated with a role in innate immunity until the mid-1990s (52,53), when mutant mice deficient in the receptor were shown to be nonresponsive to fungal infection. Subsequently, analogs have been discovered in many other animals. The "discovery indicated immediately how mammalian innate immune sensing might operate in relation to other microbes and other inducing molecules" (54). The number of TLRs discovered since has grown, and the number of PAMPs has grown even more. The tag "pathogen-associated" seems somewhat of a misnomer as the given molecular patterns are associated with all the organisms of a class, pathogen or not, such as LPS, which is associated with all gram-negative bacteria. Indeed, the conserved nature of the PAMP is the reason it is used as a marker in multicellular hosts, as any mutation in this necessary microbial sequence would render the organism nonviable (again, as in the case of LPS in gram-negative bacteria), as contrasted with the ever-changing structure of various specific virulence factors. Interestingly, the list of PAMPs has grown to include a plethora of microbial artifacts, reading as a "who's who" of microbial culprits (Table 1 and Fig. 7).

The basic pattern of innate response to endotoxin, therefore, can be characterized as (*i*) microbial intrusion (gram-negative invasion), (*ii*) host recognition by either a soluble PRR (LPS binding protein, LBP) or cell-embedded PRR (CD14) or both (as in binding by LBP and presentation to CD14), and indeed sometimes an intracellular PRR, (*iii*) activation of Toll/TLR via cross bridging of the dual receptor host cell, (*iv*) resulting transcription (via NF-κB) of response factors as in production of cytokines and antimicrobial peptides (the latter particularly significant in invertebrates), and (*v*) (eventual) activation of an adaptive immune response via TLR expressed on antigen presenting cells (APCs) culminating in the activation of intruder-specific (differentiated) T cells (in vertebrates). Innate immunity in response to bacterial endotoxin infection (in *L. polyphemus*) will be described in Chapter 10 in great detail (as it is well characterized). In this regard, innate immunity is highly pertinent to a detailed discussion of endotoxin, whereas adaptive immunity is better left out of the discussion due to its complexity, limited relevance to the host response to endotoxin, and applicability predominately to vertebrates.

TOLL-LIKE RECEPTOR 4 AND THE ENDOTOXIC PRINCIPLE

TLR4 is the principal receptor for endotoxin in man; however, three extracellular receptors are needed in conjunction with it to carry out this task. These three are LBP, CD14, present in both soluble form in the blood stream, and as a protein anchored on the surface of circulating cells, including macrophages and monocytes, and myeloid differentiation-2 (MD-2). The interaction of TRL4, LBP, CD14, and MD-2 forms the necessary participants to respond to endotoxin. In *Drosophila*, unlike vertebrates, Toll receptors do not directly bind PAMPs (56) but rather are detected via circulating binding proteins which begin a serine protease cascade. *Limulus* shares this characteristic with *Drosophila* although via a different mechanism and is the basis for the LAL reaction. So, although obviously related, the functions have diverged significantly over time in man and within Arthropoda (i.e., *Drosophila* vs. *Limulus*). Spätzle is the protein that bridges the gap in *Drosophila*

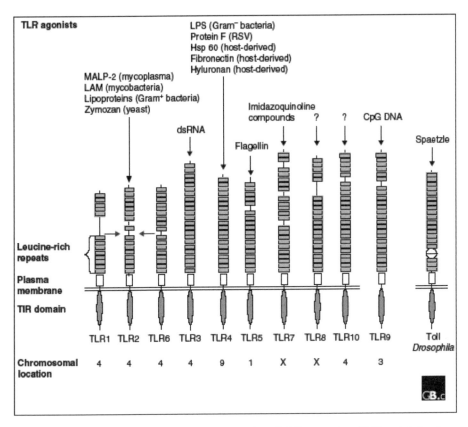

FIGURE 7 Structural features of human members of the Toll-like receptors (TLR) protein family and the archetypal *Drosophila* Toll protein. Toll and its relatives are characterized by an amino-terminal extracellular leucine-rich repeat domain, which is probably involved in ligand binding, and an intracellular Toll/interleukin-1 receptor domain required for signal transduction. Known ligands of different TLRs and chromosomal locations of the human TLR genes are indicated. Arrows indicate a possible dimerization between TLR1, TLR2, and TLR6. TLR9 is normally expressed intracellularly. *Abbreviations*: LAM, lipoarabinomannan; LPS, lipopolysaccharide; MALP-2, macrophage-activating lipopeptide-2; TIR, Toll/IL-1 receptor; details of other ligands mentioned in the figure are discussed in the text. *Source*: From Ref. 55.

whereas man and mouse do not encode spätzle or spätzle-like proteins. *Drosophila* encodes five homologs of spätzle (57). Current theory holds that both spätzle and MD-2 serve ultimately to cross-link two different TLR4 molecules to induce the endotoxic signaling event resulting in the transcription factor NF-κb and resulting cytokines and antimicrobial peptide production.

Given the rather complex orchestration of multiple partners required to span the Toll-bridge, it is not surprising that there is a very specific geometric configuration required to bring about the event (Chapters 3 and 6). It is given that LPS induces the endotoxic event, but it is also true that non-LPS constituents with the appropriate geometry have been successfully manufactured and used to elicit the event as well. Therefore, the endotoxic principle has been theorized by

Seydel et al. (58) to be as follows: (note, however, the lengthening of the sugar chain of endotoxin confounds easy predictions)

> "... prerequisites for agonistic action are amphiphilic molecules with clearly separated polar and apolar moieties and a conical conformation of the molecules with a larger cross-section of the hydrophobic than of the hydrophilic moiety."

Conversely, antiendotoxin competitors or antagonists can be described thus:

> "... a cylindrical rather than a conical conformation of the molecules, usually guaranteed by a less acylated apolar moiety. For both, agonism as well as antagonism, the presence of at least two negative charges in the polar headgroup is an important prerequisite, no matter whether these groups are provided by phosphate or carboxylate groups."

Mutations in arthropod TLR resulting in reduced immunity against pathogens (β-glucan and peptidoglycan) predated and predicted their recognition as culprits in human disease causation, including asthma, periodontal disease (59), sepsis (60), immunodeficiencies (61), and atherosclerosis (62). It stands to reason and has recently been shown that the disruption of this Toll-bridging capacity via genetic polymorphism (genetic variability with deleterious phenotypic results) also prevents or impairs the endotoxic host response, which at first glance would seem a blessing but actually results in an impaired ability to fight gram-negative infection and is most often associated with higher rates of mortality (63). Chapter 19 contains a more expert and detailed discussion of the role of Toll polymorphisms in bacterial sepsis.

ARTHROPODA AS MICROBIAL VIRULENCE-FACTOR RESERVOIRS IN EMERGING, RE-EMERGING DISEASE

Given the hundreds of millions of years of intimate interaction between Arthropoda and the microbial world that higher organisms do not share, it is not surprising that, in addition to being prime tools for modeling and understanding the inner workings of innate immunity (glad tidings), they also are harbingers of microbial death (bad tidings).

> Recent advances in our understanding of the molecular basis of pathogenicity have highlighted the fluidity of the prokaryotic genome and the interchangeable nature of many virulence factors. This study of invertebrate-associated pathogens reinforces that view. *Y. pestis, B. anthracis,* and *P. asymbiotica* seem to have each evolved from insect-associated ancestors relatively rapidly, and with only minor genetic changes. In *Y. pestis*, for example, the reliance on transmission by fleas seems to have selected for increased virulence in mammals compared with its soil-borne ancestor (64).

Waterfield et al. (64) have described the drama between metazoan immunity and prokaryotic virulence as an "arms race":

> ...as multicellular animals evolved, so did the complexity and effectiveness of their immune response. This "arms race" has driven the evolution of bacterial strategies and virulence genes that are optimized for survival against a coordinated immune response. The insect immune system closely resembles the innate immune system of mammals on both the molecular and cellular levels.

One of the most destructive of diseases from an historical human vantage has been the bubonic plague, a product of *Yersinia pestis*. The gram-negative rod is passed from rodent to man by an arthropod host, namely the flea (65). Since antiquity, many diseases have been arthropod-borne, and many diseases that are today considered "emerging infectious diseases" employ arthropod hosts as vectors; therefore, arthropods serve as major reservoirs for increasing virulence when manifested in mammalian hosts. These diseases include (*i*) tick/mite-borne diseases: "arenavirus hemorrhagic" fevers including Lassa fever, hantavirus pulmonary syndrome, which also involves rodent intermediates, Lyme disease spirochete Borrelia, Ehrlichioses, and various spotted fevers and (*ii*) insect-borne diseases: malaria, via the mosquito, typhus, via the louse (66). Note in Table 2 the number of emerging diseases that are fever-causing (typically gram negative or viral) and those that are arthropod-borne.

In plague, the literal choking of the flea[l] via a plasmid-encoded (two plasmids actually) biofilm in the feeding tube of the flea causes it to regurgitate the blood it is trying to feed upon back into the human host along with an unwelcome guest: *Y. pestis.* Morbid but fascinating, thus *Y. pestis* is able to "kill two birds with one stone" and propagate itself at the expense of arthropod and human alike.

There are seemingly two parallel stories involving the arthropod host system as a link to our interaction with gram-negative bacterial pathogens and their

TABLE 2 Emerging/Re-Emerging Infectious Diseases

Location	Arthropod-borne	Vector	Not arthropod-borne
North America	Lyme disease West Nile virus Dengue	Ticks Mosquitoes Mosquitoes	Cryptosporidiosis Vancomycin-resistant *S. aureus* *E. coli* O157:H7 Human monkeypox Whitewater arroyo virus[a] Hantavirus pulmonary syndrome[a] Anthrax bioterrorism
South America	Dengue Yellow fever Drug-resistant malaria	Mosquitoes Mosquitoes Mosquitoes	Multidrug-resistant tuberculosis Hepatitis C Human monkeypox HIV Cholera Hantavirus pulmonary syndrome[a]
Africa	Drug-resistant malaria Yellow fever Plague Rift Valley fever	Mosquitoes Mosquitoes Fleas Mosquitoes	Cholera Marburg hemorrhagic fever Ebola hemorrhagic fever
Europe	N/A		Multidrug-resistant tuberculosis vCJD Cryptosporidiosis Diptheria
India/Asia	Typhoid fever Drug-resistant malaria	Mosquitoes Mosquitoes	Vancomycin-resistant *S. aureus* H5N1 influenza *E. coli* O157:H7 SARS Cholera
Australia	N/A		Hendra virus[b]
Indo-China	N/A		Enterovirus 71 Nipah virus[b]

[a]Via rodent excrement; arthropod vector unknown.
[b]Mammal to mammal transmission.
Source: From Ref. 55.

associated endotoxins. The first is within man's power and described here as a contrast of the tools and models that Arthropoda provides man, on the one hand, with their presence as ubiquitous harbingers of disease-bearing prokaryotes on the other. The second story is ancient, written in man's genes, and beyond his reach in that his innate efforts (via Toll etc.) to counter the infections brought by the (sometimes arthropod-borne) prokaryotes represents a formidable task. The study of arthropod (phylo)genetics and inner workings of innate immunity serve to illustrate the advances, intricate complexities, and remaining work to be done in the study of host-pathogen interaction, of which humans, *Limulus*, and *Drosophila* share the common metazoan goal of repelling endotoxin-bearing invaders. This rudimentary exploration of the relevance of *Limulus* to our modern world suggests that what pertains to *Limulus* can often pertain to us all.

REFERENCES

1. Hedges SB. The origin and evolution of model organisms. Nature 2002; 3:838–849.
2. Tzou P et al. How *Drosophila* combats microbial infection: a model to study innate immunity and host-pathogen interactions. Curr Opin Microbiol 2002; 5:102–110.
3. Woese C. A new biology for a new century. Microbiol Mol Biol Rev 2004; 68(2):173–186.
4. http://www.ucmp.berkeley.edu/arthropoda/arthropoda.html.
5. Jeram AJ. Book-lungs in a lower carboniferous scorpion. Nature 343,360–361 (25 January 1990); doi 10.1038/343360a0; 343(25).
6. Siveter DJ. A Silurian sea spider. Nature 2004; 431(21):978–980.
7. Scholtz G, Edgecombe GD. Heads, Hox and the phylogenetic position of trilobites. In: Koenemann S, Jenner R, eds. Crustacea and Arthropod Relastionships. Crustacean Issues 2005; 16:139–165.
8. Kingsley JS. The embryology of *Limulus*, Part II. J Morphol 1893; VIII(2):35–68.
9. Blaxter M. Sum of the arthropod parts. Nature 2001; 413:121–122.
10. Boore JL. Deducing the pattern of arthropod phylogeny from mitochondrial DNA rearrangements. Nature 1995; 376:13.
11. Xia X. Phylogenetic relationship among horseshoe crab species: effect of substitution models on phylogenetic analyses. Syst Biol 2000; 49(1):87–100.
12. Damen WGM et al. Diverse adaptations of an ancestral gill: a common evolutionary origin for wings, breathing organs, and spinnerets. Curr Biol 2002; 12:1711–1716.
13. Negrisolo E et al. The mitochondrial genome of the house centipede Scutigera and the monophyly versus paraphyly of Myriapods. Mol Biol Evol 2004; 21(4):770–780. doi:10.1093/molbev/msh078.
14. Robinson R. Earliest-known uniramous arthropod Nature 1990; 343(11):163–164.
15. Angelini DR, Kaufman TC. Comparative developmental genetics and the evolution of arthropod body plans. Annu Rev Genet 2003; 93:95–125.
16. Kamenz C et al. Characters in the book lungs of Scorpiones (Chelicerata, Arachnida) revealed by scanning electron microscope. Zoomorphology 2005; 124(2):101–105.
17. Lemaitre B et al. The dorsoventral regulatory gene cassette spatzle/Toll/cactus controls the potent antifungal response in *Drosophila* adults. Cell 1996; 86:973–983.
18. Anderson KV et al. Establishment of dorsal-ventral polarity in the *Drosophila* embryo: the induction of polarity by the Toll gene product. Cell 1985; 42:791–798.
19. Ferrier DEK, Minguillón C. Evolution of the Hox/ParaHox gene clusters. Int J Dev Biol 2003; 47:605–611.
20. Baguna J, Garcia-Fernandez J. Evo-Devo: the long and winding road. Int J Dev Biol 2003; 47:705–713.
21. Gellon G, McGinnis W. Shaping animal body plans in development and evolution by modulation of *Hox* expression patterns, Bioessays 20.2. John Wiley & Sons Inc., Huboken, N.J. 1998:116–125.
22. Hoegg S, Meyer A. *Hox* clusters as models for vertebrate genome evolution. Trends Genet 2005; 21(8):421–424.

23. Girardin SE et al. Intracellular vs extracellular recognition of pathogens—common concepts in mammals and flies. Trends Microbiol 2002; 10(4):193–199.
24. Ferrier D, Holland PWH. Ancient origin of the *Hox* gene cluster. Nature Rev Genet 2001; 2:33–38.
25. Wang L et al. Transcriptional regulation of *Limulus* factor C. J Biol Chem 2003; 278(49):49428–49437.
26. Grenier JK et al. Evolution of the entire arthropod *Hox* gene set predated the origin and radiation of the onychophoran/arthropod clade. Curr Biol 1997 Aug 1, 7(8):547–553.
27. Averof M, Akam M. Letters to nature: *Hox* genes and the diversification of insect and crustacean body plans. Nature 376,420–423 (03 August 2002); doi 10.1038/37642a0.
28. Edelman ME, Jones FS. Outside and downstream of the homeobox. J Biol Chem 1993; 268(28):20683–20686.
29. Carroll SB. Homeotic genes and the evolution of arthropods and chordates. Nature 1995; 376:479–485.
30. Bier E, McGinnis W. Model organisms in the study of development and disease. In: Charles J, Epstein MD, eds. Inborn Errors of Development. Vol. 49. Oxford Press, New York, 2004:1082.
31. Zhang J, Nei M. Evolution of Antennapedia-class homeobox genes Genetics 1996; 142:295–303.
32. Lavrov DV, Boore JL, Brown WM. The complete mitochondrial DNA sequence of the horseshoe crab *Limulus polyphemus*. Mol Biol Evol 2000; 17(5):813–824.
33. Cook CE et al. *Hox* genes and the phylogeny of the arthropods. Curr Biol 2001; 11: 759–763.
34. Averof M. Origin of the spider's head. Nature 1998; 395:436–437.
35. Jeram AJ. Book-lungs in a lower carboniferous scorpion. Nature 1990; 343:360–361.
36. Hughes NC. Trilobite body patterning and the evolution of arthropod tagmosis Bioessays 25.4. New York, NY: Wiley Periodicals, Inc, 2003; 25:386–395.
37. Jaenicke E, Decker H. Functional changes in the family of Type 3 copper proteins during evolution. Chem BioChem 2004; 5:163–169. doi: 10.1002/cbic.200300714.
38. Ehret-Sabatier L et al. Characterization of novel cysteine-rich antimicrobial peptides from scorpion blood. J Biol Chem 1996; 271(47):29537–29544.
39. Lavrov DV, Boore JL, Brown WM. The complete mitochondrial DNA sequence of the horseshoe crab *Limulus polyphemus*. Mol Biol Evol 2000; 17(5):823–824.
40. Boore JL. Animal mitochondrial genomes. Nucleic Acid Res. 1999; 27(8):1767–1780.
41. Staton JL, Daehler L, Brown W. Mitochondrial gene arrangement of the horseshoe crab *Limulus polyphemus* L: conservation of major features among arthropod classes. Mol Biol Evol 1997; 14(8):867–874.
42. Hughes CL, Kaufman TC. Exploring the myriapod body plan: expression patterns of the ten *Hox* genes in a centipede. Development 2002; 129:1225–1238.
43. Maxmen A et al. Neuroanatomy of sea spiders implies an appendicular origin of the protocerebral segment. Nature 2005; 437(20). doi:10.1038/nature03984.
44. Rock FL et al. A family of human receptors structurally related to *Drosophila* Toll. Proc Natl Acad Sci Dev Biol 1998; 95:588–593.
45. Takeda K et al. Toll-like receptors. Annu Rev Immunol 2003; 21:335–376. doi: 10.1146/annurev.immunol.21.120601.141126.
46. Kairies N et al The 2.0-Å crystal structure of tachylectin 5A provides evidence for the common origin of the innate immunity and the blood coagulation systems. PNAS 2001; 98(24):13519–13524.
47. Melchior R, Quigley JP, Armstrong PB. Alpha2, alpha2-macroglobulin-mediated clearance of proteases from the plasma of the American horseshoe crab, *Limulus polyphemus*. J Biol Chem 1995; 270(22):13496–13502.
48. Suckale J. Evolution of innate immune systems. BAMBED 2005; 33(3):177–183.
49. Hoffmann JA, Reichhart JM. *Drosophila* innate immunity: an evolutionary perspective. Nat Immunol 2002; 3(2):121–126.
50. Anderson KV et al. Establishment of dorsal-ventral polarity in the *Drosophila* embryo: genetic studies on the role of the Toll gene product. Cell 1985; 42:779–789.
51. Gay NJ, Keith FJ. *Drosophila* Toll and IL-1 receptor. Nature 1991; 351:355–356.

52. Lemaitre B et al. The dorsoventral regulatory gene cassette spatzle/Toll/cactus controls the potent antifungal response in *Drosophila* adults. Cell 1996; 86:973–983.
53. Lemaitre B. The road to Toll. Nat Rev Immunol 2004; 4:521–527.
54. Buetler B, Reitschel ET. Innate immune sensing and its roots: the story of endotoxin. Nat Rev Immunol 2003; 3:169–176. doi:10.1038/nri1004.
55. Armant MA, Fenton MJ. Toll-like receptors: a family of pattern-recognition receptors in mammals. Genome Biol 2002; 3(8):3011.1–3011.6
56. Beutler B, Poltorack A. Sepsis and evolution of the innate immune response. Crit Care Med 2001; 29(7):52–56.
57. Gangloff M et al. Evolutionary relationships, but functional differences, between the *Drosophila* and human toll-like receptor families. Biochem Soc Trans 2003; 31(3):659–663.
58. Seydel U et al. The generalized endotoxic principle. Eur J Immunol 2003; 33:1586–1592.
59. Schröder NWJ et al. Chronic periodontal disease is associated with single-nucleotide polymorphisms of the human TLR-4 gene. Genes Immun 2005; 6. doi:10.1038/sj.gene.6364221.
60. Holmes CL et al. Genetic polymorphisms in sepsis and septic shock. Chest 2003; 124(3):1103–1115, doi:10.1378/chest.124.3.1103.
61. Schwartz DA, Cook DN. Polymorphisms of the Toll-like receptors and human disease. Clin Infect Dis 2005; 41:S403–S407.
62. Cook DN et al. Toll-like receptors in the pathogenisis of human disease. Nat Immunol 2004; 5(10). doi: 10.1038/ni1116.
63. Dahmer MK et al. Genetic polymorphisms in sepsis. Pediatr Crit Care Med 2005; 6(3 suppl):S61–S73.
64. Waterfield NR et al. Invertebrates as a source of emerging human pathogens. Nat Rev Microbiol 2004; 2:833–841.
65. Lowell JL et al. Identifying sources of human exposure to plague. J Clin Microb 2005; 650–656. doi:10.1128/JCM.43.2.650-656.2005.
66. Morens DM. The challenge of emerging and re-emerging infectious diseases. Nature 430, 242–249 (8 July 2004); doi 10.1038/nature02759; published online 8 July 2004.
67. Walls, EA, Berkson J, Smith SA. The horseshoe crab, *Limulus polyphemus*: 200 million years of existence, 100 years of study. Rev Fisheries Sci 2002; 10(1): 39–73.

6 Microbial Biodiversity and Lipopolysaccharide Heterogeneity: from Static to Dynamic Models

Kevin L. Williams
Eli Lilly & Company, Indianapolis, Indiana, U.S.A.

The history and biodiversity of prokaryotes is accumulated, expressed and propagated in the prokaryotic genome ... and prokaryotic biodiversity includes LPS heterogeneity ...

INTRODUCTION

This chapter is an overview of the recent changes in the way prokaryotes are viewed, particularly correcting the static models of the past with regard to the heterogeneity, community, and interaction of bacteria and their endotoxins, especially the way they interact with host systems. As Chapter 4 presented the static model for lipopolysaccharide (LPS) as a function of its existence in a model organism: *Escherichia coli* (EC), this chapter presents examples of the overwhelming diversity that has been found in various organisms. Nothing is quite sacred anymore as the conspiracy of contaminants has blurred the lines of demarcation between the members of Prokaryotes, the weapons at their disposal, and their interaction with one another as well as with their hosts and various environments. The changes include a continuum of heretofore-unknown capacities of individual species to modify the structure of their endotoxins and evade and overpower host defenses.

Curious also is the discovery of endotoxin in an apparently gram-positive anaerobe, *Pectinatus*, a beer fermentation contaminant that occurred almost simultaneously around the world as oxygen-excluding technology improved (1). Helander et al. question whether it is an intermediate between gram-positive and gram-negative organisms, as it does not form a classical gram-negative outer membrane structure (i.e., has some gram-positive features) and is susceptible to drugs, such as Vancomycin and Bacitracin, that are usually too large to penetrate gram-negative membranes. On the other hand, the bacterium's LPS is fully endotoxic. Prior to genomic studies it had been considered a gram-negative bacteria, but is now placed in the low gas chromatography (GC) gram-positive group of the anaerobic class Clostridia.

There are many fascinating aspects of phylogenetics and biodiversity but those discussed here are relative to endotoxin-bearing gram-negative bacteria in regard to LPS heterogeneity involved in the complex interplay of host and pathogen during invasion and infection. This chapter posits the following particulars regarding to bacterial biodiversity and LPS heterogeneity:

1. the extent of prokaryotic relatedness and biodiversity is only beginning to be recognized
2. the history and biodiversity of prokaryotes is accumulated, expressed, and propagated in the prokaryotic genome

3. prokaryotic biodiversity includes LPS heterogeneity
4. specific bacteria use LPS heterogeneity as a virulence factor
5. the host response to LPS heterogeneity via Toll-like receptors (TLR) is the ultimate arbiter of endotoxicity[a] and TLRs contain heterogeneity of their own that varies not only between species but also between individuals of the same species

PROKARYOTIC BIODIVERSITY AND PROKARYOTIC PHYLOGENETICS

The number and types of prokaryotes that have been studied are very few in comparison to the total number present in the biosphere. Some have been exhaustively studied (*EC*), whereas others are only inferred from environmental gene sequence recoveries (2) and some, if not most (3), cannot be cultured at all. Given that most bacteria occurring in nature are "unculturable" and thus remain as "virtual," almost hypothetical, genetically inferred ghosts (4), and are therefore "unknowable" in a traditional sense, the classification of bacteria can hardly be viewed as being at an advanced state, even with phylogenetic methods. Fredricks and Relman describe the current situation:

> The emergence of technology that grants ready access to nucleic acid sequences and the conceptual advances that allow inference of evolutionary relationships from certain sequences have brought about the identification and detection of novel, previously uncharacterized microorganisms. The Petri dish and traditional tissue stains have been supplanted by nucleic acid amplification technology ... and in situ oligonucleotide hybridization ... for "growing" and "seeing" some microorganisms. The power of these techniques has opened a new window on the diversity of environmental and human-associated microorganisms ... (4).

One such study, by Paster et al. (5), revealed an estimated 500 to 600 species or "phylotypes" residing in the human mouth. The samplings were taken from a variety of individuals, some with dental disease. Studies like this, from one small host environment, demonstrate the unknown prokaryotes residing[b], as roughly a third of those detected were new phylotypes that could not be cultivated, and shows that even the word "species" has become ill-defined and subject to interpretation in a way that it has not been before.

> The definition of a species is controversial, particularly when only molecular sequence data exist. Therefore, we have used the term "phylotype" in place of species for referring to novel clusters of clone sequences. In most cases, a 2% difference in 16S ribosomal RNA (rRNA) sequences does indicate separate species status, but there are exceptions. Formal naming of a species also requires a full description of the phenotypic characteristics of an organism. It is probable that the majority of the phylotypes identified in this report will eventually be validated as species. In the meantime, DNA probes can be designed to identify phylotypes and to assess their roles in disease or health. If a phylotype proves to be associated with disease, then efforts can be made to isolate and characterize the new species...

---

[a]Rather than the LPS conformation, albeit this is a circular argument and true in vertebrates but apparently less so in Arthropoda where the extent to which TLR is a true pattern recognition receptor is debated.
[b]Under our very noses.

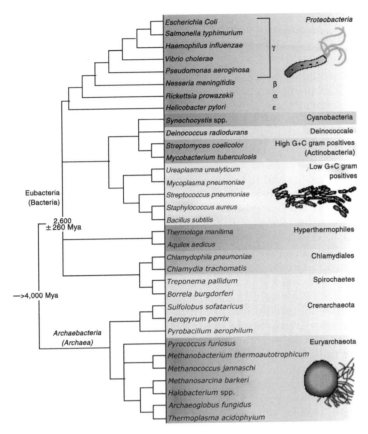

FIGURE 1 A phylogeny of prokaryotes. The relationships of selected prokaryote model organisms based on recent studies. Times of divergence (million years ago (Mya) ± one standard error) are indicated at nodes in the tree. Branch lengths are not proportional to time. Phyla and phylum-level groupings are indicated on the right. *Abbreviation*: G+C ——. *Source*: From Ref. 55.

Excluding Bergey's Manual[c], which is predominately used for diagnostic purposes, most publications, including the "The Prokaryotes,"[d] have adopted the phylogenetic system of classification of prokaryotes and associated renaming of many endotoxin-bearing organisms that Woese began (Fig. 1). The schism that has opened between the traditional and phylogenetic classification methods points to a relevant corollary in that the historical study of the "culturables" may have misled us as to the nature of prokaryotes (a term also debated) in general and is, in fact, nullifying a host of previous assumptions, in that the "unculturables" often differ radically from the "culturables" (6) in attributes. The hypothetical that directly arises from the culturable/unculturable "schism" is that the endotoxin

---

[c]http://www.bergeys.org/publications.html "The arrangement of the book is strictly phenotypic, with no attempt to offer a natural higher classification. The arrangement chosen is utilitarian and is intended to aid in the identification of bacteria."
[d]Changed in 1992 to phylogenetic classification.

that is so ubiquitous in nature has been characterized predominately in the "culturables," namely, enterobacteria such as *Escherichia* and *Salmonella*, and reveals little about the state of endotoxin in the "unculturables." If it turns out that the endotoxin of "unculturables" is significantly different and relevant to clinical states of infection, that would help explain the difficulty that has been presented to researchers exploring therapeutic strategies. This would be a significant paradigm shift, and one can see some instances of it coming to pass in various studies of the heterogeneity of endotoxin in several organisms, to be discussed in this chapter.

The system of classifying organisms was invented by Carl Linnaeus in 1753 (Systema Naturae) and began the binomial (genus/species) system, still in use today. In regard to bacteria, it became a matter of grouping suspects into classes based upon simple morphology and their consumption of various substrates, and so on. More recently, Woese and others have pioneered a new view of biology that posits genealogy as the true purpose of classification. The so-called phylogenetic grouping based upon 16S rRNA similarity wound up tossing of the phenotypic methods of classification in favor of genetic homology. Out of these studies came the grouping of three great domains of life: Archaebacteria (now Archaea), Eubacteria, (both prokaryotes), and Eucarya (protists and everything multicellular). The gene-based system seeks to weed out artifacts of morphology. Consider as an analogy the fact that an octopus and a spider both have eight legs. Phenotypically, this might appear a basis of classification, but further examination would reveal that the underlying genetics producing the two clearly have little in common.

More recently, Doolittle (7) and others have suggested that the idea of a phylogenetic tree may be untenable due to the massive amount of horizontal gene transfer that has occurred [said to be 18% of the *EC* genome (8)], recognizing that the tree one gets depends upon the data set one uses (i.e., which gene sequence or protein is used to construct a phylogeny etc.). They have suggested a net or reticulated tree, looking somewhat like the roots of the mangrove tree, [see Martin (9)] that incorporates the various chaos resultant from prokaryotic vertical and lateral gene transfer. Mayr (10) took issue with Woese for not strictly sticking to a single method of classification hierarchy (Darwinian versus Hennigian) and did not consider archaebacteria sufficiently different holistically from the eubacteria, which is, broadly, what many have protested. In return, Woese (11) took issue with Mayr for his formalism in the face of genomic's "explanatory power" and reiterated that there is, in the end, only one right answer if, as he contends and currently most agree, it is true that living nature is a continuum, a lineage from A to Z with, an albeit a difficult to decipher, chronological flow, tumbling forward in a frenzied, promiscuous fall that is actually a climb up a mountain of complexity. Guest (12) makes the point that some are less interested in phylogenetics than in classification as a means of division for public health purposes: "... determinative keys are very important in practical matters (for example, in medical microbiology, public health microbiology, and plant pathology) this tends to be forgotten by those probing evolutionary relations using molecular markers. The later press for revised taxonomic schemes and this inevitably leads to proposals for changing names of bacteria." However, one must wade humbly into the discussion for, as Tudge says, "The discussion continues but is immensely technical, and only a few people in the world are qualified to take part in it. It would be absurd for, a nonspecialist to comment." (13)

Of course the phenotypic display of an organism's enzymes and proteins, and so on is not as irrelevant as the trivial spider/octopus example might suggest, and indeed what Woese began by using rRNA, others have continued via expanded methods of classification, including the cataloging and comparison of proteins and so-called "signature sequences"[e] contained within prokaryote genomes. By these methods (identification and comparison of signature genetic sequences surrounded by highly conserved sequences), Gupta (14) maintains that Gram had it right in the nineteenth century (1886) when he divided the prokaryotes into those that stain purple and those that do not:

> The results of studies reviewed here indeed point to a very different evolutionary picture from the currently widely accepted one. In this review I present evidence based on molecular sequences that archaebacteria exhibit a close and specific relationship to gram-positive bacteria and that the primary division within prokaryotes is not between archaebacteria and eubacteria but, rather, between organisms that have either a monoderm cell structure (i.e., prokaryotic cells surrounded by a single membrane, which includes all archaebacteria and gram-positive bacteria) or a diderm cell structure (i.e., prokaryotic cells surrounded by an inner cytoplasmic membrane and an outer membrane, which includes all true gram-negative bacteria...). The sequence data also strongly indicate that the ancestral eukaryotic cell is not a direct descendant of the archaebacterial lineage but is a chimera that resulted from a unique fusion event involving two very different groups of prokaryotes-a thermoacidophillic archaebacterium (monoderm) and a gram-negative eubacterium (diderm), followed by integration of their genomes. Thus all eukaryotic organisms, including the amitochondriate and aplastidic cells, received and retained gene contributions from both lineages.

Another protein phylogeny study by Brown et al. at GlaxoSmithKline (15) used 23 different proteins, representing 45 species from all domains, to construct a universal tree, the results of which they consider closely aligned with Woese's rRNA–based conclusions. A caveat here being that the characterization determined the spirochaetes to be the earliest derived bacterial group using all the data. But when they removed nine of the 23 proteins that they reasoned were "likely candidates for horizontal gene transfer," the tree showed thermophiles (Arachaea) as the earliest bacterial lineage. They conclude: "... combined protein universal trees are highly congruent with SSU rRNA trees in their strong support for the separate monophyly of domains as well as the early evolution of thermophilic bacteria."

Genetic stuides with rRNA have provided a means of classification that can be applied with some rigor, albeit not without caveats. Perhaps the most significant caveat is the predilection of bacteria to exchange information in a horizontal manner that tends to upset the vertical inheritance applecart (9). And with that in mind Palleroni et al. have claimed that "Lateral gene transfer is far more pervasive than was once thought and for populations undergoing even limited recombination a phylogeny based on 16S rRNA may reflect little more than the phylogeny of the 16S rRNA gene" (16). Others have proposed a "net" instead of a "tree" to represent the prokaryotes (17). Therefore, perhaps, as in all organisms that are "endotoxin" in nature, the more the organisms seemingly change the more they

---

[e] ... regions in the alignments where a specific change is observed in the primary structure of a protein in all members of one or more taxa but not in the other taxa. The changes in the sequence could be either the presence of particular amino acid substitutions or specific deletions or insertions (i.e., indels). In all cases, the signatures must be flanked by regions that are conserved in all the sequences under consideration. These conserved regions serve as anchors to ensure that the observed signature is not an artifact resulting from improper alignment or from sequencing errors (14).

remain the same. The early Gram stain remains a true descriptor of a valid structural difference between bacteria that contain endotoxin (gram-negative) and those that do not (gram-positive).[f]

Some of the difficulties in classification can be seen in a single example. In 1982, the submarine Alvin brought back a sample from a Pacific deep thermal vent. It was sent to the lab and eventually categorized as a (primordial[g]) methane-producing Archaea. Lewis (18) describes it:

> The organism is a curious mix of prokaryote and eukaryote-and then some. The genes encoding its surface features and most of its metabolic enzymes resemble those of run-of-the-mill-bacteria, yet its DNA replication and protein synthetic machinery are more like those of eukaryotes. The lipids in its membranes and cell walls are unique. The biggest surprise was that 56% of its 1738 protein-encoding genes were at that time completely unknown in any prokaryote or eukaryote. On a whole-genome level, *Methalanococcus jannaschii* very much appeared to be a third form of life.

Relman et al. point out that an entire domain of prokaryotes, Archaea[h], has been found to colonize the human gut, oral, and vaginal cavities, but no association with disease causation has been found (19,20), presumably because, until recently, it has not been searched for with the right tools. According to Mayer, Archaea do not contain LPS (21) but rather are held together via peptidoglycan or some chemical variant thereof. One can also gather this from Gupta's claim that the Archaea are actually gram-positive organisms. At any rate, after being studied with advanced tools, they are being implicated in disease causation (22–24). Similarly, it is only in a host vector that many prokaryotes have made themselves known by causing disease in humans. Arthropod-borne gram-negative bacteria including *Rickettsia* (25), *Borrelia*, and *Bartonella*, the causative agents of typhus, relapsing, and trench fevers, respectively, are examples (26) for the numerous, newly emerging arthropod-borne diseases (see Chapter 5) that are becoming more prevalent, given the newly acquired means to detect their presence. These examples demonstrate the shift from static to dynamic models of prokaryotic existence. The bold, overt pathogens have made themselves readily known historically but the subtle, enigmatic bacteria have largely remained under the human radar,[i] and it is this huge, unknown bio-realm that is changing the view of the simplistic little "machines" called "bacteria" that have been modeled heretofore.

Another "dynamic" that has come to alter the view of prokaryotes is their communal way of life. Biofilms have been defined as "matrix-enclosed microbial accretions that adhere to biological or non-biological surfaces" (27). Just as "unculturables" are thought to predominate the biosphere, so too is the communityliving the more natural state of being for prokaryotes, in nature: "Hence, although microorganisms can have an independent planktonic existence, an interdependent lifestyle in which they function as an integral part of a population or community is also possible and is, in fact, more typical"; (27) and our perception of bacteria as

---

[f]Now with the apparent exception of the anaerobic genus *Pectinatus*...

[g]Tudge, Pg. 126 "... in the beginning living systems were not divided into different organisms. There was just a living 'syncytium,' which Woese has called the 'progenote'; a more-or-less continuous living slime that spread all over the globe wherever hot rocks met water, and in practice such a nexus was ubiquitous."

[h]Many so-called "extremeaphiles" for their ability to grow in extreme environments...

[i]Some while residing in the human body.

unicellular life forms is deeply rooted in the pure-culture paradigm. Since bacteria can, in a strict sense, be diluted to a single cell and studied in liquid culture, this mode of operation has been exploited and used to study many bacterial activities. Although this traditional way of culturing bacteria in liquid medium has been instrumental in the study of microbial pathogenesis and enlightening as to some of the amazing facets of microbial physiology, pure culture "planktonic" means of growth is rarely the means how bacteria exist in nature" (28).

After all, it is in their sheer numbers, not as individuals, that they are overwhelmingly effective, and it is by virtue of their numbers that their attributes are so quickly selected for, as demonstrated by an example of antibiotic resistance, briefly discussed in section "Heterogeneity Conclusions." Therefore, the historical model of the prokaryote as a static, freestanding being is, more often than not, misleading as an aide to understanding prokaryotes and points to the fact that their boundaries and borders with one another maybe more dynamic and in flux than previously believed. The "fortress" format of bacterial growth can provide a formidable defense against both pharmaceutical manufacturing contaminant containment (i.e., in water systems) and against host-defense mechanisms.

LIPOPOLYSACCHARIDE HETEROGENEITY IN BACTERIAL PATHOGENESIS

There is, of course, a prototypical or model type of endotoxin structure represented by that occurring in *EC* and *Salmonella* and other Enterobacteriaceae. However, variations are being found in the prototypical structure, which was once thought to be fairly static, at least within the Lipid A portion. Variations are being found not only in different organisms but also within species that have adapted different LPS presentations as a means of aiding host invasion or to remain undetected while residing inside the host. The differences in O-chain, core, and Lipid A acyl chain structures are referred to as the "heterogeneity" or subsets of the (proto) typical structure (29), which is the most studied and among the most toxic of structures (as described in Chapter 4).

Enterobacterial endotoxins were initially studied and modeled as hostreactive and this served to encourage researchers to lump together the mode of action of all LPS moieties—until the discovery of the various "exceptions to the rule" which now appear to be as common as the "rule." Both intra and interspecies polymorphisms in LPS TLR have also been discovered. This brings with it the realization that the host reaction is far more complex, even for the prototypical pathogen-associated microbial patterns (PAMP) LPS, than previously believed. Perhaps of more practical significance is the difference that can arise in the *Limulus* amebocyte lysate (LAL) activity of various organisms for some of these (heterogeneity) reasons. *EC*, for example, is a hundred-fold more LAL reactive[j] than *Shigella flexneri* and greater than two-fold less active than *Pseudomonas testosterone* (30). Even different strains of organism used as the standard, *EC*, have shown exaggerated swings in endotoxicity via a variety of measures including LAL testing, with a range of six hundred-fold using a variety of serotypes (31).

---

[j]The great utility of the LAL test here can be seen in that the biosensor, factor C, in *Limulus* is not a cell-bound TLR but rather a free hemolymph protease cascade initiator.

It is also interesting to note that although the presence or absence of LPS is an absolute (as are the presence of other features such as sporulation and flagella formation), it has become clear that this simple trait is not so simple when viewed from the genetic level. Consider that the genome of Archaea, *Thermoanerobacter tengcongensis* (isolated from a freshwater hot spring in China), does not contain LPS but contains some of the enzymes used in the biosynthesis of LPS (32):

> *T. tengcongensis*, as a gram-negative rod by staining, shares many genes that are characteristic of gram-positive bacteria but lacks some characteristics of gram-negative bacteria .... The *T. tengcongensis*, though having a few coding sequences (CDS) for LPS biosynthesis (TTE0652 and TTE0199), does not possess three of the key genes: the one related to LPS biosynthesis (LPS: glycosyltransferase, COG1442), and the two related to LPS transport (i.e., a periplasmic protein involved in polysaccharide export, COG1596) and an ATPase component of ABC-type polysacharide/polyol phosphate transport system COG1134. At least one of these three CDS is present in most of the gram-negative prokaryotes, such as *Pseudomonas aeruginosa*, *V. choleraserotype*, *Neisseria meningitidis*, *X. fastidiosa*, and EC ... none of the four CDS involved in Lipid A synthesis are found in the *T. tengcongensis* genome ...

The following subsections describe the efforts of some pathogens to inhabit the host by means of changing their LPS and other surface structure presentations, typically either to hide or disguise their presence upon gaining entry to the host or to alternatively ramp up their ability to effect a change in the host system status quo to favor their proliferation. Table 1 gives an overview of some LPS modification mechanisms and Table 2 gives the result or effect(s) upon the host.

Two interesting mechanisms that serve to demonstrate the utility of LPS heterogeneity occurring in the oligosaccharide-antigen (O-antigen) region are *host mimicry* and *phase variation*. The next section focuses on the LPS of a pathogen, *Nesseria meningitides*, that employs both methods and is followed by two additional sections that describe various other means of LPS heterogeneity in host occupation: *Yersinia pestis*, and *Porphyromonas gingivalis*. *Nesseria meningitides* contains truncated O-antigens referred to as lipooligosaccharides (LOS). They are able to add sialic acid residues to the short chains to create structures mimicking host cell constituents (33).

TABLE 1 Lipopolysaccharide Heterogeneity in Pathogens

Heterogeneity mechanism	Sub-mechanism(s)	Example organism(s)	Comments
O-antigen structural variation	Antigenicity (i.e., typical adaptive host response)	All gram-negative orgs.	~1,000 O-antigenic variants in *Salmonella* and ~200 in *E. coli*
	Host mimicry	*Nesseria meningitides*, *H. pylori*	See section "O-antigenic Variation–Phase variation..."
	Phase variation	*Nesseria meningitides*, *H. pylori*	See section "O-antigenic Variation–Phase variation..."
Lipid A acyl group variation/phase variation		*Bordetella*, *Yersinia pestis*	Arthropod-borne pathogens, many of which cause fevers via gram-negative pathogens. See Chapter 5
Escape of TLR4 pathway activation		*Helicobacter Pylori*	Activates TLR2 which is not typically a LPS toll pathway
Production of agonistic and antagonistic LPS		*Porphyromonas gingivalis*	Atypically activates TLR2 and TLR4

Abbreviations: LPS, lipopolysaccharide; TLR, Toll-like receptors.

TABLE 2 Summary of the Response of Each TLR4-MD-Z Combination to Various Ligands. Phenotype Relative to *Escherichia coli* Lipopolysaccharide[a]

	hMDMD-2				mMD-2			
	CF	LA	Lipid IVA	Taxol	CF	LA	Lipid IVA	Taxol
hTLR4	4 +	4 +	− −	− −	3 +	− −	2 +	1 +
mTLR4	4 +	4 +	− −	− −	4 +	4 +	4 +	2 +

[a]Responses were classified as 70–95% (4+), 50–70% (3+), 25–50% (2+), 1–25% (1+) and <1% (− −) of the response of the same receptor to EC LPS at 100 mg/mL
Abbreviations: CF, cystic fibrosis; EC, *Escherichia coli*; LA, laboratory-adapted PAK strain; LPS, lipopolysaccharide; TLR, Toll-like receptors.
Source: From Ref. 36.

They also demonstrate "phase variation" which is a form of hypervariability in the part of the genome that generates a key surface structure. *Nesseria* is a particularly virulent inducer of endotoxicity, which it exports via membrane vesicles resulting in massive stimulation of TLR4 in circulating macrophages and other cells via LOS, leading quickly to intravascular coagulation related events culminating in death. *Yersinia pestis* produces two different forms of LPS depending upon the temperature of the host environment, 27°C for the flea and 37°C for man. *Porphyromas gingivalis* produces two types of LPS, which vary drastically in that one is fully endotoxic and the other is actually an LPS agonist. Interestingly, *H. pylori* and *P. gingivalis* appear to share a unique property in their LPS activation of host immune response via TLR2 instead of (*H. pylori*) or in addition to (*P. gingivalis*) the typical LPS TLR activiation via TLR4 (34). An additional example can be seen in *Pseudomonas aeruginosa*, which has been shown to synthesize a more acylated LPS structure during adaptation to cystic fibrosis airways. Hajjar et al. showed that humans but not mice recognize the difference (hexa vs. penta-acylated LPS) (35).

Oligosaccharide-antigenic Variation—Phase Variation and Host Mimicry in *Neisseria meningitides*

The presence of O-antigens on bacterial endotoxins is responsible for the antigenic response the host generates to LPS, which is apparently less effective than the innate, TLR-mediated response (i.e., as evidenced by the lack of efficient immunity against endotoxemia). There are at least 20 sugars used in bacterial LPS O-antigens, of which many are "characteristically unique dideoxyhexoses such as abequose, colitose, paratose, and tyvelose, which are rarely found elsewhere in nature" (36) and these may occur in chain lengths up to 40 sugar residues. Therefore, the potential for variability is great indeed. There are several mechanisms by which specific pathogens vary their O-antigens in order to colonize hosts. Lerouge and Vanderleyden list four changes to O-antigens within a given strain that can bring about LPS heterogeneity (in addition to the most obvious differences in polysaccharide-chain constituents evident in different strains):

1. O-polysaccharides can be modified nonstochiometrically with sugar moieties
2. Addition of noncarbohydrate substituents, that is, acetyl or methyl groups
3. Positional or anomeric change in the linkage between sugars in the chain
4. Variation of the length of the chain

   Neisseria meningitides is found only in the "naso-oropharyngeal" mucosa of man. It is said to reside in one out of ten people, and one of the ten strains of those residing is said to be a noninvasive, noninfectious type (37). Van Deuren et al. cite four requirements to be achieved by the bacteria in order to infect the host:

> At least four conditions have to be met before invasive disease can occur.... These conditions are (*i*) exposure to a pathogenic strain, (*ii*) colonization of the naso-oropharyngeal mucosa, (*iii*) passage through that mucosa, and (*iv*) survival of the meningococcus in the bloodstream. These processes are influenced by bacterial properties, climatological and social conditions, preceding or concomitant viral infections, and the immune status of the patient.

Almeida-González (38) summarize the microbiology and heterogeneity generation capability of *Neisseria meningitides*:

> *Neisseria meningitides* is a gram-negative, aerobic, immobile, nonsporulated bacterium; it is usually encapsulated and has pilli ... It is classified in serogroups according to the immune reactivity of its capsular polysaccharide, which is the basis of the polysaccharide vaccines currently available .... Thirteen[k] serogroups are known, but most cases of meningococcal disease worldwide are caused by serogroups A, C, and B. The polysaccharide vaccine is effective for the first two. Serogroup B contains a polysaccharide of low immunogenicity, probably due to its polysialic acid content. This acid is also present in human fetal neurons ... Capsular polysaccharide is made up of homopolymers or heteropolymers of repetitive polysaccharide, disaccharide, and polysaccharide units. The component to which the bacterium owes its invasive properties is the molecular products of sialic acid present in the meningococcal capsule ... Meningococcus has the ability to exchange genetic material that controls capsule production. Therefore, it can change from serogroup B to C or vice versa.

Van der Woude and Baumler (39) describe the use of host mimicry and antigenic variation in *Neisseria meningitidis*:

> Analysis of meningococcal LOS biosynthesis provides an intriguing example of how phase variation (i.e., a heritable on/off switch of gene expression) can be used to generate antigenic variation (i.e., changes in the chemical composition) of a surface structure. In this case, expression of several genes (*lgt* genes) encoding glycosyltransferases shows phase variation. These glycosyltransferases are required for the expression of terminal LOS structures known as α-chain and β-chain extensions. Variation of α-chain and β-chain extensions dramatically changes the antigenic properties of LOS, thereby forming the basis for its classification into 14 immunotypes, L1 to L14. In many meningococcal isolates, individual genes are missing from the *lgt-1* locus (*lgtABCDE*) and/or the *lgt-3* locus (*lgtG*), thus representing meningococci capable of expressing only a small subset (often two or three) of the 14 known LOS immunotypes . It is difficult to envision how switching between a limited repertoire of LOS structures can be sufficient to allow continued immune evasion during chronic infection of the nasopharynx. A mechanism that may contribute to immune evasion is the concealment of antigens by LOS sialylation. The sialylation of α-chain extensions carrying terminal galactose residues (present in the LOS of immunotypes L2, L3, L4, L7, and L9) gives rise to LOS carbohydrate moieties mimicking carbohydrates present in glycosphingolipids of human cells.... In addition to a possible role in immune evasion, LOS variation has been postulated to be a mechanism that facilitates the adaptation of the meningococcus to environmental changes during its transition from the mucosa of the nasopharynx into the blood.

Given the severity of the host response to the particular form of endotoxin presented by *Neisseria meningitid1s*, referred to as LOS, Zaghaier et al. (40)

---

[k]Fourteen more recently as noted below.

studied the mechanism and structural variations that occur. They used defined structural variations of *Neisseria meningitidis* mutants to define the role of the CD14/TRL4-MD-2 pathway to deduce the endotoxin structure required for activation of both human and mouse macrophage cells. Their findings support the classical activation of TLR4 via lipid A.

> Meningococcal LOS is a major inflammatory mediator of meningococcemia and meningococcal meningitis. Meningococcal LOS levels in serum of ≥ 1 ng/ml are associated with shock and death in meningococcemia. The interaction of meningococcal LOS with the CD14/TLR4–MD-2 receptor complex is predicted to result in macrophage activation and subsequent release of cytokines, chemokines, nitric oxide, and ROS. The goal of this study was to define the relationship of meningococcal LOS structure with the biological activity initiated through the human CD14/TLR4–MD-2 receptor. The importance of CD14 and TLR4–MD-2 in macrophage activation by meningococcal LOS was demonstrated. When CD14 was efficiently blocked with specific monoclonal antibody, tumor necrosis factor-α (TNF-α) production was markedly reduced. When TLR4–MD-2 was blocked and CD14 was available, a significant reduction in cytokine release was also observed. Further, highly purified meningococcal LOS did not stimulate TLR2 in our experimental models when C3H/HeJ (TLR4$-/-$) cells were induced, supporting the model that CD14/TLR4–MD-2 is the meningococcal endotoxin receptor.

and

> In conclusion, meningococcal LOS is a potent activator of the macrophage TLR4 pathway. This may help explain the role of meningococcal endotoxin in acute meningococcal sepsis and meningitis. Meningococcal oligosaccharide α or β chain structure or length was not a contributor to human or murine TLR4 activation. KDO2 linked to lipid A was structurally required. ...

Thus, one can surmise that while the LOS chain is an active participant in the bacterial mechanism of infection and aids the bacterium to this end by manner of host mimicry and phase variation, which helps favor its survival in various host environs (nasopharlnynx and blood), it is not a factor in activating the classical innate immune response as was shown to occur by the typical TLR4 pathway via lipid A.

Jennings et al. (41) emphasize the importance of understanding the mechanisms of generating surface structure heterogeneity on the most basic, genetic, level, specifically in the *Neisseria meningitidis* example:

> ... the advantage of examining LPS expression in *Neisseria meningitidis* genetically rather than immunologically is the ability to classify strains by their phase variation repertoire, based on a combination of gene content and phase variation potential (homopolymeric tract presence and/or length). This is far more informative than determining the immunotype, which happens to be expressed by a single colony picked at the time of isolation, and has the potential to reveal new relationships between aspects of meningococcal disease and this important virulence factor.

Lipid A Acyl Group Heterogeneity Demonstrated by *Yersinia pestis*

Some gram-negative organisms have long been known to contain a great variety of O-antigenic variants while others do not contain an O-antigen, including some pathogens such as *Neisseria, Pasteurella, Campylobacter, Bordetella*, and *Bacteroides* (42), but more recently a great deal of variability has been found in the lipid A portion of the LPS molecule, which was not previously suspected. For example, *Bordetella* has been found to harbor an array of different LPS forms; of eight species, half have different acyl group formations (43). Previously, it was assumed that LPS was typically conserved within a given genus. Even more surprisingly, others such as *Yersinia pestis* and *Porphyromonas gingivalis* display an interesting ability to alter their LPS structure as a means of evading host immune system detection. *Yersinia pestis*, the causative agent of bubonic plague, brings about, through a somewhat circuitous route, one of the most devastating diseases in the history of mankind. In plague, the literal choking of the flea via a plasmid-encoded (two plasmids actually) biofilm in the feeding tube of the flea causes it to regurgitate the blood it is trying to feed upon back into the human host along with an unwelcome guest: *Yersinia pestis*. Morbid but fascinating, thusly *Y. pestis* is able to "kill two birds with one stone" and propagate itself at the expense of arthropod and human alike.

The LPS of *Yersinia pestis* is a part of the mechanism of the bacteria's virulence and has been studied extensively for this reason. The LPS has no O-antigenic polysaccharides (i.e., "rough type" LPS) and contains 3-hydroxy-myristic acid (3-OH-$C_{14:0}$) as the predominate fatty acid in the lipid A molecule. The prototypical structure shared among *Enterobacteriaceae* contains "four 3-OH-$C_{14:0}$, one myristic acid ($C_{14:0}$), and one $C_{12:0}$, with two nonhydroxy fatty acids bound to the hydroxyl group of 3-OH-$C_{14:0}$ in the nonreducing GlcN molecule to form an acyloxyacyl structure" (44). However, Kawahara et al. showed that the *Yersinia pestis* LPS structure at 37°C differed from the bacteria grown at 27°C. The group grew cultures at both temperatures and analyzed the resulting LPS using matrix-assisted laser description/ionization-time of flight (MALDI-TOF). Their study showed that at 27°C *Y. pestis* produces $C_{12:0}$ and $C_{16:0}$ as well as $C_{14:0}$. They used TNF induction studies using murine macrophages to gauge the relative endotoxicity of the two LPS structures referred to as A-27 and A-37. A-27 activity resembled synthetic lipid A and A-37 revealed weaker activity, only one-tenth that of A-27. Furthermore, using human macrophages A-27 was 100-fold stronger than A-37. The authors speculate that the shift from 27°C to 37°C that corresponds to the shift from arthropod (flea) to human is a benefit to *Y. pestis* survival and subsequent host infection in that the reduced virulence of the LPS at 37°C allows the bacterium to escape a vigorous initial innate immune response that a strong LPS would surely elicit. Thus, seemingly the *Y. pestis* is able to alter[1] its LPS biosynthesis in order to evade different host innate immunity mechanisms, in effect disguising its weapons until it gains firm entry into enemy territory.

Production of Agonistic and Antagonistic Lipopolysaccharide in *Porphyromonas gingivalis*

Porphyromas gingivalis is the causative agent of adult periodontitis and has the capacity to produce both agonistic and antagonistic types of LPS. Truly, this is night and day in the same organism with regard to provoking the host to respond to the bacterium's presence and, alternatively, seeking to remain hidden within the host. *Porphyromas gingivalis* releases large amounts of membrane vesicles (as does *Neisseria*) and these have the ability to release "copious amounts of outer membrane vesicles containing LPS, which can penetrate periodontal tissue and thus participate in the destructive innate host response associated with disease. The potential contribution of *P. gingivalis* LPS to the disease process is not clear, however, due to complex innate host responses to this cell wall component." (45).

---

[1]Probably more correctly stated as *Yersinia* being able to produce two genomic variations that are selected and propagated in response to the particular environment.

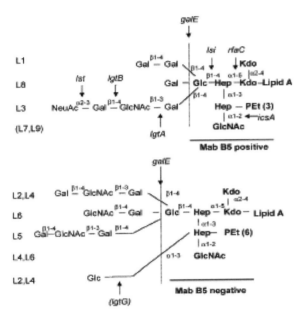

FIGURE 2 Representation of the structure of meningococcal lipopolysaccharide oligosaccharides of immunotypes L1 to L9. Immunotypes are indicated to the extreme left. The vertical line marks the junction between the inner core structures to the right and outer core structures to the left. The epitope recognized by MAb B5 is indicated in boldface (MAb B5 positive). Arabic numerals indicate the linkage between sugars or amino sugars. Alpha and beta indicate the carbon 1 linkage at the nonreducing end of the sugar. Genes for incorporating each of the key sugars or amino sugars into the LPS oligosaccharide in the biosynthetic pathway are indicated with arrows indicating where in the pathway the gene product is required. *Abbreviations*: Gal, galactose; Glu, glucose; Hep, heptose. lcNAc, *N*-acetylglucosamine; Kdo, 2-keto-2-deoxyoctulosonic acid. Immunotype L5 has no PEtn on the second heptose. The gene that adds the glucose to the second heptose (*lgtG*) is phase variable. *Source*: From Ref. 56.

Yoshimua et al. (46), studied the antagonistic properties of *P. gingivalis* and determined that

> ... LPS from two of four periodontopathic bacteria worked as antagonists for human TLR4. Although the precise effect of the antagonistic LPS on bacterial growth in the gingival sulcus and the prevalence of these unique bacteria in patients remain to be elucidated, the antagonistic activity would be a great advantage for the microorganisms to escape from the innate immune system. In spite of the potent proinflammatory activity of LPS, gram-negative bacteria predominate in moderate to severe periodontal lesions. The antagonistic LPS may play a role in this paradoxical situation and may be associated with the progression of periodontal diseases.

Darveau et al. (47) surmise that *P. gingivalis* activates host cells through both TLR2 and TLR4, which is unusual, and that the lipid A heterogeneity demonstrated (Fig. 2) is involved with the dual capability of both chronic colonization and active inflammatory induction:

> The results of HEK cell transfection assays and bone marrow cell activation experiments demonstrate that certain *Porphyromas gingivalis* LPS preparations have the ability to interact with either TLR2 or TLR4. Another related implication is that the

lipid A heterogeneity observed in *Porphyromas gingivalis* LPS preparations may reflect an ability of this bacterium to synthesize and express multiple, structurally different forms of lipid A. Alterations in the lipid A structural composition and utilization of multiple TLRs may affect host cell signaling, contributing to the ability of *Porphyromas gingivalis* to remain a persistent colonizer of the oral cavity as well as to induce inflammatory disease.

Tanamoto et al. (48) used LPS-unresponsive C3H/HeJ mice to verify that the inflammatory agent was indeed LPS and not LPS associated protein.

Host Recognition Heterogeneity of Various *Pseudomonas aeruginosa* LPS Structures

Recently it has been determined that host cells have complex signaling pathways for LPS recognition that differ both from species to species and also between individuals of a species, with some species recognizing or ignoring certain forms of LPS that bring about the opposite responses in others. Much of this heterogeneity is brought about by the differences in the Toll-like pattern recognition receptors, which are genetically encoded and conserved albeit with some variability between individuals (Fig. 3).

Human but not mice hosts recognize variations among *P. aeruginosa* (PA) LPS structures (hexa but not penta-acylated LPS). Hajjar et al. (35) determined that an 82-amino-acid region of TLR4 hypervariable across species is responsible for the heterogeneity between species.

> To determine whether human and murine cells differed in their ability to recognize PA LPS, we stimulated human monocystic THP-1 cells and murine macrophage RAW 264.7 cells with either penta-acylated LA or hexa-acylated cystic fibrosis (CF) LPS (Fig. 4). CF LPS was more than 100-fold more active in stimulating the production of both TNF-α and interleukin 8 (IL-8) in THP-1 cells than was LA LPS (Fig. and data not shown), whereas LA and CF LPS induced equivalent production of TNF-α in RAW 264.7 cells at all concentrations tested (Fig. not shown). EC LPS, a prototypical highly acylated LPS (hexa-acylated; Fig. 4A), was a potent stimulator of both human and murine cells and resulted in the production of higher levels of TNF-α at lower concentrations (Fig. not shown). These results show that human cells are deficient specifically in their ability to recognize penta-acylated PA LPS, whereas mouse cells recognize both forms of PA LPS (49).

and

> Comparison of the predicted amino acid (aa) sequences of mTLR4 and hTLR4 showed that the middle 330 aa, which lie in the extracellular domain, are the most variable (Fig. 5). This is a region in which human polymorphisms exist. When we analyzed this middle region further, we found that the first 82 aa (aa 285 − 366 in mTLR4 and aa 287 − 368 in hTLR4), which are predicted to lack leucine-rich repeats (LRRs), are the least conserved. Pair-wise alignment of hTLR4 with TLR4 proteins of other species available in GenBank showed that the first 82 aa of the middle region are hypervariable across species, whereas the remaining 248 aa have the same degree of sequence divergence as the remainder of the extracellular domain (Fig. 5) (49).

Mice have been found to be more "promiscuous" (49) in recognizing various lipid A structures via their TLR4 than human. A number of disease-causing organisms have been implicated as "poorly recognized" by human TLR4 including *H. pylori, L. pneumophilia, Yersinia Pestis,* and *Francisella* spp. Miller et al. conclude

m/z 1450

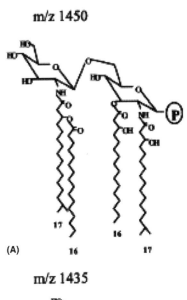

(A)

m/z 1435

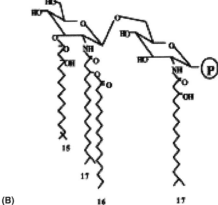

(B)

FIGURE 3 Structure of *Porphyromas gingivalis* lipid A mass ions at *m/z* 1435 and 1450 found in purified *Porphyromas gingivalis* LPS preparations. Kumada et al. (57) have eluci dated the structures of several of the major lipid A mass ions, including the mass ion at *m/z* 1450 (**A**) and *m/z* 1435 (**B**). *Source:* From Ref. 47.

that These lipid A species typically consist of only four or five acyl chains, some of which are 16 to 18 carbons in length. It seems likely that the potential for these pathogens to cause severe disease in humans is attributable, at least in part, to their relative lack of TLR4 signaling, as Th-4-null mice are highly susceptible to infection with gram-negative microorganisms (49).

It is interesting to note from Figure 4, the differences in the TLR/MD2 protein sequences and surmise that the rabbit and human differences, 68/100% and 85/100%, respectively, would likely have LPS microstructure or heterogeneity recognition differences just as do the mice versus human that have been discussed here (i.e., the rabbit vs. mice hypervariable regions are 68/63% and 85/85% relative to humans). This would lead one to predict differences in rabbit versus human in regard to pyrogen test reactivity in response to selected gram-negative organisms.

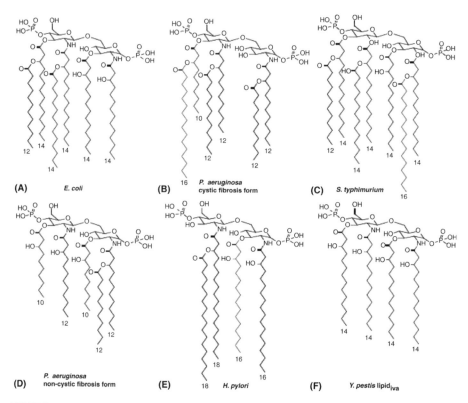

FIGURE 4 The structural diversity of lipid A in gram-negative microorganisms. Chemical structures of hexa-acylated *Escherichia coli* (**A**) and *Pseudomonas aeruginosa* (**B**), hepta-acylated *Salmonella enterica* serovar Typhimurium (**C**), penta-acylated *Pseudomonas aeruginosa* (**D**), tetra-acylated *Helicobacter pylori* (**E**) and lipidIVa, a precursor of enteric lipid A or isolated from *Yersinia pestis* grown at 37°C (**F**). Numbers indicate different fatty-acid carbon lengths at the bottom of each associated chain. (a) Chemical structures of the dominant hepta- and hexa-acylated lipid A from EC, the lipid A precursor, lipid$_{IVA}$ (which has four 3-OH C_{14} acyl groups) and the penta-acylated RS lipid A (which has two 3-OH C_{10} and C_{14} acyl groups and an unsaturated acyloxyacyl side chain (C_{14}) attached at the 2′ position). (b) Chemical structures of the dominant hexa- and penta-acylated lipid A from, respectively, cystic fibrosis (CF) and bronchiectasis (BR) clinical isolates, and the penta-acylated LPS from the laboratory-adapted PAK strain (LA). Note that colors are not reproduced but acyl chain lengths are shown numerically at the bottom of each associated chain. *Source*: From Ref. 49.

HETEROGENEITY CONCLUSIONS

Netea et al. (50) have postulated that it is the complex interplay of heterogeneity in not only various forms of lipid A from various organisms but also in various forms of TLR in various hosts (even of the same species) that is responsible for the myriad of host responses to a dizzying array of both overtly infectious, chronically infectious, and commensal organisms. Figure 6 serves to summarize their thinking. Thus, it appears that the conical shape shared by *EC* and *Salmonella* is the most endotoxic (left in Fig. 6) followed by intermediary forms that would fall between that of *EC* and *P. gingivalis* (center) and also perhaps additional intermediary

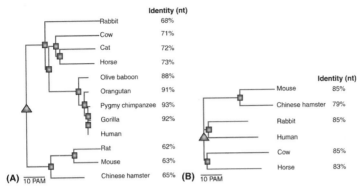

FIGURE 5 A hypervariable region of the toll-like receptors 4 (TLR4) extracellular domain and the C-terminus of the accessory protein MD2 evolved across species. Results are shown from pairwise alignments of human TLR4 (**A**) or MD2 (**B**) with those from other species. *Source*: From Ref. 49.

forms that would fall between *P. gingivalis* and *R. sphaeroides*, which appears to "clog up" the TLR system to actually block or otherwise restrict its use (or perhaps compete for it's soluble or cell-bound external co-receptors). The fine detail for the later being unavailable as of yet.

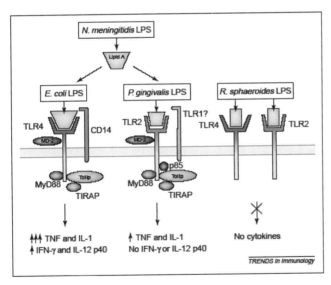

FIGURE 6 Hypothesis linking the structure of various lipid A species with their proinflammatory characteristics. Lipid A adopting a strong conical shape (e.g., from *EC*) induces a strong proinflammatory signal through Toll-like receptor4 (TLR4); lipid A adopting a slightly conical form (e.g., from *Porphyromonas gingivalis*) induces a less efficient synthesis of proinflammatory cytokines through TLR2; and strictly cylindrical lipid A (e.g., from *Rhodobacter sphaeroides*) has antagonistic properties. Lipid A from *Neisseria meningitidis* engages both TLR2–TLR1 and TLR4, probably by adopting an intermediary shape between *EC* and *Porphyromas gingivalis* lipid A. *Abbreviations*: IFN-γ, interferon-γ; IL, interleukin; LPS, lipopolysaccharide; TIRAP, toll/IL-1-receptor-domain-containing adaptor protein; TNF, tumor necrosis factor; TLR, toll-like receptor. *Source*: From Ref. 50.

It is interesting to tease out the distinctions between the TLR of *Limulus* and *Drosophila* and those of higher organisms (mouse/human) in that, as serine proteases they may not be pattern-recognition receptors to the extent of the TLRs of higher organisms and thus cannot recognize all the nuances of LPS microstructure heterogeneity, at least by the same mechanism. They do, however, recognize the broad PAMP structural differences (i.e., LPS versus peptidoglycan) and tailor their responses accordingly (51). The *Limulus* model shows that it is via the serine protease cascade that endotoxin is initially recognized, which triggers the LAL coagulation cascade in the blood. However, at least in the animal [as opposed to the in vivo LAL test, in which the granules have been lysed (i.e., the "lysate" in LAL)] there must be an initial recognition of endotoxin on the granular hemocyte surface as they are activated to release the constituents of the cascade in an increased concentration (see Chapter 11).

> Horseshoe crabs' granular hemocytes respond specifically to LPS stimulation, inducing the secretion of various defense molecules from the granular hemocytes. Here, we show a cDNA which we named tToll, coding for a TLR identified from hemocytes of the horseshoe crab *Tachypleus tridentatus*. tToll is most closely related to *Drosophila* Toll in both domain architecture and overall length. Human TLRs have been suggested to contain numerous PAMP-binding insertions located in the LRRs of their ectodomains. However, the LRRs of tToll contained no obvious PAMP-binding insertions. Furthermore, tToll was non-specifically expressed in horseshoe-crab tissues. These observations suggest that tToll does not function as an LPS receptor on granular hemocytes (52).

And indeed the same factor (C) that begins the LAL cascade has been found to function on the hemocyte surface as a pattern recognition receptor:

> Using a previously uncharacterized assay for exocytosis, we clearly show that hemocytes respond only to LPS and not to other pathogen-associated molecular patterns, such as β-1,3-glucans and peptidoglycans. Furthermore, we show that a granular protein called factor C, an LPS-recognizing serine protease zymogen that initiates the hemolymph coagulation cascade, also exists on the hemocyte surface as a biosensor for LPS (53).

MICROBIAL POPULATIONS AND RESISTANCE TO ANTIBIOTICS

Antimicrobial resistance is an example of how bacterial traits are selected by the environment and incorporated into the prokaryotic genome. LPS, as a necessary constituent of the bacterial cell, cannot be eliminated from viable cells as can antibiotic resistance genes, but as we have seen, LPS can be presented in alternating alternative forms. In similar fashion, the introduction of antibiotics into a population of bacteria creates an arena in which those mutations that can best survive, thrive, and perpetuate their survival traits and often do so due to an acquired resistance to the antibiotic in question. This topic fits into the subject of "biodiversity" because antibiotic resistance is a prime and significant example of such genomic "sharing" via plasmids that bring about and perpetuate the diversity that is generated.

> The introduction of a new antibiotic molecule into widespread human use carries with it an inevitable progression to select for resistant bacteria and to have diminished utility... The development of resistance accrues from two facets of bacterial populations—the large number of bacteria in an infection and their mutation frequency.

There may be 10^9 to 10^{10} bacteria in a fulminate infection in an animal or a person. A typical rate of spontaneous mutation that is observed is about one mutant cell in 10^7. At these frequencies there would be about a thousand mutants in a bacterial population of 10^{10}. If each of these mutants had occurred randomly they might be distributed one per gene in each of a thousand genes in the bacterial population. When the bacteria are now exposed to an antibiotic, most will die off. However, if one or more mutants in a particular gene alter the gene product to confer resistance, they will give a selective advantage for the mutant to survive and then grow up in the space vacated by their dying (sensitive) neighbors, and dominate the bacterial population. Bacterial resistance to antibiotics is a matter of when, not if, and is almost independent of the structure and type of antibiotic. The resistance could be conferred by the mutation of a single gene or multiple mutations may have to accumulate before significant growth advantage and resistance accrues (54).

The ability to modify LPS and other surface structures, to acquire resistance factors and otherwise change to accommodate host system defense mechanisms show that bacteria today are highly evolved organisms just as are higher organisms, sometimes amazingly so given the more limited complexity of their machinery.

REFERENCES

1. Helander IM et al. Lipopolysaccharides of anaerobic beer spoilage bacteria of the genus *Pectinatus* – lipopolysaccharides of a Gram-positive genus. FEMS Microbiol Rev 2004; 28:342–552.
2. Hugenholtz P et al. Impact of culture-independent studies on the emerging phylogenetic view of bacterial diversity. J Bacteriol 1998; 180(18):4765–4774.
3. Pace NR. A molecular view of microbial diversity and the biosphere. Science 1997; 276:734–740.
4. Fredricks DN, Relman DA. Sequence-based identification of microbial pathogens: a reconsideration of Koch's postulates. Clin Microbiol Rev 1996; 9(1):18–33.
5. Paster BJ. Bacterial diversity in human subgingival plaque. J Bacteriol 2001; 183(12):3770–3783, doi: 10.1128/JB.183.12.3770–3783.2001.
6. Handelsman J. Metagenomics: application of genomics to uncultured microorganisms. Microbiol Mol Biol Rev 2004; 68(4):669–685, doi: 10.1128/MBR.68.4.669–685.2004.
7. Doolittle WF. Phylogenetic classification and the universal tree. Science 1999; 284(5423):2124–2128.
8. Lawrence JG, Ochman H. Molecular archeology of the Escherichia coli genome, Evolution. Proc Nat Acad Sci 1998; 95:9413–9417.
9. Martin W. Mosaic bacterial chromosomes: a challenge en route to a tree of genomes. Bioessays 1999; 21:99–104.
10. Mayr E. Two empires or three? Proc Natl Acad Sci 1998; 95(17):9720–9723.
11. Woese CR. Default taxonomy: Ernst Mayr's view of the microbial world. Proc Natl Acad Sci 1998; 95(19):11043–11046.
12. Guest H. Bacterial classification and taxonomy: a 'primer' for the new millennium. Microbiol Today 1999; 26:70–72.
13. Tudge C. The Variety of Life, New York: Oxford University Press, 2000.
14. Gupta RS. Protein pylogenies and signature sequences: a reappraisal of evolutionary relationships among archaebacteria, eubacteria, and eukaryotes. Microbiol Mol Biol Rev 1998; Dec:1435–1491.
15. Brown JR et al. Universal trees based on large combined protein sequence data sets. Nat Genet 2001; 28:281–285, doi:10.1038/90129.
16. Palleroni NJ. Prokaryotic diversity and the importance of culturing. Antonie Leeuwenhoek 1997; 72:3–19.
17. Kunin et al. The net of life: Reconstructing the microbial phylogenetic network. Genome Res 2005; June. online publication.
18. Lewis R. Discovery, Windows on the Life Sciences, Blackwell Publishing, 2000:304.

19. Relman DA. Mining the natural world for new pathogens. Am J Trop Med Hyg 2002; 67(2):133–134.
20. Relman DA. The search for unrecognized pathogens. Science 1998; 284(5418):1308–1310.
21. Mayer F. Biology of the Prokaryotes. Ch 2. Lengeler JW, Drews G, Schlegel HG, eds. Blackwell Publishing, 999:31.
22. Eckburg PB, Lepp PW, Relman DA. Archaea and their potential role in human disease. Infect Immun 2003; 71(2):591–596.
23. Lepp PW et al. Methanogenic Archaea and human periodontal disease. PNAS 2004; 101(16):6176–6181, doi: 10.1073/pnas. 0308766101.
24. Eckburg PB. Diversity of the human intestinal microbial flora. Science 2005; 308(5728):1635–1638.
25. Roux V, Raoult D. Rickettsioses as paradigms of new or emerging infectious diseases. Clin Microbiol Rev 1997; 10(4):694–719.
26. Roux V, Raoult D. Body lice as tools for diagnosis and surveillance of reemerging diseases. J Clin Microbiol 1999; 37(3):596–599.
27. Hall-Stoodley L et al. Bacterial biofilms: from the natural environment to infectious diseases. Nat Rev Microbiol 2004; 2:95–108.
28. Davey ME, O'Toole GA. Microbial biofilms: from ecology to molecular genetics. Microbiol Mol Biol Rev 2000; 4(4):847–867.
29. Caroff M et al. Structural and functional analyses of bacterial lipopolysaccharides. Microbes Infect 2002; 4:915–926.
30. Laude-Sharp M et al. Dissociation between the interleukin 1- inducing capacity and limulus reactivity of lipopolysaccharides from Gram-negative bacteria. Cytokine 1990; 2:253–258.
31. Koyama S et al. The potential of various lipopolysaccharide to release IL-8 and G-CSF. Am J Physio 2000; 278:L658–L666.
32. Bao Q et al. A complete sequence of the T. tengcongensis genome. Genome Res 2002; 12:689–700.
33. Lerouge I, Vanderleyden J. O-antigen structural variation: mechanisms and possible roles in animal/plant-microbe interactions. FEMS Microbiol Rev 2001; 26:17–47.
34. Mandell L et al. Intact Gram-Negative *Helicobacter pylori*, *Helicobacter felis*, and *Helicobacter hepaticus* Bacteria Activate Innate Immunity via Toll-Like Receptor 2 but Not Toll-Like Receptor 4. Infect Immun 2004; 72(11):6446–6454, doi: 10.1128/IAI.72.11.6446–6454.2004.
35. Hajjar AM et al. Human Toll-like receptor 4 recognizes host-specific LPS modifications. Nat Immun 2002; 3(4), doi:10.1038/ni777.
36. Lerouge I, Vanderleyden J. O-antigen structural variation: mechanisms and possible roles in animal/plant-microbe interactions. FEMS Microbiol Rev 2001; 26(1):17–47.
37. Van Deuren M et al. Update on meningococcal disease with emphasis on pathogenesis and clinical management. Clin Microbiol Rev 2000; 13(1):144–166.
38. Almeida-González L, Franco-Paredes C, Pérez LF, Santos-Preciado JI. Enfermedad por meningococo, *Neisseria meningitidis*: perspective epidemiológica, clínica y preventiva. Salud Publica Mex 2004; 46:438–450.
39. Van der Woude MW, Baumler AJ. Phase and antigenic variation in bacteria. Clin Microbiol Rev 2004; 17(3):581–611, doi: 10.1128/CMR.17.3.581–611.2004
40. Zaghaier SM et al. *Neisseria meningitides* Lipopolysaccharide structure-dependent activation of the macrophage CD14/Toll-like receptor 4 pathway. Infect Immun 2004; Jan:371–380.
41. Jennings MP et al. The genetic basis of the phase variation repertoire of lipopolysaccharide immunotypes in *Neisseria meningitides*. Microbiol 1999; 145:3013–3021.
42. Mayer H et al. Bacterial lipopolysaccharides. Pure Appl Chem 1989; 61(7):1271–1282.
43. Caroff M et al. Structural and functional analysis of bacterial lipopolysacharides. Microb Infect 2002; 4:915–926.
44. Kawahara K et al. Modification of the structure and activity of lipid A in Yersinia pestis lipopolysaccharide by growth temperature. Infect Immun 2002; Aug:4092–4098.
45. Darveau RP et al. *Porphyromonas gingivalis* lipopolysaccharide contains multiple lipid A species that functionally interact with both Toll-like receptors 2 and 4. Infect Immun 2004; 72:5041–5051.

46. Yoshimura A et al. Lipopolysaccharides from Periodontopathic Bacteria *Porphyromonas gingivalis* and *Capnocytophaga ochracea* Are Antagonists for Human Toll-Like Receptor 4 2002; 70(1):218–225, doi: 10.1128/IAI.70.1.218–225.2002.

47. Darveau RP et al. *Porphyromonas gingivalis* lipopolysaccharide contains multiple lipid a species that functionally interact with both toll-like receptors 2 and 4. Infect Immun 2004; 72(9):5041–5051, doi: 10.1128/IAI.72.9.5041–5051.2004.

48. Tanamoto K et al. The lipid A moiety of *Porphyromonas gingivalis* lipopolysaccharide specifically mediates the activation of C3H/HeJ mice. J Immun 158(9):4430–4436.

49. Miller SI. LPS, TLR4 and infectious disease diversity. Nat Rev 2005; 3:36–45.

50. Netea MG et al. Does the shape of lipid A determine the interaction f LPS with Toll-like receptors? Trends Immunol 2002; 23(3):135–139.

51. Royet J. Infectious non-self recognition in invertebrates: lessons from *Drosophila* and other insect models. Mol Immunol 2004; 41:1063–1075.

52. Inamori K et al. A Toll-like receptor in horseshoe crabs. Immunol Rev 2004; 198(1):106, doi:10.1111/j.0105–2896.2004.0131.x.

53. Ariki S et al. A serine protease zymogen functions as a pattern-recognition receptor for lipopolysaccharides. PNAS 2004; 101(4):953–958, doi:10.1073/pnas.0306904101.

54. Hubbard BK, Walsh CT. Vancomycin assembly: nature's way. Angew Chem Int Ed 2003; 42(7):731–765.

55. Hedges SB. The origin and evolution of model organisms. Nat Rev Genet 2002; 3:838–849.

56. Plested J S et al. Conservation and accessibility of an inner core lipopolysaccharide epitope of *neisseria meningitides*. Infect Immun 1999; 67(10):5417–5426.

57. Kumada H, Haishima Y, Umemoto T, Tanamoto KI. Structural study on the free lipid A isolated from lipopolysaccharide of *Porphyromonas gingivalis*. J Bacteriol 1995; 177:2098–2106.

Nonendotoxin Microbial Pyrogens: Lesser Endotoxins and Superantigens

Kevin L. Williams
Eli Lilly & Company, Indianapolis, Indiana, U.S.A.

Membranes have a jealous nature. Their function as a boundary in a given cell is to separate what is "mine" from what is "yours" in the single-celled organism and what is "ours" from what is "theirs" in the multicellular organism. What is truly amazing is the variety of microbial cellular envelope structures capable of eliciting a deleterious host response of some kind.

SIGNIFICANT NONENDOTOXIN MICROBIAL PYROGENS

Significant nonendotoxin microbial pyrogens include cellular wall/membrane components from both gram-negative and gram-positive bacteria, fungi, virus, mycobacteria, mycoplasma, and spirochetes, as well as exotoxins from *Staphylococcus* and *Streptococcus*, notably enterotoxins from *Staphylococcus aureus* and exotoxins from *Streptococcus pyogenes*. Significant microbial constituents capable of producing a host response that may include fever are listed in Table 1. The dose (or level of infection) is a determinant of both host activity and pyrogenicity, and the potency of various microbial components vary widely. The entire list of microbial cellular constituents capable of cytokine stimulation in host cells is very large and growing, and no attempt will be made to name or describe them all. Note that the term "pyrogen" is largely being superseded by terms more in keeping with advances in the understanding of host cell activation and inflammatory response at the cellular level. While "microbial pyrogen" describes a systemic response to levels of biologically active compounds capable of eliciting such a response, many host active compounds have the capability to be pyrogenic if their dose or level of infection is high enough (Chapter 13). Because it is not altogether common for some of the microbial products discussed in this chapter to reach such levels in humans, given the reasons discussed in Chapter 2 (i.e., growth requirements) except perhaps via infection, they are not historically considered pyrogens. Furthermore, for some the ability to activate macrophage to produce tumor necrosis factor (TNF)-α and other cytokines that are prerequisites to fever has only recently been determined. One must wonder if, in the future, the idea of pyrogenicity [based as it is more in history than in the severity of adverse effects it is intended to signify (1)] will not give way altogether to new tests capable of detecting a broader class of deleterious host modulins [to use the Henderson et al. term (2)].

Some low molecular weight proteins (20–30 kDa) have been grouped together as a class of potent T-cell activators called "superantigens" (SAg). The group of SAg includes not only gram-positive enterotoxins and exotoxins but also viral and mycoplasma products. The chemical structure, function, and effects of a diverse group of microbial cell wall constituents and SAg have been greatly expanded upon recently and many have come to be implicated as bringing about adverse endotoxin-like host effects. SAg occur in both cell-associated and

TABLE 1 Wide Range of Nonendotoxin Host Active Microbial Components

Mycobacteria (5–10)	Lipoarabinomannan present in *Mycobacterium leprae* and *M. tuberculosis*
Yeast/fungal (11,12)	Cellular surface components: α-(1,3) glucans and β-glucans
Spirochetes (13–15)	LPS and lipopeptides from *Treponema pallidum* (Syphilis) and *Borrelia burgdorferi* (tick-borne Lyme disease pathogen). *Borrelia spp.* causes relapsing fever. *Borrelia burgdorferi* DNA incorporated into the genome of arthritic mice points to the role of microbial by-products as agents of diseases not previously associated with microbial causes. Relman lists six additional microbial pathogens that have been identified using a genotypic approach including: *Helicobacter pylori* (peptic ulcer disease), Hepatitis C virus (non-A, non-B Hepatitis), *Bartinella henselae* (bacillary angiomatosis), *Trophreryma whippereli* (Whipple's disease), Sin Nombre virus (Hantavirus pulmonary syndrome), and Karposi's sarconoma associated herpes virus (Karposi sarcoma).
Rickettsia (16): GNB strict intracellular parasites passed from an arthropod vector to humans	Arthropod-borne rickettsial diseases include: Murine typhus (a milder form of typhus borne by rats and transmitted to humans by fleas), rocky mountain spotted fever (borne by ticks), Mediterranean spotted fever, and Siberian tick typhus. Typhus is carried by lice.
OMP (2, 17–20): OMPs bring about inflammatory cytokine synthesis	Mangan et al. demonstrated that lipid-associated proteins from *S. typhimurium* is three to four times more active in inducing IL-1 from monocytes than protein-free LPS
	Porins, present in virtually all gram-negative bacteria, contain a 1 nm pore to allow passage of molecules <600 Da
	Flagella of *Salmonella* have been shown to restore the TNF induction capacity upon addition of flagellin protein (FliC) to nonflagellated mutant Salmonella strains as well as *Escherichia coli.*
	Pili or fimbrial proteins contain a specific adhesin allowing bacterial attachment to host receptors and have been shown to be proinflammatory
	Variable major LP of *B. recurrentis*, which produces Louse-borne relapsing fever. Scragg et al. claim that "this is the only human infectious disease in which anti-TNF therapy has been conclusively demonstrated to have a beneficial role."
Glycosphingolipids (21)	From the LPS-free GNB *Sphingomonas paucimobilis* have been shown to occur as per an endotoxin-like mechanism involving CD14
Mycoplasma (22,23) Lipopeptides/LPs	Causative agents of inflammatory reactions to mycoplasmas are opportunistic pathogens associated with arthrits, AIDS, and atypical pneumonia
LP (24) from GNB membranes stimulate cytokine induction	Zhang et al. developed a "dot blot assay" (using a monoclonal antibody specific for LP) capable of detecting 100 ng/mL of LP (and not LPS). Using this assay, the authors estimated that *E. coli* K12 released 1 mg/mL after 4 hr culture compared with 5.7 mg/mL LPS as measured by LAL

(Continued)

TABLE 1 Wide Range of Nonendotoxin Host Active Microbial Components (*Continued*)

Chlorella-like green algae (25)	Suspect LPS from an algae
PG[a] and LTA (26–28): induce cytokine production, arachidonic acid metabolism in monocytes, muted reaction with LAL	Renzi and Lee found that purified LTA from *S. aureus* was most LAL reactive yet still fell 1500 & multi below LPS for LAL activity. LTA was 1500 to 870,000 × less potent than LPS (via LAL). Renzi and Lee found that LTA was 1500 to 870,000 × less LAL reactive than *Salmonella* LPS with *S. aureus* being most reactive followed by *Step. Sanguis, Strep. yogenes, Strep. faecalis, Strep. mutans*, and *Bacillus subtilis*. LTA stimulation of blood monocytes to secrete TNF-α was only minimally active at 10 mg/mL versus 0.1 ng/mL for LPS. Wildfeuer et al determined that PG was 100,000 to 400,000 × less LAL reactive than *E. coli* LPS

[a]And its subunits mucopeptide, murein, glycopeptide, or glycosaminopeptide.
Abbreviations: GNB, gram-negative bacteria; LAL, *Limulus* amebocyte lysate; LP, lipoprotein; LPS, lipopolysaccharide; LTA, lipoteichoic acid; OMP, outer memberane proteins; PG, peptidoglycan; TNF, tumor necrosis factor.

secreted forms (3). Chapter 2 purports that microbial pyrogens that are not endotoxin are not significant to modern pharmaceutical contamination control mostly due to the low likelihood of occurrence in such an environment, excluding that of the cell culture-derived products. Nevertheless, as significant pyrogens (and/or host defense system activators) arising from infection, the presence of non-gram-negative pathogens and nonlipopolysaccharide (LPS) by-products should be considered. Significant pathogens that are not noted for pyrogenicity (or host defense activation by mechanisms that may include pyrogenicity) will not be considered (i.e., neurotoxins: botulism, tetanus, anthrax, diptheria, and pore forming toxins). Capsular polysaccharides generated by gram-positive and gram-negative organisms have been shown to be vital to bacterial pathogenicity, but the capsular material has not in itself been found to be proinflammatory or pyrogenic, and will be only briefly mentioned here (4). See Figure 1 for a summary of the relative biological activity of nonendotoxin components and a notation on the type of mechanism employed (i.e., like or not like endotoxin).

MICROBIAL CELL WALLS AND MEMBRANES

Membranes have a jealous nature. Their function as a boundary in a given cell is to separate what is "mine" from what is "yours" in the single-celled organism and what is "ours" from what is "theirs" in the multicellular organism. What is truly amazing is the variety of microbial cellular envelope structures capable of eliciting a deleterious host response of some kind. Many mimic aspects of LPS in their bioactivity, although often via a different mechanism and, except in a few cases, in a more muted manner. Given the long list of such cellular components, one is tempted to generalize that microbial cellular surface constituents are all culprits in activating host defenses and this generalization makes a strong argument for ideally excluding all cellular residues from parenteral products. Common sense dictates that cellular residues are by nature contaminants and the body recognizes them as such. Consider the list of non-gram-negative and uncommon gram-negative bioactive cellular surface-associated substances found in bacteria and nonbacterial microbes in Table 1. The fact that most non-LPS products have only very recently been

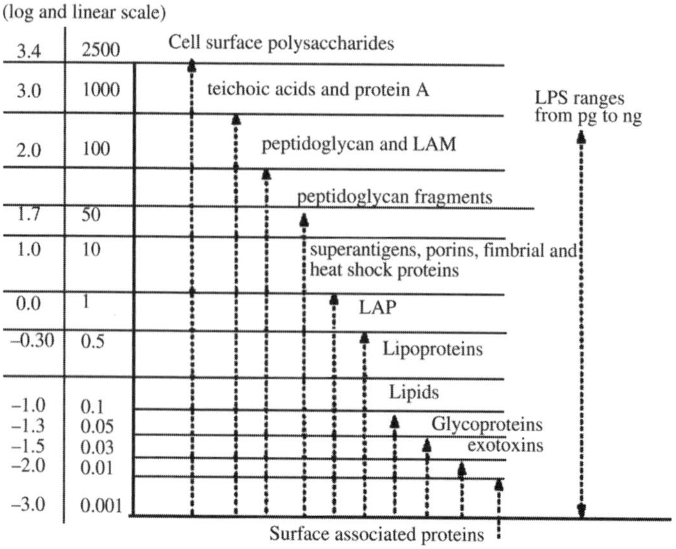

(log and linear scale)

FIGURE 1 The relative biological activity of cytokine-inducing microbial components compared with lipopolysaccharide. *Abbreviations*: LAM, lipoarabinomannan; LAP, lipid-associated proteins; LPS, lipopolysaccharide.

identified as macrophage activators and that many are associated with devastating diseases supports the underlying theme of this chapter in that there is a wide variety of potential modulators of adverse host effects (including fever) that are not endotoxin, but that may proceed by endotoxin-like mechanisms and with endotoxin-like potencies when presented by infecting organisms (not from a parenteral manufacturing perspective).

A relevant note concerning the lack of attention given to nonendotoxin cellular components in pareneteral manufacturing is the degree of difficulty researchers often encounter in obtaining the materials in a pure state devoid of endotoxin. The presence of endotoxin overrides many efforts to study nonendotoxin components due to its potency and can affect research study end points at almost undetectable background levels (fg/mL) as compared with the levels necessarily used in the study of non-LPS substances (typically in μg–mg/mL).

PEPTIDOGLYCAN AND LIPOTEICHOIC ACID

Peptidoglycan (PG) and lipoteichoic acid (LTA) are the two major cellular wall constituents of gram-positive bacteria and comprise the major inflammatory inducing components of gram-positive cellular walls (29). Like endotoxin, these cellular constituents may induce cytokine production, arachidonic acid metabolism in monocytes, and some can even react with LAL in a muted manner[a] (30). Renzi

---

[a]Baek et al. cite that "positive LAL tests have been reported with lipoteichoic acid from *Streptococcus faecalis*, lipoglycans from different strains of mycoplasma, cell wall fractions from *Micropolyspora faeni* and *Chlamydia psittaci*, hot phenol–water extracts of *Listeria monocytogenes*, and pure preparations of *Plasmodium berghei*."

and Lee (26) found that purified LTA from *S. aureus* was most LAL reactive yet still fell 1500-fold below the LAL activity of LPS. PG is a heteropolymer formed from β-1,4 linked N-acetylmuramic acid and N-acetyl-D-glucosamine residues cross-linked by peptide bridges. The glycan backbone does not vary, whereas the cross-linking peptides linking the sugars vary. PG is a constituent of all bacteria except mycoplasmas and some halophilic arachaebacteria, and contains unique molecules not found in eukaryotic organisms including N-acetylmuramic acid and D-amino acids. Gram-negative bacteria also contain PG, although in much lesser amounts. According to Dijkstra and Keck (31), "the multilayered peptidogly-can of gram-positive bacteria is located on the outside of the cell and can be up to 10 times as thick as the peptidoglycan of gram-negative bacteria, which is located in the periplasm." It is said to have the properties of a "viscous gel" (32). The PG composition is known completely for many gram-negative organisms and some gram-positives, notably *S. aureus* and *S. pneumoniae* (33). The smallest polymeric subunit of PG retaining its host response induction capacity was initially believed to be N-acetylmuramyl-L-alanyl-D-isoglutamine, but now over 300 synthetic glycopeptides have been synthesized that have macrophage activation and/or immunomodula-tion capabilities (34). See Figure 2 for the general structure of PG as compared with the structure of LPS.

Teichoic acids are polyglycerol or polyribitol phosphates occurring only in the "glycopeptide network" of gram-positve bacteria (33). Each type of gram-positive bacteria contains a variety of glycoproteins in the cellular wall that, much in the manner of LPS, may be shed into the environment, especially during cell lysis. The host cell response is determined by the types of glycopeptides pre-sented by invading microbes.

Though PG is usually described only in association with gram-positive infec-tion, recently PG has been found to be released into hosts during infection along with a number of gram-negative components.

1. In a manner analogous to that of endotoxin, PG is released by gram-positive bacteria during infection and can reach the systemic circulation (33).
2. Muramic acid has been used as a sensitive marker for GC-MS detection of gram-positive cellular residues in clinical specimens (septic synovial fluids) at levels of >30 ng/mL (35).
3. The release of PG and LTA has been shown to be induced and enhanced by β-lactam antibiotics from *S. aureus* (4–9-fold and 60–85-fold, respectively) (36).
4. Potency increases when acting in synergy with other bacterial components including LTA (37,38) and endotoxin (39).

Sensitive methods of quantifying PG and its subunits in a clinical setting have yet to be developed [or at least widely accepted as the silkworm larvae plasma (SLP) method discussed in Chapter 16 is a sensitive detection method for PG], leaving the levels associated with gram-positive sepsis largely unknown.

PYROGENIC EXOTOXINS AND SUPERANTIGENS

Pyrogenic exotoxins of group A streptococci [streptococcal pyrogenic exotoxin (SPE)] and enterotoxins of *S. aureus* [*Staphylococcus* enterotoxin (SE)] comprise a group of structurally and functionally related toxins that activate T-cells by a unique mechanism (40,41). The SEs are known to cause staphylococcal food

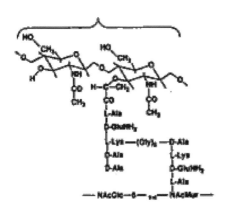

Peptidoglycan

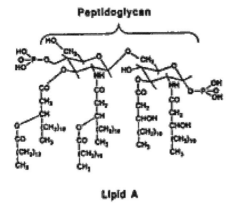

Lipid A

FIGURE 2 Chemical structures of *S. aureus* peptidoglycan (PG) and enterobacteriaceae lipid A. Similar structures in PG and lipid A are indicated by brackets. *Source*: From Ref. 29.

poisoning (enterotoxins) and toxic shock-like syndrome. The streptococcal exotoxins cause the syndrome of scarlet fever and toxic shock-like syndrome as well. These proteins are close in size and homology at approximately 230 amino acids long [toxic shock syndrome toxin-1 (TSST-1) is 194] and are highly heat and protease resistant and, therefore, (in the case of food poisoning) are capable of inducing diarrhea and vomiting via the release of histamines from gut-associated mast cells and may also release inflammatory mediators (cytokines) (42). The pyrogenic exotoxic SAg also elicit strong inflammatory cytokine host responses and enhance susceptibility to endotoxin shock (42).

According to Kotb (3), most of the "secreted pyrogenic superantigens are globular proteins that range from 20 to 30 kDa in size and, with few exceptions, many have obvious sequence homology." Though the pyrogenic exotoxic SAg differ widely from SAg arising from non-*Staphylococcus* sources, (mouse mammary tumor virus, *Mycoplasm arthriditis*, streptococcal M proteins), nevertheless, they apparently share some specific regions of sequence homology. A given structural feature predictive of superantigenicity has not been identified, but it has been postulated that SAg may share conformational features, allowing them to interact broadly with T-cell receptors (TLRs) and major histocompatibility complex (MHC)-II molecules (3). Here is an apparent commonality between SAg and LPS, that is, specific conformational requirements to fit (a) specific receptor(s).

Such biochemical conformations separate toxic LPS from nontoxic forms and common exotoxins from SAg.

Both *Staphylococcus* (staph TSS) and *Streptococcus* (strep TSS) derived TSSs have been identified. staph TSS manifests itself in high fever, rash, hypotension, and potentially multiple organ failure. Most menstrual Staph TSS illness is associated with strains of *S. aureus* that produce the superantigen TSST-1. The term "toxic shock syndrome" was coined and considered a specific affliction in 1978, when it was associated with high absorbency tampons, but today only about half of the staph TSS incidents are said to be menstrually related (43).

Strep TSS and invasive group A streptococcal infections are more often associated with disseminated infections, severe pain, invasion of tissues, and bacteremia (as opposed to dissemination of the exotoxin alone as in staph TSS). The speed and severity of certain streptococcal group A infections has lead to their recent description as "flesh-eating bacteria" (40).

The minority of gram-positive bacteria that do produce exotoxins can be exceedingly pyrogenic, including those arising from *S. aureus* (enterotoxins) and *S. pyogenes* (exotoxins). The Staph enterotoxins derive their name from their association with gastrointestinal illness (42). The toxins are low molecular weight (20–30 kDa) proteins and include TSST-1 and SPE-A, SPE-B, and SPE-C (43). SPE-A and SPE-C have been implicated in streptococcal TSS (44). Some of the toxins are structurally related and have been called "SAg" due to their potent and indiscriminant activation of T-cells, which in turn results in the massive release of cytokines and consequent disease pathology, such as TSS. SAg also originate in microbes other than *Staphylococcus* and *Streptococcus*, including *Mycoplasma* species, *Pseudomonas aeruginosa*, *Yersinia pseudotuberculosis* and *Y. enterocolitica* (45), and *Clostridium perfringens* (3). Certain viruses [Rabies, EBV, MMTV, CMV (46)] and *Mycoplasma* lipoproteins (22) have also been classified as SAg also that are structurally different from the *Staphylococcus* and *Streptococcus* exotoxins. Ulrich (47) states that the SAgs of *S. aureus* and group A Strep have common genetic origins, and also underscores the "mobile nature of their (SAgs) genetic elements."

The unique property of SAgs is their ability to interact with a large number of T-cells that share specific sequences within the variable region of the T-cell receptor (TCR). Normal antigens bind only a small number of T-cells and do not recognize the specific-like sequences (invariant regions) in the otherwise variable region. See Figure 3 for a diagram of proposed SAg structure and function. By their indiscriminant attachment mechanism, SAgs connect antigen-presenting cells (APC) and T-cells, thereby escaping the need to be processed by APC, a rate-limiting step in antigen processing (43). Conventional antigens are processed into small peptides in lysosomal compartments of APCs where they complex with MHC molecules. This results in the aberrant proliferation of T-cells with specific ($V\beta$) subsets (42). In contrast to normal antigens in which binding to MHC is determined by five variable regions of TCR: $V\beta$, $D\beta$, $J\beta$, $V\alpha$, and $J\alpha$, the interaction of SAg is dictated primarily by the $V\beta$ area. Therefore, the contrast in ability to combine with MHC (APC) and TCR is stark (3).

1. Antigens: one cell in 104 to 106 T-cells (0.0001–0.000001%).
2. SAg interact with 5% to 20% of T-cells.

The end result of SAg host interaction is the stimulation of large numbers of T-cells, which in turn trigger the initiation of defensive cellular events including cytokine gene expression. It is relevant to remember the different general routes

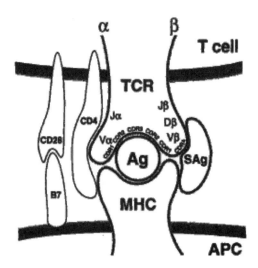

FIGURE 3 Bridging of T-cells and antigen-presenting cells: a schematic model of superantigen (SAg) interaction with T-cell receptor and class II molecules. Ag is the normal antigen-binding site whereas SAg is the superantigen-binding site on the variable region that this particular SAg is specific for. *Abbreviations*: Ag, antigen; APC, antigen-presenting cells; MHC, major histocompatibility complex; SAg, superantigen. TCR, T-cell receptor; *Source*: From Ref. 3.

of invasion associated with gram-positive versus gram-negative organisms. As noted by Sriskandan and Cohen (28), gram-negatives typically arise from within (i.e., via parenteral, gastrointestinal, humoral, urologic entry) whereas gram-positives typically arise from without (i.e., via invasive medical procedures such as catheters, intravenous tubes, food borne, etc.), and often from a locus of infection (skin, wound, muscle injury). Gram-positive organisms more often have large anti-phagocytic capsules that are not susceptible to the lytic action of complement. In host systems, they may multiply rapidly and cause bacteremia if they do gain entry systemically.

Kotb (3) lists three criteria of a protein to be designated as SAg:

1. Reproducible pattern of selective $V\beta$ interaction (i.e., it interacts with a $V\beta$ region common to a subpopulation of T-cells)
2. Dependence of the response on APC that express class II molecules
3. Ability to bypass APC complex processing

In addition to $V\beta$ interaction, exotoxic pyrogenic SAg also induce inflammatory cytokine production and enhanced susceptibility to endotoxin shock. Although there are structural similarities among many SAg, there has not been a specific structure identified as a predictor of superantigenicity.

The pathogenisis of SAg, as in the case of endotoxin, is mediated by the body's aberrant immune response. Diseases known to be caused by SAg include food poisoning, menstrual and nonmenstrual, staph TSS and strep TSS. Suspect but not proven diseases associated with SAg include a host of diseases including Lyme disease, Kawasaki disease, rheumatoid arthritis, and multiple sclerosis (3). See Tables 2 and 3 for known and suspected human diseases associated with SAg. Most recently, SAg have been associated with a number of autoimmune disorders

TABLE 2 Known and Suspected Human Diseases Associated with Superantigens

Disease	Superantigen[a]
Acute diseases	
Food poisoning	SEs
Staph TSS	
Menstrual	TSST-1
Nonmenstrual	SEB, SEC, TSST-1
Strep TSS	SPEs
Sudden infant death syndrome	SEs?, SPEs?
Autoimmune diseases	
Rheumatic fever, rheumatic heart disease	M proteins, SPE's?
Kawasaki disease	TSST-1?, SPE's?
Lyme disease	*Borrelia burgdorferi* SAg?
Rheumatoid arthritis	SAg?, MAM?
Multiple sclerosis	SAg?
Sjogren's syndrome	SAg?
Autoimmune thyroiditis	SAg?
AIDS	HIV SAg?
Silicone-induced autoimmunity	SAg?
Lymphoproliferative diseases	EBV SAg?

[a]A question mark indicates a highly suspected but not yet proven role of superantigen in disease.
Abbreviations: EBV, Epstein-Barr virus; HIV, human immunodeficiency virus; MAM, M. arthriditis mitogen; SAg, superantigen; SE, *Staphylococcus* enterotoxin; SPE, Streptococcal pyrogenic exotoxin; TSST-1, toxic shock syndrome toxin-1.
Source: From Ref. 3.

including rheumatic heart disease, rheumatoid arthritis, multiple sclerosis, and Graves' disease, and have even been implicated in sudden death syndrome (48). In the latter case, it has been hypothesized that pyrogenic exotoxins may induce cytokines that induce sleep and the associated failure of proper breathing.

SAg are potent inducers of inflammatory cytokines and it is this phenomenon that is believed to be responsible for the group's capability to induce shock. Though the end result of cytokine production is similar to the action of endotoxin (albeit via a different mechanism), the specific cytokine profile (the kinds and amounts) has been shown to differ when endotoxin and SAg are compared. This fact has led to the study of the relative cytokine profiles produced by different initiators as a means of distinguishing gram-positive and gram-negative sepsis (49). As with endotoxin, there appears to be a strong host state factor associated with superantigen susceptibility, as identical SAg recovered from different patients have been associated with widely varying disease states (3). SAg also have been shown to synergize with endotoxin to form "lytic complexes" lethal to immune cells (50), and to augment the release of cytokines and thereby exacerbate endotoxic shock (51).

CONVERGENCE OF PYROGENIC MECHANISMS

There is some convergence in the understanding of host mediator activation that includes microbial cell envelope components including LPS, PG, secreted toxins (including the streptococcal pyrogenic exotoxins), and enterotoxins (*Staphylococcus*). The modes of activation of host defenses overlap in some cases. Although endotoxin is the most potent in its activity (i.e., active at the lowest concentrations), it

TABLE 3 Known and Suspected Human Diseases Caused by Superantigens

Superantigens and pyrogenic exotoxins	Food-borne	Non-staph and Non-strep SAg	Emerging pathogens
Staphylococcus: TSS[a] (SAg: TSST-1) SSSS[b] (Exfoliative toxins)	*Clostridium perfringens*	Mycoplasma lipopeptides and lipoproteins	Spirochetes[f] Rickettsia[f]
Staphylococcus enterotoxins[c] *Staphylococcus aureus*	and	*Gram-negative SAg*: Pseudomonas aeruginosa	
Streptococcus: TSS[a] invasive group A[d] Scarlet-fever	Staphylococcus enterotoxins[c]: *Staphylococcus aureus*	Yersinia *pseudotuberculosis/ enterocolitica* α-1,3 and β-1,3 glucans[e]: *Histoplasma capsulatum*	Neonatal associated Staphylococcus and Sterptococcus diseases: SSSS[b] (Staph) GBS[g] (Strep)
		Viruses: Rabies, EBV, MMTV, CMV	

[a]Toxic shock syndrome.
[b]Staphylococcus scalded skin syndrome.
[c]Associated with food-borne illness.
[d]"Flesh-eating bacteria."
[e]Virulence factor in pathogenic yeast.
[f]Many tick-borne pathogens/pyrogens.
[g]Group B streptococcus.

is not alone in its mode of action or in its resulting effects, including mediator activation ending in TNF (and other cytokine) production and complement activation at higher doses (or levels of infection).

An increase in antibiotic-resistant gram-positve infections such as vancomycin-resistant enterococci and methicilin-resistant Staphylococci combined with the increasing use of invasive procedures, as discussed in Chapter 4, have lead to an increased frequency of sepsis due to gram-positive bacteria. The relative incidence of the two different types of septicemia is now thought to be roughly 50/50 (2). Gram-positive bacteria and many of their by-products can induce a similar proinflammatory cascade of events as gram-negative bacterial LPS. The PG and LPS pathways of activation have been found to share a common macrophage receptor (CD14), and are believed to be capable of synergistic activity. Some researchers have proposed a "two-hit" theory of sepsis, which involves a cycle of gram-negative infection with subsequent septic shock, particle recovery, gram-positive insult, and intractable septic shock followed by death (42).

Some molecules on the membranes of host white blood cells have the assignment of receiving or detecting specific molecules in the environment, and eliciting a specific and appropriate response from the inner cell. This is known as a "transmembrane signal event." CD14 is one such molecule present on the cell and also in soluble form (sCD14) that responds to LPS and has been identified as also binding to PG, MDP (synthetic PG fragments), LTAs, and the disaccharide GlcNAc-MDP (34). Various microbial polysaccharides from a diverse sampling of flora have been shown to elicit deleterious host effects mimicking those of endotoxin and sometimes approaching the potency of endotoxin.

Only recently has it been determined the degree to which non-LPS cell constituents and products produce many of the effects previously ascribed only to endotoxin. Non-LPS constituents are routinely compared with LPS in their mode of action (like or unlike) and potency (Fig. 1). Gram-positive cell walls and SAg have been shown to activate white blood cells to produce cytokines, thereby resembling the method by which endotoxin is known to work. Some similarities as well as dissimilarities include the following:

Similarities

1. Inducement of many of the same inflammatory mediators (TNF, IL-1β, IL-6, IL-8, IL-12, arachidonate metabolites, etc.) by LPS, PG, and some SAg (52).
2. Irrespective of the receptor used to activate the mediator transcription cascade by endotoxin, gram-positive cell walls, or superantigen (TSST-1), each has been shown to bring about the production of the nuclear transcription factor NF-κB as a result of a transmembrane signal event.
3. Cell activation via CD14 receptor is common to LPS and PG (but not to SAg) in similar but not identical regions of the receptor (53,54).

Dissimilarities

1. SAg predominately activate T-cells, whereas LPS and PG activate monocytes/macrophages.
2. PG and LPS activate host defenses by binding CD14 (and other) receptors, whereas SAg link major histocompatability II proteins [on APC (including macrophages)] to T-lymphocytes.
3. Profiles may differ in endotoxin versus superantigen T-cell-derived cytokines (i.e., different specific cytokines are produced in response to SAg and LPS). Some have proposed that this may prove helpful in distinguishing between gram-positive and gram-negative sepsis (52).

At least in part, a nexus in the convergence of microbial host recognition appears to be the LPS receptor CD14. Due to its wide-ranging recognition spectrum, CD14 is said to be a "pattern recognition" protein (55). Alternatively, CD14 has been proposed to recognize microbial antigens indiscriminately (as opposed to broadly but selectively). In addition to acting as a bound receptor, CD14 is also expressed as a soluble protein (sCD14) in serum (2). According to Ingalls et al. (55), "... CD14 also binds to several other microbial products, including, mycobacterial lipoarabinomannan (LAM), peptidoglycan, other cellular wall components of *Staphylococcus aureus, Streptococcus* rhamnose glucose polymers, mannuronic acid polymers, and Yeast WI-1 antigen. It is not clear, however, how these diverse bacterial products generate intracellular signals through CD14."

Dziarski (34) demonstrated the subtle though potentially significant differences in CD14 binding involving PG and LPS, and described the importance of the convergence of various mechanisms as related to devising treatments: "The concept of receptor agonists and antagonists is well-established in pharmacology and it may also prove clinically useful in regard to LPS and PG, if effective and nontoxic antagonists of LPS and PG can be found. This would be of great significance because a single compound could block or diminish the toxic effects associated with infections by both gram-positive and gram-negative bacteria." LPS antagonists have thus far had the unfortunate side effect of high associated toxicity.

ADVENTITIOUS ORGANISMS AND BIOTECHNOLOGY

Modern methods of biotechnology-based manufacturing often utilize cell culture media in the manufacture of drug products or reagents to be used in drug products. Cell cultures are necessary to grow the eukaryotic cells necessary to process today's more complex biological molecules. Given the greater associated nutritional requirements and fragility of the resultant products, precautions are required to ensure that mycoplasmas and other potential contaminants (such as exotoxins or viruses) are excluded and that such adventitious[b] contamination cannot affect either the product or the expression system used to manufacture it. Major components of the outer cellular walls of many different kinds of microscopic organisms (even intracellular parasites such as mycoplasmas that have no cell walls) not likely to be found in traditional pharmaceutical manufacturing can produce pyrogenic responses and thus can be a concern in such a manufacturing environment. Many have been shown to produce pyrogenic or other host active responses and (like endotoxin) may be capable of surviving such manufacturing processes should they occur as contaminants. A casual reading of the different components shown to be bioactive in higher organisms reinforces the idea of a constant tension between the higher and lower life forms.

Yeast and Fungi

Yeast and fungi may contain α-1,3 and β-1,3 glucans in their outer cellular walls. Glucan has been proposed as a virulence factor in pathogenic yeast (*Histoplasma capsulatum*) since most avirulent strains have 1000 times less α-1,3 glucan in their cell walls (56). Glucans form larger sugar polymers, but in solution they may form disaccharides. Disaccharides have also been found in LAL reactive material (LAL-RM) (cellobiose from cellulose-based hemodialyzers that are disaccharides covalently bound through β(1–4) linkages (57). Additionally, the aggregate size has also been shown to be critical to the biological effects elicited. The LAL activity of glucans correlates to the molecular weight of the polymer. Moderate chain glucans mimic endotoxin in the LAL reaction (actually proceeding by an alternate pathway), whereas longer or shorter chains of the polysaccharide do not react with LAL (11).

In some cases, virulence has been found to be inversely related to β-glucan content in yeasts (58). Silva and Fazioli (59) made intraperitoneal injections into mice that contained β-glucan, which resulted in their deaths. Peritonitis and inflammatory exudate was found upon autopsy. β-glucans have demanded considerable attention from pharmaceutical manufacturers and the FDA due to their ability to react with LAL, which was previously thought to be an activity specific to endotoxin. While not considered pyrogenic, β-glucans have been found to be LAL reactive and to induce a number of host responses reminiscent of endotoxin and

---

[b]*adventitious* (adj.) (1) Added from another source and not inherent or innate, (2) arising or occurring sporadically or in other than the usual location. (*Source*: Webster 9th Collegiate Dictionary)

gram-positive cellular components. The presence of glucans in some parenteral products has been widely discussed, but has not been found to be a widespread occurrence. What has occurred is the isolation of cellobiose (generally referred to as LAL-RM) from cellulose-based hemodialyzer rinses (57). β-glucans are apyrogenic (do not bring about temperature rises in the rabbit pyrogen test even at doses 2000 times above endotoxin threshold levels). Glucans and the alternate pathway of LAL activation will be discussed with the conventional LAL endotoxin reaction in Chapter 10.

As a major polysaccharide derived from microbial cellular walls, glucan can be expected to be bioactive in mammalian hosts and in fact has been shown to cause immunomodulatory responses in a number of cases including:

1. Interaction with macrophages through β-glucan receptors, resulting in the release of TNF-α (11);
2. Maximal TNF-α release from alveolar macrophages stimulated with fungal β-glucans was obtained at moderate concentrations of 100 to 200 μg/mL, whereas higher concentrations >500 μg/mL were inhibitory for TNF-α production [compare this with pg–ng/mL activities obtained with LPS (60)];
3. Injection of β-glucan gives a dose response curve of TNF induction (58).

Therefore, while glucans are not considered pyrogenic, they have been found to promote cytokine production and arachiodonic acid liberation, precursors to fever, the historical symptom of microbial contamination being guarded against in pyrogen testing. On the other hand, though cellulosic glucans have been associated with some ill effects when present in long-term hemodialysis equipment (61,62), others have found that they may actually have anti-LPS modulation capabilities (63).

According to Cooper et al. (57), the glucan substances that have been associated with alternate pathway activity to date are: zymosan from a yeast, laminarin from an algae, lentinan from a fungus, and curdlan from a bacterium. Each of these β-glucans contains (1–3)-β-D-glycosidic linkages and some (1–4) and (1–6) side linkages. Interestingly, the alternate (G factor) pathway may be blocked by solutions of low molecular weight glucans that competitively block the LAL alternate pathway as larger MW structures are needed to activate the reaction. This fact has proved useful to LAL manufacturers in preparing solutions to be used by pharmaceutical manufacturers in parenteral testing for use with products and in-process testing that require it. Solutions of laminarin from *Laminarin digitata* (>1 μg/mL) and Curdlan from *Alcaligenes faecalis* are used in pharmaceutical quality control testing to block the alternate pathway (as necessary) (64). Pearson et al. (65) used cellulase to demonstrate the cellulobiose nature of LAL-RM from hemodialyzers that utilizes β(1–4) glucan linkages. The LAL reactivity of human plasma has been found to be due to the alternate pathway reaction (54). Differing manufacturing processes used by LAL manufacturers has led to a number of reagents that differ in their LAL-RM reactivity. Some are unreactive while most remain able to detect both endotoxin and LAL-RM. Initially, the unreactive LAL was believed to be an artifact of chloroform extraction, but is now believed to be attributed to the addition of zwittergent. Zwittergent is a sufobetaine amphoteric surfactant that is added to this formulation to increase sensitivity to endotoxin acts to reduce the sensitivity of LAL to glucans (66).

The yeast *Cryptococcus neoformans* has long been known to produce a capsular polysaccharide with proinflammatory characteristics. Retini et al. (67) showed that the degree of cytokine release was a function of the yeast capsule size as well as facilitated by a suspected soluble mediator. The major capsular polysaccharide in *C. neoformans* has been identified as glucuronoxylomannan, which has been found to inhibit leukocyte migration to sites infected. Thus, *Cryptococcus neoformans*, an encapsulated yeast, is capable of causing deadly meningitis in immunocompromised patients (68).

Mycobacteria

Mycobacteria have historically been considered to cause some of the most devastating of human diseases. *Mycobacterium tuberculosis* is the causative agent of pulmonary tuberculosis in humans and produces several substances that have been shown to be significant pyrogens. *M. leprae* is another infamous member of the genus. More recently, the acquired immune deficiency syndrome (AIDS) epidemic has brought about the emergence of another Mycobacterium of clinical significance: *M. avium* (69). Mycobacteria are lipid-rich (up to 60% of the dry weight of the cell) and a host of lipids, glycolipids, and lipoproteins have been isolated from mycobacterial cell walls, including the unique acid: mycolic acid (3). LAM has been widely studied due to its immunoregulatory and anti-inflammatory effects as well as macrophage activation and subsequent significant release of TNF-α at low levels (100 ng/mL). Furthermore, suggesting an LPS-like mode of action, polymixin B (a well-known LPS binding molecule) and anti-CD14 antibodies (again, an LPS receptor) have been shown to bind to and inactivate LAM as well (3). *M. tuberculosis* is notable for its use by Koch in the formulation of his postulates of disease causation in that he visualized the organism in diseased tissue, grew it in culture, and reproduced it in animals (70).

Mycoplasmas

Mycoplasmas are the smallest of all self-replicating cells. They contain no cell walls and have been associated with a number of diseases (mainly involving mucosal surfaces of respiratory, urogenital tracts, and joints) including atypical pneumonia, nongonococcal urethritis, arthritis, and AIDS (71). They have been shown to contain numerous lipopeptides and lipoproteins in their cellular membrane that are potent macrophage stimulators. Muhlradt et al. (22) propose that macrophage-activating lipopeptide-2 "may be one of the most potent natural macrophage stimulators besides endotoxin." The entire genomes have recently been sequenced for a couple of species (*Mycoplasma genitalium* and *M. pneumoniae*), notable as the smallest of self-replicating organisms.

Mycoplasmas have been found to be a significant source of contamination in cell cultures. Estimates of contamination by mycoplasma testing are used to monitor aspects of drug-manufacturing processes that employ the use of cell cultures (72,73). Many mycoplasmas produce a potent class of immune stimulators called mitogens (some of which carry more than one kind of mitogen and SAg as well). In host systems, mitogens are able to activate lymphocytes in a nonspecific polyclonal manner and cause excess cytokine production. Mycoplasmas rival endotoxin in that they possess potent (*i*) mitogenic, (*ii*) superantigenic activities, and (*iii*) their by-products are very heat-resistant.

Virus as Pyrogen

Viruses are probably responsible for more pyrogenic episodes in humans than any other single disease agent. These diminutive pathogens are protein-covered nucleic acid particles ranging between 20 and 350 nm. Two major groups of viruses exist: those composed of only deoxyribonucleic acid (DNA) and those composed of only ribonucleic acid (RNA). These groups are simply called DNA or RNA viruses; for example, influenza virus is an RNA virus and herpes is a DNA virus.

Fever is one of the most notable clinical signs of the common cold, a rhino-virus infection. Although these infections are local, they elicit a systemic response as evidenced by the induction of fever. Some systemic viral infections, such as Coxsakie and ECHO, cause only fever. Though many viral infections are self-limiting, they can sometimes result in dangerous secondary bacterial infections. According to Pollard et al. (74), infections associated with common chickenpox (varicella zoster viral infection) are increasing, including serious septic disease associated with *Streptococcus* (group A) and *Staphylococcus* toxic shock.

Several uncommon febrile illnesses have been recently associated with new viral diseases such as hantavirus pulmonary syndrome (13). Fredricks and Relman describe the fascinating microbial detective work via the use of PCR-based assays, thus allowing parallels to be drawn between the genetic sequences found in infected host tissues and suspected pathogens, particularly intracellular pathogens such as mycoplasma, rickettsia, and viral infections. The authors cite the detection of genetic sequences from *M. paratuberculosis* in 72% of Crohn's disease patients compared with 29% of other gastrointestinal disease patients, and wonder if the finding points to causation or opportunistic infection. Other examples include "a number of infectious diseases ... associated with dormant or latent organisms," including chronic Lyme arthritis, virus-associated cancers (70), and polycystic kidney disease (PKD), (previously thought to be purely heredi-tary) (75). The LAL assay ("differential activation protocol") was used on fluids derived from PKD infected human kidney cysts to reveal both endotoxins and fungal $(1-3)$-β-D glucans. Miller-Hjelle et al. (75) speculate that PKD may be a "genetic disease promoted by microbial influences" and state that "the ubiquitous and highly potent bacterial endotoxin is again one of the usual suspects examined as the provocateur of disease...."

Viral infections have been found to result in effects both reminiscent of and contrary to those of endotoxin (proinflammatory), and some have labeled common cold infections as basically a "cytokine disease" (76). Common viral infec-tions by rhinovirus can result in anti-inflammatory cytokine production (IL-10) that contrasts with the proinflammatory cytokines known to be produced in the nasal mucosa. TNF-α inhibition has been shown to mitigate most of the effect of infection involving members of the flavivirus group that includes dengue and yellow fever (77).

TRADITIONAL VERSUS BIOLOGICS MANUFACTURE

Why are traditional, as opposed to biologics, pharmaceutical manufacturers not more concerned with virus contamination in drug products? The most obvious reason is that the growth requirements for viable viral particles are even more strin-gent than those of bacteria in that they require a living host to reproduce. Only viable virions have been shown to induce fever via infection. Given the aseptic con-ditions associated with pharmaceutical manufacturing, the necessity of removing any living organisms prior to contact with the aseptic environment precludes the concern for viral contamination. However, the use of tissue culture growth media in the production of biologicals[c] from living organisms such as bacteria (e.g., *E. coli*), yeast (e.g., *Saccharomyces cervisiae*), or mammalian[d] cells (e.g., Chinese hamster ovary) bring with them the requirements for adventitious organism testing including virus and mycoplasmas. Indeed, viral contamination of several early biological products resulted in fatalities including (78):

1. Yellow fever vaccine contaminated with avian leucosis virus in the 1940s;
2. SV40 virus and inactivated polio virus in polio vaccine in the 1950s;
3. Creutzfeldt Jakob agent in human growth hormone in the 1980s (a prion, not a virus).

Relevant to a discussion of nonendotoxin microbial contaminants is the use of monoclonal antibodies (mAb) in the manufacture of drug substances and products. The Food and Drug Administration's (FDA) draft guidance on "Monoclonal Antibodies Used as Reagents in Drug Manufacturing" (72) addresses the overriding concerns:

> The predominant concern with the use of a mAb in drug substance and drug product manufacture is the introduction of contaminants and adventitious agents (e.g., bacteria, fungi, viruses, mycoplasma, protein contaminants) that are not removed by the manufacturing steps subsequent to the introduction of the mAb reagent in the process stream. These subsequent steps may vary widely depending on the manufacturing processes ... They may range from those which involve direct final drug formulation and filling without much processing to those that may include extensive processing steps ... that are likely to remove and/or inactive potential microbial contaminants introduced by the mAb reagents... In addition, the type of the manufacturing facility (e.g., biological versus pharmaceutical) where the mAb reagents are used should be considered and evaluated for the possibility of cross-contamination with adventitious agents which may be in the cell lines and reagents. Consequently, appropriate biological safety characterization for individual mAb reagents should be determined on a case-by-case basis. Because most biotechnology-derived and biological therapeutic products are heat labile by nature and easily degradable by a range of chemical treatments, processing steps such as autoclaving or chromatography with organic solvents are unlikely to be successfully incorporated in the manufacturing process of a biologic. Therefore, CDER and CBER[e] anticipate that most reagents used in producing biotechnology products or biologics will be processed to minimize microbial contaminants and will be rigorously tested for adventitious agents.

---

[c]"The risk of viral contamination is common to all biologicals. The production of biologics requires the use of raw materials derived from human or animal sources, and that poses a threat of pathogen transmission. Potential contamination may arise from the source material (such as a cell bank of animal origin) or as adventitious agents introduced by the manufacturing process ... Evaluating the safety of a biological product begins at the level of the source material, such as the manufacturer's working cell bank ..." (73).

[d]The use of mammalian cell lines enables the complex glycolylation patterns (posttranslational modifications) used by complex recombinant proteins (74).

[e]Center for Drug Evaluation and Research (CDER) and Center for Biologics Evaluation and Research (CBER).

REFERENCES

1. Levin J. The Limulus test and bacterial endotoxins: some perspectives. In: Watson SW, Levin J, Novitsky TJ, eds. Endotoxins and Their Detection with the Limulus Amebocyte Lysate Test. New York: Alan R. Liss, 1981.
2. Henderson B, Poole S, Wilson M. Bacterial modulins: a novel class of virulence factors which cause host tissue pathology by inducing cytokine synthesis. Microbiol Rev 1996; 60(2):316–341.
3. Kotb M. Bacterial pyrogenic exotoxins as superantigens. Clin Microbiol Rev 1995; 8(3):411–426.
4. Tuomanen E et al. The Induction of meningeal inflammation by components of the pneumococcal cell wall. J Infect Dis 1985; 151:859–868.
5. Alberts B et al. Chapter 10: Membrane structure. Molecular Biology of the Cell. Vol. 3. Garland Publishing, 1994; 8(2):217–225.
6. Barnes PF et al. Tumor necrosis factor production in patients with leprosy. Infect Immun 1992; 60(4):1441–1446.
7. Chatterjee D et al. Structural basis of capacity of lipoarabinomannan to induce secretion of tumor necrosis factor. Infect Immun 1992; 60(3):1249–1253.
8. Silver RF, Li Q, Ellner JJ. Expression of virulence of mycobacterium tuberculosis within human monocytes: virulence correlates with intracellular growth and induction of tumor necrosis factor alpha but not with evasion of lymphocyte-dependent monocyte effector functions. Infect Immun 1998; 66:1190–1199.
9. Riedel DD, Kaufmann SH. Chemokine secretion by human polymorphonuclear granulocytes after stimulation with *Mycobacterium tuberculosis* and lipoarabinomannan. Infect Immun 1997; 65:620–4623.
10. Schluger NW, Rom WN. The host immune response to tuberculosis. Am J Respir Crit Care Med 1997; 157:679–691.
11. Olson EJ et al. Fungal β-glucan interacts with vitronectin and stimulates tumor necrosis factor alpha release from macrophages. Infect Immun 1996; 64(9):3548–3554.
12. Czop JK, Kay J. Isolation and characterization of beta-glucan receptors on human mononuclear phagocytes. J Exp Med 1991; 173:1511–1520.
13. Radetsky M. The emerging spectrum of tickborne infections. Curr Opin Infect Dis 1998; 11:313–318.
14. Yang L et al. Heritable susceptibility to severe *Borrelia burgdorferi*-induced arthritis is dominant and is associated with persistence of large numbers of spirochetes in tissues. Infect Immun 1994; 64:492–500.
15. Relman DA. The search for unrecognized pathogens. Science 1999; 284:1308–1310.
16. Raoult D, Roux V. Rickettsioses as paradigms of new or emerging infectious diseases. Clin Microbiol Rev 1997; 10(4):694–719.
17. Ciacci-Woolwine F et al. *Salmonella flagellin* induces tumor necrosis factor alpha in a human promonocytic cell line. Infect Immun 1999; 66(3):1127–1134.
18. Wyant TL, Tanner MK, Sztein MB. *Salmonella typhi* flagella are potent inducers of proinflammatory cytokine secretion by human monocytes. Infect Immun 1999; 67:3619–3624.
19. Scragg IG et al. Structural characterization of the inflammatory moiety of a variable major lipoprotein of *Borrelia recurrentis*. J Biol Chem 2000; 275:937–941.
20. Giambartolomei GH, Dennis VA, Lasater BL. Induction of pro- and anti-inflammatory cytokines by *Borrelia burgdorferi* lipoproteins in monocytes is mediated by CD14. Infect Immun 1999; 67:140–147.
21. Krziwon C et al. Glycosphingolipids from *Sphingomonas paucimobilis* induce monokine production in human mononuclear cells. Infect Immun 1995; 63(8):2899–2905.
22. Muhlradt PF et al. Isolation, structure elucidation, and synthesis of a macrophage stimulatory lipopeptide from *Mycoplasma fermentans* acting at picomolar concentration. J Exp Med 1997; 185(11):1951–1958.
23. Mühlradt PF et al. Structure and specific activity of macrophage-stimulating lipopeptides from *Mycoplasma hyorhinis*. Infect Immun 1998; 66:4804–4810.
24. Zhang H et al. Lipoprotein release by bacteria: potential factor in bacterial pathogenesis. Infect Immun 1998; 66:5196–201.

25. Royce CL, Pardy RL. Endotoxin-like properties of an extract from a symbiotic, eukaryotic chlorella-like green alga. J Endotoxin Res 1996; 3(6):437–444.
26. Renzi PM, Lee CH. A comparative study of biological activities of lipoteichoic acid and lipopolysaccharide. J Endotoxin Res 1995; 2:431–441.
27. Wildefer A et al. Outer membrane protein a, peptidoglycan-associated lipoprotein, and murein lipoprotein are released by *Escherichia coli* bacteria into serum. Infect Immun 2000; 28:867.
28. Sriskandan S, Cohen J. Gram-positive sepsis. In: Opal SM, Cross AS, eds. Bacterial Sepsis and Septic Shock. Philadelphia: W.B. Saunders Company, 1999:397–412.
29. Navarre WW, Schneewind O. Surface proteins of gram-positive bacteria and mechanisms of their targeting to the cell wall envelope. Microbiol Mol Biol Rev 1999; 63:174–229.
30. Baek L et al. Interaction between *Limulus* amoeboctye lysate and soluble antigens from *Pseudomonas aeruginosa* and *Staphylococcus aureus* studied by quantitative immunoelectrophoresis. J Clin Microbiol 1985; 22(2):229–237.
31. Dijkstra AJ, Keck W. Peptidoglycan as a barrier to transenvelope transport. J Bacteriol 1996; 178(19):555–5562.
32. Thwaites JJ, Mendelson NH. Mechanical behaviour of bacterial cell walls. Adv Microb Physiol 1991; 32:173–222.
33. Idanpann-Heikkila I, Tuomanen E. Gram positive organisms and the pathology of sepsis. In: Fein AM et al., eds. Sepsis and Multiorgan Failure. ch. 7. Williams and Wilkins, 1997:62–73.
34. Diziarski R. Peptidoglycan and lipopolysaccharide bind to the same binding site on lymphocytes. J Biol Chem 1991; 266(8):4719–4725.
35. Fox A et al. Absolute identification of muramic acid, at trace levels, in human septic synovial fluids in vivo and absence in aseptic fluids. Infect Immun 1996; 64(9): 3911–3915.
36. van Langevelde P et al. Antibiotic-induced release of lipoteichoic acid and peptidoglycan from *Staphylococcus aureus*: quantitative measurements and biological reactivities. Antimicrob Agents Chemother 1998; 42(12):3072–3078.
37. Kengatharan KM et al. Mechanism of gram-positive shock: identification of peptidoglycan and lipoteichoic acid moieties essential in the induction of nitric oxide synthase, shock and multiple organ failure. J Experimental Med 1998; 188(2):305–315.
38. De Kimpe SJ et al. The cell wall components peptidoglycan and lipoteichoic acid from *Staphylococcus aureus* act in synergy to cause shock and multiple organ failure. Proc Natl Acad Sci 1995; 92:10359–10363.
39. Takada H et al. Structural characteristics of peptidoglycan fragments required to prime mice for induction of anaphylactoid reactions by lipopolysaccharides. Infect Immun 1996; 64(2):657–659.
40. Stevens DL. Invasive group a Streptococcal disease. Infect Agents Dis 1996; 5:157–166.
41. Marrack P, Kappler J. The Staphylococcal enterotoxins and their relatives. Science 1990; 248:705–711.
42. Bannan J, Visvanathan K, Zabriskie JB. Structure and function of streptococcal and staphylococcal superantigens in septic shock. In: Opal SM, Cross AS, eds. Infectious Disease Clinics of North America. Philadelphia: W. B. Saunders Co, 1999:387–412.
43. Rago JV, Schlievert PM. Mechanisms of pathogenesis of staphylococcal and streptococcal superantigens. In: Vogt PK, Mahan MJ, eds. Bacterial Infections: Close Encounters at the Host Pathogen Interface. Berlin: Springer, 1998.
44. Muller-Alouf H et al. Human pro- and anti-inflammatory cytokine patters induced by *Streptococcus pyogenes* erythrogenic (pyrogenic) exotoxin A and C superantigens. Infect Immun 1996; 64(4):450–1453.
45. Stuart PM, Woodward JG. *Yersinia enterocolitica* produces superantigenic activity. J Immunol 1992; 148:225–232.
46. Huber BT, Hsu PN, Sutkowski N. Virus-encoded superantigens. Microbiol Rev 1996; 60(3):473–482.
47. Ulrich RG. Evolving superantigens of *Staphylococcus aureus*. FEMS Immunol Med Microbiol 2000; 27:1–7.

48. Sawitzke AD, Mu H, Cole BC. Superantigens and autoimmune disease: Are they involved? Curr Opin Infect Dis 1999; 12:213–219.
49. Muller-Alouf et al. Comparative study of cytokine release by human peripheral blood mononuclear cells stimulated with *Streptococcus pyogenes* superantigenic erythrogenic toxins, heat-killed Streptococci, and lipopolysaccharide. Infect Immun 1994; 62(11):4915–4921.
50. Leonard B, Scheibert P. Immune cell lethality induced by strep pyrogenic exotoxin A and endotoxin. Infect Immun 1992; 60:3747–3755.
51. Roggiani M et al. Analysis of toxicity of streptococcal pyrogenic exotoxin A mutants. Infect Immun 1997; 65(7):2868–2875.
52. Norrby-Teglund A et al. Similar cytokine induction profiles of a novel streptococcal exotoxin, MF, and pyrogenic exotoxins A and B. Infect Immun 1994; 62:3731–3738.
53. Reitschel E et al. Lipopolysaccharide and peptidoglycan: CD14-dependent bacterial inducers of inflammation. Microb Drug Resist 1998; 4(1):37–44.
54. Gupta D et al. CD14 is a cell-activating receptor for bacterial peptidoglycan. J Biol Chem 1996; 271(38):23310–23316.
55. Ingalls R et al. Lipopolysaccharide recognition, CD14, and lipopolysaccharide receptors. In: Opal SM, Cross AS, eds. Infectious Disease Clinics of North America. Philadelphia: W. B. Saunders Co, 1999:341–353.
56. Klimpel KR, Goldman WE. Cell walls from avirulent variants of histoplasma capsulatum lack a-(1,3)-glucan. Infect Immun 1988; 56:2997–3000.
57. Cooper JF, Weary ME, Jordan FT. The impact of non-endotoxin LAL-reactive materials on *Limulus* amebocyte lysate analysis. PDA J Pharm Sci Technol 1997; 51(1).
58. Hogan LH, Klein BS, Levitz SM. Virulence factors of medically important fungi. Clin Microbiol Rev 1996; 9(4):469–488.
59. Silva CL, Fazioli RA. A *Paracoccidioides brasiliensis* polysaccharide having granuloma-inducing toxic and macrophage-stimulating activity. J Gen Microbiol 1985; 131:1497–1501.
60. Maier RV et al. Endotoxin requirements for alveolar macrophage stimulation. J Trauma Injury Infect Crit Care 1990; 30(suppl 12):S49–S57.
61. Hemmendinger S et al. Mitogenic activity on human arterial smooth muscle cells increased in the plasma of patients undergoing hemodialysis with cuprophane membranes. Nephron 1989; 53:147.
62. Bergamo Collaborative Dialysis Study Group. Acute intradialytic well-being: results of a clinical trial comparing polysulfane with cuprophan. Kidney Int 1991; 40:714.
63. Soltys J, Quinn MT. Modulation of endotoxin- and enterotoxin-induced cytokine release by in vivo treatment with (1,6)-branched-(1,3)-glucan. Infect Immun 1999; 67(1):244–252.
64. Zhang GH et al. Differential blocking of coagulation-activating pathways of *Limulus* amebocyte lysate. J Clin Microbiol 1994; 32:1537–1541.
65. Pearson FC et al. Characterization of *Limulus* amoebocyte lysate-reactive material from hollow-fiber dialyzers. Appl Environ Microbiol 1984; 48:1189.
66. Roslansky PF, Novitsky T. Sensitivity of *Limulus* amebocyte lysate (LAL) to LAL-reactive glucans. J Clin Microbiol 1991; 29(11):2477–2483.
67. Retini C et al. Capsular polysaccharide of *Cryptococcus neoformans* induces proinflammatory cytokine release by human neutrophils. Infect Immun 1996; 64(7):2897–2903.
68. Ellerbroek PM et al. Cryptococcal glucuronoxylomannan inhibits adhesion of neutrophils to stimulated endothelium in vitro by affecting both neutrophils and endothelial cells. Infect Immun 2002; 70(9):4762–4771.
69. Sepkowitz KA et al. Tuberculosis in the AIDS era. Clin Microbiol Rev 1995; 8:180–199.
70. Fredricks DN, Relman DA. Sequence-based identification of microbial pathogens: a reconsideration of Koch's postulates. Clin Microbiol Rev 1996; 9(1):18–33.
71. Rawadi G, Roman-Roman S. Mycoplasma membrane lipoproteins induced proinflammatory cytokines by a mechanism distinct from that of lipopolysaccharide. Infect Immun 1996; 64(3):637–643.
72. Draft Guidance for Industry. Monoclonal Antibodies Used as Reagents in Drug Manufacturing, U.S. Dept. of Health and Human Services, FDA, CDER, CBER, May 1999:1–4.

73. Montgomery SA, ed. The BioPharm Guide to Fermentation and Cell Culture. Eugene OR; Advanstar Communications, 2000:1–50.
74. Pollard AJ et al. Lesson of the week: potentially lethal bacterial infection associated with *Varicella zoster* virus. BMJ 1996; 313:283–285.
75. Miller-Hjelle MA et al. Polycystic kidney disease: an unrecognized emerging infectious disease? Emerg Infect Dis 1997; 3(2):1–19.
76. Pitkaranta A, Hayden FG. What's new with common colds? pathogenesis and diagnosis. Infect Med 1998; 15:50–59.
77. Jacobs MG, Young PR. Dengue: a continuing challenge for molecular biology. Curr Opin Infect Dis 1998; 11:319–324.
78. Aleman MDR et al. Some methods for contamination testing of a master cell bank. BioPharm 2000; 13(6):48–56.

8 Risk Assessment in Parenteral Manufacture

Edward Tidswell

Eli Lilly & Company, Indianapolis, Indiana, U.S.A.

In contrast to the swift, systematic and inherent assessment of risk routinely performed by all sentient organisms, the wide spread implementation of rigorous risk assessment in pharmaceutical manufacture has been slow, fraught with interpretive difficulty and cumbersome. As with any newly pioneered process its gradual evolution is addressing these shortfalls.

INTRODUCTION

The analysis of hazard is a routine subconscious process inherent to all sentient creatures. Subconscious risk assessment has likely evolved as a part of survival strategy; performed on a continuous basis to preserve and sustain the quality of existence. Understanding hazards and the evaluation of any potential harm are fundamental processes facilitating swift decision-making permitting the continuance of our state of health and survival. It should therefore be of no surprise that the concept of risk assessment is favored in the management of hazards and risk to product quality in pharmaceutical manufacture—assuring patient safety. In contrast to the swift, systematic, and inherent assessment of risk routinely performed by all sentient organisms, the wide spread implementation of rigorous risk assessment in pharmaceutical manufacture has been slow, fraught with interpretive difficulty and cumbersome. As with any newly pioneered process its gradual evolution is in addressing these shortfalls.

Over the last few decades risk management and risk assessment (1) have been successfully embraced by a variety of industry sectors. Application of effective risk assessment and risk management in the manufacture of pharmaceutical products remains at a rudimentary stage compared to the financial (2), food (3–6), aerospace, and automotive industries. Ironically, there is no greater potential than within pharmaceutical manufacture for the application of salient tools and techniques to assess and address risks to product quality; ultimately benefiting the vulnerable patient population. Within pharmaceutical manufacturing aseptic processes are themselves uniquely prone to a variety of acute and chronic risks. Risk assessment and risk management is essential to devise and implement appropriate controls commensurate with the perceived quantitative estimates of risk. In this field Whyte and Eaton (7) have pioneered simple and effective techniques to assess the risk of microbial ingress into products during aseptic manufacture. Tidswell and McGarvey (8) developed these techniques further to model risk using quantitative simulations and reduce inherent assumptions and subjectivity. Aside from particulates and microorganisms, aseptically manufactured parenteral product presentations are vulnerable to risks from the presence of endotoxins. The risk to product quality from endotoxins is not only inherently linked to the presence of viable bacteria but also nonviable bacteria and their residues; necessitating a slightly different approach to risk assessment. Assessments for the purpose of evaluating the risk to parenteral manufacture from endotoxins are therefore deserving of special consideration and are the focus of this chapter.

REGULATORY GUIDANCE

Formal risk assessment of manufacturing processes to assure product quality posed by a hazard during parenteral manufacture is not as yet a mandatory requirement by the global regulatory authorities. In recent years the FDA and European Pharmaceutical Inspection Convention/Cooperation Scheme (PIC/CS)[31] have clearly recognized the many benefits that it affords the manufacturer. The regulatory agencies terminology within guidance documents has significantly changed reflecting this paradigm shift to risk management and risk-based approaches. Within the PIC/S "Guide to Good Manufacturing Practice for Medicinal Products" (9) there is the following frequency of use of terms: bioburden 2, endotoxin 3, hazard 14, risk 78, and contamination 143 times. The frequency of use of these terms illustrates current and future intent. The regulatory authorities actively encourage adoption of risk-based approaches and, although not mandatory, these terms are appearing within guidance documents. For example, Annex 15 of the European Union good manufacturing practices (GMPs) (9) clearly states that "a risk assessment approach should be used to determine the scope and extent of validation." In 2004 the FDA published two documents: "Guidance for Industry. Sterile Products Produced by Aseptic Processing—Current Good Manufacturing Practice," (10) and "Process Analytical Technology (PAT)—A Framework for Innovative Pharmaceutical Development, Manufacturing and Quality Assurance" (11). These two documents have set the future trend and course for the FDA's regulatory and inspectional strategy. Both incorporate the new paradigm; incorporating a risk-based approach both to inspections and the opportunities for manufacturers. Perhaps the most helpful publication in recent years concerning risk management is Q9: "Quality Risk Management" (12) published by the International Conference on Harmonization of Technical Requirements for Registration of Pharmaceuticals for Human Use (ICH). This resource document describes the principles and tools for the consistent application of risk management within the pharmaceutical industry. This guidance document also provides a recommended process flow for successful assessment and management of risks. Indeed, as previously anticipated, risk management and risk assessment are rapidly becoming the next phase in the continued evolution of GMPs (13).

OBJECTIVE AND PURPOSE OF RISK ASSESSMENT

According to ICH Q9: "Quality Risk Management": "Effective quality risk management can facilitate better and more informed decisions...." Moreover appropriate risk management permits the utilization of information to leverage resource in areas which can realize the greatest improvement in product quality assurance. All risk assessment techniques and tools may be regarded as decision tools; the sole objective of any risk assessment should be to facilitate and assist in decision-making. Prior to embarking upon any assessment of risk it is imperative that the precise purpose and intention is understood and clearly defined; a single risk assessment is unlikely to answer all possible questions or appropriately address all potential scenarios. Although there is a single unifying objective for all risk assessments (to facilitate decision), the precise purpose for each risk assessment is likely to be unique. With respect to the control of endotoxins in parenteral manufacturing risk assessments applied within the aseptic manufacturing environment can be used to achieve a variety of purposes, these include, but are not limited to:

1. *Prospective analysis of proposed process designs.* Performed at the early stages of a process design risk assessment can be used to drive the design philosophy. Repeated, consecutive cycles of risk assessment upon conceptual models evolve the design to refine one with the appropriate level of risk. This form of prospective risk assessment allows the identification and adoption of processes and control strategies that are truly commensurate with the magnitude of estimated risk (14). Due to the likely absence of any data concerning the conceptual designs this application of risk assessment relies upon a greater number of assumptions and a greater level of uncertainty.

2. *Comparative analysis of current processes.* The levels of risk associated with current established processes may be compared to permit identification of those more prone to higher levels of risk. Historical data are usually available and facilitates this process. Decision regarding the utilization or preference of all available process within a manufacturing strategy can be easily made. In this application risk analysis identifies those positive elements of processes and systems permitting their exploitation (15).

3. *Identification of process improvements.* In this context, risk analysis is most usually applied throughout a multistep process; evaluating consecutive steps to highlight those steps most prone to risk.

4. *Determination of worst-case conditions.* Throughout the operational life cycle of aseptic processes validation exercises have traditionally incorporated worst-case conditions. Here, risk assessment permits the data-driven and informed choice of those conditions, which truly represent the greatest challenge. One area where this could be effectively accomplished is in equipment cleaning validation (16).

5. *Identification of the scope of validation activities.* Over the last two decades it has been fashionable to commit to validation activities without a thorough assessment of the appropriate scope. Risk assessment does permit the identification of whether a "realistic" risk truly exists and necessitates appropriate validation activities.

INTRINSIC AND EXTRINSIC ENDOTOXIN HAZARD—A RISK MODEL

All conceivable risks to parenteral manufacturing processes are dependent upon the presence of at least one recognizable and tangible hazard. In this context hazards have been described as "any circumstance in the production, control, and distribution of a pharmaceutical, which can cause an adverse health effect" (17). Within this definition hazards can be distinguished as either intrinsic or extrinsic (18); intrinsic hazards are integral or inherent elements of processes or systems, extrinsic hazards are those entities which originate externally and are therefore not predesigned constituents of the process. The adverse health effects elicited by endotoxins within parenteral products are well recognized; endotoxins are thus regarded as a hazard. The risk to product quality realized by endotoxins may be achieved as when manifested as an intrinsic or an extrinsic hazard. An example of endotoxins representing an intrinsic hazard includes the "natural" load typically found within active pharmaceutical ingredient derived from a recombinant gram-negative bacterial fermentation. In contrast, endotoxin contaminating a parenteral product presentation component (e.g., vial or stopper, sealing ring or plunger) originates externally and therefore typifies extrinsic hazards.

Endotoxin within a parenteral product presentation can jeopardize patient health by eliciting a pyrogenic affect. This affect can be elicited by endotoxins existing within product presentations in several potential forms. In its "purest" form endotoxins may exist as packets of molecules, most likely as micelles within a fluid or coating as a layer upon substrate (equipment or presentation) surfaces. Endotoxin may also similarly have a detrimental affect upon patient safety when associated with the cellular form either as nonviable, dormant, or nonreplicating microorganisms or as viable, animate, replicating microorganisms. Here, endotoxins are released as fragments or the vestiges of these whole microbial cells. To thoroughly evaluate the risk to product quality posed by endotoxins it is essential to recognize the various forms in which endotoxin hazard may present itself and eventually pose a risk to patient safety. It is therefore possible to define a conceptual model for the possible risks posed by endotoxin hazard; any evaluation of risk must consider and evaluate all these risks, wherever necessary. Table 1 summarizes those risks to parenteral product manufacture, which must be considered when evaluating endotoxin hazard. Furthermore, manufacturing processes are consecutive sequences of diverse stages or operations and therefore require the application of the risk model to each individual step.

All parenteral manufacturing processes are susceptible to varying degrees of risk from intrinsic endotoxin hazard; all at some point are reliant upon a formulation process which combines many potential sources of endotoxins (e.g., active pharmaceutical ingredient, water for injection). Appropriately designed manufacturing processes include mechanisms (either fortuitous or purposefully designed), which control the intrinsic or inherent endotoxins hazard. In aseptic manufacture of parenterals the risks posed to product quality from the intrinsic endotoxin hazard is therefore almost solely associated with the risk of the physical retention of endotoxins. If the endotoxin exists in the form of viable whole cells (all nonsterile parenteral constituents will posses a level of bioburden), then the potential of cellular proliferation and increased risk also exists. Irrespective of the nature of these two distinct forms of risk they both can be interpreted and assessed as the failure of control mechanisms.

TABLE 1 Risks which Must be Considered when Assessing the Risk to Product Quality by Endotoxins During Parenteral Manufacture

Hazard		Ingress	Risks proliferation	Retention
Extrinsic	Endotoxin	Yes	No	Yes
	Viable gram-negative microorganisms	Yes	Yes	Yes
	Nonviable gram-negative microorganisms	Yes	No	Yes
Intrinsic	Endotoxin	No	No	Yes
	Viable gram-negative microorganisms	No	Yes	Yes
	Nonviable gram-negative microorganisms	No	No	Yes

In contrast, an extrinsic endotoxin hazard may manifest as a sequence of risks; initially as a risk of ingress (accessing and contaminating) and secondly, as with intrinsic hazard, a risk of retention (the physical maintenance or juxtaposition of endotoxin or microbial cells) within the manufacturing process. The latter is further complicated with consideration of viable microorganisms as sources of endotoxins. Inevitably, all pharmaceutical manufacturing processes are continually vulnerable to varying degrees of ingress risk posed by extrinsic hazards.

All risk assessments must be based upon a risk model, which defines the mechanism of risk to a manufacturing process (8). Here recognition and consideration of the model for possible risk posed by endotoxin determines the choice of risk assessment tool, the structure and content of a risk assessment. Failure to recognize any of these facets of the risk model may result in misinterpretations and ultimately diminish the effectiveness of any risk assessment.

QUANTIFYING RISK FROM ENDOTOXIN IN PHARMACEUTICAL MANUFACTURE

A number of well established risk assessment tools and techniques are available and have been effectively used to discern risks of bioburden ingress, retention, and proliferation within pharmaceutical manufacturing processes (7). These also lend themselves to assessing the risks of endotoxins ingress and retention and include:

1. Failure Mode and Effect Analysis (FMEA) (19–21)
2. Failure Mode Effects and Critical Analysis (FMECA) (22)
3. Hazard Analysis and Critical Control Points (HACCP) (23,24)

Ubiquity has been demonstrated in the application of HACCP in the pharmaceutical and medical device manufacturing (25–27). HACCP is particularly relevant in that it drives analysis toward the examination and establishment of control points. As illustrated previously, the precise nature of the risks within the risk model may guide the choice of technique; the risk of endotoxin retention is possibly best assessed via a form of failure mode analysis (28).

Regardless of the risk assessment tool elected, each is based upon the consensus among professional bodies and international standards (29–32) that risk is purely defined by two dimensions; probability of occurrence (representing the uncertainty of a potential event) and the severity of occurrence (consequential impact of the event). Quantification of risk can therefore be achieved using the Fundamental Risk Equation 1:

$$\text{Risk} = \text{Severity of occurrence} \times \text{Probability of occurrence} \qquad (1)$$

The dimension of severity in the assessment of risks from endotoxin in parenteral manufacture can be defined by the quantity of endotoxin within the process stream or product. Similarly the dimension of probability should likewise consider the quantity of endotoxin either challenging or within the process or product. Although the risks exacted from bioburden and endotoxin hazard to parenteral manufacturing process have previously been quantified simultaneously (14), this is not always appropriate. For example, in aseptic fill and finish of a product the ingress of bioburden into product results in the loss of sterility. The result of one microorganism gaining access to the product has the same result or degree of severity, as would multiple microorganisms; therefore, in aseptic manufacture the severity of occurrence will always be invariable and will always have a numerical contribution to the overall risk of bioburden ingress of unity.

For bioburden ingress into product during aseptic manufacture the Fundamental Risk Equation 2 must therefore be:

$$\text{Risk} = \text{Probability of occurrence} \tag{2}$$

Clearly the fundamental equations quantifying risk associated with bioburden, and endotoxin hazards may be quite different for different stages in parenteral manufacture.

The risk model for endotoxin hazard (Table 1) describes a number of discrete risks, however each are potentially complex, multifactorial, and are quantitatively the sum of a number of contributing risk components. Risk components reflect those contributing but quite distinct elements, which have no interdependency, influence, or propensity to influence each other; therefore contributing purely in an additive manner to any quantitative estimate of risk. Each risk component is itself defined by the numerical product of risk factors representing the Fundamental Risk Equation 1. These operate in concert with direct influence upon each other to numerically define the magnitude of risk; therefore, the numerical values of these are multiplied together. This hierarchical relationship relating hazards, risks, risk components, and risk factors (18) provides an appropriate architecture for the assessment of risk that is applicable irrespective of risk model, process, or risk tool adopted (Fig. 1). Several contemporary approaches describe formulaic and quantitative risk assessment processes for aseptic manufacture, (33,34) each based upon a similar form of risk hierarchy.

Risks only represent possible future events; the predictive nature of risk assessments are dependent upon specified criteria and assumptions deemed appropriate to achieve a realistic quantitative enumeration of risk. Contemporary risk assessment tools and techniques all necessarily incorporate the following assumptions:

- All risk components and risk factors are appropriate. Risk components must include risk factors, which represent accurately to define the likely occurrence and severity of that event consistent with the general definition of risk and the risk model. Choice of salient risk factors and components is ultimately discretionary based upon expert opinion (i.e., consensus of the personnel responsible for the risk assessment) to genuinely represent the event.
- Assigned numerical values sufficiently represent risk factors. Risk factors are either assigned a numerical value or a surrogate descriptor such as "low," "medium," or "high" (22). The designation is most usually empirical, based upon informed expert opinion or the perceived appropriate magnitude by those personnel responsible for the risk assessment. Subjectivity in assigning risk factor values may instill significant bias and makes the quantitative estimation of risk less reliable (35). Where feasible, the initial designation of risk factor scores should be based upon known data, specifications, or accepted standards. For example, when considering the quantity of endotoxin (severity risk factor) scoring might be gauged relative to the *U.S. Pharmacopeia* (USP) level for endotoxin in water for injection, as in Table 2. Alternatively, the risk factor values could be derived in relation to the actual weight of endotoxin. Similarly, criteria for risk factor values for viable or nonviable microorganisms could be

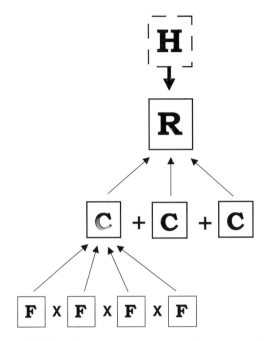

FIGURE 1 The risk hierarchy describing the relationship between hazards (H), risk (R), risk components (C), and risk factors (F) as previously described by Tidswell. *Source*: From Ref. 18.

based upon the amount of bioburden required to significantly impact product quality. Assuming that an endotoxin quantity exceeding that for the water for injection specification (0.25EU/ml) represents a significant impact to product quality, this would equate to approximately 0.05 ng of endotoxin. The amount of bioburden required to generate this quantity of endotoxin would be approximately 1.25×10^3 *Escherichia coli* cells (36).

■ It is recommended that the lowest risk factor value is never zero. If zero is used then the risk score will always be zero. This is never the case as if there is a hazard present there will always be an attendant risk. Removal of as much subjectivity as possible and consistency is essential to make the assessment as meaningful and beneficial as possible.

■ Invariable risk factor values are adequate. All contributing risk factors are likely to posses an inherent variability. Contemporary methodologies of risk

TABLE 2 Examples of Risk Factor Scoring Criteria for the Quantity of Endotoxin: Values Are Based on the *U.S. Pharmacopeia* Specification for Water for Injection

Amount of endotoxin	Quantity of endotoxin	Amount of bioburden[a]	Risk factor value
≤0.25 EU	≤0.05 ng	1.25×10^3 cfu	0.5
0.25–0.75 EU	0.05–0.15 ng	1.25×10^3–3.75×10^3	1.0
0.75–1.25 EU	0.15–0.25 ng	3.75×10^3–6.25×10^3	1.5
≥1.25EU	≥0.25 ng	≥6.25×10^3	2.0

[a]These values relate to cfu of *Escherichia coli*; however, for simplicity these bioburden values are applied to all microorganisms irrespective of species.
Abbreviation: EU, endotoxin unit; cfu, colony forming units.

assessment cannot easily account the stochastic nature of risk factors. Designation of an appropriate risk factor value might therefore be perplexing and forces a crucial decision—how best to numerically represent these risk factors? Herein lies a dilemma: Is it more appropriate to consider average data, worst-case data, or even specification limits?

- A single maximum risk score is sufficient. To compare different process scenarios or process steps, a single universally applied maximum risk score has to be employed. This demands that the same number of risk components and risk factors must be employed in each assessment together with an identical means of scoring. Sources, opportunities, and mechanisms for bioburden ingress frequently vary from scenario to scenario or between process steps, therefore it is unlikely that each circumstance can be adequately described by an identical set of risk components and risk factors.

- An arbitrarily designated maximum level of acceptable or tolerable risk is appropriate. Evaluation of risk using scores based upon representative numerical values provides a suitable frame of reference and means of assessment, however the designation of a numerical level above which the risk is deemed "intolerable" (14) and requires responsive risk reduction is purely subjective. Risk is never zero nor is it an absolute certainty, but rather exists along a continuum extending from a very low level of possibility, through, to a high level of certainty (37). An alternative modus operandi of distinguishing unacceptable levels of risk or criticality is to generate a risk profile. The numerical risk scores derived from risk components and risk factors for each process step are simply plotted in process-ordered sequence. This gives an overall chart or profile for the risks posed by hazards from start to finish of the process under scrutiny. A simple contextual evaluation of risk is permitted; furthermore the shape, location, and spread of the risk profile can provide additional information concerning the risk to the process (14).

Contemporary risk assessment techniques evaluating bioburden ingress during aseptic manufacture (23,33) have provided appropriate models for wide application, and these can be used for assessing risk from endotoxin hazard. However, in comparison to the financial (2), food (3–6), aerospace, and automotive industries these risk assessment methodologies remain rudimentary. The continued evolution of appropriate techniques has escalated sophistication to a level comparable to those used in other industry sectors. Tidswell and McGarvey (8) innovatively applied quantitative risk modeling incorporating Monte Carlo (38) simulations (39) for assessing bioburden risks in aseptic manufacture. Many of the constraints and assumptions inherent to contemporary risk assessments, mentioned earlier, are removed or reduced using this technique.

RISK IN ASEPTIC PARENTERAL MANUFACTURE

A generalized scheme for the aseptic manufacture of parenteral product presentations (within a stoppered vial) is illustrated in Figure 2. The left-hand box (defined by a broken line) encompasses nonsterile operations and materials within the formulation and preparation process steps and operational stages. This box therefore includes all those processes, which actively control or remove endotoxins. Processes and operations in this area of the schematic are vulnerable to challenge from both intrinsic and extrinsic endotoxin hazards. The right-hand box (defined

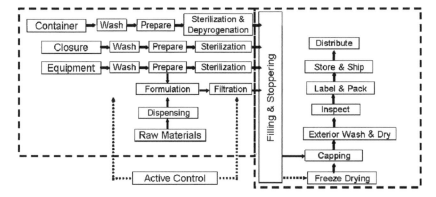

FIGURE 2 Generalized schematic for the aseptic manufacture of parenteral product presentations (vial). Those process steps and operations, which actively reduce or remove endotoxin, are identified.

by a broken line) encompasses aseptic fill and finish processes; bringing together sterile and depyrogenated product, component and closure to generate product presentations. Here there is no intrinsic endotoxin hazard present, by virtue of the active control (depyrogenation and sterilization) processes upstream; therefore, there is no attendant risk. Fill and finish processes are performed within cleanroom environments in which there should be a complete absence of viable gram-negative microorganisms, nonviable gram-negative microorganisms, and endotoxin all of which would constitute extrinsic hazard. Therefore, there is no risk in aseptic fill and finish operations due to the complete absence of endotoxin hazard.

CASE STUDY: VIAL STOPPER PREPARATION PROCESS

To illustrate how risk assessment and risk profiling of endotoxin hazard can be used to benefit parenteral manufacturing processes a case study is presented herewith. A vial stopper preparation process within a parenteral manufacturing facility was subject to a HACCP-based risk assessment. The purpose of the risk assessment was to facilitate the improvement in a vial stopper preparation process. The objective was to prioritize those process steps and characteristics which when improved would have the greatest benefit on product quality. A HACCP risk assessment team who completed the evaluation and who collectively decided through consensus:

- Risk factors used within the Fundamental Risk Equation 1
- Criteria for assigning risk factor values
- Risk factor values
- Level of criticality, above which risk factor scores indicate an obligation for process improvement

The risk model (Table 2) was used to distinguish the risks evaluated at each step of the vial stopper preparation process, for simplicity only the risk assessment for endotoxin ingress is reported here. The risk factors chosen to quantitatively estimate risk of endotoxin ingress were identified as:

1. Amount of endotoxin
2. Likelihood of endotoxin ingress

3. Proximity of endotoxin to vial stoppers during the preparation process
4. Effectiveness of the method of control

Table 3 summarizes the criteria stipulated by the HACCP team to score the individual risk factors. In this risk assessment many of the risk factors could be regarded as subjective and arguably open to interpretation when assigning numerical values. Exacting data assisting in the scoring of risk factors such as quantitative transfer coefficients, previously employed by Tidswell and McGarvey (8), to enumerate bioburden ingress in aseptic manufacture were unavailable for endotoxin ingress. Informed expert opinion of the HACCP team in considering known and documented data salient to the vial stopper preparation process was necessary to reach consensual decision of risk factor values. Where consensus could not be reached or in scenarios where available data were inconclusive, risk factors were automatically scored at the highest possible value. Risk factor values for each process step were multiplied together to generate risk scores in the usual fashion. Risk scores for endotoxin ingress determined for each process step were plotted in process ordered sequence to generate the risk profile as displayed in Figure 3. Table 4 summarizes the data from the risk assessment and risk profile. The shape of the risk profile is acceptable with a general exponential decrease in risk scores with processing steps. Although no single processing step exceeded the level of criticality, five did demonstrate higher risk scores (meeting the level of criticality). These steps required some form of risk mitigation or risk reduction. Further evaluation and analysis of the risk assessment discerned that several of these steps involved the stopper-cleaning agent. These steps were given the maximum risk

TABLE 3 Criteria Adopted to Assign Numerical Values to Risk Factors

Amount of endotoxin-severity	
Amount of known or likely endotoxin	**Numerical risk factor value**
<0.05 EU/mL or cm^2	0.5
0.05–0.25 EU/mL or cm^2	1.0
>0.25 EU/mL or cm^2	2.0

Likelihood of ingress-probability	
Likelihood of ingress	**Numerical risk factor value**
Very low	0.5
Low	1.0
Medium	1.5
High	2.0

Proximity of endotoxin to product-probability	
Proximity of endotoxin	**Numerical risk factor value**
Remote	1.0
Indirect contact	1.5
Direct contact	2.0

Effectiveness of control-probability	
Perceived effectiveness of control	**Numerical risk factor value**
Very good	0.5
Good	1.0
Some control	1.5
No control	2.0

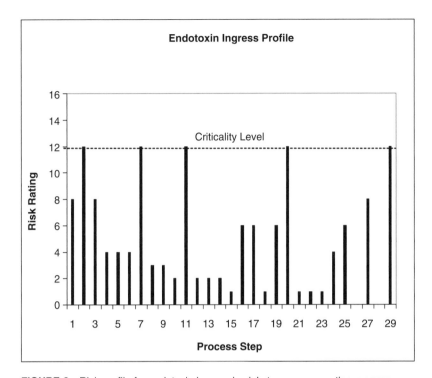

FIGURE 3   Risk profile for endotoxin ingress in vial stopper preparation process.
Key to process steps: 1) Stopper storage, 2) manual removal of bags of stoppers from box, 3) manual transfer of bags of stoppers to cart, 4) move cart to air lock, 5) sanitize bags of stoppers and cart in air lock, 6) transfer bags of stoppers to UAF in cleanroom, 7) fill detergent feed tank, 8) visual inspection of washer for stoppers and debris, 9) preparation of the stopper washer for operations, 10) washer operation checks, 11) detergent volume dispensing checks, 12) filter function and operation checks, 13) rinse fill pressure check, 14) water temperature check, 15) visual check wash bucket, 16) transfer of stoppers from sealed bag into wash bucket, 17) visual check stoppers for debris, strangers and so on, 18) check wire basket of stopper washer for strangers or debris, 19) transfer wash bucket to stopper washing machine wash basket and lock in place, 20) initiate washing of stoppers, 21) spin washer basket to remove excess water, 22) remove wash bucket from stopper washer, 23) check cylinders for strangers, 24) manually transfer washed stoppers into cylinders, 25) addition of silicone oil or emulsion, 26) blending of stoppers, 27) preparation of cylinders for stopper sterilization, 28) autoclave sterilization, and 29) declumping of stoppers.

factor scores for the amount of endotoxin (severity). These values were assigned due to the absence of appropriate data assuring the HACCP team of the endotoxin level within the cleaning agent. A simple exercise of acquiring this data and appropriate assurance of endotoxin control in the cleaning agent results in a significant

TABLE 4   Summary of Risk Assessment Data and Risk Profile for
Endotoxin Ingress During Vial Stopper Preparation

No. of steps exceeding criticality level	0
No. of steps meeting or exceeding criticality level	5
Process steps meeting criticality level	2, 7, 11, 20, 29
Average risk rating (all steps)	4.9
General shape of risk profile	Exponential decrease

reduction of the risk scores. This point illustrates that it is essential to be aware of the assumptions and criteria used to derive risk factor scores, moreover, how and why risk factor values were assigned. The absence of data or a level of uncertainty associated with available data can have profound influence upon subsequent risk mitigation and reduction activities.

CONCLUSION

Commercial manufacturing environments will inevitably impose ever-increasing pressure to achieve improved efficiencies for less resource and less expenditure. Risk assessment offers not only a pragmatic means of managing pharmaceutical processes to benefit product quality and the patient population, but additionally the means of directing finite resources to those areas to realize maximum benefit. The various global regulatory agencies have realized the merit in using risk-based approaches to complete their obligations in assuring the supply of quality medicines to patients. Furthermore, the regulatory bodies have begun to encourage pharmaceutical manufacturers to adopt similar strategies in the production and supply of medicines. Although the regulatory guidance has to date been in the form of active encouragement it is likely that risk-based approaches, risk-management, and risk assessment will form part of future GMPs. A cautionary note; although these risk-based approaches are well accepted and encouraged, they do not provide a means of obviating the pharmaceutical manufacturer from compliance obligations.

The applications of risk assessment tools and techniques have the special merit in deterministically forecasting risks associated with endotoxin hazards potentially challenging parenteral manufacturing processes. Frequently, when evaluating or quantitatively estimating the impact or significance of endotoxin hazard upon a process, the data can be both variable and uncertain. Risk assessment can account for a lack of perfect knowledge and therefore assist in making informed decisions.

Contemporary risk assessment techniques have several shortfalls, notably the amount of assumptions made or the degree of subjectivity which inevitably instill a degree of inexactitude. Nevertheless, thorough documentation and careful consideration of the details within a risk assessment may mitigate this. Thorough analysis of the quantified estimates of risk is also necessary to permit the most appropriate interpretation of the analysis— risk profiling can assist here. Quantitative risk modeling and simulation does represent the next stage in the evolution of risk assessment in pharmaceutical manufacture permitting swift quantification, fewer assumptions, and a greater amount of more easily interpreted data. Future needs of quality assurance of parenteral manufacture will likely demand such sophisticated techniques not only to assess the status quo but also to more adeptly assess new designs or predicatively anticipate scenarios for contingency. Quantitative risk models and simulations allow for this; models can be perturbed in a fashion to simulate high levels of hazards or possible failure modes and predicatively quantify the risk. With the advent of PAT and implementation of real time process, monitoring for the likes of endotoxin and then the amount of data available in pharmaceutical manufacture facilities will significantly increase. It is likely that this new flow of data will require appropriate consideration and interpretation through risk assessment to make expedient and informed evaluation.

REFERENCES

1. Hillson DA. Risk management: the case for including opportunity. APM Yearbook 2004/2005, 2005:3–4.
2. Winston W. Financial models using simulation and optimization II: investment valuation, options, pricing, real options, and product pricing models. West Drayton, UK: Palisade Corporation Europe, 2001.
3. Nauta MJ. Separation of uncertainty and variability in quantitative microbial risk assessment models. Int J Food Microbiol 2000; 57:9–18.
4. Cassin MH, Lammerding AM, Todd ECD, Ross W, McColl S. Quantitative risk assessment of Escherichia coli O157:H7 in ground beef hamburgers. Int J Food Microbiol 1998; 41:21–44.
5. Thompson KM, Burmaster DE, Crouch EAC. Monte Carlo techniques for quantitative uncertainty analysis in public health risk assessments. Risk Anal 1992; 12:53–63.
6. Lammerding AM, Paoli GM. Quantitative risk assessment: an emerging tool for emerging foodborne pathogens. Emerg Infect Dis 1997; 3(4):483–487.
7. Whyte W, Eaton T. Risk management of contamination (RMC) during manufacturing operations in cleanrooms. Parenetral Society Technical Monograph 14, 2005.
8. Tidswell EC, McGarvey B. Quantitative risk modeling in aseptic manufacture. PDA J Pharm Sci Technol 2006; 60(5):267–283.
9. Anon. Guide to good manufacturing practice for medicinal products (PE 009-3), 2006. http://www.picscheme.org/indexnoflash.php?p = guides#
10. Anon. Guidance for Industry. Sterile products produced by aseptic processing – current good manufacturing practice, 2004a. http://www.fda.gov/cder/guidance/
11. Anon. PAT-a frame work for innovative pharmaceutical development, manufacturing and quality assurance, 2004b. http://www.fda.gov/cder/guidance
12. Anon. ICH Q9 Quality risk management, 2005. EMEA/INS/GMP/157614/2005-ICH. http://www.emea.eu.int/pdfs/human/ich/15761405en.pdf#search = 'ich%20q9'
13. Anon. GMP Movement to risk management seen. Gold Sheet 2000a; 34(5):1.
14. Tidswell EC. Risk profiling pharmaceutical manufacturing processes. Eur J Pharm Sci 2004; 9(2):49–55.
15. Hillson D. Business uncertainty. Threat or opportunity. Ethos 1999; 13:14–17.
16. Tidswell EC. Bacterial adhesion: considerations within a risk-based approach to cleaning validation. PDA J Pharm Sci Technol 2005a; 59(1):10–32.
17. Anon. WHO Technical Report Series. Vol. 908. World Health Organization 2003:99–112.
18. Tidswell. Risk-based approaches facilitate expedient validations for control of microorganisms during equipment cleaning and hold. Am Pharm Rev 2005b; 8(6):28–33.
19. Anon. Analysis techniques for system reliability—Procedures for failure mode and effect analysis (FMEA). International Electronic Commission Geneva, Switzerland, ICE 812-1985, 1985.
20. Kieffer RG, Bureau S, Borgmann A. Applications of failure mode effect analysis in the pharmaceutical industry. Pharm Technol Eur 1997; September:36–49.
21. Sandle T. The use of risk assessment in the pharmaceutical industry application of FMEA to a sterility testing isolator: a case study. Eur J Parent Pharm Sci 2003; 8(2):43–49.
22. Whyte W, Eaton T. Microbiological contamination models for use in risk assessment during pharmaceutical production. Eur J Par Pharm Sci 2004; 9(1):11–15.
23. Whyte W. A cleanroom contamination control system. Eur J Parent Sci 2002; 7(2):55–61.
24. Anon. Hazard Analysis Critical Control Point Principles and Application Guidelines. National advisory committee on microbiological criteria for foods, US Food and Drug Administration, 1997.
25. Jahnke M. Use of the HACCP concept for risk analysis of pharmaceutical manufacturing process. Eur J Parent Sci 1997; 2(4):113–117.
26. Lovtrup S. Risk assessment in the manufacture of medical products based on design and barrier assessment (daBa). Eur J Parent Sci 2001; 6(2):53–57.
27. Jahnke M, Kuhn KD. Use of hazard analysis and critical control points (HACCP) risk assessment on a medical device for parenteral application. PDA J Pharm Sci Technol 2003; 57(1):32–42.

28. Lee PS, Plumlee B, Rymer T, Schwabe R, Hansen J.Using FMEA to develop alternatives to batch testing. Med Dev Diag Ind 2004; Jan: 148.

29. Simon PW, Hillson DA, Newland KE, eds. Project risk analysis and management (PRAM) guide. Bucks, UK: APM Group, 1997.

30. Anon. Risk management. Australian/New Zealand Standard AS/NZS 4360:1999. New Zealand: Standards Australian/Standards New Zealand. Homebush NSW, 1999.

31. Anon. Project management—part 2: vocabulary. British Standard BS6079-2:2000, British Standards Institute, London, UK, 2000b.

32. Anon. A Risk Management Standard. London, UK: Institute of risk management, 2002.

33. Eaton T. Microbial risk assessment for aseptically prepared products. Am Pharm Rev 2005; 8(5):46–51.

34. Ackers J, Agalloco J. Risk analysis for aseptic processing: the Ackers-Agalloco method. Pharam Technol 2005; 29(11):74–88.

35. Hillson DA. Assessing risk probability: alternative approaches. Proceeding of PMI global congress, Prague Czech Republic, 2004.

36. Williams KL. Endotoxins, Pyrogens, LAL Testing and Depyrogenation, ch 2. New York: Marcel Dekker Inc., 2001.

37. Vesper JL. Assessing and managing risk in a GMP environment. BioPharm Int 2005; 18(3):46–58.

38. Metropolis N, Ulam S. The Monte Carlo method. J Amer Stat Assoc 1949; 44:335–341.

39. Vose D. Quantitative Risk Analysis: a Guide to Monte Carlo Simulation Modeling. New York: John Wiley and Sons 1996.

9 Endotoxin as a Standard

Kevin L. Williams
Eli Lilly & Company, Indianapolis, Indiana, U.S.A.

If ever a material seemed ill suited for standardization, it is endotoxin. As a standard it has been domesticated, but not entirely tamed; captured from the wild, grown up in captivity on rich media; chemically groomed (by solvent extraction), and trained to behave in a somewhat civilized manner in modern assays. But, still it prances like a caged lion, back and forth, unable to escape its dual ampiphilic nature; unable to decide on the direction it should go in aqueous solution.

OVERVIEW AND DISCUSSION

If ever a material seemed ill-suited for standardization, it is endotoxin. As a standard, it has been domesticated, but not entirely tamed; captured from the wild, grown up in captivity on rich media, chemically groomed (by solvent extraction), and trained to behave in a somewhat civilized manner in modern assays. But still it prances like a caged lion, back and forth, unable to escape its dual amphiphilic nature; unable to decide on the direction it should go in aqueous solution. The hydrophobic end would much rather aggregate with ends of its own kind or stick to the plastic or glass of a test tube or container in which it resides (or parenteral closure to which it has been applied for depyrogenation validation) rather than mingle with water. Furthermore, the biological activity of endotoxin derived from different bacteria run the gamut from apyrogenic to highly pyrogenic (the extremes in variability holds true for endotoxicity also). Henderson et al. (1) claim that lipopolysaccharide (LPS) from commercial suppliers can contain up to 60% protein, which puts those preparations more in the realm of endotoxin than LPS. Indeed, laboratories select different endotoxins for different purposes (i.e., product testing standards vs. depyrogenation validation applications) given varying empirical recovery experiences.

The *United States Pharmacopeia* (USP) defines reference standards as "... substances selected for their high purity, critical characteristics, and suitability for the intended purpose" (2) and recognizes that "heterogeneous substances, of natural origin are also designated 'Reference Standards' where needed. Usually these are the counterparts of international standards." Furthermore, "as a rule, an International Standard for a material of natural origin is discontinued once the substance responsible for its characteristic activity has been isolated, identified, and prepared in such forms that it can be completely characterized by chemical and physical means"[a] (3). The process of international harmonization has currently borne fruit in that a single International Standard (IS) has been prepared and

---

[a]Though physical and chemically well characterized, endotoxin may be considered as less than completely characterized due to aggregation, heterogeneity, and the need for biological potency determination. A chosen lipid A standard might be considered better characterized, but its insoluble nature precludes its use as a standard in the water-based LAL method.

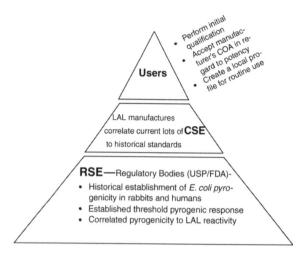

FIGURE 1 Foundation of endotoxin standardization.

accepted by the USP/FDA (USP G/EC-6), EP (European Pharmacopoeia Standard for Endotoxin called BRP-2), and World Health Organization (WHO[b]) (IS-2) as a single reference standard.[c] The harmonized standard along with the harmonized USP/Pharm Europa/JP Bacterial Endotoxin Test [USP Chapter 85, Second Supplement USP 24-NF 19, pp. 2875–2879 (effective July 1, 2000)] has greatly clarified the testing requirements for multinational pharmaceutical manufacturers who must meet what were previously multiple requirements.

Implied in the definition of a reference standard is the idea that the material serving as the standard broadly represents the material being referenced. However, with endotoxin this is not possible, as the endotoxic potency of different bacterial LPSs is known to vary widely. This does not mean that standard endotoxin poorly serves its purpose as a means of comparing the relative activity of unknown endotoxins in solution. It does mean, however, that (given the diversity of endotoxins in nature and their associated relative bioactivity and even the presence of nonendotoxin, but endotoxin-like active substances of microbial origin) the *Limulus* amebocyte lysate (LAL) test serves as an indicator of the presence of bioactive (almost exclusively gram negative) cellular residues and not an absolute predictor (or quantifier) of endotoxin content as a chemically defined mass. It seems somewhat incongruent that the specifications for product endotoxin concentrations can be mathematically determined to three decimal places (as can the test result), but the potency of any given standard (even the reference standard) is a composite value of a sometimes wide range of individual readings (i.e., refer to standard recovery range shown in Fig. 3 for IS-2).

In the early 1970s, when endotoxin standards were first used for LAL testing, LAL use was limited to industry in-process testing, with each company employing its own in-house standard. This standard was set by direct comparison with the established pyrogen assay being run routinely at the time as an FDA requirement.

---

[b]The laboratory for WHO is the National Institutes for Biological Standards and Controls (NIBSC) located in London.

[c]Dawson M. Harmonization of endotoxin standards and units. LAL User Group Meeting Minutes, Wilmington, Delaware, Oct 9, 1997 referred to IS-2 as "a harmonized standard for the Western world where USP = WHO = BP."

Such practices made it difficult for the FDA to compare result uniformity across different labs and to establish appropriate limits (4). Also confounding early attempts to produce meaningful and consistent LAL test results was the use of endotoxin weight as the unit of measurement. Concerned with the early confusion (1982) created by the continued use of an endotoxin's weight as a unit of activity, Outschoorn (5) of the USP urged users to switch to the more relevant unit of activity established with his help: the endotoxin unit (EU). The following paragraph underscores the ultimate importance of the establishment of the endotoxin official standard to the validity of the LAL assay results (6):

> The Bureau of Biologics, with long experience in the measurement of potency of various biologics, early defined an Endotoxin Unit. This can only mean, by definition, the activity contained in a stated amount of a particular preparation designated the U.S. Standard. It is amazing that in this day and age there are still endeavors to express endotoxin activities in weight of endotoxin. It is inescapable that equal weights of any two endotoxins are not necessarily possessed of equal potency, i.e., endotoxin activity, whether on lysates or in producing fever in rabbits or humans. Unfortunately, ... different types of articles have been evaluated with different endotoxin references. This is of little value unless the potency of these references is known in relation to their effects on humans. The least that might have been done was for any candidate references to have been compared with different lysates. The most logical way to express their relative potencies would be in relation to a single reference, i.e., in terms of the legal, defined U.S. Endotoxin Unit. The contention that valid comparisons of these different endotoxin references cannot be done with different lysates is not acceptable. If that is so, then the results of estimating endotoxin levels of pharmaceutical articles with lysate and in comparison with any endotoxin references is also not acceptable. This means that the test would then not be a valid alternative to the pyrogen test with rabbits ... The essential requirement of the official USP Bacterial Endotoxins Test for the application of the procedure for determining endotoxin limits was the provision of a characterized reference standard endotoxin (RSE).

The EU was, therefore, established as the activity of a specific endotoxin preparation (EC-2) (6) defined as one-fifth the amount of *Escherichia coli* (EC-2) endotoxin required to bring about the threshold pyrogenic response [1 ng/kg was already historically established as the threshold response level using *E. coli* in several studies beginning with Greisman and Hornick (7)] when injected into man and rabbits on a per kilogram basis. The EU thus established and defined as 0.2 ng of EC-2 expressed the biological activity of any given solution under test in terms of *E. coli* similarity. EC-2 became the measuring stick labeled as an EU against which any sample showing activity in the LAL test would be compared from here forward.

Since the days of widespread, pyrogen assay use a number of factors have served to redefine endotoxin (though endotoxin has not changed) as both a standard and natural phenomenon, including:

1. Development of an in vitro (LAL) test as a replacement of pyrogenicity as an in vivo test
2. The 10- to 1000-fold greater sensitivity[d] of the LAL assay as compared to the pyrogen assay (8)

---

[d]Consider the 5.0 EU/kg rabbit threshold pyrogenic response level of the assay multiplied by a 4 kg rabbit weight divided by a 10 mL dose of drug product as the "sensitivity" (2.0 EU/mL) of the pyrogen assay. Compare this value with LAL assay detection limits (lambda) of 0.06 to 0.001 EU/mL. This comparison gives an approximate range of 33- to 200-fold greater sensitivity for LAL testing.

3. The formation of units of measurement [EU; Insulin Unit, IU] based upon the standardized reactivity of endotoxin to the in vitro test in lieu of the weight (in nanograms) of the reactive material
4. The chemical definition of LPS: partial structures capable of bringing about a range of biological host responses (9,10)
5. The recognition of both natural and synthetic partial LPS structures that are not biologically active (11,12)
6. The identification of nontoxic "endotoxins" from some gram-negative bacteria (13,14)
7. The description of *Legionnella* bacteria that are highly endotoxic as gauged via LAL and only very weakly pyrogenic (15,16), thus further refining or clouding (depending on one's view) the practical definition of "endotoxin"
8. The determination that some partial LPS structures and nontoxic endotoxins can act as competitive antagonists of toxic LPS (13,14,17) [glucan has also been found to be capable of attenuating LPS toxicity (18)]
9. The identification of microbial substances with "endotoxin-like" activity (at least in LAL reactivity) including β-glucan, peptidoglycan (Chapter 5), and even an algae mentioned previously (19) as having LAL activity

Different extraction methods of LPS yield varying mixtures in terms of purity and biological activity (20). Each extraction yields impurities to some extent including a mixture of nucleic acids, glycans, and proteins and phospholipids from the cellular wall. In contrast to Outschoorn, Jack Levin weighs the dilemma created by the necessity of calling a specific endotoxin or a specific assay, "the standard":

> The variety of bioassays for endotoxins, and the variability of endotoxins, i.e., their physical structure, chemical composition, solubility, and particulate nature, should prepare us to anticipate that different assays may produce different results (21).

This is a surprising admission to what many believe to be true in practice but are reluctant to admit openly with much confidence. Levin points out that the very definition of endotoxin has relied upon the use of different methods of its detection. By such practical definitions, the term "pyrogen" has become (erroneously) synonymous with the term "endotoxin":

> ... definitions are operational. Pyrogenicity is the way endotoxin has been defined in the past because of the assay that was used, but we now (1981) have to seriously consider that a new definition of endotoxin as necessarily being pyrogenic may not always be appropriate (21).

The importance of a positive test in the model being used (pyrogen, LAL assay, or a cytokine assay) should be its ability to predict the occurrence of the adverse biological effects for which the assay was designed to guard against rather than serving to restrict the definition of a deleterious host response. Levin says it best:

> It is possible that the *Limulus* test measures a more important function of bacterial endotoxin, i.e., its ability to activate various enzymatic systems (other examples are the mammalian coagulation, complement, and kallikrein systems), inappropriate activation of which can produce pathophysiological effects and cause death. A definition of endotoxin based on a positive Limulus test may be of greater importance than whether it is pyrogenic. One is often bound by historical precedent; diseases and materials previously have been inappropriately defined by the first available test (21).

Along those lines, a more currently appreciated difference between the concept of a "pyrogen" and that of a nonpyrogenic substance may be only a matter of degree in that the pyrogen produces a level of systemic change that affects the entire organism whereas a nonpyrogen may produce the very same effects on a local (cellular or molecular) level (absent one indicator of a systemic response: fever).

Cooper relates a story of an international meeting held in Brussels many years ago to consider the then daunting task of replacing the rabbit pyrogen test with the LAL test. After much-heated debate, a French spokesman and LAL proponent commented that the rabbit pyrogen test would still be only a *proposal* if it had been subjected to the same degree of scrutiny as the LAL test was incurring (22). An apparent contradiction in the historical opposition to the adoption of LAL as a substitute for the rabbit pyrogen assay lies in the argument that LAL fell short as a parenteral assay due to the lack of coverage of the all classes of pyrogens, yet today the LAL assay is criticized because it is not wholly specific to endotoxin but can also react to β-glucans and other carbohydrates of microbial origin (23). This raises the question, should a parenteral assay for pyrogens be a general assay to include as wide a variety as possible of potential pyrogens or should it be specific for what is believed to be the "worst case" pyrogen: endotoxin? Clearly, the question is a dormant one in that the LAL test has fully assumed the role.

The definition of endotoxin has been and most likely will be further modified by newer methods of testing. Such a change from the "old" endotoxin to the "new" endotoxin will always beg the question (as it had in the switch from the rabbit pyrogen to LAL assay) in the case of a dispute "which is the real endotoxin?" Asked in another way, which test of those becoming more practically available (Chapter 12) will provide the truest predictor of the human responses that are being guarded against and, perhaps more importantly, exactly which of the many responses now recognized are being guarded against if not just fever? Here again there are no definitive answers.

Although elaborate methods have been developed in some cases to circumvent the β-glucan pathway (24,25), it has not been found to be a necessary precaution (or a widespread occurrence) in day-to-day pharmaceutical quality control testing. Perhaps manufacturers of drugs targeting specific indications such as hemodialysis and AIDS (26) patients, or patients with systemic fungal infections (27,28) in which β-glucan is a specific disease marker may find the exclusion of β-glucan a desirable (if not necessary) goal. Various researchers have explored the use of sensitive (though time consuming and costly) biotechnology tests to detect contaminants that induce cytokine production as an alternative to pyrogen or LAL reactivity (29). Here is another instance in which the information becoming available in performing a test (given the explosion of immunological and biotechnology techniques) may outgrow, if it has not already, industry and regulatory ability to assimilate and apply the information meaningfully.

THE CHANGING FACE OF ENDOTOXIN

Historically implied in the very definition of endotoxin is the fact that it is derived from gram-negative organisms. While this is still true, there have been recent discoveries of both nontoxic gram-negative LPS and toxic, endotoxin or endotoxin-like molecules isolated from other, sometimes distinctly unrelated (to gram negatives) organism types, such as the eukaryotic *Chlorella*-like green algae (19). A few recent discoveries serve to illustrate the point that the concept of endotoxin as a functional structure is subject to revision. LPS from many gram-negative photosynthetic bacteria have Lipid A structures differing significantly from the typical structure (Enterobactereaceae). These photosynthetic bacterial structures lack endotoxicity and Galanos (30) has considered that these structures may be excluded from the class of "endotoxins" simply because they are not toxic. Therefore, to complicate our early definitions we now know that all endotoxins are LPS, but not all LPSs are endotoxins due to the lack of associated toxicity. (See Chapter 6 on LPS heterogeneity.)

Royce and Pardy (19) determined that the (rare nongram negative) extracted LPS isolated from the eukaryotic, unicellular, symbiotic algae (*Chlorella*) was as endotoxic as enteric LPS as determined by LAL gelation and otherwise indistinguishable from endotoxin by a battery of confirmatory tests including the presence of 2-keto-3-deoxyoctonic (an unusual core sugar in gram-negative LPS). The LPS or LPS-like material was extracted via hot phenol–water treatment followed by acid hydrolysis of the purified extract to yield a precipitate with characteristics of lipid A including the tell-tale acyl groups: 3-hydroxylauric and 3-hydroxymyristic acids identified by gas chromatography. LAL reactivity was greatly reduced by incubation with polymyxin B sulfate and *Limulus* endotoxin-neutralizing protein, two proven neutralizers of gram-negative bacterial endotoxin. Extreme precautions were taken to prevent the likelihood of endotoxin contamination in these studies.

The increased number of choices available to identify and quantitate various host responses and the compounds that bring them about [including cytokine tests and gas chromatography and mass spectroscopy (GC-MS)] point to the luxury of refining and choosing more accurate predictors of adverse host events in parenteral solutions (as specific events dictate), either by (*i*) including nonendotoxin markers of potential contamination (such as peptidoglycan and β-glucan) or (*ii*) by excluding LAL reactive components believed to be insignificant (also β-glucan) for a given drug application. In the former case, an experimental method using silk worm (*Bombyx mori*) larvae plasma (SLP) (31,32) has shown some early promise as a sensitive (ng/mL) indicator of peptidoglycan in both gram-positive and gram-negative organisms. SLP is reminiscent of the LAL test in that it is a blood product derived from the blood of a primitive animal. SLP is being looked at as a rapid method in diagnosing meningitis, which was one of the early uses of the LAL test (33). In the case of β-glucan, LAL activity serves as a current example of the refinement of the working definition of endotoxin.

The LAL-active, nonendotoxic substance, β-glucan, has generated some controversy (33). The reactivity of LAL previously believed to be specific to endotoxin has been shown also to react to β-glucans, though LAL-β-glucan interactions have been found to be quantitatively inconsistent as compared to endotoxin in the LAL reaction. Zhang et al. (25) demonstrated that different LAL preparations show much greater variation in assaying β-glucan than in assaying endotoxin. The FDA has left it largely up to the user to accept or reject the occurrence of β-glucans in their product (Chapter 10), but has stated that it is incumbent on the user to prove that such activity is not the result of endotoxin. β-glucan has served here as an example of a nonendotoxin LAL active exception that has been discovered, but it is proving to be only one of many microbial substances now known to evoke mammalian host responses (34–41) (Chapter 5, Table 1).

The point of exploring such exceptions in a discussion of endotoxin standards is that they may serve to refine our concept of "endotoxicity" to include substances that are not endotoxin but the activity of which may be observed via the LAL test (host active microbial membranes) and may lead to the further exploration into alternate methods to encompass such changing definitions. However, such exceptions may, in the end, serve primarily to illuminate the existence of the general rule: endotoxicity generally relates to pyrogenicity and both the rabbit and LAL models correlate as predictors of human febrile and inflammatory response and primarily associated with the presence of the major pyrogen: endotoxin. Such a rule has served industry and the public health faithfully for decades and, though exceptions are being discovered, the rule is in no immediate danger of failing due to an explosion in knowledge of the details. Perhaps, the knowledge of the details can be used to the advantage of certain patient groups.

Short of testing every vial leaving the parenteral manufacturing facility in human subjects, some assumptions (compromises) must be accepted in arriving at a given quality control assay. Assumptions inherent in any chosen endotoxin test include:

1. The endotoxin used as a standard bridges the gap (i.e., can be realistically related to the biological activity brought about by endogenous endotoxin) from potential environmental contaminants to the threshold pyrogenic dose (TPD) as defined by a reference bacterial endotoxin (*E. coli*).
2. The method chosen as an assay correlates as an appropriate predictor of the appropriate deleterious host effect(s), be it fever, cytokine production, etc.
3. The appropriate biological host response is being selected, analytically detected, and thus guarded against in parenteral manufacturing.

As a team of parenteral scientists at Genentech found (42), a situation can conceivably occur in which an "atypical" parenteral solution contains an "atypical" endotoxin or responds "atypically" to a given assay (pyrogen, LAL, or both), but provides a "typical" pyrogenic response in human subjects. This particular instance involved the chemical modification of endotoxin by lyophilization in glycine–phosphate buffer that reduced by 10- to 20-fold the in vivo and in vitro model recovery but not the system being modeled (i.e., recovery in humans) during a clinical trial. In this manner, the redefining of what constitutes "endotoxin" perhaps will be modified in the future to prevent the occurrence of hazards yet poorly understood.

THRESHOLD PYROGENIC DOSE

Closely tied to the concept of a "standard" endotoxin is the idea of a TPD for such a standard endotoxin. The establishment of a defined, specific endotoxic level has allowed the concept to be established that a certain amount of endotoxin is allowable and a certain amount of endotoxin should not be delivered into the bloodstream or cerebrospinal fluid. The advent of LAL allowed the quantitation of endotoxin as a contaminant. In turn, quantitation has allowed for the creation of specific and relevant endotoxin limits for manufactured drug products, raw materials, active ingredients, devices, components, depyrogenation processes, and in-process samples that constitute the legal requirement for releasing to market products that are not considered "adulterated" by the US FDA.

Today's user of the LAL test rightly views such concepts as the bread and butter of endotoxin testing, but it is good to appreciate the degree to which today's system of endotoxin quantitation has progressed, in that

1. "Quantification" in the rabbit assay was limited to a pass/fail response (rabbit response = 0.6°C temperature rise);
2. The pyrogen test was initially established without attempting to quantify the amount of endotoxin necessary to produce a febrile response;
3. Early LAL testing used the weight of dried bacterial endotoxins in nanograms first with various gram-negative organisms, then with a specific strain of *E. coli*.

None of the early tests could have been used effectively to develop product specific tolerance limits (TLs) as they exist today, much less provide the degree of in-process control needed for modern pharmaceutical and biotechnology manufacturing contamination control. In some respects, the 10- to 1000-fold greater sensitivity of the LAL test created the "luxury" of controversy on several fronts. A whole new system of relating the new assay to the existing test had to be developed to avoid unnecessary product test failures due to the greater sensitivity of the LAL assay (43). The "system" included the formation of or association with:

1. The EU as a measure of relative biological activity
2. The TL (endotoxin limit concentration)
3. The maximum valid dilution to relate the product dose to the allowable endotoxin content (realizing that a positive LAL response in any given solution as in the pyrogen assay would be inappropriately stringent)
4. The lysate sensitivity (lambda) to standardize the relative reactivity of each LAL to each control standard endotoxin (CSE) (Fig. 2)

Prior to this "system" several of the principals of the early LAL assay expressed concern that the greater sensitivity of the assay would end up becoming an apparent disadvantage used by some to confound industry efforts to develop the assay as a replacement for the rabbit pyrogen test. ["I hope that we do not turn the advantage provided by the greater sensitivity of the Limulus test into a problem"—Jack Levin (21)].

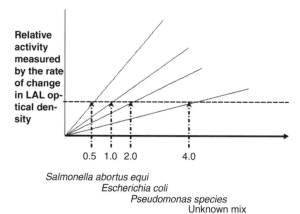

Relative activity measured by the rate of change in LAL optical density

0.5 1.0 2.0   4.0

Salmonella abortus equi
Escherichia coli
Pseudomonas species
Unknown mix

FIGURE 2   Relative pyrogenicity/endotoxicity (threshold pyrogenic dose) of various gram-negative bacteria as compared to the chosen standard (*E. coli*) on a weight basis (ng/kg). *Abbreviation:* LAL, *Limulus* amebocyte lysate.

HISTORICAL PYROGEN STANDARDS

Although, the TPD per kilogram body weight is virtually identical for human and rabbit, the dose–response relationship for the human is steeper than it is for the rabbit. At doses considerably higher than the threshold dose, humans respond to endotoxin more vigorously than do rabbits. This premise allowed the USP rabbit pyrogen test to be used as a valid predictor of pyrogenic risk for humans. Historically, there have been four widely used endotoxin (pyrogen) preparations including *Shigella dysenteriae, E. coli* 0113:H10: KO(EC), *E. coli 055:B5*, and *Salmonella abortus equi* (Table 1). Researchers realized early on that bacterial endotoxins from different species differed greatly in potency on a weight basis (44). The TPD in humans and rabbits was first shown to be between 0.1 and 0.14 ng/kg for *S. typhosa*, 1.0 ng/kg for *E. coli*, and 50 to 70 ng/kg for *Pseudomonas* by Greisman and Hornick (7) (Fig. 3). The low pyrogenic dose reported in this study for *S. typhosa* (as well as other studies on purified endotoxin) was based on a highly purified endotoxin preparation that bears little, if any, resemblance to the muted pyrogenicity encountered with naturally occurring endotoxins found in pharmaceutical manufacturing environments. Pearson in the first edition of this book gives a detailed history of the development of the early pyrogen standards, which has been summarized in Table 1.

ENDOTOXIN STANDARDS SINCE THE ADVENT OF LAL TESTING

In the early 1970s, the medical community began using LAL to diagnose septicemia, meningitis, and urinary tract infections (44) without regulatory guidance around the time the pharmaceutical industry began to use LAL for in-process testing. Because LAL was a blood product, Bureau of Biologics (BoB), a branch of the FDA, published the first reference to the LAL test in the *Federal Register* (1973) (45). The referenced made clear that LAL was a blood product subject to license requirements and drugs must continue to tested by the pyrogen test (i.e., the LAL test had not been shown to be a suitable replacement). The 1973 *Federal Register* reference allowed the use of nonlicensed LAL with the following preconditions:

1. Testing with LAL be limited to in-process testing of drugs and other products
2. Those using it would do so voluntarily
3. The LAL label state that it was not a suitable replacement for the rabbit pyrogen test

The FDA was aware of the variable potencies associated with different endotoxin preparations and decided that a suitable standard endotoxin was needed. A bulk endotoxin, *E. coli* 0113:H10K from Dr. J.A. Rudbach at the University of Montana (44), was prepared by Westphal extraction, and lyophilized with 0.1% normal serum human albumin and called "EC-1" (44). The particular strain chosen (*E. coli* 0113, Braude strain) was important for several reasons.

1. It did not contain dideoxyhexose present in many enteric endotoxins, thus allowing (if necessary) it to be quantified by a chemical test in which ketodeoxyoctulosonic acid is detected directly with periodate-thiobarbituric acid in the absence of interfering chromogen generated from dideoxyhexoses (46).

TABLE 1 Historical Pyrogen Standards

Standard organism	*Shigella dysenteriae*	*E. coli* 055 : B5	*E. coli* 0113 : H10 : KO (EC)	*Salmonella abortus equi*
Extraction method	Acetone-dried cells extracted with diethylene glycol and ppt. by fractional treatment with ammonium sulfate Phospholipids removed with acidic ether ethanol. Sediment collected between 25,000 and 105,000×g	Extracted from *E. coli* as per Boivin (trichloro-acetic) or Westphal extraction) Commercially available from Difco Labora-tories	Rudbach et al. (65) prepared initially using Westphal phenol-extraction; KO = capsule negative	Extracted using Westphal phenol–water and re-extracted using phenol, chloroform, and petroleum ether. End product is a uniform sodium salt (66)
Pros	Highly purified and chemically characterized	Low lot-to-lot variability in LAL test; homogeneous Same biological activity as official standard	Extensively studied in various biological systems	Relatively water soluble; more purified than the *E. coli* standards
Cons	Potency variable from 1 : 1 to 20 : 1 (67)	Not selected as the USP/FDA reference standard	Contains additives of 2% lactose and 2% polyethylene glycol 6000 (68)	Significantly more potent than EC standards
Notable	Developed in 1956 for WHO by Davies of Microbiological Research Dept., England (67) National Institute for Medical Research (London) used to create the world's first pyrogen standard in 1957	Selected by the HIMA as its first standard for devices after a collaborative study (4); replaced in 1987 by EC-5 as per FDA Guideline on Validation.	Used to define EU in 1981 by assigning a unit value of 5.0 EU/ng to EC-2 (69)	Salmonella O-antigens are the most extensively studied Distributed as Novo Pyrexal by Hermal Chemie, Kurt Hermann, Hamburg, West Germany
Relative potency[a]	3.28 EU/kg (70)	1 ng/kg (71)	1 ng/kg	0.56 ng/kg (72)
Comment	Not now used	Common CSE	USP/FDA EC line	Formerly "Pyrexal"

[a]As measured by the amount producing a marginal USP rabbit pyrogen failure.
Abbreviations: CSE, control standard endotoxin; EC, *Escherichia coli*; EU, Endotoxin Unit; FDA, Food and Drug Administration; LAL, *Limulus* amebocyte lysate; USP, *United States Pharmacopeia*.
Source: From Ref. 73.

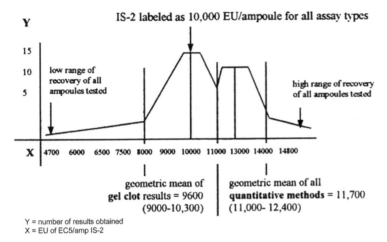

FIGURE 3 The range of geometric means and the grouping of results for all valid gelation and photometric assays as *n* (number of assays) versus Endotoxin Unit (EU) of EC5 per ampule of candidate standard in an approximate manner is shown.

2. The given strain is K negative and, therefore, incapable of forming capsular protein that could end up contaminating the lot.
3. The strain was already known to remain stable for decades (47).

Firca and Rudbach describe the criteria that were used at the time to select a suitable "reference standard endotoxin." It was decided that such an endotoxin should be from a "typical" bacterial species (47). Other properties deemed desirable included:

1. A dry preparation
2. Available in large quantities
3. Stable at room temperature
4. Only slightly hygroscopic
5. Readily soluble in water
6. A clear solution
7. Potency tested in man and rabbits

A number of criticisms were put forward at the time. The major criticisms included the fact that the standard was not "pure" lipid A for which the chemical formula had been defined and the fact that other, more potent endotoxins, were available. The criticism concerning the purity of the endotoxin was discounted due to the need for a readily soluble standard (lipid A being insoluble). The goal of obtaining a reference endotoxin free of biologically active proteins, peptides, polynucleotides, and polysaccharides had been achieved (47). As for the potency of the new endotoxin reference standard, it was believed that an "average" potency would be more relevant to the testing of a wide range of endotoxins, with a range of potencies, likely to be encountered in real world testing.

EC-1 was established in 1976. A larger batch was prepared after EC-1 consisting of vials containing 1 μg of endotoxin. This lot (1500 vials), designated EC-2, was assigned a potency of 5 EU/ng or 5000 EU/vial (40,47,48) based on a collaborative study undertaken by the Office of Biologics and the three LAL manufacturers that existed then. At this time, the EU was defined as 0.2 ng of EC-2. EC-2 was stabilized with albumin in an attempt to decrease the variable potency observed with EC-1 and served as the official reference for the United States until July 1, 1980. The convention of using EUs has endured in LAL testing usage as has the use of the TPD to determine end product release limits of 0.5 EU/mL or 5.0 EU/kg for devices and drugs, respectively. The exceptions are intrathecals and radiopharmaceuticals, which involve more restrictive limits. The use of EUs has enabled the replacement of an original reference lot with subsequent lots (secondary standards or control standards) that can be related to the original reference by the assignment of an appropriate potency value.

Lots EC-3 and EC-4 later filled in 1979 and 1980, respectively, were small lots prepared without fillers in response to hypothetical concerns that the serum albumin might bind endotoxin in some products (44). EC-3 was thrown out altogether because of insufficient activity. EC-4 was filled and significant variation from EC-2 was noted by a number of researchers and LAL manufacturers. Preliminary results of a collaborative study conducted by Health Industry Manufacturers Association (HIMA) indicate that EC-4 was four times less potent than EC-2. However, for both EC-2 and EC-4, pooled vial-to-vial variance was insignificant. Because most EC-4 vials presented problems to lysate and pharmaceutical manufacturers, an EC-5 preparation was filled during the first quarter of 1981 (44).

EC-5 was contracted for production by a licensed LAL manufacturer according to USP and BoB criteria, which included lactose and polyethylene glycol (44). The 28,000 to 30,000 vials of EC-5 were determined to be 2.1 times more potent than EC-2. The labeled potency was rounded to 10,000 EU/vial and divided between the USP and the Office of Biologics (OB) (now called Center for Biologics Evaluation and Research). The EC-5 preparation was evaluated by 14 laboratories in a collaborative effort to establish its relative potency as compared with EC-2. The geometric mean ratios of end points of EC-5 to EC-2 were calculated for each LAL reagent used. Data from only nine of the laboratories was deemed suitable to be included in the study tabulations. For each of the lysate groups, the results from all laboratories were combined and a ± 25.0 range (95% confidence limits) was established. The overall relative potency was determined to be 2.10. This figure was rounded to 2.0, providing EC-5 an assigned potency of 10,000 EU/ vial, a potency two times that established for EC-2 (44). The USP labeled and sold EC-5 as USP-F. EC-5 has lasted until 1997 when the current endotoxin reference standard was produced (EC-6, USP-G).

CORRELATION OF THE RABBIT PYROGEN AND LAL
TEST STANDARD ACTIVITY

An underlying assumption of the modern LAL test lies in its acceptable correlation to its historical predecessor: the rabbit pyrogen test (Chapter 12). Not much time has been taken here to draw up a convincing argument for accepting such a correlation because it seems moot at this point given that the bacterial endotoxin testing is referenced in some 500-plus USP monographs (see Outschoorn's comments). Furthermore, as Levin has said, perhaps LAL reactivity is not necessarily equivalent (in every way) but is a truer measure of a more significant host response (especially given that the sensitivity allows for the subsystemic detection of endotoxin contamination-unlike pyrogenicity). Some poor correlation exceptions have been alluded to but the rule of equivalence at the threshold level using *E. coli* endotoxin is well established. For review, some references include papers by Cooper (49), Tomasulo (50,51), Elin (52), Weary (53), Muller-Calgan (54), and Pearson (55).

MEDICAL DEVICE STANDARDS

Prior to the current (1987) FDA Guideline on Validation (45), the endotoxin standards used for drugs and devices were different. The designation of different endotoxins as standards resulted from administrative determinations made by the two different FDA bureaus involved. The choice of the *E. coli* 055:B5 preparation by the Bureau of Medical Devices was the result of a cooperative effort between the bureau and the members of the medical device industry for the express purpose of developing guidelines for using the LAL test with medical devices. At a later date, the Bureaus of Drugs, Veterinary Medicine, and Biologics initiated their combined effort to develop LAL guideline for human drugs, veterinary drugs, and biologicals. These bureaus later decided to use the U.S. RSE developed by the OB. The decision was based on available data and experience with RSE use by the OB. After sufficient experience with the RSE was gained, the EC-5 standard was applied to devices (as a single agency became responsible for both drugs and devices). However, regardless of the RSE assignment, *E. coli* 055:B5 preparations continued (and continue still) to be commonly used as CSEs in gel-clot and kinetic assays for both drugs and devices. The only caveat is that of successful qualification as a CSE against the RSE.

Another difference in the guidelines for drugs and devices is that endotoxin limits are expressed in different terms. The endotoxin limit for human and veterinary drugs is expressed as a concentration of endotoxin per unit of product as per the route of administration. The limit for devices is expressed as a concentration of *E. coli* endotoxin per milliliter of rinse. When both limits are expressed in terms of the rabbit dose of endotoxin allowed per kilogram of body weight or in terms of total EUs per person (5 EU/kg × 70 kg/person = 350 EU/person), they are predicated upon the same threshold pyrogenic response values (depending again upon the route of drug or device administration).

The test solution employed in the LAL test procedure contributes to the difference in how the limits are expressed. In the case of drugs, the test solution is either the actual drug product or a dilution of the drug product. In this situation, the amount of endotoxin allowed can always be related to some quantity of the drug product, such as milligram, milliliter, or drug unit (i.e., IU). This is not the case for devices for which the test solution represents a composite of rinsings from a number of production devices. Due to the diversity of devices involved, the volume of the rinse solutions and the number of units represented in the composite vary. To specify an endotoxin limit that could be applied to all devices, the Bureau of Medical Devices adopted the TPD of 1.0 ng/kg (5 EU/kg). This relates to the test dose volume of 10 mL/kg for the rabbit test, which is the common factor for all devices.

The FDA Guideline on Validation of the LAL Test (45) describes the standard recommendations of the HIMA Collaborative Study in the section "General Requirements":

> The CDRH has reviewed the results of the HIMA Collaborative Study for the Pyrogenicity Evaluation of a Reference Endotoxin by the USP Rabbit Test. This study recommends 0.1 ng/mL (10 mL/kg) of *E. coli* 055:B5 endotoxin from Difco Laboratories as the level of endotoxin, which should be detectable in the LAL test when used for end

product testing of medical devices. This sensitivity (0.1 ng/mL given 10 mL/kg) is sufficient for LAL testing and for retest of devices in rabbits. According to recent collaborative studies in the rabbit pyrogen and LAL tests, 1 ng of *E. coli* 055:B5 endotoxin is similar in potency to 5 EU of the USP Endotoxin Reference Standard. The endotoxin limit for medical devices has been converted to EU and is now 0.5 EU/mL using the rinse volume recommended in Section 2 .... Liquid devices should be more appropriately validated and tested according to the requirements for drugs by taking the maximum human dose per kilogram of body weight per hour into consideration ....

Manufacturers may retest LAL test failures with the LAL test or a USP rabbit pyrogen test. If the endotoxin level in a device eluate has been quantitated by LAL at 0.5 EU/mL endotoxin or greater, then retest in rabbits is not appropriate. Medical devices that contact cerebrospinal fluid should have less than 0.06 EU/mL of endotoxin. These values correspond to those set by the CBER for intrathecal drugs. Manufacturers shall use an LAL reagent licensed by OBRR in all validation, in-process, and end product LAL tests.

HARMONIZATION: THE SECOND INTERNATIONAL STANDARD FOR ENDOTOXIN

As recently as the late 1990s, there have been as many as five different official international standards (IS) active at once (56). For an international manufacturer, this meant either the construction of a singe test designed to overlap all the test requirements, including the use of a control standard calibrated against each official reference standard or the performance of multiple testing of each lot of drug material. An initial IS for endotoxin testing was established by the WHO's Expert Committee on Biological Standardization (ECBS) in 1987 (57). The first IS was calibrated against the U.S. national standard, EC5. However, the potency assignments for the semiquantitative LAL gel-clot and photometric tests did not agree. Most of the collaborative data consisted of gel-clot testing; therefore, the ECBS of WHO assigned IS-1 as a gel-clot standard (58). The assigned potency was 14,000 IU/ampule.

In 1994, the ECBS of WHO acknowledged that the use of the photometric tests (end point and kinetic chromogenic and turbidimetric) had greatly grown in terms of the number of LAL users since IS-1 was established and recognized the need for a common standard for both gelation and photometric tests (59). The USP made available 4000 vials of a batch of USP-G/EC-6 for the proposed WHO Second International Collaborative Study. The stage was, therefore, set for a comprehensive study organized by the WHO involving the United States, European, and Japanese pharmacopoeias.

Poole et al. (59) describe the ambitious aims of the study.

1. Calibrate the IS as compared to EC5 (USP-F) (although superseded by EC6 it was the primary calibrant for IS-1 and the JP reference standard) and assign a single IS unit for all endotoxin applications.
2. Compare the current IS (IS-1), EC5, and the candidate standard (CS) using LAL gelation, kinetic, and end point assays (chromogenic and turbidimetric).
3. Determine the relationship of IU to EU.
4. Compare the CS to the United States, European (BRP-2), and Japanese reference standards.

TABLE 2 Results of World Health Organization International Standard-2 Collaborative Study

Assay type	Mean recovery	No. of tests (n)
Gelation assay	10,300 EU/vial	103
Kinetic chromogenic assays	11,700 EU/vial	13
Kinetic turbidimetric assays	11,800 EU/vial	11
Chromogenic end point assays	11,200 EU/vial	3
All assays (gel and photometric)	10,400 EU/vial	68
IS-2 assigned value	10,000 IU/vial	

Abbreviations: EU, Endotoxin Unit; IS, International Standard.

A common lysate (supplied by Associates of Cape Cod) was used in 24 laboratories using the for two assays and an "in house" lysate (i.e., whatever was already being used in that laboratory). In all, the 24 laboratories performed a total of 108 gel-clot assays (620 individual preparations) and 133 photometric assays were performed using end point chromogenic (three labs), kinetic chromogenic (13 labs), and kinetic turbidimetric (12 labs). In the gel-clot tests, the geometric mean for the CS sublots did not differ significantly from one another from laboratory to laboratory or from LAL to LAL reagent source (59).

The CS geometric mean result for each assay type obtained in terms of EC5 is shown in Table 2.

RELATING CONTROL STANDARD ENDOTOXIN TO REFERENCE STANDARD ENDOTOXIN

LAL manufacturers, who correlate the current control standard to the current lots of LAL they routinely manufacture, supply certificates of acceptance (COA) to support the use of specific CSE/LAL combinations. The certificates demonstrate that the CSEs have been tested and shown to agree with the appropriate reference standard(s). Drug manufacturers may either accept the COAs supplied by performing an acceptable qualification test as per the appropriate method (i.e., gel-clot, kinetic turbidimetric, etc.) or confirm the RSE/CSE test by comparison with the current reference standard(s) followed by an acceptable qualification test. Agreement of a CSE within a two-fold of the lambda label-claim in the gel-clot test confirms the label claim. For routine reference, a local reference standard protocol (LRSP) is created in the Lilly laboratory to reference the qualification test documentation and to document the correct standard dilutions to be performed on a routine basis (see Appendix B). Kinetic testing requires recovery of a valid standard control curve using the Initial Qualification reader software template that does not average standard values in determining curve point acceptability (as do routine and inhibition/enhancement standard curves) to meet the requirements of the 1991 Interium Guideline. The complexity of standardizing a CSE against multiple reference standards has recently been greatly reduced by the adoption of a single harmonized standard.

STANDARDS OF THE FUTURE

The two most significant changes in the past 15 years in terms of the standardization of endotoxin has been (*i*) the production of more consistent successors to the originally standardized preparations of RSE, CSE, and LAL and (*ii*) the recent agreement on an international scale of an official harmonized endotoxin test and RSE. A significant drawback to purified LPS has always been the stickiness of the preparation given its hydrophobic nature. The fact that such solutions stick tenaciously to glass and plastic tubing is a presumed cause of much variation and can limit the utility of automation applications and confound attempts to validate depyrogenation processes. The stickiness of LPS also contrasts in this regard with naturally occurring endotoxin that remains in solution better due to a variety of attached cellular residues. One LAL manufacturer (Cambrex, Inc.) has developed a proprietary CSE that they supply in liquid form [Liquid Endotoxin Standards, LES™ (60)]. Presumably, Cambrex has employed LES or some resulting version of it in their PyroSense™ in-line water-testing robot as well (Chapter 16).

If new methods of endotoxin detection gain acceptance they will bring with them their own standards, however, none are clearly in sight at this time and the PyroGene® rFC application uses the existing CSE. An original objection to the choice of *E. coli* endotoxin as an LAL test reference standard was that its structure was not entirely known and it was not wholly purified down to the part of the structure that was known to be endotoxic (lipid A). Another complaint, curiously and diametrically opposed to the first, was that it was not of a broad enough spectrum to represent the whole of endotoxins and, alternatively, was not the most potent endotoxin found. Given the advances in defining the "endotoxic complex" (the necessary components of lipid A required to bring about the host effects of endotoxin) by Reitschel (Chapter 4) and others (as well as the characterization of nontoxic endotoxins) it is possible that other "markers" (peptidoglycan as a constituent of gram-positive and gram-negative cellular envelope residues) or "submarkers" (lipid A itself being a marker) could be used in the future for sophisticated endotoxin screening by chemical or alternate biomarker detection methods.

As an example, β-hydroxymyristic acid (among other lipid A 3 OH-fatty acids) has been identified as a constituent present in endotoxic LPS molecules and can be detected (to levels comparable to the LAL assay) by GC-MS detector (Chapter 16) [even the use of a double MS detector, GC-MS-MS, used for the detection of muramic acid as a marker for peptidoglycan (61)]. Researchers have made use of the β-hydroxymyristic acid marker (with its known molecular weight of 315.4 Da) to confirm the presence of endotoxin in ambiguous solutions such as those suspected of causing nonspecific LAL activation (61) or in clinical applications such as the detection of meningococcal endotoxin in plasma, which often provides a complex interfering matrix for the LAL test (62). A purely chemical marker (as opposed to an activity based assay) can give the user definitive confirmation of the presence of endotoxin at sensitive levels. Markers detected thus have been described as finding a specific "needle in a haystack" of microbial components (J. Patrick, personal communication, 2000) or, alternatively, as finding a specific needle in a haystack of needles.

Laude-Sharp et al. (63) have expressed open distrust of using LAL solely as a means of determining the presence of endotoxin in a clinical setting based upon their studies. The researchers used organisms (LPS purified from *Neisseria meningitidis*, *Pseudomonas cepacia*, and *P. testosteroni*) isolated from clinically used bicarbonate dialyzate. They demonstrated a lack of correlation between LAL testing results and interlukins-1 (IL-1) induction capacity in serum-free cultured human monocytes. The molecular weight of the endotoxin aggregates was a critical parameter of both IL-1 induction and LAL reactivity. Only LPS that exceeded 8000 Da were detectable by LAL assay, whereas LPS monomers with molecular weights below 3000 induced IL-1 production. The study is significant because the LAL test is used, according to the authors, to provide proof that fever and IL-1 production after hemodialysis is not caused by passage of LPS through dialysis membranes. Their study points out that LAL used previously in some studies to demonstrate that LPS cannot pass through such filters perhaps cannot detect the LPS most likely to pass through, that of low molecular weight aggregates (<8000 Da). In the context of standard LPS, the chosen reagent and method (LAL) used to demonstrate or validate the testing of these filters was clearly inappropriate and, in retrospect, should have included some low molecular weight endotoxins combined with alternative mechanisms of detection.

APPENDIX A

This appendix is an extract from the FDA's Guideline on Validation (73).

Determination of the Relationship Between the Control Standard Endotoxin and the Reference Standard Endotoxin

If a manufacturer chooses to use an endotoxin preparation (CSE) other than the United States Pharmacopeia Reference Standard Endotoxin (RSE), the CSE will have to be standardized against the RSE. If the CSE is not a commercial preparation which has been adequately characterized, it should be studied and fully characterized as to uniformity, stability of the preparation, etc. The relationship of the CSE to the RSE should be determined prior to use of a new lot, sensitivity, or manufacturer of the LAI or a new lot source or manufacturer of the CSE.

Gel-Clot Technique

The following is an example of a procedure to determine the relationship of the CSE to the RSE:

At least 4 samples (vials) for the lot of CSE should be assayed. State in ng/mL the end point for the CSE and in EU/rnL of the RSE. The values obtained should be the geometric mean of the end points using a minimum of 4 replicates.

Example: LAL end points for the RSE and CSE are as follows:

RSE = 0.3 EU/mL
CSE = 0.018 ng/mL

The EUs per ng of CSE are calculated as follows:

RSE = 0.3 EU/mL = 16.7 EU/ng
CSE = 0.018 ng/mL

This indicates that 0.018 ng of the CSE is equal to 0.3 EU of the RSE. Thus, the CSE contains 16.7 EU/ng.

Chromogenic and End Point: Turbidimetric Techniques

At least four samples (vials) for the lot of CSE should be assayed. In addition to a water blank, assay dilutions of RSE which fall in the linear range and dilutions of the CSE. Linear regression analysis is performed on the absorbance values of the RSE standards (y axis) versus their respective endotoxin concentrations (x axis). Calculate the EU/ng of the CSE by inserting the average CSE O.D. readings for each concentration which falls in the RSE standard range into the RSE straight line equation. The resulting CSE values (in EU) are then divided by their corresponding concentrations (in ng/mL). These values are then averaged to obtain the potency of the CSE lot.

Reference Standard Endotoxin Standard Curve

Concentration O.D.	RSE (EU/mL)
0.1	0.11
0.25	0.26
0.5	0.49
1.0	1.06
y-intercept $= -0.008$	slope $= 1.056$; $r = 0.999$

Straight line equation $(y) = -0.008 + (1.056 * x)$.

Control Standard Endotoxin Standard Curve

Corresponding EU/ng	CSE conc. (ng/mL)	Average D. RSE (EU/mL)	RSE/CSE
0.01	0.12	0.119	11.9
0.025	0.31	0.301	12.0
0.05	0.60	0.626	12.5
0.1	1.23	1.291	12.9

Mean EU/ng $= 12.3$.

Kinetic Turbidimetric Technique

In order to assign EUs to a CSE, the following should be performed on four vials from the same CSE lot.

Two-fold dilutions of the RSE should be made in the range of 1.0 EU/mL to 0.03 EU/mL. Determine the time of reaction (T) for at least duplicates of each standard concentration. Construct a standard curve ($\log_{10} T$ versus $\log_{10}$ endotoxin concentration (E). Calculate the mean T for 1.0 and 0.03 EU/mL. These Ts define the RSE standard range.

For each of the four vials of CSE make twofold dilutions such that the T values for at least three concentrations of the CSE are within the RSE standard range. Determine the T values for at least duplicates of each endotoxin concentration. Calculate the EU/ng of CSE by inserting the log mean CSE T values for each endotoxin concentration which falls in the RSE standard range into the RSE straight line equation. The resulting CSE values (in EU) are then divided by their corresponding concentrations (in ng/mL). These values are averaged to obtain the potency of the CSE lot.

Example
Reference Standard Endotoxin Standard Curve

Straight line equation $(y) = 3.03 + (-0.181^*x)$

RSE standard range $= 1037 - 2235$ seconds $(17.3 - 37.3 \text{ minutes})$

Control Standard Endotoxin Standard Curve

	Endotoxin concentration (ng/mL)					
Vial	0.1	0.05	0.025	0.0125	0.006	0.003
1	1018.8	1114	1218.6	1402.7	1548.7	1740.7
2	990.7	1090.6	1249.8	1406.4	1586.0	1780.0
3	998.2	1116.8	1227.8	1411.0	1554.1	1800.9
4	1003.4	1086.1	1198.5	1415.6	1593.9	1781.0

Note: Each *T* in the above table is expressed in seconds and represents the mean of at least duplicate determinations.

Mean *T* (sec)	1002.8*	1101.9	1223.7	1408.9	1570.7	1775.7
Log mean *T*	3.001	3.042	3.088	3.149	3.196	3.249

Calculations

Solving for EU/mL equivalent by substituting onset times generated with CSE (ng/mL) into the above RSE standard line equation, $x = (y - 3.03)/-0.181$, where $y = $ log mean onset time and $x = $ log EU/mL equivalent.

CSE (ng/mL)	Endo. Conc.	Log Mean *T*	EU/mL (RSE Std. Line) Log	Equivalent EU/ng Antilog
0.1[a]	3.001	0.16	1.45	14.5
0.05	3.042	−0.066	0.859	17.2
0.025	3.088	−0.32	0.479	19.2
0.0125	3.149	−0.657	0.22	17.6
0.006	3.196	−0.917	0.121	20.2
0.003	3.249	−1.210	0.062	20.6

Mean EU/ng = 19.0 (SD = 1.52)
[a]Outside the RSE standard range—not used in calculation of mean.

The values for the *y*-intercept and slope of the four CSE curves used for the EU/ng determination may be stored for use in routine testing (archived standard curve) instead of running a series of standards each day. Using the EU/ng conversion factor, CSE standards within the range of the RSE curve can be made up in EUs. Standards outside this range require the use of RSE and a new RSE standard curve. If CSE standards outside the RSE standard range are required the EU/ng conversion factor must be determined for the new range as described above.

APPENDIX B

This appendix is an extract from Local Reference Standard Profile (LRSP) Example for CSE.

Local Reference Standard Profile: Gel-Clot Method

Endotoxin (CSE):	Associates of Cape Cod 74 expires 02/06/2003
Lysate (LAL):	Associates of Cape Cod 597-11-041 expires 11/25/2002
Lysate sensitivity:	0.06 EU/mL
Acceptance test:	Confirmation of Labeled LAL Sensitivity test performed confirmed the sensitivity of the lysate within 2-fold of lambda (0.06 EU/mL). Refer to LRSP Package.
Date established:	10/19/98 (in lab)
Preparation:	Reconstitute LAL with 5 mL SWI, proceed per GP8010
CSE potency:	10 USP EU/ng
RSE:RSE ratios:	1 EU (USP): 1 IU (BRP)
1 EU (USP):	1 EU (JP)
Acceptance test:	See Certificate of Analysis
Date established:	04/16/98 (by manufacturer)
Preparation:	Reconstitute CSE with 5 mL SWI
Stock:	1000 EU/mL [(500 ng/vial x 10 EU/ng)/5 mL/vial]

Control Standard Endotoxin Spike Preparation

	Endotoxin concentration in EU/mL
S1.) 0.5 ml of STOCK into 4.5 ml of SWI.	100
S2.) 0.5 ML OF (S1) INTO 4.5 ML OF SWI	10
S3.) 3.0 ML OF (S2) INTO 3.1 ML OF SWI	4.92
S4.) 0.5 ML OF (S3) INTO 4.65 ML OF SWI	0.48
S5.) 0.24 mL of (S3) INTO 9.6 mL of SWI	0.12

Standard Curve Preparation

	Endotoxin concentration in EU/mL
C1.) 1.0 mL of (S4) into 1.0 mL of SWI.	0.24
C2.) 1.0 mL of (C1) into 1.0 mL of SWI	0.12
C3.) 1.0 mL of (C2) into 1.0 mL of SWI	0.06
C4.) 1.0 mL of (C3) into 1.0 mL of SWI	0.03
C5.) 1.0 mL of (C4) into 1.0 mL of SWI	0.015
C6.) 1.0 mL of SWI.	negative control

SWI—Sterile Water for Injection Handling:

 Storage Conditions: Keep Refrigerated

1—slight; 4—extreme

Purchased combination of CSE/LAL reagents used only for quantitation of bacterial endotoxin as per gel-clot method.

Local Reference Standard Profile: GMP Library
Written by: —————————Date: ———
Supervisor's Signature: ————Date: ———
Revision: 1.0

REFERENCES

1. Henderson B, Poole S, Wilson M. Bacterial modulins: a novel class of virulence factors which cause host tissue pathology by inducing cytokine synthesis. Microbiol Rev 1996; June:316–341.
2. Reference Standards. ch 11. USP 24, 2000.
3. USP Reference Standard Catalog, 2000.
4. Weary ME. Understanding and setting endotoxin limits. J Parenter Sci Technol 1990; 44(1):16–18.
5. Outschoorn AS. The new USP reference standard endotoxin-A collaborative project. Pharm Forum 1982; 8:1743–1745.
6. Outschoorn AS. Characterization of the USP Reference Standard Endotoxin, in Endotoxins and Their Detection With the Limulus Amebocyte Lysate Test. Watson SW, Levin J, Novitsky TJ, eds. New York: Alan R. Liss, Inc., 1982:115–119.
7. Greisman SE, Hornick RB. Comparative pyrogenic reactivity of rabbit and man to bacterial endotoxin. Proc Soc Exp Biol Med 1969; 131:1154–1158.
8. Mascoli CC, Weary MB. Limulus amebocyte lysate (LAL) test for detecting pyrogens in parenteral injectable products and medical devices: advantages to manufacturers and regulatory officials. J Parenter Drug Assoc 1979; 33:81.
9. Loppnow H et al. IL-1 induction-capacity of defined lipopolysaccharide partial structures. J Immunol 1989; 142(9):3229–3238.
10. Pedron T et al. New synthetic analogs of lipid a as lipopolysaccharide agonists or antagonists of b lymphocyte activation. Int Immunol 1992; 4(4):553–540.
11. Nowotny A. Review of the molecular requirements of endotoxic actions. Rev Infect Dis 1987; 9(suppl 5):S503–S511.
12. Johnson AG et al. Characterization of a nontoxic monophosphoryl lipid A. Rev Infect Dis 1987; 9(suppl 5):S512–S516.
13. Rose J et al. Agonistic and antagonistic activities of bacterially derived rhodobacter sphaeroides lipid A: comparison with activities of synthetic material of the proposed structure and analogs. Infect Immun 1995; 63:833–839.
14. Loppnow H et al. Cytokine induction by lipopolysaccharide (LPS) corresponds to lethal toxicity and is inhibited by nontoxic Rhodobacter capsulatus LPS. Infect Immun 1990; 58(11): 3743–3750.
15. Wong KH et al. "Endotoxicity" of the legionnaires' disease bacterium. Ann Intern Med 1979; 90:624–627.
16. Neumeister B et al. Low endotoxic potential of legionella pneumophila lipopolysaccharide due to failure of interaction with the monocyte lipopolysaccharide receptor CD14. Infect Immun 1998; 66(9):4151–4157.
17. Lynn WA, Golenbock DT. Lipopolysaccharide antagonists. Immunol Today 1992.
18. Soltys J, Quinn MT. Modulation of endotoxin- and enterotoxin-induced cytokine release by in vivo treatment with -(1,6)-Branched -(1,3)-Glucan. Infect Immun 1999; 67:244–252.
19. Royce and Pardy. Endotoxin-like properties of an extract from a symbiotic, eukaryotic Chlorella-like green alga. J Endotoxin Res 1996; 3(6):437–444.
20. Galanos C et al. Chemical, physicochemical and biological properties of bacterial lipopolysaccharides. In: CE, ed. Biomedical Applications of the Horseshoe Crab (Limulidae). New York: Alan R. Liss, 1979:321–332.
21. Levin J. The Limulus Test and Bacterial Endotoxins: Some Perspectives. In: Watson SW, Levin J, Novitsky TJ, eds. Endotoxins and Their Detection With the Limulus Amebocyte Lysate Test. New York: Alan R. Liss, Inc. 1982:7–24.
22. Cooper JF. Is FDA Modification of the Pyrogen Test Justified? P&MC Industry, Jan/Feb, 1983.
23. Cooper J, Weary M, Jordan F. The impact of nonendotoxin LAL-reactive materials on Limulus amebocyte lysate analyses. PDA J Pharm Sci Technol 1997; 51:2–6.
24. Kambayashi J et al. A novel endotoxin-specific assay by turbidimetry with Limulus amoebocyte lysate containing beta-glucan. J Biochem Biophys Methods 1991; 22:93–100.
25. Zhang G et al. Differential blocking of coagulation-activating pathways of Limulus amebocyte lysate. J Clin Microbiol 1994; 32:1537–1541.

26. Delfino D et al. Tumor necrosis factor-inducing activities of Cryptococcus neoformans components. Infect Immun 1996; 64(12):5199–5204.
27. Yasuoka A et al. (1– > 3) beta-D-glucan as a quantitative serological marker for Pneumocystis carinii pneumonia. Clin Diagn Lab Immunol 1996; 3(2):197–199.
28. Miyazaki T et al. Plasma (1– > 3)-beta-D-glucan and fungal antigenemia in patients with candidemia, aspergillosis, and cryptococcosis. J Clin Microbiol 1995; 33(12): 3115–3118.
29. Werner-Felmayer G et al. Detection of bacterial pyrogens on the basis of their effects on gamma interferon-mediated formation of neopterin or nitrite in cultured monocyte cell lines. Clin Diagn Lab Immunol 1995; 2(3):307–313.
30. Galanos C. Encyclopedia of Immunology. Roitt IM, ed. Academic Press, 1992.
31. Tsuchiya M et al. Reactivities of gram-negative bacteria and gram-positive bacteria with Limulus amebocyte lysate and silkworm larvae plasma. J Endotoxin Res 1994; 1(suppl 1):70.
32. Tsuchiya M et al. Detection of peptidoglycan and b-glucan with silkworm larvae plasma test. FEMS Immunol Med Microbiol 1996; 15:129–134.
33. Khan W. New rapid test for diagnosing bacterial meningitis. In 36th Interscience Conference on Antimicrobial Agents and Chemotherapy, New Orleans, Louisiana: ICAAC, 1996.
34. Muhlradt P, Frisch M. Purification and partial biochemical characterization of a Mycoplasma fermentans-derived substance that activates macrophages to release nitric oxide, tumor necrosis factor, and interleukin-6. Infect Immun 1994; 62(9):3801–3807.
35. Mühlradt PF et al. Structure and specific activity of macrophage-stimulating lipopeptides from mycoplasma hyorhinis. Infect Immun 1998; 66:4804–4810.
36. Kaufmann A et al. Induction of cytokines and chemokines in human monocytes by mycoplasma fermentans-derived lipoprotein MALP-2. Infect Immun 1999; 67: 6303–6308.
37. Giguère S, Prescott JF. Cytokine induction in murine macrophages infected with virulent and avirulent Rhodococcus equi. Infect Immun 1998; 66:1848–1854.
38. Fenno JC et al. Cytopathic effects of the major surface protein and the chymotrypsinlike protease of treponema denticola. Infect Immun 1998; 66:1869–1877.
39. Zhang H et al. Lipoprotein release by bacteria: potential factor in bacterial pathogenesis. Infect Immun 1998; 66:5196–5201.
40. Retini C et al. Capsular polysaccharide of Cryptococcus neoformans induces proinflammatory cytokine release by human neutrophils. Infect Immun 1996; 64:2897–2903.
41. Norrby-Teglund A et al. Similar cytokine induction profiles of a novel streptococcal exotoxin, MF, and pyrogenic exotoxins A and B. Infect Immun 1994; 62:3731–3738.
42. Dinarello C et al. Human leukocyte pyrogen test for detection of pyrogenic material in growth hormone produced by recombinant E. coli. J Clin Microbiol 1984; 20(3):323–329.
43. Cooper J. Formulae for maximum valid dilution. In: Watson SW, Levin J, Novitsky TJ, eds. Endotoxins and Their Detection With the Limulus Amebocyte Lysate Test. New York: Alan R. Liss, 1982:55–64.
44. Hochstein HD. Review of the bureau of biologic's experience with limulus amebocyte lysate and endotoxin. In: Watson SW, Levin J, Novitsky TJ, eds. Endotoxins and their Detection with the Limulus Amebocyte Lysate Test. New York: Alan R. Liss, 1982:141–151.
45. FDA. Guideline on Validation of the Limulus Amebocyte Lysate Test as an End-Product Endotoxin Test for Human and Animal Parenteral Drugs, Biological Products, and Medical Devices. Rockville, MD, 1987:1–48.
46. Karkhanis YD et al. A new and improved microassay to determine 2-keto-3-deoxyoctanoate in lipopolysaccharide of gram-negative bacteria. Anal Biochem 1978; 85: 595–601.
47. Firca JR, Rudbach JA. Reference endotoxin: a practical rationale. In: Watson SW, Levin J, Novitsky TJ, eds. Endotoxin and Their Detection with the Limulus Amebocyte Lysate Test. New York: Alan R. Liss, 1982.
48. Dawson ME. Endotoxin Standards and CSE Potency. LAL Update, 11(4):2–5.

49. Cooper JF, Levin J, Wagner HN Jr. Quantitative comparison of in vitro and in vivo methods for the detection of endotoxin. J Lab Clin Med 1971; 78(1):138–148.
50. Tomasulo PA et al. Biological activities of tritiated endotoxins: correlation of the Limulus lysate assay with rabbit pyrogen and complement activation assays for endotoxin. J Lab Clin Med 1977; 89:308.
51. Tomasulo PA. Correlation of the Limulus amebocyte lysate assay with accepted endotoxin assays. In: CE et al., ed. Biomedical Applications of the Horseshoe Crab (Limulidae). New York: Alan R. Liss, 1979:293.
52. Elin RJ, Sandberg AL, Rosenstreich DL. Comparison of the pyrogenicity, Limulus activity, mitogenicity and complement reactivity of several bacterial endotoxins and related compounds. J Immunol 1976; 117:1238.
53. Weary M et al. The activity of various endotoxins in the USP rabbit test and in three different LAL tests. In: Watson SW, Levin J, Novitsky TJ, eds. Endotoxins and Their Detection with the Limulus Amebocyte Lysate Test. New York: Alan R. Liss, Inc., 1982:365–379.
54. Muller-Calgan H. Experiences with comparative examinations for pyrogens by rabbit pyrogen test versus the LAL test. In: Watson SW, Levin J, Novitsky TJ, eds. Endotoxins and Their Detection with the Limulus Amebocyte Lysate Test. New York: Alan R. Liss, Inc., 1982:343–356.
55. Pearson FC et al. Relative potency of environmental endotoxin as measured by the Limulus amebocyte lysate test and the USP rabbit pyrogen test. In: Watson SW, Levin J, Novitsky TJ, eds. Endotoxins and Their Detection with the Limulus Amebocyte Lysate Test. New York: Alan R. Liss, Inc., 1982a:65–77.
56. Novitsky TJ. Selection of the Standard. LAL Update, 1996; 17(1):1–4.
57. World Health Organization. Technical Report Series. 1987; 760:29.
58. Poole S, Das REG. Report on the collaborative study of the candidate second international standard for endotoxin. Expert Committee on Biological Standardization, 1996.
59. Poole S, Dawson P, Das REG. Second international standard for endotoxin: calibration in an international collaborative study. J Endotoxin Res 1997; 4(3):221–231.
60. Berzofsky RN. Liquid Endotoxin Standards. LAL Review, 1997; Summer:1–4.
61. Maitra S, Nachum R, Pearson FC. Establishment of beta-hydroxy fatty acids as chemical marker molecules for bacterial endotoxin by gas chromatography-mass spectrometry. Appl Environ Microbiol 1986; 52(3):510–514.
62. Brandtzaeg P et al. Meningococcal endotoxin in lethal septic shock plasma studied by gas chromatography, mass-spectrometry, ultracentrifugation, and electron microscopy. J Clin Invest 1992; 89(March):816–823.
63. Laude-Sharp M et al. Dissociation between the interleukin 1-inducing capacity and limulus reactivity of lipopolysaccharides from gram-negative bacteria. Cytokine 1990; 2(4):253–258.
64. Guideline on Validatioin of the Limulus Amebocyte Lysate Test as and End-Product Endotoxin Test for Human and Animal Parenteral Drugs, Biological Products, and Medical Devices. Appendix. C. FDA, Dec. 1987.
65. Rudbach JA et al. Preparation and properties of a national reference endotoxin. J Clin Microbiol 1976; 3:21.
66. Galanos C, Luderitz O, Westphal O. Preparation and properties of a standardized lipopolysaccharide from Salmonella abortus equi (Novo-Pyrexal). Zentralbl Bakteriol [Orig A] 1979; 243:226.
67. Humphrey JH, Bangham DR. The international pyrogen reference preparation. Bull WHO 1959; 20:1241.
68. Cooper JF. New reference endotoxin ends uncertainty in LAL reagent labeling. Partic Microb Cont 1982; 1(1):43.
69. Hochstein DH. The LAL test versus the rabbit pyrogen test for endotoxin detection. Pharm Technol 1981; 5(8):35.
70. Weary ME et al. Relative potencies of four reference endotoxin standards as measured by the Limulus amoebocyte lysate and USP rabbit pyrogen test. Appl Environ Microbiol 1980; 40:1148.

71. Dabbah R et al. Pyrogenicity of *E. coli* 055:B5 endotoxin by the USP rabbit test-a HIMA collaborative study. J Parenter Drug Assoc 1980; 34:212.
72. Garratt DC, Hartley RE, Mussett MV. Reproducibility of the Limulus amoebocyte lysate test in UK laboratories. Pharm J 1981; January:112–116.
73. Pearson F. Pyrogens, Endotoxins, LAL Testing and Depyrogenation. Marcel Dekker, Inc., 1984.

10 *Limulus* Amebocyte Lysate Discovery, Mechanism, and Application

Kevin L. Williams

Eli Lilly & Company, Indianapolis, Indiana, U.S.A.

While attempting to demonstrate Koch's postulates of disease causation, Bang subsequently showed that the "disease" was brought about by the organism's own defense mechanism in response to a heat stable by-product of the isolated bacterium.

ORIGIN AND IMPORTANCE OF LAL

The rabbit pyrogen assay served as the only official pyrogen test for 37 years. However, during the early 1960s, several events occurred that would eventually lead to the development of a seemingly unlikely replacement—a blood product (lysate) derived from the horseshoe crab *Limulus polyphemus*. The importance of the changes brought about in the pharmaceutical industry by the switch from the in vivo based rabbit pyrogen test to the in vitro bacterial endotoxin test are often underappreciated for a couple of reasons. First, the labor intensity inherent in the rabbit pyrogen assay served limited the amount of in-process testing that could realistically be performed (from a cost and resource perspective) to support the manufacture of parenteral lots (100 rabbit pyrogen tests a day would be a colossal effort). The advent of *Limulus* amebocyte lysate (LAL) testing allowed the broad application of current good manufacturing practices (cGMPs) as they relate to the detection of endotoxins across the entire manufacturing process. Quality control testing of only the latter forms of a parenteral drug provides a greatly reduced probability of detecting a contaminated unit of that material from a statistical standpoint, and would make it impossible to preclude the use of contaminated materials prior to the manufacture of an expensive biological[a] lot.

Today's modern pharmaceutical manufacturing processes include sampling and LAL testing of not only the finished (beginning, middle, and end of lot), bulk, and active pharmaceutical ingredient material but also in-process materials including containers and closures, sterile water, bulk drug materials, and more recently, excipients. Such testing, using the pyrogen assay, was very expensive and its expansion unlikely, given the cost and other resource constraints.

Second, the inability to quantify endotoxin associated with pyrogen testing acted as a "blind spot" to restrict the improvement of processes that are now readily monitored given the sensitivity and quantification associated with the LAL test. It is difficult to work toward lower specifications when performing an

---

[a]From Scott (1993): Macromolecular (>500 kd) substances either composed of, or extracted from, a living organism. The products bring with them increasing complexity and associated "tertiary structure, location, and extent and type of glycosylation" and tend to be less well defined in terms of analytical characteristics, activity, and utility.

assay that has an inherent invisible pass/fail result. Modern biopharmaceuticals may indeed contain trace amounts of endotoxin or may have activities (i.e., interferon) mimicking endotoxin, and in such cases the accurate and reproducible quantification of these minute levels, as well as the differentiation of interference and endotoxin content, become paramount in demonstrating that allowable levels are present.

FIRST APPLICATIONS OF LAL

The first application of the clotting reaction discovered by Levin and Bang was made by Cooper et al. (1) in their use of the "pregel" to determine the endotoxin content in radiopharmaceuticals in 1970. According to Hochstein (2), Cooper was a graduate student at Johns Hopkins in 1970 and worked for the Bureau of Radiological Health. That summer Cooper persuaded the Bureau of Biologics (BOB) group led by Hochstein that a lysate from the horseshoecrab's blood would be useful in detecting endotoxins in biological products. Given the short half-life and stringent pyrogen requirements associated with radiopharmaceutical drugs, Cooper believed that LAL could be used to accomplish the improved detection of contaminated products. Though Cooper left the BOB to finish his graduate studies, Hochstein continued the Bureau's efforts to explore the use of LAL in the testing of drug products.

The potential for improvement in the area of pharmaceutical contamination control was evident in Cooper, Hochstein, and Seligman's very first application of the LAL test involving a biological (3): the results of 26 influenza virus vaccines included as a subset of a 155 sample test using LAL varied from lot to lot by up to 1000-fold and revealed endotoxin in the 1 µg range in the 1972 study. Cooper and Pearson (4) later pointed out that newer vaccines used in mass inoculation of Americans for A/swine virus were subsequently required to contain not more than 6 ng/mL of endotoxin, a level that could not be demonstrated with pyrogen testing. Suspected adverse reactions were reported prior to the inception of the LAL assay and were an expected part of some drug reactions such as that associated with L-asparaginase antileukemic treatment as a product of *Escherichi coli* (5).

Another early application on radiopharmaceuticals and biological vaccines mentioned earlier involved the detection of endotoxin in intrathecal injections into the cerebrospinal fluid of drugs. Cooper and Pearson (4) reported that ten such samples implicated in adverse patient responses were obtained and tested by LAL, and all ten reacted strongly. The rabbit pyrogen test was negative for all samples when tested on a dose-per-weight basis. They concluded that the rabbit pyrogen test was not sensitive enough for such an application given that endotoxin was determined to be at least 1000 times more toxic when given intrathecally.

THE HORSESHOE CRAB

In 1885, Howell (6) observed that the blood of *L. polyphemus*, the horseshoe crab, formed a solid clot when withdrawn from the animal. A year later, Loeb (7) reported that, when the blood of Limuli were collected and exposed to a foreign substance, they underwent liquefaction followed by coagulation. This was the first in a series of papers (8,9) that Loeb published detailing various aspects of coagulation with particular reference to amebocytes, the only circulating cell found in the blood of *Limulus*. Subsequently, Shirodkar et al. (10) reported that an unidentified marine gram-negative bacterium (GNB) caused a fulminating disease of the horseshoe crab characterized by extensive intravascular clotting and death. A heat-stable derivative of this bacterium, as well as a number of heat-stable derivatives from other GNB, caused intravascular clotting in otherwise normal Limuli. Using an in vitro maintenance system for amebocytes, Shlrodkar et al. were able to demonstrate the degranulation and destruction of cells exposed to pathogenic *Vibrio* or their thermostable toxins.

Horseshoe crabs have served several uses to people through the ages (loosely speaking they have always been around) including food for Asian-Pacific and Native American inhabitants; spears (their tails) for early Native Americans of Roanoke Island, North Carolina; fertilizer for some tide water farmers; and bait for fishermen's traps (11). There remain today only four species, three inhabiting the eastern shores of Asia and one scattered along the North American Atlantic ranging from Maine to Mexico.

Limulus, Latin for "sidelong," was named after the one-eyed giant of Greek mythology (11). *Limulus* has nine eyes: one oval, lateral eye on each side, two small center eyes and five light sensitive receptors under its shell. *Limulus* has one more leg than it has eyes, (five pairs). The crabs live on worms and mollusks. The spike tail allows the crab to right itself if flipped over (unlike the turtle). The blood of the horseshoe crab has been an area of interest because of its blue color, which is due to a copper-based oxygen acceptor rather than the iron-based receptor seen in mammals and other animals. The amebocyte, the only blood cell of the animal, does not contain the hemocyanin (which remain in the plasma after centrifugation of the cells) and contains all the elements of the coagulation system for *Limulus*. Besides its blood, the animal's unique "lateral compound eye" has been the most studied aspect of *Limulus*. These studies have yielded insight to the workings of the human eye.[b]

DISCOVERY: THE BIG BANG

In 1956 Frederik Bang at the Marine Biological Laboratories in Massachusetts was studying the effects of what he initially believed to be a bacterial disease causing the intravascular coagulation (coagulopathy) of the blood of a horseshoe crab in a group that he was observing. He isolated the bacterium from ill *Limuli*, believing it to be a marine invertebrate pathogen such as (he cites) the marine bacterium *Gaffkia*, which kills lobsters.

He described the basic observation that prompted him to publish the landmark study in "A Bacterial Disease of *L. polyphemus*" (12) as follows:

> Bacteria obtained at random from fresh seawater were injected into a series of horseshoe crabs (*L. polyphemus*) of varying sizes. One *Limulus* became sluggish and apparently ill. Blood from its heart did not clot when drawn and placed on glass, and yet instant clotting is a characteristic of normal *Limulus* blood. ... The bacteria caused an active progressive disease marked by extensive intravascular clotting and death. Injection of a heat-stable derivative of the bacterium also caused intravascular clotting and death. Other gram-negative bacteria or toxins also provoked intravascular clotting in normal Limuli. When these same bacteria or toxins were added to sera from normal limuli, a stable gel was formed.

---

[b]The 1967 Nobel Prize for studies of the *Limulus* optical system went to Dr. H. Keffer Hartline of Rockefeller University (11).

Even in this very early paper (12) Bang was able to draw parallels to the human vascular system by referring to an existing study by Koch:

> In one recent case report (13), an acutely ill patient was found to have a failure of blood clotting due to lack of fibrinogen associated with bacteremia with *E. coli* and acute yellow atrophy.

While attempting to demonstrate Koch's postulates of disease causation, Bang subsequently showed that the "disease" was brought about by the organism's own defense mechanism in response to a heat stable by-product of the isolated bacterium: "To our surprise we found that bacterial suspensions, which had been boiled for five or ten minutes still killed the Limuli" (11). Furthermore, he showed that a suspension of the bacterium reacted to form a distinctive clot when combined with the *Limulus'* amebocyte cells (or washings of the cells).

Following Bang's initial observations, he paired up with a hematologist, Jack Levin, at the suggestion of another colleague. Together they explored the requisite coagulate factors of *Limulus* and published a paper entitled: "The Role of Endotoxin in the Extracellular Coagulation of *Limulus* Blood" (14) in an effort to "study the mechanism by which endotoxin affects coagulation in the *Limulus*, and to elucidate the mechanism by which endotoxin exerts its effect in a biological system that may be less complex than that found in mammals." In this study they made a number of observations:

1. The amebocyte is necessary for clotting
2. Clotting factors are located only in the amebocytes and not in the blood plasma
3. The formation of a gel-clot reaction occurs by the conversion of a "pre-gel" material upon addition of gram-negative bacteria.

Levin and Bang suspected that the causative agent of the observed intravascular coagulation was endotoxin (Levin had some previous experience with endotoxin) and that its effect on the host *Limulus* was similar to the previously described generalized Shwartzman reaction, which they described:

> ... as the occurrence of renal cortical necrosis in rabbits following appropriately spaced injections of endotoxin. During the course of this reaction, there is a fall in the numbers of circulating platelets and granulocytes; and there may be an abrupt decrease in the level of circulating fibrinogen and shortening of the clotting time. Intravascular coagulation may be an important part of this phenomenon, and the mechanism by which endotoxin affects the coagulation system appears to be mediated through the platelet (14).

Levin and Bang demonstrated that extracts of the amebocytes gelled in the presence of gram-negative bacterial endotoxin. In the introduction of that early paper they describe the phenomenon that would later become the basis for the LAL assay:

> *Limulus* blood contains only one type of cell called the amebocyte. When the whole-blood is withdrawn from the *Limulus*, a clot quickly forms. Thereafter, this clot shrinks spontaneously, and a liquid phase appears. Under appropriate conditions, this liquid material has the capability of gelling when it is exposed to bacterial endotoxin, and is defined here as pre-gel .... The results (of the study that served as the basis for their April 1964 publication) demonstrate that cellular material from the amebocyte is necessary for coagulation of *Limulus* plasma, and that plasma free of all cellular elements does not clot spontaneously nor gel after addition of endotoxin.

Levin and Bang not only used the initial bacterial isolate (they had now identified it as a *Vibrio* species) to bring about gelation, but they also used *E. coli* since they now believed that endotoxin common to gram-negative bacteria was bringing about the gelation phenomenon. Their study revealed that agitation of the amebocytes (amebocyte disruption) aided in the production of the pregel (i.e., in the production of gel precursor most susceptible to subsequent endotoxin clotting), and that the rate of gelation of pre-gel was directly related to the concentration of endotoxin in the mix. In their third paper Levin and Bang (15) describe the "striking similarities between *Limulus* amebocytes and mammalian platelets . . ." during cellular coagulation upon exposure to endotoxin.

Like Pasteur, who worked from general observation and curiosity ("chance prefers the prepared mind"), Bang turned a general observation into a series of productive experiments and successful collaboration based upon his initial intuition. He later described the "serendipity" that brought about the discovery and subsequent utilization of LAL for the detection of bacterial endotoxin in an address that he called: "Rules and Regulations Regarding Serendipity" (16).[c]

EARLY CHARACTERIZATION OF LAL

The ability of hemocytes to coagulate in the presence of gram-negative bacteria or their endotoxins is not restricted solely to *Limulus* and has been demonstrated in the lobster, crab, and oyster (17) as well as insects (18) (although getting enough blood volume for a lysate from an oyster might prove difficult). In a subsequent study, Levin et al. (19) developed a sensitive assay for endotoxin in human plasma using the material lysed from *Limulus* amebocytes. As little as 0.0005 µg (0.5 ng) of endotoxin per milliliter could be detected, and the rate of reaction was shown to be dependent on the concentration of endotoxin. Yin et al. (20) refined Levin's original endotoxin assay to detect picogram amounts of endotoxin and demonstrated that the lipid A portion of lipopolysaccharide (LPS) was responsible for lysate gelation.

After Levin and Bang demonstrated that the clotting activity of *Limulus* hemolymph resided in the amebocyte, work by Young et al. established the enzymatic nature of the endotoxin-induced reaction. Using Sephadex G-50 and G-75 column chromatography, these workers isolated three peaks. One fraction contained a clottable protein that had a molecular weight of 27,000 and was heat stable. The second fraction was comprised of a high molecular weight, heat-labile substance that was activated by endotoxin and formed a gel with the clottable protein. Concentrations of both the heat-labile fraction and endotoxin indicate that the rate of reaction is dose dependent.

The heat-labile fraction was affected by a number of enzyme inhibitors, suggesting that activity was based on serine hydroxyl and sulfhydryl groups. The authors concluded that the reaction of LAL with endotoxin is dependent on endotoxin activation of the high molecular-weight enzyme, which in turn gels the lower molecular weight clottable protein. This reaction is critical for providing an end point in the conventional LAL gel-clot test. Sullivan and Watson (21) further characterized the high-molecular-weight clotting enzyme. The purified enzyme

---

[c]Prepared for publication posthumously by J. Levin from the notes from Bang's address at an International Conference (14).

was isolated from endotoxin-activated lysate by using gel filtration, ion-exchange chromatography, and disk gel electrophoresis. The purified and activated enzyme in fresh LAL induced gel-clot formation, as it would when endotoxin was added to LAL. The clotting enzyme had a molecular weight of 84,000 and contained two subunits, each with a molecular weight of 43,000. The enzyme was heat labile and pH sensitive and had an isoelectric point of 5.5.

Further studies by Tai and Liu (22) demonstrated that activation of the clotting enzyme zymogen (proclotting enzyme) depended not only on endotoxin but also on Ca^{2+}. In contrast to the studies of Sullivan and Watson, the work of Tai and Liu showed that the proclotting enzyme had a molecular weight of at least 150,000, determined by using sodium dodecyl sulfate (SDS) gel electrophoresis, and appeared to consist of a single peptide chain. Exposure of the reduced and carboxymethylated enzyme to 6 M guanidine hydrochloride failed to disassociate it into subunits. Because the enzyme was affected by soybean trypsin inhibitor, this study also suggested that the proclotting enzyme was a serine protease, confirming the findings of Young et al. Trypsin, a serine protease, had been shown to induce the gelation of LAL (23–24).

The low-molecular-weight clotting protein was studied by Solum (23,24), who named it coagulogen. Using an acidification procedure to inactivate the proclotting enzyme, he was able to purify coagulogen by chromatography, using Sephadex G-75 and 1.7 M acetic acid as an eluent. Clotted coagulogen was produced, using endotoxin as a gelation activator, and was purified by the same method employed for the nonclotted substance. Molecular weights of approximately 23,000 and 17,000 daltons were determined for coagulogen and the clotted material, respectively. The author concluded that the 6000 dalton loss in molecular weight was caused by the proclotting enzyme splitting a portion of the coagulogen polypeptide. This conclusion was consistent with the observation that trypsin promoted clot formation of untreated as well as acid-treated preparations. Nakamura et al. (26,27) demonstrated that including coagulogen with the activated proclotting enzyme obtained from the blood of *Tachypleus tridentatus*, the Japanese horseshoe crab, produced a gel clot protein consisting of two peptide chains and accompanied by the release of low molecular weight peptide C.

OVERVIEW OF HEMOLYMPH COAGULATION IN *LIMULUS* AND *TACHYPLEUS*

Invertebrates lack adaptive immune systems and rely on innate immunity to antigens common to pathogenic organisms. Nakamura et al. have extensively studied the hemolymph (blood) system of the Japanese horseshoe crab (*T. tridentatus)* and found amebocytes contain two types of granules: large (L) and small (S), which contain the clotting factors, proteins, and antimicrobials that are released into the crab's plasma via a process called degranulation (28,29). Regardless of the relative simplicity of the crab's defense system (the amebocyte), Nakamura et al. consider it to be "a complex amplification process comparable to the mammalian blood coagulation cascade" and "very similar to those of mammalian monocytes and macrophages . . ." (30). The ability of *Limulus* and *Tachypleus* blood to clot and form webs of fibrin-like protein serve as a means of entrapping and facilitating the deactivation of both invading organisms and endotoxin by the release of additional anti-endotoxin and antimicrobial factors. The clotting action also serves to prevent leakage of hemolymph at external sites of injury. Many research efforts have focused on delineating the mechanism of action, among the most advanced originating and ongoing in Japan using *Tachypleus*.

Upon gram-negative bacterial invasion of the hemolymph, hemocytes detect LPS on their surface and release their granule contents (degranulate). The known biosensors consist of coagulation factor C and factor G, which serve as the triggers for the coagulation cascade that converts soluble coagulogen to the insoluble coagulin gel. These two serine protease zymogens are autocatalytically activated by LPS and (1,3)-β-D-glucan, respectively. The LPS initiated cascade (via activation of the proclotting enzyme) involves three serine protease zymogens: factor B, factor C, and proclotting enzyme (Fig. 1). The final step of the clotting reaction involves the creation of coagulin from coagulogen by the excision of the midsection of the protein, called peptide C. Without peptide C, the monomers form AB polymers, consisting of the NH2-terminal A chain and the COOH-terminal B chain covalently linked via two disulfide bridges (31) (Fig. 2).

Coagulogen has been referred to as a "fibrinogen-like" invertebrate protein as the soluble form and coagulin in its (post-enzyme-activated) gelled form (32). The conversion of coagulogen to coagulin is mediated by the sequential activation (cascade) of several zymogens arising from the single blood cell of *Limulus* or

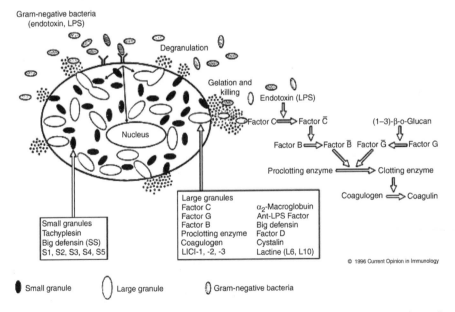

FIGURE 1 Domain structures of horseshoe crab clotting factors. Coagulogen is a much smaller protein than the mammalian homolog, fibrinogen. Arrowheads indicate cleavage sites for zymogen activations. The potential carbohydrate attachment sites are indicated by closed diamonds. Hypothetical mechanism of coagulogen gel formation. Upon gelation of coagulogen by a horseshoe crab clotting enzyme, peptide C is released from the inner portion of the parent molecules. The resulting coagulin monomer may self-assemble to form the dimer, trimer, and multimers. *Source:* From Refs. 32,33.

TABLE 1   Selected Defense Molecules Found in Hemocytes of the Horseshoe Crab

Proteins and peptides	Mass (kDa)	Function/specificity	Location
Coagulation factors			
Factor C	123	Serine protease	L-granule
Factor B	64	Serine protease	ND
Factor G	110	Serine protease	L-granule
Proclotting enzyme	54	Serine protease	L-granule
Coagulogen	20	Gelation	L-granule
Antimicrobial substances			
Anti-LPS factor	12	GNB	L-granule
Tachyplesins	2.3	GNB, GPB, FN	S-granule
Big defensin	8.6	GNB, GPB, FN	L & S-granule
Factor D	42	GNB	L-granule
Lectins			
Tachylectin-1	27	LPS (KDO), LTA	L-granule
Tachylectin-2	27	GlcNAc, LTA	L-granule
Tachylectin-3	15	LPS (O-antigen)	L-granule
Tachylectin-4	470	LPS (O-antigen)	LTA, ND

Abbreviations: FN, fungus; GlcNAc, GNB, gram-negative bacteria; GPB, gram-positive bacteria; KDO, 2-keto-3-deoxyoctonic acid; LAF, *Limulus* 18-kDa agglutination-aggregation factor; LPS, lipopolysaccharide; LTA, lipoteichoic acid; ND, not determined.
Source: From Ref. 33.

Tachypleus (the amebocyte or granulocyte) (Fig. 3). The L-granules contain all the clotting factors for hemolymph coagulation, protease inhibitors, and anti-LPS factor, as well as several tacylectins with LPS binding and bacterial agglutinating activities. L-granules contain in excess of 20 proteins ranging from 8 to 123 kDa in size (32). The small granules contain about six proteins, each less than 30 kDa,

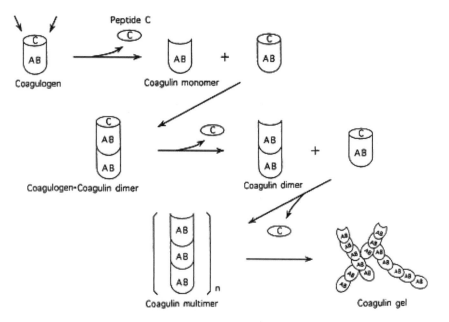

FIGURE 2   Spectrum of glucan reaction via factor G with *Limulus* amebocyte lysate.

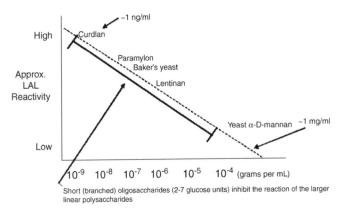

FIGURE 3 The conversion of coagulogen to coagulin is mediated by the sequential activation (cascade) of several zymogens arising from the single blood cell of *Limulus* or *Tachypleus*. *Source*: From Ref. 18.

which possess antimicrobial or bacterial agglutinating activities. See Table 1 for a summary of the major constituents.

The specific coagulation enzymes of LAL have been fractionated and recombined minus factor G to produce endotoxin specific LAL (34). The group performed a similar preparation for use as a chromogenic assay (35). Such preparations may have utility in specific interference problems through the factor G pathway, but the problem is rarely encountered in parenteral testing and can easily be overcome by the use of diluents containing glucans in concentrations, appropriate to block the LAL reaction with factor G. The LAL-specific reagents foreshadowed the use of recombinant LAL (rFC) in that they were separated and recombined minus factor G.

More recently, further detail of the reaction has been proposed (35). The detail of this can be seen in Figure 3 and as described in the attached figure description.

INDIVIDUAL CONSTITUENTS OF THE LAL CASCADE
Factor C Biosensor
At the front end of the cascade (coagulin being the end result), the most significant protein in the clotting system is factor C. It has been referred to as a "biosensor," "LPS-mediated initiation factor," "affinoligand to LSP," and an "initial activator of the clotting cascade." factor C is a 123,000 dalton glycoprotein that is transformed to an activated form in the presence of femtogram amounts of LPS (37). The activation of factor C occurs autocatilytically with no change in molecular weight (approximately 130,000 daltons) (32). The two disulfide bridged polypeptide chains consist of heavy and light chains ($\sim$80,000 and $\sim$40,000 daltons respectively). The specific site of affinity between factor C and LPS has been investigated and characterized as an approximately 38,000 dalton fragment (37).

Factor B
Initially factor B was believed to be sensitive to endotoxin but after further purification it was determined that only factor C is biosensitive to endotoxin. Factor B is

similarly made up of two chains joined by disulfide linkages to form a 64,000 dalton serine protease (31).

Proclotting Enzyme

The proclotting enzyme is insensitive to endotoxin as a single chain glycoprotein, but is activated by activated factor B, denoted –B. The activated clotting enzyme has two polypeptide chains of 27,000 and 31,000 daltons. After the clotting enzyme has been activated, it in turn catalyzes coagulogen to coagulin gel (32) via the removal of peptide C. It is noteworthy to mention that it is at this step that the clotting enzyme also hydrolyzes the chromogenic substrate [t-butyloxycarbonyl (BOC)-Leu-Gly-Arg-p-Nitroanilide], to release p-Nitroanilide, which forms the basis of the kinetic chromogenic color formation (31).

Coagulogen and Coagulin

Coagulogen has been isolated, purified, and characterized as a single polypeptide with a molecular weight of 19,700 ($\pm$50) (33), which corresponds to 175 amino acids. The amino acid sequences of three coagulogens present in the American (*L. polyphemus*), Japanese (*T. tridentatus*), and Southeast Asian (*T. gigas*) crabs are very similar but not identical in amino acid sequence (32). Coagulogen consists of a single peptide chain but contains three regions termed the A chain, peptide C, and the B chain, consisting of 18, 28, and 129 amino acid residues, respectively. The conversion of soluble coagulogen by *Limulus* clotting enzyme to insoluble coagulin is instigated by the removal of a large peptide (peptide C) from the middle of the parent coagulogen. The resulting gel consists of the two chains, A and B joined by two disulfide linkages. Both A and B chains of the three *Limulus* crabs have great homology with similar conformation, which is not surprising given their similar functions. Factor C is the serine protease zymogen that initially responds to the presence of LPS (called a biosensor) and is converted into the active form (factor C), which subsequently activates factor B in converting the proclotting enzyme to the active clotting enzyme, used to finally convert coagulogen to coagulin gel. Coagulin is formed via the aggregation of AB monomers to form the gel-like, AB polymeric substance (Fig. 1). The monomers have been measured to be approximately 60 $\times$30 $\times$20 Angstroms (32).

Additional Antimicrobial Constituents: Factor G and Tachyplesins

In addition to the factors ascribed to bringing about LAL gelation, the crab's hemolymph defense system has been found to contain additional antimicrobial factors including (32):

1. Factor G-biosensor in the detection of *b*-glucans
2. Anti-LPS (in L-granules)
3. Tachyplesins (in S-granules)
4. A host of other factors [tachylectins (1–5), big defensin, 18K-LAF, TCRP (1–3), LCRP (*Limulus* C-reactive protein), and TCRP (*Tachypleus* C-reactive protein)].

Anti-LPS factor inhibits the growth of gram-negative bacteria by binding to LPS lipid A, whereas tachyplesins inhibit the growth of gram-negatives, gram-positives, and fungi by increasing the potassium permeability of the microbes, presumably due to its highly amphipathic nature (33). One LAL manufacturer has made use of the anti-LPS factor to provide a novel LPS removal mechanism employing an immobilized endotoxin affinity ligand (endotoxin neutralizing protein or ENP) (38). The anti-LPS factor is supplied, bound to a resin bead, and the sample is added and incubated (at room temperature) with gentle agitation (for as little as four hours or as long as overnight). After treatment, the beads are centrifuged out taking 99% of the LPS with it bound to the endotoxin neutralizing protein (ENP)-coated resin bead. Generally, moderate amounts of endotoxin are removed to undetectable levels. The product removes LPS from solutions containing up to 2000 EU of various gram-negative bacteria and purified lipid A. Interestingly, the product does not claim to remove LPS associated with *Vibrio* species (40), the very bacterium that led to Bang's discovery and Levin and Bang's development of LAL.

THE ALTERNATE (1,3)-β-D-GLUCAN PATHWAY (FACTOR G PATHWAY)

In 1981 Iwanaga et al. discovered an alternate LAL activation pathway initiated by the factor G zymogen. This additional factor in LAL is activated in the presence of both (1,3)-β-D-glucan, a constituent of the cell walls of fungi, yeast, and algae and LAL-reactive material (LAL-RM), a β-(1,4)-D-glucan from "hollow-fiber hemodialyzer with saponified cellulose acetate of cuprophan membranes" and "cotton wool and in certain cellulose-based filters used in the processing of medicinals" (42), and are also LAL reactive via factor G.

Factor G, once activated into factor-G, activates the proclotting enzyme directly. Purified factor G is activated by other various glucans containing (1,3)-β linkages of different origins, but not by LPS. The G pathway is activated most efficiently by linear (1,3)-β-D-glucans (curdlan and paramylon), whereas chains containing branches are less effective, and short oligosaccharide chains (two to seven glucose units) do not activate factor G at all (33). As seen in Figure 4, as little as a nanogram of curdlan activates the factor G pathway. Shorter oligopolysaccharides not only inhibit the activation of factor G, but they have been found to block the reaction with larger oligopolysaccharides and have been formulated and made available by LAL manufacturers to use as diluents in the testing of solutions that may contain (1,3)-β-D-Glucan. Curdlan is obtained from the culture of *Alcaligenes faecalis var myxogenes* and has been used as a "standard" glucan in studies of the effect of structure and molecular weight on factor G activity. LAL activation by (1,3) β-D-glucan depends on the type of glucan as well as the concentration in solution. Curdlan and paramylon activate the LAL reaction with as little as 1 nanogram, serving to activate factor G to G. Figure 4 shows the concentration of various glucans required for the activation of factor G zymogen. In the Chapter on Method Development (Chap. 11), some means of determining and overcoming glucan reactivity will be further described.

Roslansky and Novitsky (40) studied the relative reactivity of both raw LAL (no additives) and some commercial LALs with the following concentrations needed to bring about gelation as shown in Table 2.

The extraction of formulated (commercial) LAL with chloroform increased LAL sensitivity (minimum concentration demonstrating a positive test) to endotoxin and lipid A as well as to glucans as can be seen in the results in Table 3, using a lot of LAL that was *not* chloroform extracted. For example, sensitivity increased from 25 to 3.125 pg/mL in the case of endotoxin and Associates of Cape Cod (ACC)-formulated LAL. Furthermore, all LAL reagents used were >1000 times more reactive with

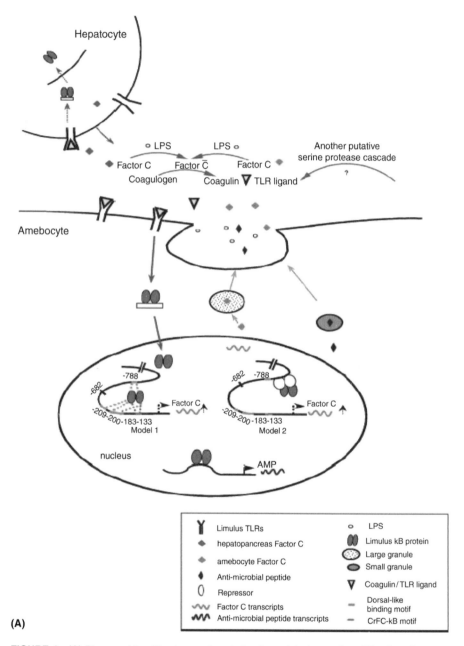

FIGURE 4   (**A**) Phases of the *Limulus* amebocyte lysate-endotoxin reaction. (*Continued*)

endotoxin than with glucans. In each case the authors showed that the addition of the detergent, Zwittergent®, decreased sensitivity of LAL reactive materials (LAL-RM) to LAL. They also studied the effect of enzyme digestion on glucans and LAL-RM using laminarinase and cellulase. Treatment of laminarin with laminarinase revealed a

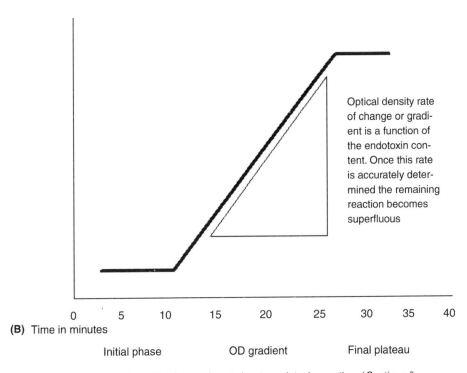

Optical density rate of change or gradient is a function of the endotoxin content. Once this rate is accurately determined the remaining reaction becomes superfluous

(B) Time in minutes		
Initial phase	OD gradient	Final plateau

FIGURE 4 **(B)** Phases of the *Limulus* amebocyte lysate-endotoxin reaction. (*Continued*)

concomitant six to eight-fold loss of LAL reactivity. Treatment of LAL-RM with cellulase gave an almost 100-fold reduction (10 mg/mL to 0.125 mg/mL showing positive LAL reactivity) in LAL reactivity. These results support the contention that LAL-RM contains mostly β-(1,4) linked glucans as opposed to laminarin's predominantly β-(1,3) linked glucans (41).

TABLE 2 Raw and Commercial *Limulus* Amebocyte Lysate Sensitivity: Concentrations Needed to Bring About Gelation (All units are pg/mL)

Reaction sensitivity with raw LAL			LAL with no chloroform extraction		
Curdlan	63,000		32,000		
Laminarin	100,000,000		1,300,000		
LAL-RM	6,300[a]		630[a]		
Lipid A	3,100		50		
Endotoxin	1,000		25		
Commercial LAL (pg/mL):	Endotoxin	Lipid A	Laminarin	Curdlan	LAL-RM
ACC	3.125	3.1	2,600	2,600	35
Whittaker Bioproducts[b]	6.25	250	1,300,000	1,300,000	0
Mallinkrodt	12.5	2,000	1,000,000	130,000	0

Note: The extraction of formulated LAL with chloroform increased LAL sensitivity to endotoxin and lipid A as well as to glucans as can be seen in Table 4 using a lot of LAL that was not chloroform-extracted (as compared to those above).
[a]No verifiable concentration. Arbitrary initial concentration of 100 ng/mL used;
[b]Now Cambrex.
Source: From Ref. 41.

TABLE 3 Standard Curve Values Obtained from a Kinetic Chromogenic Assay ($\lambda = 0.05$ Eu/Ml) Tested on a Commercial Reader/Software System.

Slope (m):	-0.265	
Coefficient of Correlation (r):	-0.997	
Y-intercept:	2.943	
Blank:	**** (no reaction)	average = ****
Standard 1 (0.05 EU/mL):	1984, 1995, 1996, 1984	average = 1989
Standard 2 (0.5 EU/mL):	1007, 997, 999, 1001	average = 1001
Standard 3 (5.0 EU/mL):	594, 591, 593, 575	average = 588

Note: These are the data from which the kinetic reader software uses the formulas referenced in Attachment A for the result calculations given unknown sample reaction times.

While the presence of glucans in pharmaceutical preparations has not been forbidden by the Food and Drug administration (FDA) interpretations (see Attachment A at the end of this chapter), they are nevertheless of microbial origin (except in the case of cellulosic LAL-RM) and have been found to have bioactive properties. The FDA has stated that the presence of glucans will be considered on a case-by-case basis. According to Muta and Iwanaga (18), purified factor G is also activated by sulfatides and cholesterol sulfates. Some known bioactive properties of $\beta(1,3)$-D-glucans are as follows:

1. Radioprotective (43)
2. Immunological adjuvants (44)
3. Inhibitors of tumor growth (44)
4. Synergistic contributors of endotoxicity in septicemia and septic shock (45,46)
5. Cytokine induction capability.

Porperties of LAL-RM (47):

1. Antigenic
2. Activate complement by alternate pathway
3. Implicated in hypersensitivity reactions in dialysis patients
4. Linked atherosclerosis in dialysis patients using cuprophane filters.

PREPARATION AND STANDARDIZATION OF LAL

The first commercial, large-scale production of LAL was in 1971 by Mallinckrodt, Inc. LAL is prepared by placing horseshoe crabs in restraining racks and inserting a sterile, nonpyrogenic 18-gauge needle through the muscular hinge between the cephalothorax and abdominal region. Hemolymph can then flow freely from the cardiac chamber into an appropriate container half-filled with an anticlotting agent, such as 0.125% N-ethylmaleimide (NEM) in 3% sodium chloride solution. These substances are thought to stabilize the rather fragile membrane of the amebocyte (48,49). After collection, the amebocytes are centrifuged for ten minutes, and the blue, hemocyanin-containing supernatant is discarded. Amebocyte harvests are then washed two to three times in 3% sodium chloride to remove residual anticlotting chemicals and serum components. The cell yield is subjected to osmotic shock by addition of nonpyrogenic distilled water, thus releasing intracellular lysate. Other methods of lysis have also been employed successfully (50,51). The aqueous raw product is then lyophilized and remains stable at 4°C for at least three years.

Hochstein's description of the standardization of LAL contrasts to the protracted attempts to devise a suitable endotoxin standard described in Chapter 9. The BOB purchased a large lot of the first LAL submitted for license application and labeled it "Reference Lysate Lot 1"(2). Nevertheless, one of the early criticisms of the use of LAL for detection of endotoxin was the lysate's variability from season to season and lot to lot. It was not uncommon to experience a difference of one order of magnitude in sensitivity among lots produced at various times of the year, or from crabs collected in different locations. Sullivan and Watson (50) were the first to successfully deal with the issue of lysate sensitivity, postulating an inhibitor in lysate that was thought to be responsible for lot-to-lot variability. Their efforts led to the development of a chloroform treatment that decreased variability and increased sensitivity. The addition of divalent cations had no effect on variability, but substantially increased the sensitivity of lysate, which could thus be increased from clot formation at 6 ng/mL of endotoxin to formation at 0.04 ng/mL.

The FDA Office of Biologics recognized the critical nature of endotoxin detection by LAL in pharmaceutical products. As a result, the organization was instrumental in establishing standards governing the production and potency of LAL. The Office established an endotoxin reference standard to be used by manufacturers in potency testing each lot of lysate. To further ensure that lysate was standardized for end point sensitivity and to support label claims, a gel-clot potency test was established using limits for positive and negative responses. In 1977 the Office introduced a standard reference lysate to be used in establishing the sensitivity of each lot of commercial lysate. They also published guidelines detailing the laboratory procedure for comparing each lot of lysate to the standard (53). The first Bacterial Endotoxins Test (i.e., nonpyrogen test) was outlined in the twentieth edition of the *United States Pharmacopeia* (USP).

The LAL model of endotoxin concentration determination relies on the measure of relative biological effectiveness (not an absolute amount present) in an assay subject to its own inherent variables, including the variable ability of different bacteria to initiate gelation and the use of an *E. coli* standard that also varies batch to batch (54). The addition of yet another variable in the equation, that of the LAL (crab and preparation variability), requires further controls and consistency in both the manufacture of LAL and in the proper laboratory confirmation of the labeled lysate sensitivity (label claim verification). LAL standardization ensures that the 5 EU/kg, 0.2 EU/kg, 0.5 EU/mL, and 0.06 EU/mL endotoxin limit concentrations (threshold limits) for parenteral, intrathecal, medical device eluates, and devices that come into contact with cerebrospinal fluid, respectively, are accurately correlated (55) with the results obtained from such testing.

OVERVIEW OF PROMINENT LAL TESTS

According to a Parenteral Drug Association (PDA) survey "Current Practices in Endotoxin and Pyrogen Testing in Biotechnology" (55), as of 1990 the gel-clot assay was the most used assay (77%) with the remainder, the kinetic chromogenic and turbidimetric LAL assays, representing less than one-third of users responding. Most of respondents (71%) indicated for the continued use of the rabbit pyrogen test for at least some final product testing; however, was very seldom indicated for any other sample tests. With that survey now over fifteen years old, current indications are that the use of the kinetic methods have ballooned while the end point, pyrogen and gel-clot tests have diminished significantly. It also seems fair to say that the recombinant factor C test will have to climb a fairly steep learning curve but that eventually it may end up the primary test. Albeit, in laboratories with fewer samples, the simplicity and elegance of the gel-clot assay may still be preferred.

Assay Characteristics of the General LAL
Reaction with Endotoxin

Early on, Levin and Bang (56) described three critical properties of the gelation of LAL in the presence of LPS that formed the basis for subsequent assays, including:

1. The increase in optical density (OD) that accompanies coagulation is due to the increase of clottable protein
2. The concentration of LPS determines the rate of the OD increase
3. The reaction occurs in the shape of a sigmoid curve (i.e., a plateau, a rapid rise, and a final plateau).[d]

Each of these factors is demonstrated graphically (Fig. 4).

The total amount of clotted protein formed depends upon the initial LAL concentration. An excess of LAL is provided for LAL testing and the amount of clotted protein eventually ends up the same, regardless of the amount of endotoxin in the sample. The end result of the enzymatic cascade is the formation of a web of clotted protein. The gel-clot and end point tests take a single time point reading from the data to determine if the reaction reached an assigned level during the assigned time, whereas the kinetic tests are "watching" (at the appropriate wavelength) throughout the entire course of the reaction. The endotoxin concentration determines the rate of protein clot formation and thus the OD change over time as determined by measuring the time to reach an assigned mOD value. The rate of OD formation is then related to the standard curve formed using control standard endotoxin. It can be seen from a plate that sits out that all wells containing endotoxin will eventually form a dark colorimetric or turbidimetric solution regardless of the endotoxin concentration.

Besides the basic gelation of LAL in the presence of LPS, the two methods of observing the assay include the end point and kinetic assays. In the end point test, the reaction proceeds until it is stopped by the user via the addition of a stop reagent (such as acetic acid) at which point the OD readings are recorded for all sample and standard curve points. The drawbacks associated with the end point method of observing the reaction are (*i*) necessity of the user attention at the end of data collection (typically 30 minutes) and (*ii*) the limited standard curve range (a single log). In the kinetic assay, the spectrophotometer records the OD reading continuously [as often as the operator determines via the software settings, but within the manufacturer's recommendations—typically 1:30 to 2:00 minute intervals (due to the amount of internal data that can otherwise needlessly accumulate thus creating very large files to backup)]. Kinetic testing measures the rate of the OD change, by recording the time it takes to reach a preset OD setting called the "onset"

---

[d]See Hurley's paper on methods of endotoxemia detection: Endotoxemia: methods of detection and Clinical Correlates. Clin Microbiol Rev 1995; 8(2):268–292.

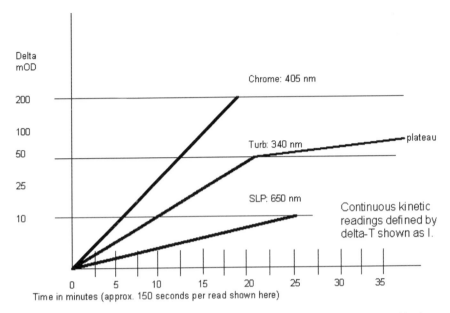

FIGURE 5 Time to reach mOD as a measure of the rate of change of three kinetic assays: chromogenic, turbimetric, and silk worm plasma. *Abbreviation*: OD, optical density.

or "threshold" time (Fig. 5). The kinetic assay plots the log of the resulting reaction time in seconds against the log of the endotoxin concentration of the known standards and can span several logs (typically two to four) and proceeds unattended, thus overcoming the two disadvantages presented by the end point tests.

The Gel-Clot Assay
The gel-clot assay is a simple test not far removed from Levin and Bang's original observations. Until recently it has been the most widely used procedure for the detection of endotoxin in solutions. When equal parts of LAL are combined with a dilution of sample containing endotoxin, one can expect to see gelation in the amount equivalent to the endotoxin sensitivity [called lambda (λ)] of the given lysate. A series of dilutions will reveal the approximate content of a sample with those samples containing equal to or greater than the given sensitivity being positive, and those below the sensitivity not clotting the mixture. The solutions are incubated at a temperature correlating to a physiological temperature (37°C) for one hour and clots are observed by inverting the tubes 180 degrees. In 10 mm × 75 mm depyrogenated test tubes, the clot must remain in the bottom of the tube when inverted. The method is considered semi-quantitative because the true result obtained (indicated by the last gelled sample in the series) is actually somewhere between the two serial dilutions. This is because the result cannot be extrapolated between the (usually two-fold) dilution tubes as it is in the kinetic and end point assays via the use of a mathematical standard curve extrapolated over the entire range of standards although one may continue to assay tighter and tighter dilutions to arrive at the approximate endotoxin concentration via the

gel-clot method. But such is the labor intensity of pinpointing a more approximate result via the gel-clot assay.

Because commercial lysates are available with various standardized end points (sensitivities), the assay can be used to quantify the level of endotoxin in a particular solution or product. The level of endotoxin is calculated by multiplying the reciprocal of the highest dilution (the dilution factor) of the test solution giving a positive end point by the sensitivity of the lysate preparation. For example, if the sensitivity of the LAL employed were 0.03 EU/mL and the dilution end point were 1:16, then the endotoxin concentration would be $16 \times 0.03 = 0.48$ EU/mL. For products administered by weight, the result in EU/mL is divided by the initial test solution potency (as reconstituted or as per the liquid in the vial) to give a result in EU/unit (EU/mg, EU/insulin unit, EU/mL of drug, etc.) that can then be compared to the tolerance limit specification. The geometric mean calculation is used for assays as opposed to the pass-fail limit test (that is reported as a "less-than" number if there is no activity).

Characteristics of Kinetic Methods

Given that kinetic assays continue to be the overwhelming area of growth in LAL testing (listed as a primary reason for the harmonization of endotoxin standards in IS-2), it is relevant to discuss the history and details of kinetic testing. The first kinetic chromogenic test was developed by Nakamura et al. (58). Nakamura et al. (58) tested eight different synthetic substrates and only one showed good reactivity (100%) with endotoxin [BZ (a-N-benzoyl)-Ile-Glu-Gly-Arg-PNA (p-nitroanilide)]. This substrate had previously been used with factor Xa. The development of the chromogenic assay was largely driven by the desire to accurately determine the endotoxin content for bacteremia (60), endotoxemia (61), and bodily fluids such as blood plasma and cerebrospinal fluids (62).

The first kinetic test resembling today's test was developed by Ditter et al. (62). The following passage describes the early kinetic chromogenic test:

> ... the OD is measured every minute for 100 min to obtain the complete kinetics of each reaction in the microtiter plate in a modified photometer (Titertek Multiskan, Flow Laboratories) providing a constant temperature of 37°C. As an index for each of the 96 reactions, the maximal increase in OD per minute (Odmax/min) within 100 minutes is computed. This procedure results in a standard curve that is linear over an extremely wide range, in contrast to the limited linearity of endotoxin standard curves obtained by photometric end point methods.

Urbaschek et al. (61) included an internal standardization method that is used today, namely, the practice of including known standards contained within the sample (positive product control) as described [though Uraschek used the control standard endotoxin (CSE) in a series of concentrations in the product thus mimicking the preparation of the standard curve, a method seldom used today but described in the 1987 FDA Guideline]:

> This internal standardization, based on a mathematical model, allows the quantification of the unknown endotoxin concentration in the sample and at the same time reveals the extent of sample-related interferences. Whereas an endotoxin standard curve is linear in samples not containing endotoxin, it shows a characteristic deviation of this slope when the sample contains endotoxin ... (63).

Though at the time the group could find no improved utility in this method versus the turbidimetric kinetic method for the test of bodily fluids, nevertheless, the test served as a precursor to later efforts by Lindsay et al. (57) to improve upon the kinetic methods (chromogenic and turbidimetric) as alternatives to end point tests. Current kinetic tests can be used to span up to 5 logs (i.e., 0.005 to 50 EU/mL). Moreover, whereas early chromogenic tests employed multiple reagents (LAL, chromogenic substrate, and buffer), current tests have an increased ease of use in that the LAL, substrate, and buffer are colyophilized into a single vial.

Table 4 shows standard curve values obtained from a kinetic chromogenic assay ($\lambda = 0.05$ EU/mL) tested on a commercial reader/software system. These

TABLE 4 Relative Advantages and Disadvantages of Major *Limulus* Amebocyte Lysate Test Types

Kinetic end point tests versus gel-clot method
Kinetic quantitative extrapolation of an unknown result between standards via linear or polynomial regression.
Less prone to variation due to user technique.
Provides "on board" documentation and calculation capabilities for consumables and products used in the test.
The mathematical treatment of data allows for the observance of trends and for the setting of numerical system suitability and assay acceptance criteria.
May have different interference profiles than gel-clot assays (useful if the gel-clot assay will not give a valid result at a sensitive level).
Assays may be automated.
Lambda may be varied by changing the bottom value of the standard curve (within the limits of the given LAL), thus allowing the MVD to be extended for diffifult-to-test (interfering) products.

Kinetic tests versus end point tests
Quantifies a result over a range of several logs (i.e., the difference between the highest and lowest standard curve points) versus a single log.
Tests to completion without user intervention after LAL addition—precision, speed, and accuracy improved.

Chromogenic versus turbidimetric tests (kinetic and end point)
Calculates a result over a range of several logs (i.e., the difference between the highest and lowest standard curve points) versus a single log.
Tests to completion without user intervention after LAL addition.
Turbidity determinations are made based on the physical blocking of transmitted light (like nephlometry).
Chromogenic methods (end-point and kinetic) are not limited by particulate constraints associated with Beer's Law (absorbance is directly proportional to common parameters such as well depth).
The chromogenic method may be applied to turbid samples.
The turbidimetric method may be applied to samples with a yellow tint.

Recombinant factor C (fluorescent test)
May provide sample suitability advantages as it does not contain unknown factors associated with the blood of the horseshoe crab (i.e., no glucan pathway).
Fluorescence associated with emission not absorbance as per kinetic methods.
rFC not susceptible to lot-to-lot variability as it is not a product of seasonal *Limulus* blood harvest and purification.
Considered an alternate assay by USP standards and requires validation of USP parameters including comparative study to accepted USP method.
It is not a blood product and therefore, technically, not subject to the same constraints in its manufacture and distribution; however, the converse of this is less guidance in its use to date.
Provides a much needed safeguard against catastrophic loss of *Limulus*.

Abbreviations: MVD, maximum valid dilution; LAL, limulus amebocyte lysate.

are the data from which the kinetic reader software uses the formulas referenced in Attachment A for the result calculations given unknown sample reaction times.

Among the most significant advantages of kinetic and end point testing over the gel-clot assay is that they allow for the quantitative extrapolation of an unknown result between standard points. (See Table 4 for a summary of the relative advantages presented by each major type of LAL test.) In the gel-clot test, results are limited by the dilutions that can be made, typically in a two-fold fashion. In this manner, the gel-clot assay can only reveal that the true value is between the positive and negative recovery in the given test tubes (i.e., the "break point"), whereas in the kinetic test samples are pipetted into a 96 well microtiter plate layered with LAL and read photometricallly by a spectrophotometer set on 405 or 340 nm (kinetic chromogenic and turbidimetric). The color or turbidity reaction that occurs between LAL and endotoxin is recorded in the form of the time in seconds that it takes a sample to reach a threshold OD reading as a defined setting in the reader's software (OD or mOD). The log of the time obtained for each sample is plotted against the log of the endotoxin content obtained in the same test for known standards.

The gel-clot quantification approach has been widely used to monitor in-process materials and water, but has been largely supplanted by kinetic tests due to the ability of kinetic assays to quantify and extrapolate accurate results over a wide range of endotoxin concentration. A positive control consisting of a product sample spiked with a known concentration of endotoxin and a negative control using nonpyrogenic water is used in LAL test procedure to ensure the lack of inter-ference in the sample matrix. Although a simple clot end point may be adequate for routine release testing of various pharmaceuticals, the ability to quantify endotoxin is invaluable for troubleshooting production-related pyrogen problems. Daily moni-toring of plant water and in-process testing can alert production personnel to poten-tial pyrogen problems before they become critical. Corrective action can be taken to reduce pyrogen loads and levels of endotoxin at this time. Using the gel-clot assay, one would not see the increase in activity until the sample forms a clot. Thus there is little or no warning prior to failing a given lot of water sample (or anything else).

Kinetic Turbidimetric Assay

Turbidity is a precursor to gel-clot formation and, therefore, the turbidimetric test is clearly an extension of the gel-clot assay. This LAL reagent contains enough coagu-logen to form turbidity when cleaved by the clotting enzyme, but not enough to form a clot (64). Although the solid gel-clot assay is still widely used as an LAL test, it has the disadvantage of being an "early end point" test. Consequently, if it is used, endotoxin cannot be quantified below the level at which a solid clot is formed. The LAL turbidimetric assay, on the other hand, gives a more quantitative measurement of endotoxin over a range of concentrations. This assay is predicated on the fact that any increase in endotoxin concentration causes a proportional increase in turbidity due to the precipitation of coagulable protein (coagulogen) in lysate (hence forming coagulin). Thus, the OD of various dilutions of the sub-stance to be tested are read against a standard curve obtained that has been spiked with known quantities of endotoxin in sterile water.

Kinetic Chromogenic Substrate Assay

The chromogenic assay differs from the gel-clot and turbidimetric reactions in that the coagulogen (clotting protein) is partially (or wholly) replaced by a chromogenic substrate, which is a short synthetic peptide containing the amino acid sequence at the point of interaction with the clotting enzyme. The end of this peptide is bound to a chromophore, para-nitroanilide (pNA).

Japanese workers pioneered the use of chromogenic substrates and lysate (from *Limulus* and from *Tachypleus*, the Japanese horseshoe crab) for the detection of endotoxin (65,66). The chromogenic method takes advantage of the specificity of the endotoxin-activated proclotting enzyme, which exhibits specific amidase activity for carboxyterminal glycine-arginine residues. When such sequences are conjugated to a chromogenic substance, pNA is released in proportion to increasing concentrations of endotoxin. Thus, it is possible to measure endotoxin concentration by measuring endotoxin-induced amidase activity as release of chromophore. Release of chromogenic substrate is measured by reading absorbance at 405 nm. Testing is conducted with 100 μL^e of lysate and an equal amount of sample or diluted sample. The quantitative relationship between the logarithm of the endotoxin concentration and amidase activity can be observed between 5×10^{-6} and 5×10^{-2} ng/mL of endotoxin and, therefore, can be used for the detection of picogram quantities of endotoxin, associated with medical device eluates, immersion rinse solutions, and drug products.

The early chromogenic studies of Lindsay (66) have been extended in recent years by a number of investigators. Suzuki et al. improved the chromogenic assay by using Tos-Ile-Glu-Gly-Arg as a chromophore with the lysate prepared from the amebocytes of *Tachypleus* (67). Endotoxin-induced amidase activity was optimal at a pH of 8 and at 40°C. Induction of the reaction requires Mg^{2+}. The authors concluded that the system was 50 times more sensitive than the *Limulus* gelation test. The single step chromogenic method was subsequently developed by Linday et al. Associates of Cape Cod (68) and in this form set the stage for today's simplified use of the kinetic and end point chromogenic assays. The previous chromogenic assays were all end point assays [except for that used by Urbaschek et al. (69) in 1984, which used an experimental kinetic chromogenic test for clinical endotoxemia studies] employing multiple reagent additions that introduce more variability.

The New Recombinant Factor C Reagent

The commercialization of Wang et al. and Tan et al.'s (35,37) efforts to isolate and clone the endotoxin sensitive region of the factor C biosensor has resulted in a remarkable feat: the mass production of a sensitive detector of bacterial endotoxin that is not reliant on a blood source. Interesting detail can be gained from the United States patents on the material.[f] The method employs a copy of the factor C endotoxin-binding sequence of 333 amino acids of *Carcinoscorpius rotundicauda* (i.e., Singapore horseshoe crab) DNA expressed in a baculoviral system, which is the first such expression system to preserve the "highly complex mosaic structure" (US patent 6,719,973) required to detect endotoxin. The entry of such a test was able to by pass the level of regulatory scrutiny historically reserved for LAL in that it is not the by-product of a blood system and therefore is not subject to the same type of

---

[e]The Seiku Geiku ACC package insert references the use of 50 microliters of sample and standard.
[f]Patent numbers 5,712,144 and 6,719,973.

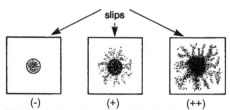

(-)	(+)	(++)

"Ring formation Decreased "cloud" "Cloud-like" spread of gel with stained with "spot" formation
cell debris

FIGURE 6   Typical reactions using the microslide *Limulus* amebocyte lysate assay. *Source*: From Refs. 75,76.

overview as LAL. This allowed rapid commercialization of a product (PyroGene™ by Cambrex Biosciences). The removal of such a barrier of entry being seemingly opens the door for eventual cost reduction once the patents expire or if other, similar, recombinant type biosensors are introduced in a competitive manner. The assay, though still relatively new, provides needed insurance against the inevitable, unfortunate decline of the most ancient of mariners (*Limulus*).

The new rFC assay is incorporated in a process analytical technology employed by the manufacturer Cambrex in their Pyrosense™ automated water testing robot (in-line system) as described in Chapter 16. Seemingly, a barrier to early user-acceptance of rFC appears to be the use of fluorescence instead of the conventional spectroscopy used in the kinetic photometric assays. The limit of detection claim is 0.01 EU/mL[g]. Though Cambrex has incorporated the test into their software platform a reader with fluorescence capability is a necessity if employing the test. Correspondingly, the validation and qualification activities do not appear as clear cut as those that have become commonplace in LAL testing, given the 1987 Guideline on LAL validation.

"CATS AND DOGS" OF LAL

The methods mentioned here are largely antiquated and would not meet compendial requirements for endotoxin testing; nevertheless, they give an appreciation for the current methods and bring with them the knowledge that today's tests are but a fraction of the number of tests that could be (and that have been) developed using the basic LAL mechanism, as discovered by Levin and Bang. Some of the assays also serve as references for reduced-reagent assays the desirability of which may increase with diminished populations of horseshoe crabs, though presumably rFC may negate such a necessity. It is also conceivable that some could be adapted to microfluidics or nanotechnology methods. This information was elaborated on in the first two editions, but has now been condensed into Table 5 given herewith.

---

[g]Cambrex Biosciences package insert for PyroGene™.

TABLE 5 Largely Superseded Methods

Diazo-Coupling of Chromogenic Reagent

A test not widely used is an extension of the chromogenic assay in that the p-nitroaniline formed by the conventional reaction is further chemically modified by the additional reagents to form the magenta colored, azo dye (62). While only an end point test, it provides one advantage in that the magenta color is read at an absorbance of 540 nm thus avoiding interference with yellow samples such as urine and culture media (71).

The Travenol Optical Density-Lowry Protein-Colorimetric Method

Like turbidimetric, it is based on the observation that increasing concentrations of endotoxin precipitate proportionally increasing amounts of lysate protein. Thus, the amount of protein (coagulin) precipitated can be quantified by performing a simple Lowry protein determination (71). Equal volumes of test sample and lysate (0.1 mL) are mixed in pyrogen-free tubes and incubated at 37°C for one hour and then centrifuged at approximately 1375×g for 10 mm. Supernatant is then removed by vacuum aspiration. The amount of lysate-specific precipitated protein is determined using the Qyama and Eagle (72) modification of the Lowry protein assay. Using a flow-through spectrophotometer, the OD is recorded at 660 nm. The results can then be related to a standard reference curve.

Nephelometric Method (NM)

NM test has found some utility (i.e., in Japan) as a means of pyrogen detection in large-volume parenterals (LVP) and testing water for production or rinses of depyrogenated components (73). The method employs a Hyland laser nephelometer. Instead of being read as OD, the nephelometer records the light scattered relative to its position at a 90° angle from the light source (Tyndall scattering of turbid liquids) (74). Sodium dodecyl sulfate (SDS) terminates the enzymatic reaction and ensures the uniformity of precipitated lysate-specific protein. Critical micellar concentration (CMC) is then added as a suspension stabilizer. The test can be completed within an hour using only 50 μL of lysate, which can readily detect picogram amounts of endotoxin.

Slide Test

Frauch (75) first suggested a simple LAL slide test. Using a calibrated capillary pipette, 10 μL of lysate was mixed with an equal volume of sample. This preparation is incubated in a moist chamber at 37°C for 30 minutes. A positive control, a negative control, and test samples were prepared on slides with black backgrounds. The controls and samples are easily differentiated on the basis of viscosity and turbidity. Another Japanese worker, Okuguchi (76), reported an improved LAL microslide method employing 10 μL of lysate. Samples are incubated in the presence of lysate on a tissue culture chamber slide for 30 minutes at 37°C. Test samples are then stained with a drop of bromophenol blue and end points determined using an inverted-phase contrast microscope. Samples forming a ring filled with cell debris are negative for endotoxin, but positive samples exhibit a cloud-like formation throughout the mixture.

Micro Assay

Gardi and Arpagaus (77) described an LAL microtechnique using 1 μL of reagent and sample. Samples are incubated in 5 μL capillary tubes, which are dipped into a dye. When a firm gel is formed, the dye cannot enter the tube and the test result is recorded as positive. The single greatest virtue of the microslide method is cost savings; the price of lysate has historically been considerably higher elsewhere than in the United States.

53. Wilson M, Harvey W. A new assay for bacterial lipopolysaccharides. Curr Microbiol 1990; 21:91–94.
54. F.D.A. Guideline on Validation of the *Limulus* Amebocyte Lysate test as an end-product test for human and animal parenteral drugs, biological prodcuts and medical devices. U. S. Dept. of Health & Human Services, Dec, 1987.
55. PDA. Current practices in endotoxin and pyrogen testing in biotechnology. PDA J Parenter Sci Technol 1990; 44(1).
56. Levin J, Bang FB. Clottable protein in *Limulus*: its localization and kinetics of its coagulatioin by endotoxin. Thromb Diath Haemorrh 1968; 19:186–197.
57. Lindsay GK, Roslansky PF, Novitsky TJ. Single-step, chromogenic *Limulus* amebocyte lysate assay for endotoxin. J Clin Microbiol 1989; 27(5):947–951.
58. Nakamura S et al. A sensitive substrate fro the clotting enzyme in horseshoe crab hemocytes. J Biochem 1977; 81(5):1567–1569.
59. Nachum R, Berzofsky R. Chromogenic amebocyte lysate assay for rapid detection of bacteriuria. J Clin Microbiol 1985; 21(5):759–763.
60. Cohen J, McConnell JS. Observations on the measurement and evaluation of endotoxemia by a quantitative *Limulus* lysate microassay. J Infect Dis 1984; 150(6):916–934.
61. Urbaschek B et al. Protective effects and role of endotoxin in experimental septicemia. Circ Shock 1984; 14:209–222.
62. Ditter B, Becker KP, Urbaschek R, Urbaschek B. Detection of endotoxin in blood and other specimens by evaluation of photometrically registered LAL-reaction-kinetics in microtiter plates. Prog Clin Biol Res 1982; 93:385–392.
63. Novitsky TJ. LAL methodology: the choice is yours. MD&DI 1984; January.
64. Morita T et al. Horseshoe crab (*Tachypleus tridentatus*) clotting enzyme: A new sensitive assay method for bacterial endotoxin. Jpn J Med Sci Biol 1978; 31:178.
65. Iwanaga S et al. Chromatogenic substrates for horseshoe crab clotting enzyme-its application for the assay of bacterial endotoxins. Haemostasis 1978; 7:183.
66. Lindsay G. Quantitative colorimetric endotoxin analysis. Parenteral Drug Association Summer Meeting, Philadelphia, June 1980.
67. Suzuki TH et al. Further studies on the chromogenic substrate as-say method for bacterial endotoxins using horseshoe crab (*Tachypleus tridentatus*) hemocyte lysate. J Biochem 1982; 92:793.
68. Lindsay GK, Roslansky PF, Novitsky TJ. Single-step, chromogenic *Limulus* amebocyte lysate assay for endotoxin. J Clin Microbiol 1989; 27(5):947–951.
69. Urbaschek B et al. Protective effects and role of endotoxin in experimental septicemia. Circ Shock 1984; 14:209–222.
70. Novitsky TJ. Diazo-coupling option with pyrochrome chromogenic LAL. LAL Update 1998; 16(2):1–3.
71. Nanden R, Brown DR. An improved in vitro pyrogen test: to detect picograms of endotoxin contamination in intravenous fluids using *Limulus* amebocyte lysate. J Lab Med 1977; 89:910.
72. Qyama VI, Eagle H. Measurement of cell growth in tissue culture with a phenol reagent (Folin-Ciocalteau). Proc Soc Exp Biol Med 1956; 91:305.
73. Dubczak J, Cotter R, Dastoli F. Quantitative detection of endotoxin by nephelometry. In: Cohen E, ed. Biomedical Applications of the Horseshoe Crab (Limulidae). New York: Alan R. Liss, 1979:403.
74. Perkampus H. Encyclopedia of Spectroscopy. Weinheim: VCH Verlagsgesellschaft mbH, 1999:389–390.
75. Frauch P. Slide test as a micromethod of a modified *Limulus* endotoxin test. J Pharm Sci 1974; 63:808.
76. Okuguchi S. Improvement of the micromethod for the *Limulus* lysate test. Microbiol Immunol 1978; 22:113.
77. Gardi A, Arpagaus GR. Improved microtechnique for endotoxin assay by the *Limulus* amebocyte lysate test. Anal Biochem 1980; 109:382.

ATTACHMENT A:

DEPARTMENT OF HEALTH AND HUMAN SERVICES PUBLIC HEALTH SERVICE

Memorandum

Date: MAY 11 1992
From: Chairman, FDA LAL Task Force

Subject: Statement Concerning Glucans and LAL-Reactive Material in Pharmaceuticals and Medical Devices

To: To Whom It May Concern

It has been reported to the LAL Task Force that information has been circulated concerning FDA's position on glucans defined LAL-reactive material (LAL-RM) in pharmaceuticals and medical devices. Glucans are defined as polysaccharides composed only of recurring units of glucose, such as, glycogen, starch, and cellulose.

FDA is not aware of data indicating that glucans or LAL-RM are common in pharmaceuticals or maybe common in medical devices or whether they may pose a health hazard to patients using these products. The only product that has been shown to contain LAL-PM is dialysis membranes made of cellulose. LAL-RM is composed of very small fragments of the cellulose which break loose from the filter matrix. Studies in animals and tissue cultures indicate that LAL-RM is non-toxic in the quantities detected in dialyzers. Some investigators have indicated that LAL-RM may be responsible for some of the adverse reactions seen in dialysis patients. However, no direct correlation has been established. LAL-RM is the only glucan that has been reported in any medical device. LAL-RM is not considered a contaminant, because its source is not extrinsic to the device. It is a breakdown product of the cellulose membrane that is a component of the device. Since the majority of medical devices do not contain natural materials, there is no source of glucans in these devices.

No cases of glucans or LAL-RM have been reported in parenteral drug products. Most parenteral drug products are manufactured from chemically synthesized components. This fact coupled with good manufacturing practices makes the possibility of contamination with glucans very remote. It appears that large amounts of glucans are required (at least 1,000 times more by weight than endotoxin) to elicit a LAL positive reaction.

At this time, FDA considers that the presence of glucans in parenteral drug products and most medical devices to be more of a theoretical than actual problem. Firms should be aware that false positive results may be possible when testing medical devices having cellulose based components. It is the responsibility of the manufacturer to conclusively establish that any positive LAL test is not due to endotoxin contamination.

FDA will consider whether parenteral drug products or medical devices are adulterated due to the presence of glucans on a case-by-case basis, until such time as more information is obtained.

Terrry E. Munson

ATTACHMENT B:

KINETIC CALCULATIONS

User Performed

A. Pass/Fail Cutoff (PFC): $\quad$ PFC $= (TL \times PP)/PD$

B. Minimum Valid Concentration (MVC): $\quad$ MVC $= (\lambda \times M)/K$

C. Maximum Valid Dilution: MVD $= (TL \times PP)/\lambda$ or PP/MVC

for equations A to C:
$\quad$ K $\;=$ Threshold level of 5 EU/kG (0.2 EU/kG for intrathecal drugs)
$\quad$ M $\;=$ Maximum dose
$\quad$ PP $=$ Product potency at 1:1 dilution (undiluted)
$\quad$ PD $=$ Product dilution
$\quad$ λ $\;\;=$ Sensitivity of assay (lowest standard concentration)

Software Performed

D. Mean Reaction Time: $\quad \bar{X}_{RT} = \dfrac{\sum X_{RT}}{n}$

E. Standard Deviation of X (S_x): $\quad S_x = \sqrt{\dfrac{N\sum x^2 - \left(\sum x\right)^2}{N(N-1)}}$

F. Standard Deviation of y (S_y): $\quad S_y = \sqrt{\dfrac{N\sum y^2 - \left(\sum y\right)^2}{N(N-1)}}$

G. Coefficient of Correlation (r): $\quad r = \dfrac{N\sum xy - \left(\sum x\right)\left(\sum y\right)}{N(N-1)SxSy}$

H. Slope (m): $\quad m = \left(\dfrac{Sy}{Sx}\right)r$

I. Y - Intercept: $\quad b = \left(\dfrac{\sum y}{N}\right) - \left(\dfrac{\sum x}{Nm}\right)$

J. Endotoxin Concentration: $\quad$ EU/mL $=$ Antilog$\left[\dfrac{Log\bar{X}_{RT} - b}{m}\right]$

For equations D to J:
$\quad$ X $=$ Log (Concentration in EU/mL)
$\quad$ Y $=$ Log mean, reaction time
$\quad$ N $=$ Number of standards used
$\quad$ ΣX $=$ Summation of individual log (Standard concentrations in EU/mL)
$\quad$ ΣY $=$ Summation of individual log (mean reaction times)
$\quad$ ΣXY $= \Sigma$X x ΣY, $\Sigma(X_{RT}) =$ Summation of all sample or standard replicate reaction
$\qquad$ times
$\quad$ n $=$ Number of replicate

11 *Limulus* Amebocyte Lysate Assay Development, Validation, and Regulation

Kevin L. Williams

Eli Lilly & Company, Indianapolis, Indiana, U.S.A.

Historically, large volume parenteral manufacturers have been foremost in developing tests for Bacterial Endotoxin assays due to the criticality of even minute endotoxin concentrations in solutions administered in large doses. However, many of today's problems revolve around the recovery of control standard endotoxin spike, the difficulty of which is exacerbated by the chemical nature of the small volume drug materials being validated rather than their dose, which is often small.

OVERVIEW: IMPORTANCE OF A GOOD TEST

For parenteral products administered in large volumes, such as saline infusions, even minute volumes of endotoxin are unacceptable. Historically, large volume parenteral manufacturers have been foremost in developing tests for bacterial endotoxin assays due to the critical need for very sensitive detection of endotoxin in their products. However, many of today's problems in developing suitable endotoxin tests are not issues of sensitivity, as doses[a] are often small, but rather revolve around the recovery of control standard endotoxin spike, the difficulty of which is exacerbated by the chemical nature of the drug materials[a]. Small-volume parenteral drugs often contain high drug concentrations which interfere both with the physiology of rabbits in the rabbit pyrogen assay and with spike recoveries in the *Limulus* amebocyte lysate (LAL) assay (1). Some common types of problem compounds encountered in developing endotoxin assays for small-volume parenterals include water-insoluble drugs, drugs containing activity that mimics that of endotoxin, drugs containing endotoxin (that it may be desirable to remove prior to method validation), bulk drugs with variable potencies, multiple drugs in a given container, and potent, highly interfering drugs such as chemotherapy drugs. Now that the science of LAL testing has been firmly established, the challenges that remain often reside in difficult, product specific applications. Perhaps the last great challenge encountered in each parenteral analytical laboratory is the development of, not just an LAL test, but also a rugged, reproducible, and perhaps automatable test that will stand the test of time in routine use.

Given all the LAL methods that have been tried or potentially could be constructed (see Chapter 10), the question remains: What characteristics must a good LAL test have?[b] A good LAL test from a legal standpoint must meet the

---

[a]And the associated stringency of the resulting limit calculation.
[b]Considering that the bacterial endotoxin testing (BET) method is well-established, one need not consider the question in terms of establishing a new method as would be required with a prospective method.

appropriate compendial requirements and need not even be quantitative except in its ability to demonstrate the detection of the endotoxin limit concentration (gel-clot). However, beyond meeting compendial requirements, the best test is the one that provides the most information on the content of the analyte: endotoxin. The regulatory question that must be answered in order to put a drug on the market is: "Does it pass the release test?"[c] The scientific and business questions that remain to be answered are "How much endotoxin does the sample contain?," "How does the result compare to previous lot measurements?," and "How close to the endotoxin limit concentration is the result?"

The objective of method development and validation is to deliver a "good test" that has the following characteristics:

1. Noninterfering (positive controls are positive and negatives are negative)
2. Appropriate product solubility if reconstituted and diluted or as diluted only
3. Does not reduce (destroy) endotoxin that may be present if harsh conditions or solvents are employed[d]
4. Performed at an appropriate level as determined by the appropriate drug dose [or as per the United States Pharmacopeia (USP) monograph tolerance limit (TL) assigned for existing drugs], potency, lambda, and proposed or dictated specification requirement
5. Unaffected by significant batch or laboratory test variability
6. Resolution of a result (well) below the specification to allow manufacturing process contamination problems to be monitored prior to rising to alert levels
7. Provides a neutral pH environment (6–8) of the inhibition/enhancement (I/E) sample dilution after being combined with LAL
8. Contains the appropriate laboratory support testing such as labware controls (endotoxin free and noninterfering), Reference standard endotoxin (RSE)/control standard endotoxin (CSE), LAL label claim (gel-clot) or initial qualification (kinetic and end point tests), and diluent interference tests (i.e., their effect on LAL senstivitity)
9. Has test events that have proper documentation
10. Endotoxin-free and noninterfering nature of articles used in the test have been documented
11. Supported by appropriate user training, instrument installation qualification/operational qualifications, preventative maintenances (PMs), and so on.

There is some basic information to be gathered prior to setting out to develop a new test (i.e., determining and applying the appropriate sample preparation

---

[c]And significantly: (a) is the manufacturing process used to produce it compliant with cGMP requirements and (b) does the sampling and testing of precursors to the end product support the contention that the product is free of endotoxin at the levels required?

[d]Validation via a series of sample dilutions in tubes containing spike demonstrates that the sample spikes endures the harsh treatment. However, if a kinetic or end point in-plate spike is used at a significant dilution, then the demonstration that the spike has acceptably endured the entire sample preparation method should be performed in the validation testing. For instance, a sample prepared in dimethyl formimide (DMF) or other suspected harsh treatment then diluted to 1:1000 in water prior to spike in the plate will not demonstrate that the DMF does not destroy potential endotoxin. After all, the goal of validation is not to destroy endotoxin that may be present in the sample prior to testing.

treatments to a specific drug compound) particularly for a new chemical entity (NEC) as opposed to an established product. A list of questions for the submitting department or developing scientist(s) may be compiled:

1. The Maximum Human Dose (MHD), which will typically allow room for the clinic to increase the doses, as needed in safety and efficacy studies. The response should be documented in a written manner for inclusion in the validation documentation.
2. The formulation should be documented to establish the appropriate excipient tests (as will be discussed), and since it will likely change.
3. The presentation should be recorded as a critical assay parameter and may be subject to change [i.e., the product potency (PP) and volume or weight (for a given indication)].
4. The approximate scheduling of the manufacture of the (at least) three lots needed for validation testing (if available)
5. A change notification mechanism to notify the laboratory of potency, dose, and/ or presentation changes
6. Solubility profile [recommended reconstitution diluent(s)]. How water soluble is it? Or what is it most soluble in?
7. pH profile. What is the expected sample pH range?
8. Interference related questions:
   - Is it a known chelator [such as ethylenediaminetetraacetic acid (EDTA)]?
   - Does it possess enzymatic activity (such as trypsin or serine proteases) likely to interfere with LAL?
   - Is the active compound likely to be inactivated by heating in a water bath at 70°C (an enzyme)?
   - Is it likely to contain cellulosic material?
   - What is the molecular weight of the compound? If there is endogenous endotoxin, it will have to be removed (via filtration or binding) for validation purposes and the MW of the sample will determine if it may be filtered and still retain the active compound in the filtrate.

THE BACTERIAL ENDOTOXIN TESTING ASSAY DEVELOPMENT PROCESS

The need for a new bacterial endotoxin test (BET) typically begins with a call from a development scientist with a new compound. Perhaps it is a compound prepared for an animal toxicology study or perhaps it is a lot prepared in the development laboratory (a so-called "lab-lot"). The early lots of drug substance or drug product will not be used in people, but there is a need to establish their safety to insure that the studies being performed are not skewed in some manner by the presence of endotoxin. Drug development is a costly endeavor and the generation of misleading results can lead developers down lengthy and costly blind alleys. Typically, compounds have been handed over to a development team from a discovery research effort that has taken years in arriving. The compound has been formulated now for parenteral use, perhaps only one of the many current or potential formulations, by combining a drug substance [bulk or active pharmaceutical ingredient (API)] solubilizers, stabilizers, preservatives, emulsifiers, thickening agents, and so on (2). The compound is in flux and may change several times in its formulation (excipients), presentation (i.e., potency, container, size), and application (e.g., dose and perhaps indication). Perhaps, if its prospects seem especially bright, it will spawn a host of sister compounds that vary in the means of drug delivery (e.g., parenteral, for inhalation, time-delay parenteral, etc.) and, therefore, in several relevant parameters required to be defined prior to developing additional suitable endotoxin tests (Fig. 1).

The development of a new assay for the BET for a given compound may be as simple as:

1. Calculating the new product's proposed TL and maximum valid dilution (MVD) based upon the clinical dose of the material (or USP monograph listed TL if it is an established drug)
2. Diluting the material in sterile reagent water
3. Testing it by either the gel-clot, end point, or a kinetic (turbidimetric or chromogenic) method at a dilution below the MVD.

Guilfoyle and Munson (3) of the FDA New York regional laboratory surveyed samples tested by the LAL method in 1980. They reported that, of 298 samples examined, 61% (181) were incompatible as tested undiluted with LAL. The second year of surveillance revealed that 84% (244/289) were not compatible without dilution. Furthermore, 7% and 5% were not compatible even after dilution out to their calculated minimum valid dilutions (MVDs). When data were compiled from four additional FDA labs, a total of 1400 samples had been analyzed consisting of 257 different drugs. Guilfoyle and Munson determined that 20% could be tested without dilution, 75% required dilution, and about 5% of the interfering samples could not be tested at all. They reported that of the 23 (1980) samples that required dilution, 11 (~50%) could be directly tested after reconstituting in 2% pyrosperse (a "metallo-modified polyanionic dispersant," Cambrex, Inc. Walkersville, Maryland, U.S.A.) (4).

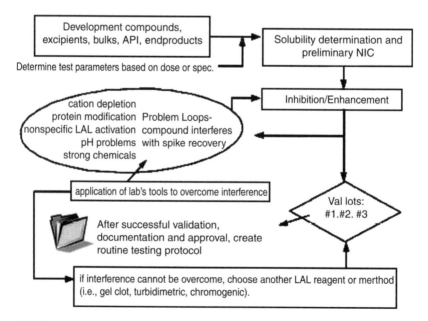

FIGURE 1 Interrelationship of parameters to be defined in validating a development compound. *Abbreviations*: API, active pharmaceutical ingredient; NIC, non-inhibitory concentration.

However, given that early drugs were much less complex than today's drugs, it seems that the days of simple validations that do not require additional sample treatment(s) have passed. Now one would not realistically expect to test most drugs in an undiluted fashion. Many compounds have mitigating factors seemingly designed to frustrate the best assay development efforts as previously described. Additional mitigating sample complications include:

1. Cost: some product candidates are so expensive that product development scientists are reluctant to supply sufficient quantities for protracted method development and validation.
2. Multiple interference properties not overcome by simple dilution whereby adjusting one causes a deterioration of another
3. Poorly characterized products: at an early stage of drug development one can expect to see drug products that vary greatly from lot to lot (i.e., they are still being adjusted by those charged with establishing their formulation).

Early laboratory method development activities revolve around finding a suitable solvent (if it is not particularly water soluble) and determining the dilution required to overcome interference preliminary non-inhibitory concentration (pNIC). The submitter may have a detailed solubility profile if the compound has complex solubility requirements.

OVERVIEW OF COMMON TESTING PROTOCOLS

The types of testing protocols used in developing a new method include (*i*) solubility protocols (see Attachments A and B to this chapter for example protocols), (*ii*) pNIC protocols, and the (*iii*) full validation protocol. The tests performed in this sequence are cumulative. In simple terms, the NIC test varies the sample concentration while keeping the endotoxin concentration fixed (none and 2λ) while the I/E test varies the endotoxin concentration (to mimic the standard curve) while maintaining a constant product concentration. The three tests for the gel-clot method and subsequent result calculation (which can be applied to the kinetic and end point methods with some adjustments) serve to establish several parameters upon which to base future routine testing:

1. One cannot perform the pNIC without having a good idea of the solubility characteristics of the material. To bridge the gap for water-insoluble compounds by dissolving the compound in a suitable solvent that does not destroy endotoxin (dimethyl sulfoxide is such a suitable diluent for many water-insoluble compounds) but that also is readily diluted with water or buffer. The right proportion will have to be found to keep the compound dissolved, but to allow enough dilution in water to overcome potential interference by both the compound and the solvent. The pH characteristics go hand in hand with the solubility. It may be necessary to acidify a given solution before a compound is added into the solution. A caveat here is that, whatever is done to the sample should be done to the CSE spike to demonstrate that the (sometimes harsh) conditions used to solubilize the compound has not destroyed any endogenous endotoxin that may be present. The full survival of the CSE will serve to document this. This is necessary to mention because of the prevalence today of adding kinetic spikes to only the final dilution of a series in the microtiter plate itself.

2. The preliminary NIC will determine where the full validation test may be successfully performed. Typically, at some point in a series of two-fold dilutions of both spiked (2λ) and nonspiked samples, a "break-point" will be determined [first positive spike (2λ) recovery of the series coexistent with no recovery in the unspiked sample at the same dilution]. If the unspiked two-fold dilution is negative and the positive is positive, then this demonstrates that the observed interference has been overcome by the dilution. Therefore, the noninhibitory concentration is somewhere between the first positive and the negative (2λ) spiked sample test directly preceding it. If it occurs at a level that is compatible with the calculated MVD [minimum valid concentration (MVC) for a bulk, excipient or API sample], then one may proceed to the full validation test.
3. The full validation test typically includes both an NIC confirmation and an I/E curve, which is simply a standard curve performed in sample solution at the concentration of the sample that one would not exceed (validated level). The I/E dilution level must not exceed the MVD (or one-third MVD for pooled vial tests) and must exceed the MVC of sample (or 3 × MVC for pooled vials) needed to detect the endotoxin limit concentration (the TL amount of endotoxin). The full validation test may include a limit test at the proposed routine test dilution, but it is not necessary because that dilution is contained within the NIC and will be greater than or equal to the I/E dilution being tested.
4. The validation reportable test result will be based upon the successful performance of the I/E test. If the I/E test agrees within a two-fold dilution with the labeled LAL label claim (and the included valid CSE curve) then the sample (test result, TR) can be said to contain:

$$TR = \frac{< \lambda X \ DF \ X \ PF^{6^e}}{PP}$$

where PP is the product potency of the active ingredient as reconstituted for a weighed sample or as labeled for a liquid sample containing a predetermined potency, DF is the dilution factor, and PF is the pool factor. A geometric mean is not necessary to determine the result calculation obtained here because the I/E is either valid at the given dilution (sample concentration) or is invalid (i.e., does not confirm the label claim).

RESOLVING TEST INTERFERENCES

Given that the LAL assay in its many forms is a water-based assay derived from a sensitive physiological environment (blood of the horseshoe crab), it is not too surprising that as one ventures farther from such an aqueous environment the results often correspondingly deteriorate. The Catch-22 of such testing resembles the contradiction presented by endotoxin itself in that an increase in water content of a

---

[e]The Lilly laboratory uses a conservative approach in that when beginning, middle, and end vials are pooled for end product testing (as required by the FDA guideline), then the result obtained is multiplied by the pool factor (usually 3) to account for the potential worst case endotoxin content of a single vial to report a numerical result. It is at least theoretically possible that all the endotoxin content in a sample could be contributed by a single vial (i.e., either the beginning, middle, or end vial of the batch); therefore when pooled samples are tested the result is multiplied by the pool factor.

hydrophobic material in solution will cause the material to precipitate (and endo-toxin to aggregate) but, conversely, as one gets away from water, the reaction of LAL and endotoxin will bring about assay interference.

Cooper's paper on interference mechanisms encountered during LAL testing is perhaps the most useful on the subject (5). Cooper lists five (the first five of the seven items listed below) major interference mechanisms to be expected when testing various parenteral drugs for BET using the LAL test and points out that often interference mechanisms result from the sample matrix's effect on the aggre-gation properties of the CSE rather than or as well as on the lipopolysaccharide (LPS)–LAL reaction itself. The broad mechanisms listed by Cooper include:

1. Suboptimal pH conditions
2. Aggregation or adsorption of control endotoxin spikes
3. Unsuitable cation concentrations
4. Enzyme or protein modification
5. Nonspecific LAL activation (sometimes an interference mechanism cannot be determined)
6. Samples containing endotoxin
7. Endotoxin masking

Each broad interference mechanism will be briefly explored along with notable (common or unique) means of overcoming the associated interference:

1. Suboptimal pH conditions are an unsurprising interference mechanism given that the LAL coagulation system is a product of a physiological system and many drugs are not. A pH of 6.4 to 8.0 is said to be optimal and a pH require-ment of 6.0 to 8.0 taken on a given sample and LAL combination (subsequent to test) is required by the USP and is listed by most LAL vendor package inserts as a requirement as well. Many LAL reagents are buffered either as lyophilized or as reconstituted and serve to help overcome minor pH problems. Alternatively, an initial pH adjustment using 0.1N or lower HCl or NaOH of a buffered sample (unbuffered solutions should not be pH'ed) will pull a sample within a suitable range for the LAL to do the remaining buffering. For more acidic or basic samples, the use of an initially stronger buffer (such as 100 mM Tris buffer) may prevent many subsequent variability problems for a user where the sample comes to the lab with a variable pH. Cooper maintains that pH pro-blems "are the most important biochemical cause of LAL-test inhibition" (6). The pH statement in the USP concerning the 6.0–8.0 requirement leaves it open to debate if the intention is that every test should be accompanied by a pH test. An FDA inspector has gone on record as saying that such testing was not routinely required for a validated method unless committed to in the firm's new drug application (7). However, the inspector continued on to imply that a failure to study the upper and lower limits of the product pH range might necessitate such routine pH testing (6).

   If a buffer is used to reconstitute an unbuffered LAL, the user must ensure that the LAL sensitivity is not changed in the process. Additionally, any diluent (or any article for that matter) used in a test that is not water must be shown to neither inhibit nor enhance the recovery of endotoxin as compared to the CSE in water standard as per the USP (8).
2. Endotoxin modification is a problem involving the amphiphilic properties of the CSE. Strong salts and other solutions causing a large increase in test sample ionic

strength will cause endotoxin aggregation and poor spike recovery. Dispersing agents such as Pyrosperse™ (Cambrex Corp., Baltimore, Maryland) along with dilution (within the MVD parameters) is often used to overcome such interference. Adsorption of endotoxin to containers made of polypropylene is a widely known interference mechanism and is therefore avoided in all types of endotoxin testing labware except pipette tips (9–11). The short time solutions encounter pipette tips have not proved to result in reduced endotoxin recovery. The demonstration of the lack of interference with each article coming into contact with the LAL test is a harmonized pharmacopoeial requirement.

3. Unsuitable cation concentrations can occur due to chelators such as EDTA that are added for the very purpose of complexing cations that may cause instability in parenteral formulations. 50 mM $MgCl_2$ is routinely used as an LAL test diluent to provide suitable levels of Ca^{+2} and Mg^{+2}. Reagents may vary in cation concentration and buffering capacity among those supplied by LAL manufacturers (12).

4. Protein or enzyme modification occurs when the enzymes (serine proteases) necessary to complete the LAL gelation reaction are denatured by strong chemicals (alcohols, phenols, oncolytic drugs, etc.). If the offending agent is itself an enzyme, it can be denatured by heating a sample or dilution of a sample at 70°C for about ten minutes prior to dilution and testing. Other offenders may be removed by ion or size filtration, though the validation requirements may be onerous and unique for each application thereby requiring extensive development work. Mallinckrodt (before their LAL business split off to become Cambrex) described a method of liquid–liquid extraction capable of pulling endotoxin into the aqueous phase, which would thereby leave an inhibitor or difficult to work with sample (oil) in the discarded oily phase[f]. Mallinckrodt maintained that the endotoxin due to its lipid nature tends to remain associated with oils, but by the use of Pyrosperse in the liquid–liquid extraction, the endotoxin can be coaxed into the aqueous page. These more complex interference removal mechanisms require considerable validation skills.

5. Nonspecific LAL activation includes the detection of LAL-reactive material and drugs that mimic endotoxin such as those containing proteases. Proteases may be heat-inactivated. Products that mimic endotoxin activity provide a more difficult challenge. A process of elimination may be employed to show that the activity that is occurring is not endotoxin. This is achieved by testing the product thereby revealing a certain level of activity followed by treatment of the sample to bind the suspected endotoxin (if the molecular weight of the product prohibits filtration removal). If the sample endotoxin content is not reduced there is a good probability that it is not endotoxin. At this point, one either needs an alternate method of testing (typically the rabbit pyrogen test will also be positive and will not help) or can lower the lambda of the test to allow sufficient dilution to overcome ("outrun") the interference. Otherwise, one may proceed to the next mechanism that follows. Some critical confirmatory information has to be gathered concerning whether the sample contains endotoxin or if the pharmacological activity of the sample is responsible for the activity and perhaps necessary for the desired pharmacological activity of the drug as a therapy as well.

---

[f]Mallinckrodt I. Testing of Oil Solutions with Pyrogen (LAL). Pyrogen Application Bulletin 2, p. 1–2.

6. Samples containing endotoxin present a problem similar to the previous mechanism if the levels are relevant to the required test levels, given the associated specifications. For development testing it may be desirous to remove endotoxin prior to performing the I/E test. Methods of removal include filtration [20,000 Sartorious filter (Sartorious AG, Goettingen, Germany) (13)] or a binding method such as End-X^{TM} (14) or Profos^{TM} (15), when the molecular weight of the sample ingredient(s) exceed the cut-off rating of the filter. See Figure 1 concerning the "problem loop" presented by situations posed in the previous mechanism and the one presented here.

7. A potentially difficult interference mechanism not on Cooper's list is called "masking." Petsch et al. (16) describe an interference mechanism involving the properties of certain cationic proteins[g] that they refer to as "masking." This phenomenon involves proteins or peptide containing drug compounds that bind endotoxin and thus reduce or prevent the ability of LAL to detect contaminating endotoxin or the CSE spike, added to determine the sample's interference properties. The types of drug products containing peptides have grown recently. Some detail of the group's (16) development work is described in Case Study 3.

ENDOTOXIN ASSAY DEVELOPMENT CASES STUDIES

A few assay development projects are noteworthy due to either the complexity of the problem presented and/or the protracted nature of the solution.

Case Study 1

Piluso and Martinez (17) developed a quantitative LAL method of testing liposome material. Piluso and Martinez (17) considered that with their particular product "there can be no assurance that endotoxin has not incorporated within the forming liposome unless specific analysis is executed," because the function of the liposome as a drug delivery vehicle is to entrap and deliver fixed amounts of pharmaceutical agent in vivo. The difficulty of testing liposomes by an LAL method is that they are insoluble in water and possess colloidal properties that interfere with spectrophotometric analysis. The solution presented by the authors was to treat the sample with various surfactants to disperse the lipids of the liposome followed by subsequent dilution. They examined a number of surfactants including triton-X, polyoxyethylene-10-lauryl ether (PELE), sodium dodecyl sulfate (SDS), and CHAPS, a zwitterionic surfactant. The introduction of a "protein-denaturing detergent such as SDS" necessitated the complete characterization of the test method. The testing of each diluent revealed that SDS provided the best recovery of spike when present at very low concentrations (<0.001% w/v). A mathematical relationship of SDS, CHAPS, and PELE concentration as related to percent endotoxin spike recovery was established. The Triton-X treated sample was not pursued because it did not disrupt the liposome. In addition to SDS, CHAPS gave acceptable recovery at concentrations at or below 0.01% w/v surfactant concentration (17). Although the absolute recoveries using SDS were closer to theory, the minimum inhibitory concentration of CHAPS was ten times greater than that of SDS (0.01 versus 0.001% w/v), implying as the researchers contend that CHAPS was ten-fold less destructive toward the lysate reagent. This study provides a good example of a method that

---

[g]Positively-charged proteins that bind negatively-charged endotoxin molecules.

can be expected to be trouble-free in routine use because the entire range of the effects of the test matrix on the endotoxin recovery was demonstrated (in sigmoidal fashion) as opposed to the "we tested it, it works, it's validated" method sometimes employed and sometimes inferred from the FDA Guideline "3 lot validation" requirement (i.e., "if it worked three times, all the problems must be solved").

Case Study 2
In this laboratory, the in-process testing of a purchased cell culture additive revealed a fairly consistent level of activity presumed to be endotoxin. Due to the lipid nature of the product the suspicion existed that there was some nonendotoxin reactivity occurring. Treatment of the early (in the development cycle of this compound) samples could not remove the low levels of activity by any means. The treatments that were tried included End-X binding, heat treatment of the sample at 70°C for ten minutes (used in case the activity was not due to endotoxin), and dilution in a glucan blocking buffer. Due to the viscosity of the material, filtration was not an option. No appreciable difference between the before and after treatment of specific samples was observed. The supplier of the material for a developmental compound was in the course of switching to an upgraded (new) manufacturing facility, the completion of which immediately reduced the counts routinely observed in newly manufactured lots. The laboratory obtained several lots possessing levels of endotoxin below the detection limit and those lots were used for the "validation" of the in-process sample test method. The new lots were consistently below a very restrictive limit imposed (somewhat arbitrarily as the additive is not a product or an excipient).

As a check of the material from the new manufacturing facility, selected lots that tested below the limit but still contained detectable activity were treated with End-X for the minimum time of four hours [the package insert recommends from four hours to preferably overnight (18)] of gentle shaking at room temperature. End-X is an Associates of Cape Cod (ACC) product created from endotoxin-neutralizing protein (the recombinant form of amebocyte-derived *Limulus* anti-LPS factor) (19) bound to a resin bead (20, 21) to facilitate endotoxin binding and removal. The endotoxin concentration was reduced this time from the pre-treated level of approximately 30 EU/mL to approximately 4 EU/mL. While one cannot be entirely certain the initially higher levels of endotoxin observed were entirely due to endotoxin (and not some artificial interference mechanism, given the lipid nature of the product), the activity that remained could now be attributed to being low levels of endotoxin with certainty based on the very specific binding activity with the End-X product. Thus, the desired goals were accomplished in that (*i*) the supplier would supply low level endotoxin materials, (*ii*) Lilly assay development would be able to verify and document those levels with confidence to ensure that the lower levels could be monitored and were in fact endotoxin [largely due to the specificity of the End-X material (22)], and (*iii*) the analytical test could be used with confidence to ensure that endotoxin cannot affect the expression system used in the manufacturing process.

Case Study 3
Petsch describes the concerns involved with developing LAL test methods for compounds that mask endotoxin:

> These two points, the uncertainty about the toxicity of protein-bound endotoxins and their impaired LAL activity, cause serious problems when cationic pharmaproteins are

assayed for endotoxins. In these cases the LAL assay is not appropriate to determine the absolute amount of residual endotoxins, that is, the biological risk of the product.

Therefore, in order to create an appropriate test, such drug compounds must be modified (treated) prior to test. Luckily, for everything living made in nature there is seemingly something else made to degrade it, for proteins these enzymes are called proteases (23)[h]. Proteases exist in all living organisms and are necessary to provide a number of diverse and critical functions. An example of this is the clotting function of blood in higher organisms. If the clotting function were always "on" it would be catastrophic. Therefore, the proteins responsible exist typically in a zymogen state and are produced only as needed and for short periods of time such as needed to stop the flow of blood from a wound. The use of proteases in commercial food preparation (cheese) and as additives in detergents are examples of their common worldwide historical application. Some of the newer uses as applied to human health include the use in polymerase chain reaction (PCR) testing, as additives to antibiotic therapy against *Helicobacter pylori* infection (24), and as methods to decontaminate surgical instruments potentially contaminated with prions (25).

Though rife with caveats[i], the use of purified, purchased proteases can overcome the effects of peptide masking. After many nonprotease attempts, Petsch et al. employed several different proteases to overcome the observed masking of protein compounds (demask). Treatment under a variety of conditions using trypsin, RNase A, chymotrypsin, pronase, and proteinase K were all tried with the most success occurring with proteinase K. Proteins used to examine the phenomenon included lysozyme, human immunoglobulin G (IgG), bFGF, bovine serum albumin (BSA), and murine IgG_1. Tests were done in pH 7 20 mM phosphate buffer at protein concentrations of 1 mg/mL. The following data insert table show the results of an initial test and a subsequent test performed by passing a culture filtrate of *Escherichia coli* (to mimic endogenous endotoxin) through a filter with and without each protein solution. The recoveries obtained demonstrate the amount of endotoxin that was bound by the protein and thus not recovered from the filtrate.

Protein	EU/mL w/o protein	EU/mL w/ protein
Lysozyme	6180	297
Rnase A	726	146
Human IgG	6180	99
b-FGF	478	9
BSA	6180	6100
Murine IgG_1	6180	5840

The authors demonstrated that the proteins with a net positive charge result in significant loss of endotoxin via binding whereas those with a net negative charge do not. Significantly, the dilution of each of the samples given in the table prior to filtration employed only protein concentrations that were noninterfering with the LAL assay thus "the reason for the poor endotoxin recoveries" are due to masking and cannot be overcome by dilution.

---

[h]Consider lipase that breaks down lipids, amylase, glucoamylase, cellulase, xylanse, laccase, phytase, and so on.
[i]Perhaps the most significant being the propensity to themselves contain endotoxin.

The authors continue their study to dissociate the endotoxin-protein complexes by using lysozyme as a model. The use of detergents and high ionic solutions did nothing to break up the masking effect. Proteinase K is used routinely to degrade proteins and peptides into their amino acids to aid in the isolation of DNA and in RNA from tissue prior to PCR. Results are shown below.

Protein	EU/mL$^{via\ LAL}$	EU/mL$^{via\ LAL\ w/protease}$
Lysozyme (6000 EU/mL)	297	6012
Lysozyme (30 EU/mL)	4.2	24
Commercial Lysozyme	3.4	18
Rnase A (726 EU/mL)	146	712
Human IgG (6000 EU/mL)	99	5496

Case Study 4

Work in this laboratory (Lilly assay development) with a problematic antibiotic revealed similar release of compound-bound CSE spikes by using Pronase (Sigma-Aldrich). Factors affecting recovery include incubation time, temperature, protease potency (proteases are rated in units/mg in regard to degradation of a common protein, typically casein[j,k]), protease concentration (mass in solution), and, of course, the specificity of the protease chosen. As Petsch et al. observed a caveat in using these enzymes is that typically they contain endotoxin. More purified, commercially available products in regard to endotoxin content would greatly aid their use in this application. To successfully employ such a method the protease necessitates screening for endotoxin content prior to use and method development to minimize the effect of adding endotoxin to the test sample by using a higher potency protease and thereby reducing the amount (mass) needed to produce the desired proteolytic effect. There is also a possibility that observed endotoxin activity in the protease could be due to serine protease activation of the LAL cascade (which employs a number of serine proteases from the horseshoe crab reagent). However, this was not observed in the specific example discussed here in that, heating at 80°C prior to test did not reduce the observed activity. Serine proteases are typically easily degraded at such a temperature. Ultimately, the use of the protease in this latter example was not needed as the test performed in purified BSA solution provided similarly excellent results without the need for pre-purification. In this case it was not necessary to cleave the compound with protease but rather the endotoxin control spikes could be unmasked using an innocuous protein that apparently changed the binding characteristics of the CSE and product combination.

Petsch et al. conclude that the use of proteases to "unmask" endotoxin-binding products may be applied to other LAL applications such as bringing the dilution necessary to test a compound without interference down in cases when the MVD is low. They also mention that proteases could be used to improve endotoxin detection in plasma or serum testing, albeit in combination with other methods since protein constituents are not the only problems involved in testing plasma or serum.

---

[j]One unit will hydrolyze casein to produce peptide equivalent to 1.0 μmole (181 μg) of tyrosine per min at pH 11.0 at 30°C. (Data from Sigma Aldrich product information.)
[k]One unit will hydrolyze casein to produce color equivalent to 1.0 μmole (181 μg) of tyrosine per min at pH 7.5 at 37°C (color by Folin-Ciocalteu reagent), unless otherwise indicated. (Data from Sigma Aldrich product information.)

SETTING ENDOTOXIN SPECIFICATIONS

The beginning of this chapter has dealt with the scientific aspects of developing a good endotoxin test; this half of the chapter will focus on the scientific-regulatory interface (LAL manufacturer's and foreign and domestic regulators) and regulatory requirements. Both the Guideline on Validation of the LAL Test (26) and the FDA Interim Guidance for Human and Veterinary Drug Products and Biologicals (27) provide detailed descriptions on the means of satisfying the agency's requirements.

While it is not the responsibility of the assay development laboratory to set specifications, the group does play a key role in verifying that the specifications set are within the appropriate bounds established by the FDA guideline calculations and pharmacopeial requirements. Practically speaking, the lab will determine the informal specification for early development testing given the clinician's dose range. At a later date project lead scientists will negotiate the specifications with a specification committee. There appear to be two divergent philosophies on setting specifications. The first is to set the most stringent specification that the laboratory can support (i.e., around the limit of detection). The second is to set the specification around the regulatory limit allowed (i.e., the TL calculated value), which is the highest legal level. See Figure 2 for the effect of dose changes on the resulting TL.

Late Clinical Dose	Validation Dose[a]	Marketed Dose
1500 mg/m^2 Max. Human Dose in FDA parameters	3600 mg/m^2 Max. Human Dose in FDA parameters	1250 mg/m^2 Max. Human Dose in FDA parameters
$\dfrac{1500 \text{ mg/m}^2 \times 1.8 \text{ m}^2}{70 \text{ kg/hr}}$	$\dfrac{3600 \text{ mg/m}^2 \times 1.8 \text{ m}^2}{70 \text{ kg/hr}}$	$\dfrac{1250 \text{ mg/m}^2 \times 1.8 \text{ m}^2}{70 \text{ kg/hr}}$
MHD = 38.57 mg/kg/hr	MHD = 92.57 mg/kg/hr	MHD = 32.14 mg/kg/hr
TL = $\dfrac{5 \text{ EU/kg} \propto}{38.57 \text{ mg/kg}}$ 0.1296 EU/mg	TL = $\dfrac{5 \text{ EU/kg} \propto}{92.57 \text{ mg/kg}}$ 0.0540 EU/mg	TL = $\dfrac{5 \text{ EU/kg} \propto}{32.14 \text{ mg/kg}}$ 0.1555 EU/mg
MVD = (AL × PP)/λ $\dfrac{-0.1296 \text{ EU/mg} \times 20 \text{ mg/mL}}{0.005 \text{ EU/mL}}$ = 1:5184	MVD = (AL × PP)/λ $\dfrac{-0.05 \text{EU/mg} \times 20 \text{ mg/mL}}{0.005 \text{ EU/mL}}$ = 1:200	MVD = (AL × PP)/λ $\dfrac{-0.1555 \text{EU/mg} \times 20 \text{ mg/mL}}{0.005 \text{ EU/mL}}$ = 1:622

The difference in the reportable results assuming no endotoxin detected at each level[b] is nmt 0.1296, nmt 0.05, and nmt 0.1555 EU/mg. Therefore, a sample tested at the MVD based upon the validated dose could fail (≥0.05 EU/mg) but still be 3X below the legal limit based upon the marketed dose in this example.

[a]equal to the tolerance limit
[b]based on early clinical dose

Important Points:
- Retest is allowed on pooled samples.
- Companies are very reluctant to update established specifications regardless of current dose parameters.
- Doses may be set high during clinical testing and may not be subsequently revised to more relevant levels as per the marketed dose.
- Resetting a specification during a failure may (of course) be inappropriate.

FIGURE 2 Effect of changing the product dose on the resulting tolerance limit calculation.

Concerning the first philosophy, setting the specification too tightly may come back to haunt the participants in the form of a test failure and subsequent destruction of an expensive lot of drug that, scientifically and from a regulatory perspective, does not exceed allowable endotoxin levels. Early clinical doses are often several-fold higher than subsequent marketed drug doses, but there does not appear to be a mechanism to ratchet specifications down as doses decrease in the clinic. When products inevitably go to market, they will do so with a dose that is sometimes significantly lower than that used to establish the endotoxin test.

The second philosophy is as poor as the first. If the specifications are set too close to the values allowed by law, then the routine examination of the drugs will not detect changes in endotoxin content until they are at failing levels. Ideally, one wants to "see" the endotoxin content well below the specification to serve as a warning that the manufacturing process is beginning to allow contamination well before it reaches a level relevant to the manufacturing process. If the specification is too high, then there will be no time for corrective action preceding a test failure.

Those that are not familiar with endotoxin limit calculations often see a value and gauge whether it is "high" or "low" simply by how large the number is. However, the specification is a function of the dose and any specification that is set appropriately will allow <350 EU/patient dose/hr. Naturally, a several gram dose will allow much less endotoxin on a per milligram basis than will a drug that is delivered in micrograms. The situation may arise in which a limit of nmt 100 EU/mg is set beside another compound with a limit of nmt 0.25 EU/mg, making the 100 EU/mg appear less "stringent" when, in fact, they both allow the same amount of endotoxin delivery as per their associated dose. A committee may scratch their collective heads and determine that the 100 EU/mg specification must be ratcheted down. The proof of this is given here in the two side-by-side calculations:

$$TL = K/M \quad 5.0 \text{ EU/kg}/(3.5 \text{ mg/70kg/hr}) = 100 \text{ EU/mg} = 350 \text{ EU/dose}^1$$

$$TL = K/M \quad 5.0 \text{ EU/kg}/(1400 \text{ mg/70kg/hr}) = 0.25 \text{EU/mg} = 350 \text{ EU/dose}^1$$

ANCILLARY ACTIVITIES TO VALIDATING THE LAL TEST

The initial process of validation may be as ongoing as the compound itself. Factors subject to change include: the product potency, presentation, included excipients, interference factors, containers, etc. Factors that are absolutely critical for establishing a test that will detect the endotoxin limit concentration include the MHD, PP, and LAL lambda (λ) to be used in the TL and MVD (or MVC) calculations. An error in calculation or failure to secure a relevant dose for the TL calculation will nullify subsequent efforts to provide an accurate result. The TL is equal to the threshold pyrogenic response (K in EU/kg) divided by the dose in the units by which it is administered (mL, Units, or mg) per 70 kg person per hour.

Factors that must be considered in performing this critical calculation include:

1. Body weight adjustments (conversion from m^2 may be necessary)
2. Delivery method clarification (bolus vs. multiple daily doses, etc.)
3. Dosage based on a method relevant to the means of administration

---

[1]By definition TL = 350 EU/dose.

4. Use the units of active ingredient (i.e., use mg instead of mL, particularly when the reconstitution may vary)
5. Product reconstitution changes (i.e., PP changes) bring about changes in the MVD formula calculation
6. Increases in the clinic dose will lower the TL of the test (as the basis of the MVD calculation)

It is the overall process that is important in the development of a new LAL assay for a drug to be used in the clinic. Establishing a process that captures all the details is critical for ensuring that the right tasks are performed in the right sequence, the right information is documented, and that the information is correctly applied to the test both in its performance and in the determination of the parameters that govern its proper performance. Such a detailed process may be difficult to capture in a standard operating procedure, and an extensive training will be necessary before an analyst is proficient in all the nuances of developing an LAL assay, particularly for a new drug candidate.

INTERNATIONAL REGULATION (METHOD CHOICES AND REGULATORY SUPPORT)

Thankfully, more and more each test (USP, FDA Guideline, PharmEuropa, JP, etc.) need not be considered in an isolated manner from a regulatory perspective. The tests have been harmonized as initially described in the June 2000 issue of *Pharmacopeial Forum* and was the first harmonized microbiology method. A common reference standard has been developed in International Standard-2 (IS-2) (at least as per USP and Pharm Europa) and is in reality the same material filled separately.

Significantly, the gel-clot, end point, and kinetic methods (photometric) are described in the new harmonized test that meets the requirements of USP, Pharm Europa, and JP BET. The previous USP chapter <85> made scant reference to the end point and kinetic tests and leaves the photometric assays as alternate tests with the associated implied requirements for the demonstration of equivalence with no description of how this should be accomplished.

Cooper (28) was one of the first to point out that the new harmonized procedure contained a few ambiguities:

1. Does not describe the use of a CSE, which could technically be interpreted as not allowing for the use thereof and not describing the qualification of it relative to the RSE, if it is allowed (though the USP does describe and allow for the use of control standards in lieu of reference standards, in general, and it is hard to imagine that the pharmacopeia would consider proposing that all users should use reference standard, which would be a great expense and would deplete the stock).
2. Does not mention the use of the MVC as a means of determining testing parameters for bulk, excipient, and other powder forms of samples. However, for those with a dilution (as opposed to concentration) mindset, this omission

can be overcome by the use of adjusted product potency.

$$MVD^{[\text{for a bulk}^m]} = \frac{TL \times PP^n}{\lambda}$$

Overall, the harmonized test gets high marks in ease of understanding and practicality when applied to real-world test conditions and as the first biological test to be harmonized. Furthermore, to multinational companies that must meet international requirements the benefits of the harmonized test cannot be overstated. In a nutshell these benefits include:

1. The harmonized test elevates of the status of non gel-clot tests, including kinetic and end point chromogenic and turbidimetric tests by including them (though the FDA already considered that if one follows the 1987 Guideline, then one is assured of meeting FDA expectations and the USP has no inspection role or capability).
2. The gel-clot assay has been split into a limit test or an assay, something that is fairly routine but not specified previously and the limit test no longer requires the confirmation of label claim with each block of tubes tested.
3. The requisite positive product control standard recovery has been widened from 50% to 150% to 50% to 200%, which is in effect the recovery associated with the gel-clot assay (one two-fold dilution). This change only allows for one's test to enhance the recovery of endotoxin all the more (200% vs. 150% recovery), which will only serve to provide an overestimation of endotoxin content.

REFERENCES

1. Tsuji K, Steindler KA, Harrison SJ. *Limulus* amoebocyte lysate assay for detection and quantitation of endotoxin in a small-volume parenteral product. Appl Environ Microbiol 1980; 40(3):533–538.
2. Nema S, Washkuhn RJ, Brendel RJ. Excipients and their use in injectable products. J Pharm Sci Technol 1990; 44(1).
3. Guilfoyle DE, Munson T. Procedures for improving detection of endotoxin in products found incompatible for direct analysis with *Limulus* amebocyte lysate. In: Watson SW, Levin J, Novitsky TJ. eds. Endotoxins and their Detection with the *Limulus* Amebocyte Lysate Test. New York: Alan R. Liss, 1982:79–90.
4. Cambrex I. Pyrosperse™. Product Package Insert.
5. Cooper J. Resolving LAL test interferences. J Pharm Sci Technol 1990; 44(1):13–15.
6. Cooper JF. Using validation to reduce LAL pH measurements. LAL Times 1997; 4(2):1–3.
7. Motise PJ. Human drug CGMP notes. PDA Lett 1996; March:12.
8. USP24. Bacterial endotoxin test. U.S. Pharmocopiea, ch. 85. 2000.
9. Novitsky TJ, Schmidt-Gengenbach J, Remillard JF. Factors affecting recovery of endotoxin adsorbed to container surfaces. J Pharm Sci Technol 1986; 40(6):284–286.
10. McCullough KZ. Variability in the LAL test. J Pharm Sci Technol 1990; 44(1):19–21.
11. Roslansky PF, Dawson ME, Novitsky TJ. Plastics, endotoxins, and the *Limulus* amebocyte lysate test. J Pharm Sci Technol 1991; 45(2):83–87.
12. Twohy CW et al. Comparison of *Limulus* amebocyte lysates from different manufacturers. J Pharm Sci Technol 1983; 37(3):93–96.

---

^{m}Or excipient, API, or in-process powder (or liquid where the weight of the liquid is used).
^{n}Where the PP is an assigned value as per the weight and reconstitution specified by a given test method.

13. www.Sartorius.com
14. www.Acciusa.com
15. www.Profos.de or www.Cambrex.com
16. Petsch D, Deckwer WD, Anspach FB. Proteinase K digestion of proteins improves detection of bacterial endotoxins by the *Limulus* amebocyte lysate assay: application for endotoxin removal from cationic proteins. Anal Biochem. 1998; 259(1):42–47.
17. Piluso LG, Martinez MY. Resolving liposomal inhibition of quantitative LAL methods. J Pharm Sci Technol 1999; 53(5):260–263.
18. ACC. END-X Endotoxin Removal Products. Technical Report, 1999.
19. Bannerman DD, et al. Endotoxin-neutralizing protein protects against endotoxin-induced endothelial barrier dysfunction. Infect Immun 1998; 66(4):1400–1407.
20. Wainwright NR, et al. Endotoxin binding and neutralizing activity by a protein from *Limulus polyphemus*. In: Nowotny A, Spitzer JJ, Ziegler EJ, eds. Cellular and Molecular Aspects of Endotoxin Reactions. Amsterdem: Elsevier Science, 1990:315–325.
21. Alpert G, et al. *Limulus* antilipopolysaccharide factor protects rabbits from meningococcal endotoxin shock. J Infect Dis 1990; 165:494–500.
22. Warren HS, et al. Binding and neutralization of endotoxin by *Limulus* antilipopolysaccharide factor. Infect Immun 1992; 60:2506–2513.
23. Maheshwari, et al. Thermophilic fungi: their physiology and enzymes. Microbiol Mol Biol Rev 2000; Sept: 461–488.
24. Jackson GS, et al. An enzyme-detergent method for effective prion decontamination of surgical steel. J Gen Virol 2005; 86 (Pt 3):869–878.
25. Gotoh A, et al. Additive effect of pronase on the efficacy of eradication therapy against *Helicobacter pylori*. Helicobacter 2002; 7(3): 183.
26. FDA. Guideline on validation of the *Limulus* amebocyte lysate assay as an end product endotoxin test for human and animal parenteral drugs, biological prodcuts, and medical devices. DHHS, Dec, 1987.
27. FDA. FDA Interim Guidance for Human and Veterinary Drug Products and Biologicals—Kinetic LAL Techniques. DHHS, July, 1991.
28. Cooper J. Harmonized BET is effective in 2001 for USP. LAL Times 2000, 7(1):1.

ATTACHMENT A:

FDA INTERIM GUIDANCE FOR HUMAN AND VETERINARY DRUG PRODUCTS AND BIOLOGICALS—KINETIC LAL TESTS

This guideline sets forth acceptable conditions for use of the *Limulus* amebocyte lysate test. It also describes procedures for using this methodology as an end product endotoxin test for human injectable drugs (including biological products), animal injectable drugs, and medical devices. The procedures may be used in lieu of the rabbit pyrogen test.

For the purpose of this guideline, the terms "lysate" or "lysate reagent" refer only to *Limulus* amebocyte lysate licensed by the Center for Biologic Evaluation and Research. The term "official test" means that a test is referenced in a United States Pharmacopeia drug monograph, a New Drug Application, New Animal Drug Application or a Biological License.

Background

In a notice of January 12, 1973 (38 FR 1404), FDA announced that *Limulus* amebocyte lysate (LAL), derived from circulating blood cells (amebocytes) of the horseshoe crab, (*Limulus polyphemus*), is a biological product. As such, it is subject to licensing requirements as provided in section 351 of the Public Health Service Act (42 U.S.C. 262). Since 1973, LAL has proved to be a sensitive indicator of the presence of bacterial endotoxins (pyrogens). Because of this demonstrated sensitivity, LAL can be of value in preventing the administration or use of products, which may produce fever, shock, and death if administered to or used in humans or animals when bacterial endotoxins are present.

When the January 12, 1973 notice was published, available data and experience with LAL were not adequate to support its adoption as the final pyrogen test in place of the rabbit pyrogen test, which had been accepted and recognized for many years. In order to establish a database and gain experience with the use of LAL, that notice permitted the introduction of LAL into the marketplace without a license. This was upon the condition that its use be limited to the in—process testing of drugs and other products, that the decision to use it be reached voluntarily by affected firms, and the labeling on LAL state that the test was not suitable as a replacement for the rabbit pyrogen test.

Since that time, production techniques have been greatly improved and standardized so that they consistently yield LAL with an endotoxin sensitivity over 100 times greater than originally obtained. Moreover, it is widely recognized that the LAL test is faster, more economical, and requires a smaller volume of product than does the rabbit pyrogen test. In addition, the procedure is less labor intensive than the rabbit test, making it possible to perform many tests in a single day.

In a notice published in the *Federal Register* of November 4, 1977 (42 FR 57749), FDA described conditions for the use of LAL as an end product test for endotoxins in human biological products and medical devices. The notice stated further that the application of LAL testing to human drug products would be the subject of a future *Federal Register* publication.

The then Bureau of Medical Devices, now FDA's Center for Devices and Radiologic Health (CDRH), issued recomiended procedures for the use of LAL testing as an end product endotoxin test on March 26, 1979. These procedures were revised as a result of the comments received from interested parties.

As a direct result of CDRH's experience in approving petitions for the use of the LAL test in place of the rabbit pyrogen test, several procedures for using the LAL test have evolved and have been adopted for devices.

In the *Federal Register* of January 18, 1980 (45 FR 3668), FDA announced the availability of a draft guideline that set forth procedures for use of the LAL test as an end product testing method for endotoxins in human and animal injectable drug products. This draft guideline was made available to interested parties to permit manufacturers, especially those who had used the LAL test in parallel with the rabbit pyrogen test, to submit data that could be considered in the preparation of any final guideline.

In response to comments received on the January 18 draft guideline, FDA made several significant changes (i.e., endotoxin limits were changed and deletion of section on Absence of Nonendotoxin Pyrogenic Substances), and many minor editorial changes. The agency also determined that a single document should be made available covering all FDA regulated products that may be subject to LAL testing. Primarily because of the addition of biological products and medical devices to the guideline, the the agency made, in the *Federal Register* of March 29, 1983 (43 FR 13096), another draft of the guideline available for public comment.

Based on the comments received on the March 29 draft guideline, FDA has made several changes in this final guideline. The comments used in support of these changes may be viewed at FDA's Dockets Management Branch, Room 4-62, 5600 Fishers Lane, Rockville, MD between 9 a.m. and 4 p.m. Monday through Friday. Briefly, the significant changes made are:

A. Inclusion of validation criteria for the chromogenic, end point— turbidimetric and kinetic-turbidimetric LAL techniques.
B. Any technique (gel-clot, chromogenic or turbidimetric) can be used in testing a product for endotoxin. However, if a gel-clot lysate is used in a different technique the results must be interpreted using the criteria for the technique being used.
C. Elimination of the requirement to test the sensitivity of a rabbit pyrogen testing colony.
D. The Center for Devices and Radiological Health (CDRH) has adopted the USP Endotoxin Reference Standard and revised the limit expressions from ng/mL to EU/rnL. The new limit for medical devices is 0.5 EU/mL except for devices in contact with cerebrospinal fluid for which the limit is 0.06 EU/mL. These limits for deices are equivalent to those for drugs for a 70 Kg man when consideration is given to the following:
    1. In the worst case situation, all endotoxin present in the combined rinsings of 10 devices could have come from just one device. A wide variation in bioburden is common to some devices.
    2. Published FDA studies indicate that less than half of added endotoxin is recovered from devices using a nonpyrogenic water rinse.
E. The Center for Drug Evaluation and Research (CDER) has added a listing of the maximum doses per Kg per hour and the corresponding endotoxin limits for most of the aqueous injectable drugs and biologics currently on the market. This listing was added to promote uniformity among companies making the same product.

This guideline is issued under section 10.90(b) (21 CFR 10.90(b)) of the FDA's administrative regulations, which provides for use of guidelines to outline procedures or standards of general applicability that are acceptable to FDA for a subject matter within its statutory authority. Although guidelines are not legal requirements, a person who follows an agency guideline may be assured that the procedures or standards will be acceptable to FDA. The following guideline has been developed to inform manufacturers of human drugs (including biologicals), animal drugs, and indical devices of procedures FDA considers necessary to validate the use of LAL as an end product endotoxin test. A manufacturer who adheres to the guideline would be considered in compliance with relevant provisions of the applicable FDA current good manufacturing practice regulations (CGMP) for drugs and devices and other applicable requirements. As provided in 21 CFR 10.90(b), persons who use methods and techniqifes not provided in the guideline should be able to adequately assure, through validation, that the method or technique they use is adequate to detect the endotoxin limit for the product.

Regulatory Provisions that Permit Initiation of End Product Testing with LAL

The regulatory provisions that a firm must meet before using the LAL test as an end product test are not the same for all categories of products because of the different applicable statutory provisions and regulations. These provisions are as follows:

Human Drugs subject to New Drug Applications (NDAs) or Abbreviated New Drug Applications (ANDAs). Antibiotic Drug Applications, and animal drugs subject to New Animal Drug Applications (NADAs), and Abbreviated New Animal Drug Application.

For these classes of drugs, manufacturers are to submit a supplemental application to provide for LAL testing. However, under 21 CFR 314.70(c) for drugs for human use and 21 CFR 514.8(d)(3) for drugs for animal use various changes may be made before FDA approval. Under these sections changes in testing of a human or animal drug that give increased assurance that the drug will have the characteristics of purity it purports or is represented to possess should be placed into effect at the earliest possible time. Therefore, if a firm validates the LAL test for a particular drug product covered by a new drug application by the procedures in this guideline using a LAL reagent licensed by the Center for Biologic Evaluation and Research (OBER) for the technique being used, the change may be made concurrently with the submission of the supplement providing for it. The supplement should contain initial quality control data, inhibition/enhancement data and the endotoxin limit for the drug product.

Biological Products for Human Use

Under 21 CFR 601.12 significant changes in the manufacturing methods of biological products are required to be reported to the agency and may not become effective until approved by the Director, OBER. Therefore, a manufacturer of a biological product shall obtain an approved amendment to its product license before changing to the use of LAL in an end product test, irrespective of the validation procedure used.

Drugs Not Subject to Remarket Approval

A manufacturer of an injectable drug for human or animal use that is not subject to premarket approval would be able to use the LAL test as an end product test for endotoxins without submitting any information to the agency. CGMPs require the manufacturer to have data on file to validate the use of the LAL test for each product for which it is being used.

Medical Devices

On the basis of extensive experience in review of LAL data on devices since November 1977, CDRH believes that the LAL test, when validated according to this guideline, is at least equivalent to the rabbit pyrogen test as an end product test for medical devices. A manufacturer labeling a device as nonpyrogenic must validate the LAL test for that device in the test laboratory to be used for end product testing before using the LAL test as an end product endotoxin test for any device.

The data discussed under Section V of this guideline may be expressed graphically or in tabular form and should be on file at the manufacturing site; no preclearance prior to use of the LAL test as an end product test is required if it is used according to this FDA guideline. Voluntary submission of LAL validation and inhibition data obtained following issuance of this guideline will be accepted for CDRH review and comment.

When a manufacturer plans to use LAL test procedures that deviate significantly from the LAL guideline, a premarket notification under section 510(k) of the Federal Food, Drug, and Cosmetic Act (the Act) or a Premarket Approval Application (PMA) supplement under section 515 of the Act should be submitted. Significant deviations would include, but not necessarily be limited to higher endotoxin concentration release criteria, sampling from fewer than three lots for inhibition/ enhancement testing, lesser sensitivity to endotoxin, rabbit retest when the LAL method shows endotoxin above the recommended allowable endotoxin dose, and a device rinsing protocol resulting in greater dilution of endotoxin than that recommended in this guideline.

CDRH will also consider submissions in the form of a premarket notification or PMA supplement for another deviation from this draft guideline; process control of endotoxin contamination with reduced end product testing, that is, a decrease in the number of devices per lot undergoing end product testing. The manufacturer must demonstrate adequate control of the production process by the use of routine checks for endotoxin at key stages of production except where it has been shown that no possibility of contamination exists.

To facilitate subsequent PMA review, providers of investigational devices subject to 21 CFR part 812 or 813 are encouraged to use this guideline when a nonpyrogenic device is to be manufactured.

General Requirement

Manufacturers shall use an LAL reagent licensed by CBER in all validation, in-process, and end product LAL tests.

Validation of the LAL Test

Validation of the LAL test as an endotoxin test for the release of human and animal drugs includes the following: (*i*) initial qualification of the laboratory, and (*ii*) inhibition and enhancement tests.

Initial Qualification of the Laboratory

Various methodologies have been described for the detection of endotoxin, using *Limulus* amebocyte lysate. Currently, commercially available licensed lysates use the gel-clot, chromogenic, end point—turbidimetric or kinetic—turbidimetric techniques. Other methods which have been reported show potential for increasing further the sensitivity of the LAL method.

Manufacturers should assess the variability of the testing laboratory before any offical tests are performed. Each analyst using a single lot of LAL and a single lot of endotoxin should perform the test for confirmation of labeled LAL reagent sensitivity or of performance criteria. Appendix A gives the procedures and test criteria for the current licensed techniques.

Inhibition and Enhancement Testing

The degree of product inhibition or enhancement of the LAL procedure should be determined for each drug formulation before the LAL test is used to assess the endotoxin content of any drug. All validation tests should be performed on undiluted drug product or on an appropriate dilution. Dilutions should not exceed the Maximum Valid Dilution (MVD) (see Appendix D). At least three production batches of each finished product should be tested for inhibition and enhancement.

Gel-Clot Technique

Inhibition/enhancement testing should be conducted according to the directions in the preparatory section of the USP Bacterial Endotoxins Test (see Appendix B). Briefly, the method involves taking a drug concentration containing varying concentrations of a standard endotoxin that bracket the sensitivity of the lysate and comparing it to a series of the same endotoxin concentrations in water alone. The drug product is "spiked" with endotoxin and then diluted with additional drug product (so that the drug concentration remains constant) to the same endotoxin concentrations in water. Results of endotoxin determination in water and the drug product should fall within plus/minus a two-fold dilution of the labeled sensitivity. If the undiluted drug product shows inhibition, the drug product can be diluted, not to exceed the MVD, with the same diluent that will be used in the release testing and the above procedure repeated. Negative controls (diluent plus lysate) should be included in all inhibition/enhancement testing.

Chromogenic and End Point-Turbidimetric Techniques

In inhibition/enhancement testing by these techniques, a drug concentration containing 4 lambda concentration of the RSE or CSE (lambda is equal to the lowest endotoxin concentration used to generate the standard curve) is tested in duplicate according to the lysate manufacturer's methodology. The standard curve for these techniques shall consist of at least four RSE or CSE concentrations in water that extend over the desired range. If the desired range is greater than one log, additional standards concentrations should be included. The standard curve must meet the criteria for linearity as outlined in Appendix A (2). The detected amount of endotoxin in the spiked drug must be within plus or minus 25% of the 4 lambda concentration for the drug concentration to be considered to neither enhance nor inhibit the assay. If the undiluted drug product shows inhibition, the drug product can be diluted, not to exceed the MVD, and the test repeated.

An alternate procedure may be performed as described above except the RSE/ CSE standard curve is prepared in LAL negative drug product, i.e. no detectable endotoxin, instead of LAL-negative water. The standard curve must meet the test for linearity, i.e. r equal to or greater than 0.980, and in addition the difference between the O.D. readings for the lowest and highest endotoxin concentrations must be greater than 0.4 and less than 1.5 O.D. units. If the standard curve does not meet these criteria, the drug product cannot be tested by the alternate procedure.

Kinetic-Turbidimetric Technique

In inhibition/enhancement testing by this technique, a drug concentration containing 4 lambda concentration of the RSE or CSE (lambda is equal to the lowest endotoxin concentration used to generate the standard curve) is tested in duplicate according to the lysate manufacturer's methodology. The standard curve shall consist of at least four RSE or CSE concentrations. If the desired range is greater than one log, additional standard concentrations should be included. The standard curve must meet the criteria outlined in Appendix A(3). The calculated mean amount of endotoxin in the spiked drug product, when referenced to the standard curve, must be within plus or minus 25% to be considered to neither enhance nor inhibit the assay. If the undiluted drug product shows inhibition or enhancement, the drug product can be diluted, not to exceed the MVD, and the test repeated.

An alternate procedure may be performed whereby the RSE/CSE standard curve is prepared in drug product or product dilution instead of water. The drug product cannot have a background endotoxin concentration of more than 10% (estimated by extrapolation of the regression line) of the lambda concentration (lambda equals the lowest concentration used to generate the standard curve). The standard curve must meet the test for linearity, that is, r equal to or less than -0.980, and in addition the slope of the regression must be less than -0.1 and greater than -1.0. If the standard curve does not meet these criteria, the drug product cannot be tested by the alternate procedure.

In those instances when the drug is manufactured in various concentrations of active ingredient while the other components of the formulation remain constant, only the highest and lowest concentration need be tested. If there is a significant difference, i.e. greater than two-fold, between the inhibition end points or if the drug concentration, per mL, in the test solutions is different, then each remaining concentrations should be tested. If the drug product shows inhibition or enhancement at the MVD, when tested by the procedures in the above sections, and is amenable to rabbit testing, then the rabbit test will still be the appropriate test for that drug. If the inhibiting or enhancing substances can be neutralized without affecting the sensitivity of the test or if the LAL test is more sensitive than the rabbit pyrogen test the LAL test can be used. For those drugs not amenable to rabbit pyrogen testing, the manufacturer should determine the smallest quantity of endotoxin that can be detected. This data should be submitted to the appropriate FDA office for review.

The inhibition/enhancement tests must be repeated on one unit of the product if the lysate manufacturer is changed. If the lysate technique is changed, the inhibition and enhancement tests must be repeated using three batches. When the manufacturing process, the product formulation, the source of a particular ingredient of the drug formulation, or lysate lot is changed, the positive product control can be used to reverify the validity of the LAL test for the product. Firms that are obtaining an ingredient from a new manufacturer are encourged to include as part of their vendor qualification the rabbit pyrogen test to determine that the ingredient does not contain nonendotoxin pyrogens.

Routine Testing of Drugs by the LAL Test

End product testing is to be based on data from the inhibition/enhancement testing as outlined in Section A(2). Samples, standards, positive product controls and negative controls should be tested at least in duplicate. For the gel-clot technique, an endotoxin standard series does not have to be run with each set of tests if consistency of standard end points has been demonstrated in the test laboratory. It should be run at least once a day with the first set of tests and repeated if there is any change in lysate lot, endotoxin lot or test conditions during the day. An endotoxin standard series should be run when confirming end product contamination. Positive product controls (two lamda concentration of standard endotoxin in product) must be positive. If your test protocols state that you are using the USP Bacterial Endotoxin Test, remember that it requires a standard series to be run with each test. The above deviation must be noted in your test protocol.

For the chromogenic and end point-turbidimetric techniques, an endotoxin standard series does not have to be run with each set of tests if consistency of standard curves has been demonstrated in the test laboratory. It should be run at least once a day with the first set of tests and repeated if there is any change in lysate lot, endotoxin lot or test conditions during the day. However, at least duplicates of a 4 lambda standard concentration in water and in each product (positive product control) must be included with each run of samples. The mean endotoxin concentration of the standard must be within plus/minus 25% of the actual concentration and the positive product control must meet the same criteria after subtraction of any endogenous endotoxin. An endotoxin standard series should be run when confirming end product contamination. If the alternate procedure is used, a standard in product series must be conducted each time the product is tested.

For the kinetic-turbidimetric test, it is not necessary to run a standard curve each day or when confirming end product contamination if consistency of standard curves has been demonstrated in the test laboratory. However, at least duplicates of a 4 lambda standard concentration in water and in each product (positive product control) must be included with each run of samples. The mean endotoxin concentration of the standard when calculated using an archived standard curve (See Appendix C), must be within plus/minus 25% of the actual concentration and the positive product control must meet the same criteria after subtraction of any endogenous endotoxin. If the alternate procedure is used, a standard in product series must be conducted each time the product is tested.

Before a new lot of lysate is used, the labeled sensitivity of the lysate or the performance criteria should be confirmed by the laboratory, using the procedures in Appendix A.

The sampling technique selected and the number of units to be tested should be based on the manufacturing procedures and the batch size. A minimum of three units, representing the beginning, middle, and end, should be tested from a lot. These units can be run individually or pooled. If the units are pooled and any endotoxin is detected, repeat testing can be performed. The LAL test may be repeated no more than twice. The first repeat consists of twice the initial number of replicates of the sample in question to examine the possibility that extrinsic contamination occurred in the initial assay procedure. On pooled samples, if any endotoxin is detected in the first repeat, proceed to second repeat. The second repeat consists of an additional

10 units tested individually. None of the 10 units tested in the second repeat may contain endotoxin in excess of the limit concentration for the drug product.

The following should be considered the endotoxin limit for all parenteral drugs to meet if the LAL test is to be used as an end product endotoxin test:

1. K/M: For any parenteral drug except those administered intrathecally, the endotoxin limit for endotoxin is defined as K/N, which equals the amount of endotoxin (EU) allowed per ng or mL of product. K is equal to 5.0 EU/Kg. (see appendix D for definition of M).

For parenteral drugs that have an intrathecal route of administration, K is equal to 0.2 EU/Kg.

Drugs exempted from the above endotoxin limits are:

1. Compendial drugs for which other endotoxin limits have been established.
2. Noncompendial drugs covered by new drug applications, antibiotic drug applications, new animal drug applications, and biological product licenses where different limits have been approved by the agency.
3. Investigational drugs or biologicals for which an IND or INAD exemption has been filed and approved.
4. Drugs or biologicals which cannot be tested by the LAL method.

A batch which fails a validated LAL release test should not be retested by the rabbit test and released if it passes. Due to the high variability and lack of reproducibility of the rabbit test as an endotoxin assay procedure, we do not consider it an appropriate retest procedure for LAL failures.

Appendix A
Quality Control Procedure
The following procedures and criteria are used for initial qualification and requalification of analysts in the laboratory, and to test new lots of lysate before use.

Gel-Clot End Point Technique
For the gel-clot technique the procedures in the USP Bacterial Endotoxins Test Monograph (see Appendix B) should be used for quality control testing.

Chromogenic and End Point-Turbidimetric Techniques
Each test should be conducted according to the specific manufacturer's methodology.

Using the RSE or CSE whose potency is known, assay 4 replicates of a set of endotoxin concentrations, which extend over the labeled linear range. The standard concentrations must include the stated lower and upper limits of the range. Linear regression analysis is performed on the absorbance values of the standards (y-axis) versus their respective endotoxin concentrations (x-axis). The coefficient of correlation, r, shall be greater than or equal to 0.980. If r is less than 0.980 the cause of the non-linearity should be determined and the test repeated. This linearity limit is also used to judge the validity of standard curves used for inhibition/enhancement tests and sample tests. In addition to meeting these requirements, any other test or requirements specified by the lysate manufacturer should also be met.

Kinetic-Turbidimetric Technique
Each test should be conducted according to the manufacturer's instructions.

Using the RSE or CSE whose potency, in endotoxin units (See Appendix C), is known, assay at least 6 concentrations in triplicate which extend over the range 0.03–1.0 EU/mL. If instrument configuration does not allow you to run all 6 concentrations at one time, the data can be obtained in multiple runs and combined. Perform regression-correlation analysis on the log of the Time of Reaction (T) versus the log of the endotoxin concentration (E). The coefficient of correlation, r, shall be less than or equal to −0.980. If r is greater than −0.980 the cause of the nonlinearity should be determined and the test repeated. In addition to meeting these requirements, any other test or requirements specified by the lysate manufacturer should also be met.

Appendix D
From Guideline on Validation of the LAL Test as an End Product Endotoxin Test for Human and Animal Parenteral Drugs
Biological Products, and Medical Devices
To determine how much the product can be diluted and still be able to detect the limit endotoxin concentration, the following two methods will determine the maximum valid dilution (MVD).

Method I
This method is used when there is an official USP limit or when the limits listed in Appendix E are used.

$$\text{MVD} = \frac{\text{Endotoxin limit} \times \text{Potency of product}}{\lambda}$$

For drugs administered on a weight-per-kilogram basis, the potency is expressed as mg or units/mL and for drugs administered on a volume-per-kilogram basis, the potency is equal to 1.0 mL/mL.

Method II
This method is used when there is no official USP limit and the limits listed in Appendix E are not used.

Step 1. Minimum Valid Concentration (MVC)

$$\text{MVC} = \frac{\lambda \times M}{K}$$

where λ = Gel-clot labeled sensitivity in EU/mL (usually 0.C6 EUI/mL) Chromogenic, Turbidimetric and Kinetic-Turbidimetric:
The lowest point used in the standard curve (Kinetic is 0.05 EU/mL)

M = Rabbit dose or maximum human dose/Kg of body weight that would be administered in a single one hour period, whichever is larger. For radiopharmaceuticals, M equals the rabbit dose or maximum human dose/Kg at the product expiration date or time. Use 70 Kg as the weight of the average human when calculating the maximum human dose per Kg. Also, if the pediatric dose/Kg is higher than the adult dose then it shall be the dose used in the formula.

K = 5.0 EU/Kg for parenteral drugs except those administered intrathecally; 0.2 EU/Kg for intrathecal drugs.

Step 2. Maximum Valid Dilution (MVD)

$$MVD = \frac{Potency\ of\ product}{MVC}$$

For drugs administered on a weight-per-kilogram basis, the potency is expressed as mg or units/mL and for drugs administered on a volume-per-kilogram, the potency is equal to 1.0 mL/mL.

Examples: Method I
Endotoxin Limit Expressed by Weight:
   Product: Cyclophosphamide Injection
   Potency: 20 mg/mL
   Lysate Sensitivity (λ): 0.065 EU/mL
   Endotoxin Limit (Appendix E): 0.17 EU/mg

$$MVD = \frac{0.17\ EU/mg \times 20\ mg/ml}{0.065\ EU/mL} = \frac{3.4}{0.065}$$

$$= 1:52.3\ or\ 1:52$$

Endotoxin Limit Expressed by Volume:
   Product: 5% Dextross Injection
   Lysate Sensitivity (λ): 0.065 EU/mL
   Endotoxin Limit (Appendix E): 0.15 EU/mL

$$MVD = \frac{0.5\ EU/mL \times 1\ mL/mL}{0.065\ EU/mL} = \frac{0.5}{0.065} = 1:7.7$$

Examples: Method II
Parenteral Drugs Except Intrathecal
Drug Administered on a Weight-per-Kilogram Basis
   Product: cyclophosphamide Injection
   Potency: 20 mg/mL
   Mamimum Dose/Kg (M): 30 mg/Kg
   Lysate Sensitivity (λ): 0.065 EU/mL

$$MVC = \frac{\lambda M}{K} = \frac{0.065\ EU/mL \times 30\ mg/Kg}{5.0\ EU/Kg}$$

$$= 0.390\ mg/mL$$

$$MVD = \frac{Potency\ of\ product}{MVC} = \frac{20\ mg/mL}{0.390\ mg/mL}$$

$$= 1:51.2\ or\ 1:51$$

Drug Administered on a Volume-per-Kilogram Basis
  Product: 5% Dextrose in Water
  Mamixum Dose/kg (M): 10.0 mL/Kg
  Lysate Sensitivity (λ): 0.065 EU/mL

$$\text{MVC} = \frac{\lambda M}{K} = \frac{0.065 \text{ EU/mL} \times 10.0 \text{ mL/Kg}}{5.0 \text{ EU/Kg}}$$

$$= 0.13 \text{ mL/mL}$$

$$\text{MVD} = \frac{\text{Potency of product}}{\text{MVC}} = \frac{1.0 \text{ mL/Kg}}{0.13 \text{ mL/mL}} = 1\text{:}7.7$$

Department of Health and Human Services
Public Health Service
Rockville MD 20857
Interim Guidance for Human and Veterinary
Drug Products and Biologicals
July 15, 1991

Kinetic LAL Techniques
Until we update the guideline the following guidance and the lysate manufacturers approved procedures can be used. The kinetic LAL techniques should be done according to the lysate manufacturers recommended procedures, that is, sample/lysate ratio, incubation temperature and times, measurement wavelength, and so on. Instrumentation other than the one recommended by lysate manufacturer can be used. The performance characteristics (slope, y-intercept and correlation coefficient), for the lysate lot, sent by the manufacturer will not be valid. New performance characteristics have to be established for each lot by performing the procedures outlined in Appendix A.

Inhibition/Enhancement Testing
In inhibition/enhancement testing of a product by kinetic techniques, test a drug concentration containing a quantity of the RSE or CSE between 0.1 and 0.5 EU/mL or 1.0 and 5.0 EU/mL depending on its Pass/Fail Cutoff (PFC) in duplicate according to the lysate manufacturer's methodology. The 4 lambda spike procedure, in the current guideline, is still valid and can be used in the kinetic techniques. This procedure should be used with caution if lambda is less than 0.01 EU/mL.

The Pass/Fail Cutoff equals the endotoxin limit of the product solution (EU/mL) times the potency of the ptoduct divided by the product dilution used for the test. For PFCs less than or equal to 1.0 EU/mL the endotoxin spike should be between 0.1 and 0.5 EU/mL, otherwise the endotoxin spike should be between 1.0 and 5.0 EU/mL.

The standard curve shall consist of at least three RSE or CSE concentrations. Additional standards should be included to bracket each log increase in the range of the standard curve so that there is at least one standard per log increment of the range. The standard curve must meet the criteria outlined in Appendix A. The calculated mean amount of endotoxin when referenced to the standard curve, minus any measurable endogenous endotoxin in the spiked drug product, must be within plus or minus 50% of the known spike concentration to be considered to neither enhance or inhibit the assay. If there is no measurable endogenous endotoxin in the product the value will usually be equal to or less than plus or minus 25% of the standard curve value. If the undiluted drug product shows inhibition or enhancement, the drug product can be diluted, not exceeding the MVD, and test repeated.

An alternate procedure may be used, in which the RSE/CSE standard is prepared in drug product or product dilution instead of water.

The drug product (at the concentration used to orepare the standard curve), cannot have an endotoxin concentration greater than the lowest concentration used to generate the product standard curve, when referenced against a standard curve prepared in water. The product standard curve must meet the test for linearity, i.e., r equal to or greater than the absolute value of 0.980, and slope of the regression line must be less than −0.1 and greater than −1.0. If the standard curve does not meet these criteria, the drug product cannot be tested by the alternate procedure.

Routine Testing

The standard curve shall consist of at least three RSE or CSE concentrations in duplicate. Additional standards should be included to bracket each log increase in the range of the standard curve so that there is at least one standard per log increment of the range. The standard curve must meet the criteria outlined in Appendix A. For the kinetic techniques, it is not necessary to run a standard curve each day if consistency of standard curves is shown in your test laboratory. Determine consistency by regression analysis of the data points from the standard curves generated over three consecutive test days (minimum of three curves). If the coefficient of correlation, r, meets the criteria in Appendix A then consistency is proven and the curve becomes the "archived curve." If r does not meet the criteria then consistency in your laboratory has not been shown and you cannot use an archived curve in routine testing. The archived curve is only valid for ~ lysate/endotoxin lot combination. If you use an archived standard curve, at least duplicates of a standard endotoxin concentration, equal to the mid-point on a log basis, between the endotoxin concentration of the highest and lowest standards in the standard curve, in water must be included with each run of samples. The mean endotoxin concentration of this standard control must be within plus/minus 25% of the standard curve concentration when calculated using the archived standard curve. ndependent of using an endotoxin standard curve, at least duplicates of a standard endotoxin in each product or product dilution (positive product control), equal to either 0.1–0.5 or 1.0–5.0 EU/mL depending on its PFC or 4 lambda, must be included with each run of samples. The mean endotoxin concentration of the positive product control when referenced to the standard curve must be within plus/minus 50% of the known concentration after subtraction of any endogenous endotoxin. An endotoxin standard series should be run when retesting to determine if end product endotoxin contamination exceeds product limit. If you use the alternate procedure, a standard curve prepared in product must be conducted with each product test.

Appendix A

Using a RSE or CSE of known potency, in endotoxin units, assay least 2 concentrations in triplicate that extend over the desired endotoxin range. Additional standards should be Included to bracket each log increase in the range of the standard curve so that their is at least one standard per log increment of the range. Do regression - correlation analysis on the log Reaction Time versus the log of the endotoxin concentration for each replicate.

Do not average the reaction times of replicates of each standard before peforming regression-correlation analysis.

The coefficient of correlation, r, shall be greater than or equal to the absolute value of 0.980. If r is less than the absolute value of 0.980 the cause of the nonlinearity should be determined and test repeated.

ATTACHMENT B:

DEPARTMENT OF HEALTH AND HUMAN SERVICES

Public Health Service

Memorandum

Date: May 11 1992
From: Chairman, FDA LAL Task Force
Subject: Statement Concerning Glucans and LAL-recactive Material in Pharmaceuticals and Medical Devices

To: To Whom It May Concern

It has been reported to the LAL Task Force that information has been circulated concerning FDA's Position on glucans defined LAL-Reactive Material (LAL-RM) in pharmaceuticals and medical devices. Glucans are defined as polysaccharides composed only of recurring units of glucose, such as, glycogen, starch, and cellulose.

FDA is not aware of data indicating that glucans or LAL-RM are common in pharmaceuticals or maybe common in medical devices or whether they may pose a health hazard to patients using these products. The only product that has been shown to contain LAL-PM is dialysis membranes made of cellulose. LAL-RM is composed of very small fragments of the cellulose which break loose from the filter matrix. Studies in animals and tissue cultures indicate that LAL-RM is non-toxic in the quantities detected in dialyzers. Some investigators have indicated that LAL-RM may be responsible for some of the advcrse reactions seen in dialysis patients. However, no direct correlation has been established. LAL-RM is the only glucan that has been reported in any medical device. LAL-RM is not considered a contaminant, because its source is not extrinsic to the device. It is a breakdown product of the cellulose membrane that is a component of the device. Since the majority of medical devices do not contain natural materials, there is no source of glueans in these devices.

No cases of glucans or LAL-RM have been reported in parenteral drug products. Most parenteral drug products are manufactured from chemically synthesized components. This fact coupled with good manufacturing practices makes the possibility of contamination with glucans very remote. It appears that large amounts of glucans are required (at least 1,000 times more by weight than endotoxin) to elicit a LAL positive reaction.

At this time, FDA considers that the presence of glucans in parenteral drug products and most medical devices to be more of a theoretical than actual problem. Firms should be aware that false positive results may be possible when testing medical devices having cellulose based cornponents. It is the responsibility of the manufacturer to conclusively establish that any positive LAL test is not due to endotoxin contamination.

FDA will consider whether parenteral drug products or medical devices are adulterated due to the presence of glucans on a case-by-case basis, until such time as more information is obtained.

Terrry E. Munson

ATTACHMENT C:

LOCAL REFERENCE STANDARD PROFILE

Kinetic Turbidimetric Method

Endotoxin (CSE):	Endosafe EX82672 Exp. Date 10/2001
Lysate (LAL):	Endosafe N1882L Exp. Date 02/2003
Lysate sensitivitv(λ):	0.05 EU/ml (assigned as per lowest point on standard curve)
Acceptance test:	Refer to initial qualification in LRSP package
Date established:	2/16/00
Preparation:	Reconstitute LAL with 5.2 ml SWI, proceed per GP 8010
CSE Potencies:	50 USP EU/ml 50 BRP IU/ml
RSE:RSE Ratios*:	1 IU = 1 EU
Acceptance Test:	Refer to Certificate of Analysis
Date Established:	2/16/00
Preparation:	Reconstitute CSE with 2.4 ML SWI, proceed per GP 8010
Stock Solution:	50 EU/ML

Endotoxin Conc. in:
Standard Curve Preparation: USP EU/ML

S1. 0.25 mL of (STOCK) into 2.25 mL of (Diluent) . . . . 5.0 EU/ML
S2. 0.25 mL of (S1) into 2.25 mL of (Diluent) . . . . 0.50 EU/ ML
S3. 0.25 mL of (S2) into 2.25 mL of (Diluent) . . . . 0.05 EU/ML
Blank 1 ml of (Diluent) . . . . NEGATIVE CONTROL

(*Diluent*): Sterile Water for Injection or LAL Reagent Water
Handling: Storage Conditions: Keep refrigerated
Safety Information: Fire: 0, Reactivity: 0, Hazard: 4, Special: 0.
Evolution: Update LRSP to comply with requirements stated in Lilly Procedure 009136. Purchased combination of CSE/LAL reagents used only for quantification of Bacterial Endotoxin according to the Kinetic Turbidimetric Method GP 8021.

Local Reference Standard Profile Package: GMP Library.

Written by: _____ Date: _____
Approved by: _____ Date: _____

ATTACHMENT D:

SOLUBILITY DETERMINATION STUDY

Compound description:_____
Item number:_____
Lot# used:_____

(A) Weigh _____ mg (document exact weight) of the sample to be solubilized (balance #: _____).
(B) Dissolve in_____mL of diluent. Note characteristics below (if applicable).
(C) Determine pH of sample _____ (document) and sample with equal parts of LAL (if needed to establish 6–8 range): _____.

Note any unusual characteristics concerning the solubility/appearance of the dissolved sample:

_____

_____

_____

Diluent used to (attempt to) solubilize compound:

_____

Diluent preparation notebook, if applicable:_____

Tested by: _____   Date: _____
Verified by: _____   Date: _____

ATTACHMENT E:

PRELIMINARY NIC PROTOCOL

Item description: Product X
Item and lot number: LY123456

ACC CSE 74 ACC LAL 597-11-041 (λ = 0.06 EU/ml)

SAMPLE PREPARATION: **DILUTION**

A. MIX WELL A SINGLE HYPORETTE 1:1

NIC TESTING—UNSPIKED DILUTIONS

B. USE 2.0 ML OF (A) ABOVE 1:1
C. 1.0 ML OF (B) INTO 1.0 ML OF DILUENT 1:2
D. 1.0 ML OF (C) INTO 1.0 ML OF DILUENT 1:4
E. 0.5 ML OF (D) INTO 1.0 ML OF DILUENT 1:8
F. 0.5 ML OF (E) INTO 1.0 ML OF DILUENT 1:16

NIC TESTING—SPIKED DILUTIONS (ALL SPIKED AT 2λ)

G. 2.0 ML OF (A) + 0.05 ML OF (S3) 1:1
H. 1.0 ML OF (R) INTO 1.0 ML OF (S5) 1:2
I. 1.0 ML OF (S) INTO 1.0 ML OF (S5) 1:4
J. 1.0 ML OF (T) INTO 1.0 ML OF (S5) 1:8
K. 1.0 ML OF (U) INTO 1.0 ML OF (S5) 1:16

Diluent: Sterile water for injection or LAL Reagent water.
Spike Preparation: Prepare spike as denoted in Local Reference Standard Profile
(Gel-Clot Method GP8010).
Control Standard Endotoxin: Prepare Control Standard Endotoxin Curve as directed
in the CSE Profile (Gel-Clot Method).
Procedure: Prepare dilutions stated above and proceed as described in General
Procedure No. GP8010, Bacterial Endotoxin Test (Gel-Clot Method) and Lilly Pro-
cedure No. 014690, Bacterial Endotoxin Test (Gel-Clot Validation Method).

Written by: _____   Date: _____
Verified by: _____   Date: _____

ATTACHMENT F:

BACTERIAL ENDOTOXIN TESTING VALIDATION PROTOCOL[a]

Example Test Protocol—Gel-Clot Validation

Item Description: Product X
Item and lot number: LY123456

ACC CSE 74 ACC LAL 597-11-041 ($\lambda = 0.06$ EU/ml)

SAMPLE PREPARATION   **DILUTION**

A. Pool three hyporets (one each from beginning, middle, and end of lot).
   Mix well. Refrigerate excess until test complete 1:1
B. 3.0 mL of (A) into 21.0 mL of diluent 1:8

INHIBITION/ENHANCEMENT (AT A 1:8 DILUTION OF PRODUCT)

C. 0.25 ML OF STOCK INTO 2.25 ML OF (B) . . . . 100 EU/ML
D. 0.25 ML OF (C) INTO 2.25 ML OF (B) . . . . 10 EU/ML
E. 1.5 ML OF (D) INTO 1.55 ML OF (B) . . . . 4.92 EU/ML
F. 0.5 ML OF (E) INTO 4.65 ML OF (B) . . . . 0.48 EU/ML
G. 1 ML OF (F) INTO 1 ML OF (B) . . . . 0.24 EU/ML
H. 1 ML OF (G) INTO 1 ML OF (B) . . . . 0.12 EU/ML
I. 1 ML OF (H) INTO 1 ML OF (B) . . . . 0.06 EU/ML
J. 1 ML OF (I) INTO 1 ML OF (B) . . . . 0.03 EU/ML
K. 1 ML OF (J) INTO 1 ML OF (B) . . . . 0.015 EU/ML
L. 1 ML OF (B) . . . .
NEGATIVE CONTROL

NIC TESTING – UNSPIKED DILUTIONS

M. Use 1.0 ML OF (A) above 1:1
N. 0.5 ML OF (M) INTO 0.5 ML OF DILUENT 1:2
O. 0.5 ML OF (N) INTO 0.5 ML OF DILUENT 1:4
P. 0.5 ML OF (O) INTO 0.5 ML OF DILUENT 1:8
Q. 0.5 ML OF (P) INTO 0.5 ML OF DILUENT 1:16

NIC TESTING – SPIKED DILUTIONS (ALL SPIKED AT 2λ)

R. 1.0 ML OF (A) + 0.025 ML OF (S3) 1:1
S. 0.5 ML OF (R) INTO 0.5 ML OF (S5) 1:2
T. 0.5 ML OF (S) INTO 0.5 ML OF (S5) 1:4
U. 0.5 ML OF (T) INTO 0.5 ML OF (S5) 1:8
V. 0.5 ML OF (U) INTO 0.5 ML OF (S5) 1:16

---

[a]Note: see Chapter 8 for the corresponding Local Reference Standard Profile for CSE ACC 74/ LAL 597-11-041.

Diluent: Sterile water for injection or LAL Reagent water.

Spike Preparation: Prepare spike as denoted in Local Reference Standard Profile (Gel-Clot Method GP8010).

Control Standard Endotoxin: Prepare Control Standard Endotoxin Curve as directed in the CSE Profile (Gel-Clot Method).

Procedure: Prepare dilutions stated above and proceed as described in General Procedure No. GP8010, Bacterial Endotoxin Test (Gel-Clot Method) and Lilly Procedure No. 014690, Bacterial Endotoxin Test (Gel-Clot Validation Method).

Written by: _____   Date: _____
Verified by: _____   Date: _____
Rev. 1.0   Reason for Rev <u>NA</u>

ATTACHMENT G:

ROUTINE BACTERIAL ENDOTOXIN TEST PROTOCOL

Lot number:_____
Item: Product X
TEST DILUTION: 1:10
MVD = (λ/TL) = 1:83

SAMPLE PREPARATION   **DILUTION**

Conc.
A. Mix individual vials well. Pool each of three vials (beginning, middle, and end of lot) and mix pool well .... 1:1 10 mg/ml

UNSPIKED DILUTION TEST

B. 0.25 mL of (A) into 2.25 mL of diluent .... 1:10 1.0 mg/ml

POSITIVE CONTROL TEST (2 λ)

C. 2.0 mL of (A) + 0.05 mL of (S3)......................... 1:1 10 mg/ml
D. 0.25 mL of (C) + 2.25 mL of (S5)....................... 1:10 1.0 mg/ml

Diluent: Sterile water for injection or LAL Reagent water.
Control Standard Endotoxin: Prepare Control Standard Endotoxin Curve as directed in the CSE Profile (Gel-Clot Method).
Procedure: Prepare dilutions stated above and proceed as described in General Procedure No. GP8010, Bacterial Endotoxin Test (Gel-Clot Method).

Written by: _____
Date: _____
Approved by: _____
Effective Date: _____
Revision No.:   _____1.0_____

ATTACHMENT H:

**KINETIC TURBIDIMETRIC BACTERIAL ENDOTOXIN
TESTING VALIDATION PROTOCOL**

**CSE/LAL Manufacturer and Lot Numbers:
Endosafe EX82672 / N1882L**

Item: Product X
Lambda: 0.05 EU/mL (lowest point on kinetic curve)
Lot number: (1) _____(2) _____ (3) _____

SAMPLE PREPARATION: **DILUTION**

A. Mix well a single vial (for validation purposes) 1:1
B. Add 0.25 mL of (A) into 2.25 mL of diluent (X). Mix well 1:10

SPIKED SAMPLE DILUTIONS (SPIKED AT 0.5 EU/ML):

Prepare each PPC well by adding 0.01 mL of 5 EU/mL to 0.1 mL to Sample B.

DILUENT:

50 mM Tris Buffer (Cambrex)

CONTROL STANDARD ENDOTOXIN:

Prepare CSE Curve as directed in the CSE profile (LRSP) for the Kinetic Turbidimetric Method.

PROCEDURE:

Prepare dilution stated above and proceed as described in General Procedure
GP8021 and 023145, Validation of Pharmaceutical products By the Kinetic Chromogenic and Turbidimentric Methods.

   Test dilution B and corresponding spiked sample dilutions (PPC's) in
quadruplicate.

Perfomed by: _____   Date: _____
Verified by: _____   Date: _____

ATTACHMENT I:

KINETIC TURBIDIMETRIC BACTERIAL ENDOTOXIN
ROUTINE TEST PROTOCOL PRODUCT X

Primary Lysate/CSE: CR Endosafe

Lot No._____

TEST DILUTION: 1 : 10
AL = <0.5 EU/mg
MVD = 1:33

UNSPIKED SAMPLE DILUTIONS: DILUTION CONCENTRATION

A. Mix well the contents of 3 hyporettes (beginning, middle,
end of lot). Pool 3 hyporettes into suitable
container. Mix well . . . . 10 mg/mL
B. Add 0.25 mL of (A) into 2.25 mL of diluent and mix well . . . . 1.0 mg/mL

SPIKED SAMPLE DILUTIONS (PPC) SPIKED AT 0.5 EU/ML

C. Prepare each PPC well by adding 0.01 mL of 5 EU/mL
standard to 0.1 mL of (B) . . . . 1 : 10   1.0 mg/mL

Diluent: Sterile Water for Injection or LAL Reagent Water
Control Standard Endotoxin: Prepare Control Standard Endotoxin Curve as directed
in the CSE LRSP profile for the Kinetic Turbidimetric method.
Procedure: Prepare dilutions stated above and proceed as described in General Procedure GP8021, Bacterial Endotoxin Test (Kinetic Turbidimetric Method).

Written by: _____   Date: _____
Approved by: _____   Effective Date: _____
Revision: 1.0

12 The Pyrogen Test

Karen J. Roberts
Eli Lilly & Company, Indianapolis, Indiana, U.S.A.

In its simplest form, the rabbit pyrogen test involves measuring the rise in temperature of rabbits following an intravenous injection of a test solution. The test is designed for products that can be tolerated by the rabbit in doses not to exceed 10 mL/kg body weight, per intravenous injection, within a period of not more than 10 minutes.

PYROGEN TEST DEVELOPMENT

In the mid-1920s, Seibert (1) completed a series of classic studies, which proved conclusively that injection fevers associated with intravenous therapy resulted from heat-stable, filterable bacterial products that are commonly referred to as pyrogens. To ascertain the presence or absence of febrile responses caused by her test solutions, Seibert selected the rabbit as her animal test model, a choice that was later proven to be fortuitous (2). Since that time, many other species have been shown to have fever reactions when injected with bacterial pyrogens. Monkeys, horses, dogs, and cats, like the rabbit, have reproducible fever responses that are similar in nature to those of humans. On the other hand, the temperature response to pyrogens in rats, guinea pigs, mice, hamsters, and chicks is irregular and unpredictable, thus rendering them unsuitable for investigations of fever (3). For reasons of convenience and economics, the final selection of an animal test model for pyrogen testing was narrowed down to the dog and the rabbit. In 1942, Tui and Schrift (4), who had extensive experience with the two species, described the relative advantages and disadvantages of both. The rabbit has a labile thermoregulatory mechanism and frequently gives false-positive tests. For this reason, a negative test in a rabbit is more significant than a positive one. The dog, on the other hand, has a much more stable thermoregulatory mechanism, but is less sensitive to pyrogen than is the rabbit. A positive pyrogen response in a dog is so characteristic, with additional symptoms of leukopenia, vomiting, and diarrhea, that it is unmistakable. Therefore, a positive test for pyrogens in a dog is much more significant than a negative one. In summary, Tui and Schrift concluded that the rabbit was the better animal to use to test for the absence of pyrogens, but the dog was better used to establish the presence of pyrogens.

The knowledge that fevers resulting after an injection were actually caused by bacterial by-products has enabled hospital pharmacies and drug companies to develop production methods to prevent pyrogen contamination of their intravenous solutions. By the early 1930s, saline and dextrose large-volume parenterals (LVP) were available for the first time from commercial manufacturers. The major advantage advertised for these products was a label claim of nonpyrogenicity. Assurance of nonpyrogenicity inevitably resulted from a finished product lot quality control pyrogen assay based on the rabbit test developed by Seibert and other researchers. World War II produced a heavy demand for LVP therapy and drew attention to the need for an official *United States Pharmacopeia* (USP) compendial test to ensure the absence of pyrogens in intravenous preparations. Thus, in 1941, the Committee of Revision of the USP authorized Subcommittee 3 on Biological Assays to carry out the first USP collaborative study of pyrogens, under the direction of Henry Welch. Using potent pyrogen filtrates of *Pseudomonas aeruginosa*, produced by Welch and his coworkers in the Division of Bacteriology of the Food and Drug Administration (FDA), the collaborative study was undertaken by the Food and Drug administration (FDA), the NIH, and 14 pharmaceutical manufacturers (5,6). The study involved 3300 rabbit tests, utilizing 253 rabbits, and included 501 control tests in which rabbits were accustomed to the procedure, 1782 tests with pyrogenic material, and 1017 tests with nonpyrogenic physiological saline solution. Results of the study, which were published in 1943, led to incorporation of the first official rabbit pyrogen test in the 12th edition of the USP in 1942. The test procedure as it stands today in USP 30 NF 25 follows the same basic format as the original USP 12 assay (7). Although refinements have been introduced from time to time, the test offers considerable freedom of choice in pyrogen test methods and equipment. The test is far from perfect, but it did provide the pharmaceutical industry with an effective and reliable means of ensuring nonpyrogenicity to the consumer of parenteral products and intravenous solutions for nearly 60 years.

DESCRIPTION

In its simplest form, the rabbit pyrogen test involves measuring the rise in temperature of rabbits following an intravenous injection of a test solution. The test is designed for products that can be tolerated by the rabbit in doses not to exceed 10 mL/kg body weight per intravenous injection within a period of not more than 10 minutes. Exceptions are given in individual product monographs or, in the case of antibiotics or biologics, in the Code of Federal Regulations. The conditions under which the test is to be conducted currently are defined in the USP, and are expanded upon here.

CORRELATION

Over the years, a number of studies have attempted to correlate the rabbit pyrogen test to pyrogenic reactions in humans. Most researchers today feel that the definitive work in this area was published in 1969 by Greisman and Hornick (8), who compared the effects of three purified endotoxin preparations on a weight basis in rabbits and healthy adult male volunteers. Results showed that for the induction of threshold pyrogenic responses, humans and rabbits require approximately the same per kilogram quantity of bacterial endotoxin. However, as the pyrogen dose is increased, humans respond more vigorously than do rabbits. For this reason, most users of the rabbit test employ the threshold pyrogenic dose in rabbits as a minimum standard for correlation with humans on a dose per weight basis and attempt to increase the test safety margin for humans by several times, if at all possible.

TEST ANIMAL

The USP lists several requirements for test animals. Pyrogen test rabbits must be both healthy and mature.

Strain

The rabbits most widely used in pyrogen testing today are albino strains, especially New Zealand Whites, which are most commonly used in the United States. They are easily handled and trained for the pyrogen test procedure. Their ears are slightly shorter than those of Belgian Whites (which are more commonly used in Europe and Canada). Upon request, animal vendors will select long-eared rabbits for pyrogen test customers. This is important because a longer marginal ear vein is useful if rabbits are to receive frequent injections. A disadvantage of the New Zealand White rabbit is its propensity to suffer several intestinal and respiratory infections; thus, good animal breeding practices among vendors are essential to ensure specific pathogen-free animals for use in the pharmaceutical industry. Adequate in-house husbandry practices to prevent widespread colony infections are also necessary. Other rabbit strains occasionally used for pyrogen testing are chinchillas and Dutch Belts. These have distinct advantages and disadvantages. Dutch Belts have a high resistance to intestinal disease, smaller size, and tendency toward slow weight gain, whereas chinchillas have good health and emotional stability, but gain weight rapidly, which limits their extended use in a pyrogen colony. These two strains also possess the disadvantage of pigmented skin, which makes it more difficult to administer intravenous injections to these animals than to albino strains (3).

Gender

Rabbits of either gender may be used for pyrogen testing. Most laboratories prefer to use rabbits of a single gender, however, to avoid emotional or hormonal stimuli that might potentially affect pyrogen test results. It has been shown, though, that rabbits of both genders can be individually caged in the same room without significantly influencing pyrogen test results (9). Female rabbits tend to be easier to manage and more docile than males, especially as they grow older. In addition, male rabbits urinate with a forceful spray, which often creates added problems of handling and sanitation. Males tend to gain weight more rapidly and sometimes demonstrate aggressive posturing and territorial behavior toward handlers. Febrile responses to endotoxin appear to be equivalent, however, regardless of the gender of the test animal.

Size

The USP specifies use of mature rabbits. Rabbits younger than seven weeks of age are 50 times less susceptible to the physiological actions of endotoxin than are older animals (10). Tennant and Ott (11) showed that rabbits weighing less than 2 kg have lower sensitivity, a lesser dose–response relationship, and more individual biological variation than rabbits above that weight. Probey and Pittman (12) also reported that rabbits weighing from 2 to 3.5 kg gave much more uniform responses than did smaller rabbits. The most practical weight range for albino New Zealand Whites appears to be 2 to 4 kg.

Length of Use

The USP refers only to frequency of use of test rabbits, not age limits or length of usefulness. Frequency of use is not to exceed once every four to eight hours or be less than two weeks following a maximum rise of temperature of 0.6°C or more during a pyrogen test or following injection of a test specimen that was judged pyrogenic. Length of use is partially dependent upon the types of solutions being assayed. Rabbits used to test nonantigenic solutions, such as saline and dextrose, can be used repeatedly over years. In fact, fluctuations of rabbit temperatures normally become less pronounced, as animals become more accustomed to routine handling. Reuse of rabbits thus contributes to the continued accuracy of pyrogen testing. If new rabbits enter a pyrogen test colony at the onset of maturity, they can be used for at least two years, and theoretically through the fourth year of age, before degenerative aging diseases begin to interfere with testing (9). There are reliable data to suggest that uterine adenocarcinoma presence is largely a function of age; tumor incidence is 4.2% in female rabbits from two to three years of age and 79.1% in rabbits over five years old (13). If, on the other hand, rabbits are to be used to test biologicals, such as protein fractions, hormones, or other antigenic compounds, reuse of these test animals is quite limited. Most contract pyrogen testing facilities use naive rabbits for every test to preclude antigenicity problems yielding questionable test results. When predominantly antigenic solutions are tested, the inability to use rabbits repeatedly becomes economically significant. On these occasions, rabbits' reuse should be defined with reference to frequency, duration, and limit of antigenic injections, provided no pyrogenicity is observed (14).

MAINTENANCE

Rabbits should be obtained from reliable breeders of research animals who have demonstrated long-term ability to provide specific pathogen-free animals. A combination of environmental stressors due to shipping or changes in housing and diet can produce illness in newly received animals; if these new animals were immediately placed in caging alongside older colony test rabbits, they might jeopardize the health of the entire colony. For this reason, a quarantine period of at least one week is usually instituted before animals are added to the colony. During this time, rabbits should be carefully observed, checked for any signs of disease or failure to adapt to the new housing, and treated appropriately, if necessary. Confidence in the vendor can be periodically reinforced through existence of a sentinel animal health program in the testing facility, to maintain colony animals as valid test subjects, capable of delivering accurate test results.

If animals are to be maintained in a colony for extended periods of time, they must be uniquely and positively identified. This may be accomplished by means of ear tattoos or the implanting of microchip transponders, which are cross referenced to cage numbers. The USP does not describe whether access to feed should be restricted or what specific kind of food should be given. Typically, a consistent type and ration of chow per day, as well as a defined feeding schedule are observed. Food is to be withheld from the rabbits during a pyrogen test, because rabbit temperatures are notably affected by ingestion of food; thus, animals require 1 to 1.5 hours for stabilization after initiation of fasting (15). Nonrestricted access to food before testing might introduce variables that could adversely affect test results. A restricted diet of 85 g of commercial rabbit pellets per day, or about 100 g of a low-fat/high-fiber chow, are adequate to permit normal growth and maintenance while preventing obesity. This diet is normally consumed within a few hours after it is offered, thus eliminating food waste and spoilage. Furthermore, if rabbit colony subjects are fed after pyrogen testing is completed for the day, animals eligible for test on the following day will be well-fasted at the appropriate time.

HOUSING

The USP requires that rabbits be individually housed in an area with a uniform temperature of between 20°C and 23°C and free from disturbances likely to excite them. Room temperatures must not vary more than ±3°C from the selected temperature. The pyrogen test area must be separated from the housing area, but maintained under similar environmental conditions. For this reason, it is most convenient to locate the pyrogen test laboratory adjacent to the housing area. Rabbits can then be transported easily from one location to the other, with minimal excitement to the animals. Individual rabbit cages should conform to the dimensions recommended by the American Association of Accreditation of Laboratory Animal Care, and the Guide for the Care and Use of Laboratory Animals by the National Research Council (16). Among the modern improvements in cage design are such useful features as: automatic watering devices, waste management systems, individually exhausted air supply from cages/racks, improved component materials, and interchangeable repair parts. Animals also benefit from being housed with enrichment devices to chew on and play with, as they spend considerable time alone in their cages.

PERFORMANCE
Sham Testing or Pretesting

Before rabbits are used for the first time in a pyrogen test, the USP requires that they be conditioned with a sham test that includes all of the actual test steps, except the injection. This sham test must be performed within seven days of the actual test. Many laboratories that keep rabbits for long periods of time use repeated sham tests, frequently including injections of sterile, pyrogen-free reference materials, to screen rabbits and keep them eligible test animals. Marcus et al. (17) recommended using at least two sham tests, followed by three injection pretests, to screen new rabbits for admission to a test colony. Any animals showing persistently high or low initial temperatures, or temperature increases over 0.6°C, should be permanently removed from the pyrogen colony.

Temperature Measurements

Rectal temperatures of rabbits may be determined in a number of ways. The USP requires the use of clinical thermometers, thermistor probes, or other probes that have been calibrated to ensure an accuracy of ±0.1°C. Probes must also be tested to determine that a maximum reading is obtained in less than five minutes. They must be calibrated/checked according to a regular schedule to ensure accurate operation. Temperature-sensing probes are inserted rectally in the rabbit at a depth of not less than 7.5 cm. When clinical thermometers are used for temperature measurements, they are usually lubricated with petroleum jelly before insertion, and the test rabbit is normally cradled in the operator's lap. The thermometer is left in place until the indicated temperature stabilizes (usually one to two minutes). Because this procedure is time consuming, it is practical only when limited numbers of pyrogen tests are to be performed. For large-scale pyrogen testing, most laboratories use electronic thermometers containing copper-constantan thermocouples or thermistors. This equipment permits the testing of more rabbits per day than would be possible with clinical thermometer use. Most electronic thermometers have flexible probes, which are inserted rectally, and secured to remain in place during the entire test period. Temperatures are usually displayed on a lighted galvanometer scale or digital monitor. Either a chart recorder or an automated scanning-recording system with a printer may be used to capture temperature responses automatically at appropriate time intervals. In addition to automated printout capacity, these recorders may possess on-line computer acquisition and data management capability. The cost of this type of equipment limits its use to high-volume industrial operations.

TEST LABORATORY

The USP requires that tests be performed in an area designated solely for pyrogen testing and under environmental conditions similar to those in which the animals are housed. The area should also be free of disturbances likely to excite the test animals. If the laboratory uses clinical thermometers for temperature recording, rabbits may be returned to their cages between recording periods. If, on the other hand, electronic recording devices are used, rectal temperature probes must remain in place throughout the pyrogen test and animals should be lightly restrained. Under these conditions, the USP states that rabbits must be fitted with loose neck stocks that allow the rabbits to assume a natural resting posture. Restraining boxes, constructed so that the rabbit's neck is placed in a comfortable, loose-fitting stock, may be placed on tables or shelves. For ease of handling, portable racks or tables are commercially available from a number of cage manufacturers. Stocks of the best design have drainage systems to handle urine and feces. Restraining boxes should be placed on shelves in such a way as to be easily accessible from the front (for injections) and also from the rear (for insertion and adjustment of rectal probes). To avoid disturbing the rabbits during the test period, the test area should be kept calm and peaceful, with a minimum amount of activity. Strangers should not be allowed into the area during testing because their presence often results in false-positive rabbit temperature responses. Even the presence or voice of a new animal handler in an area may be upsetting enough to panic established colony rabbits.

Preinjection Procedure

Rabbits selected for testing on any given test day must not have been used for testing during the preceding four to eight hours, or prior to two weeks following a maximum rise in temperature of 0.6°C or more while on test, or following use on a test specimen judged to be pyrogenic. In addition, in any group of test rabbits, control temperatures may not vary from rabbit to rabbit by more than 1°C, and no rabbit is to be used if its normal temperature exceeds 39.8°C. It, therefore, may be advantageous to establish an acceptable range of initial rabbit temperatures from 38.9°C to 39.8°C to ensure that test rabbits in a group do not vary by more than 1°C.

Before testing, the rabbits must be weighed in order to determine the correct dosage of test solution to be administered by injection. At the time of weighing, general health status should be evaluated (e.g., nails, teeth, eyes, and coat). If rabbits are weighed on the day of use, care should be taken not to excite them. Unusual noises or rough handling during weighing and transferring rabbits into restraining boxes may induce temporary hyperthermia. With a large rabbit colony, it may be more convenient to weigh all rabbits at a routine interval, such as once a week, instead of on test days. Individual weights can be recorded in logbooks or stored in electronic databases. Abrupt weight losses signal possible disease conditions or dehydration and should be immediately reported to veterinary staff personnel. Animals under observation or exhibiting health problems are not suitable test animals for laboratory use. After transferring the rabbits to restraining boxes, rectal probes are inserted. Probes are usually lubricated with petroleum jelly before insertion and are held in place by attaching a soft piece of lead wire, band, or tie to the probe; the wire or band may be twisted around the rabbit's tail to hold the probe in place throughout the test period. Test animals should be allowed to stabilize for at least 30 minutes before their "control" temperatures are taken. Control temperatures are the base values used to determine all subsequent changes and are recorded as "normal" temperatures. In accordance with the USP, test material must be administered within 30 minutes of recording the control temperature. Before injection, test solutions are warmed to 37°C. Syringes, needles, and glassware used in testing must be pyrogen-free, according to USP recommendations. To simplify this process, pyrogen-free disposable needles and syringes can be purchased for use.

Injection Procedure

A depyrogenated syringe is filled, either by aspiration or by pouring the test solution directly into the syringe barrel. With the syringe plunger in place, the needle is put into place and all air bubbles are expelled from the barrel. For injection of large volumes, a 20 G × 1 inch needle may be used. However, thin or brittle rabbit veins may necessitate the use of 22 to 25 G needles for most tests. Three rabbits are injected for each USP test. The marginal ear vein area of each rabbit is prepared appropriately; the analyst may shave the ear, rub it to warm, and dilate the vein, or moisten it with water or 70% alcohol to render the vein more visible. The needle is inserted, bevel up, as close to the tip of the ear as possible, to prolong the useful life of the vein lumen. Once the needle is in place securely, test solution is injected using steady pressure on the syringe plunger. Test solutions are injected into rabbit ear veins at a usual dosage of 10 mL/kg body weight, unless otherwise specified in individual USP monographs or regulatory committee documents. The injection is to be completed within 10 minutes. In general, neither the volume nor the rate of injection appears to influence the magnitude of the fever response (18). Most test solutions can be safely injected within a minute or two. However, slower injection rates may be necessary if the product to be tested has acute pharmacological effects that interfere with or obscure a temperature response. Severe reactions, including death, can occur from rapid infusion of solutions of high acidity, alkalinity, nonphysiological quantities of certain cations, such as Ca^{2+}, Mg^{2+}, or K^+, or markedly hypertonic or hypotonic solutions (19). Upon completion of an injection, the needle is withdrawn and firm pressure is applied to the injection site to prevent excessive bleeding. If bleeding persists, a piece of cotton is applied with pressure to the injection site to stop bleeding and promote clot formation. When rabbits are repeatedly subjected to intravenous injections, damage to their ear veins is common. Efforts should be made to reduce this trauma to a minimum, such as changing sites on an ear or alternating left and right ears. If vein scarring occurs despite all precautions, rabbits should be rested for one to two weeks before they are used again. At the conclusion of the injection, exact time is recorded and rabbit temperatures are recorded at 0.5, 1, 1.5, 2, 2.5, and

3 hours postinjection, or as required by the compendial source or the test protocol. Immediately prior to scheduled temperature recordings, the rectal probes are checked to ensure that they are properly positioned for accurate readings. At all other times, the animals should be disturbed as little as possible. After the final temperatures have been recorded, rectal probes are removed and the rabbits are returned to their cages. Rectal probes should be carefully washed in warm soapy water, dried, disinfected, and then air dried. Clinical thermometers should be similarly cleansed each time temperatures are taken with them.

TEST INTERPRETATION

USP pyrogen test specifications state that a test is positive if one rabbit in three shows a temperature of 0.6°C or greater than its control temperature, or if the sum of the three rabbits' temperature rise exceeds 1.4°C. In either case, a repeat test is done on five additional rabbits. If not more than three of the total of eight rabbits have individual increases of 0.6°C or more and if the sum of the eight increases does not exceed 3.7°C, the material under examination meets the requirements for absence of pyrogens. Fever responses in a rabbit resulting from injection of endotoxin follow a typical biphasic pattern, when all but minimal doses are administered. There is a lag phase of 15 to 18 minutes followed by a rapid rise to a peak during the first two hours. This rise is followed by a transient but incomplete temperature drop that precedes a second temperature rise, followed by a return to the baseline after six to nine hours (20). False-positive temperature rises are not uncommon and may result from a wide variety of stimuli, including: injury, upset, or illness of the animal, the presence of noise or strangers in the test area, a badly-placed rectal probe, or unique properties of the test materials.

FACTORS INFLUENCING THE TEST
Nature of the Test Sample
Drugs or solutions that cause, decrease, or arrest fever are obviously ill-suited to the rabbit pyrogen testing modality. Examples of products that arrest the fevers produced by pyrogens are acetanilide, acetophenetidin, and acetylsalicylic acid. Drugs that mask pyrogenicity by decreasing fever include some phenothiazine derivatives, hypnotics, local anesthetics (such as procaine), and strophanthin (18). Phosphate and other specific buffer solutions have been shown to elicit pyrogenic responses in rabbits, if sufficient ions are infused intravenously, even though the buffers are free of bacterial endotoxin (14). Some substances, such as steroids or antibiotics, are also known to elicit fever in most mammals; while others may be intrinsically toxic to the rabbit (21). It is, therefore, extremely important to understand the pharmacological effects of new test solutions before submitting them for rabbit pyrogen testing.

Degree of Restraint
As was discussed earlier, it is necessary to restrain pyrogen test rabbits if rectal thermometer probes remain in place throughout the test period. However, rabbits tend to become hypothermic when they are restrained (22), with the degree of hypothermia related to the degree of restraint. Sheagren and Wolff (23) injected 5 μg endotoxin into two conditioned groups of rabbits. A group of six rabbits was kept upright and restrained by loosely fitting collars in stocks that allowed

freedom of movement of their torsos and legs. The second group of five rabbits was securely restrained in a prone position with their legs extended. The upright rabbits developed fever; the others did not. Despite these differences, sera obtained from these two groups one hour after injection contained similar amounts of endogenous pyrogen. In addition, some workers have also observed that the rectal temperatures of loosely restrained rabbits were 0.2°C to 0.3°C lower than that observed in animals that had not been placed in stocks. This type of hypothermia decreases after several hours. The maximum response of rabbits to injection of pyrogens occurs when the degree of restraint is at a minimum, and rabbits which are repeatedly used in pyrogen testing soon tolerate light restraint without hypothermia (18).

Tolerance

Acquired resistance to endotoxins was first noted by clinicians who employed these substances to produce experimental hyperpyrexia. Human subjects given repeated doses of endotoxin develop remarkable resistance to its fever-producing action and require progressively increasing doses to achieve comparable febrile responses. The same resistance occurs in rabbits and poses a particular problem for pyrogen testing. It is now understood that endotoxin tolerance develops in two distinct phases, early and late. Early tolerance is most easily demonstrated when rabbits are continuously infused with endotoxin. Within hours, the animals will be totally unresponsive. This refractory state is relative and can be overcome either by increasing the rate of infusion or the dose of endotoxin delivered. Such early tolerance is specific for endotoxins as a class. There is not apparent specificity for individual endotoxins and an animal remains fully responsive to injected endogenous pyrogen. The level of antibody to endotoxin is not related to tolerance, and tolerance is not transferable with plasma (24). Similarly, early phase pyrogenic tolerance occurs when single doses of endotoxin are injected into rabbits. This early tolerance, after a single injection of endotoxin, wanes rapidly and is minimal by 48 hours post-injection. As is the case with continuously-infused endotoxin, early tolerance is specific for all endotoxins, as a class, and is not associated with incremental changes in antibody level.

It is now generally accepted that this early phase of pyrogenic tolerance is mediated by a direct effect of endotoxin on the target cells responsible for production of endogenous pyrogen (hepatic Kupffer cells). The effect is such that these cells cease releasing endogenous pyrogen in response to contact with the endotoxin molecule. In contrast to the early phase of pyrogenic tolerance to endotoxin, the second, or late-phase tolerance, possesses very different characteristics. Late-phase tolerance is seen about 72 hours after a single injection of endotoxin. It generally increases over the next several days and may persist for several weeks. In contrast to early tolerance, the late phase is unrelated to the initial febrile response, but is related to the antigenicity of the immunizing substance injected into the rabbit. In addition, it tends to be specific for the homologous endotoxin used for the initial injection. Late-phase tolerance appears to be caused by anti-endotoxin antibodies directed against both O and common-core antigens that block the release of endogenous pyrogen from hepatic Kupffer cells. The common-core antigens are masked in the presence of the O-antigenic side chains and become effective immunogens only when O side chains are lacking.

When endotoxin is administered repeatedly at closely spaced intervals, both the early (nonimmune) and late (immune) phase mechanisms may become superimposed. This phenomenon has resulted in many confusing descriptions of endotoxin tolerance in the literature. The endotoxin-tolerant state is dependent on the relative contribution of each mechanism (early and late), which in turn is dependent on the injection schedule, antigenicity of the endotoxin, dosage, and the immunological competence of the host. The USP requires rabbits that have been tested with pyrogenic solutions to be rested for two weeks before they are reused. Because the incidence of pyrogenic reactions in test laboratories is infrequent, most rabbits do not receive repeated injections of a given pyrogenic compound causing them to develop immunological tolerance. Unfortunately, the effect of repeated subfebrile doses of endotoxin is unknown, but could produce some degree of tolerance to marginally pyrogenic solutions. It is possible that this unsuspected tolerance could explain the wide range of rabbit colony febrile responses to endotoxin standards employed in intraindustry and international collaborative studies (6,25,26).

CONCLUSION

For nearly 60 years, the rabbit test was the only official test for pyrogens recognized in pharmacopoeial compendia. Despite the vast amount of knowledge gained about the chemistry and physiology of pyrogens during this period, the test has remained basically unchanged. It remains a qualitative test, subject to a "pass" or "fail" interpretation, with results dependent upon the sensitivity of three test rabbits to any pyrogenic substances contaminating a test product. In an effort to convert this in vivo test to an in vitro method, the gel-clot bacterial endotoxin method was developed, optimized, and validated for use testing waters, diluents, large volume parenterals, and pharmaceutical product testing, as well as for quality assurance validation of industrial depyrogenation processes. Advantages of the rabbit pyrogen test include: similar response to that of humans, long track record of reliability, and suitability to detect a broader spectrum of pyrogenic substances than the endotoxin method (gram-negative bacteria only). Disadvantages of the in vivo method include: expense of maintaining a rabbit colony, inability to quantitate the contaminant present, less sensitivity than the *Limulus* amebocyte lysate (LAL) method, increased time for an assay, and biological variability factors. In general, this test has worked well over the years. In only rare instances have substances proven pyrogenic in humans that have not shown evidence of pyrogenicity in rabbits. It still remains an excellent informational quality control tool that will serve as an adjunct to the LAL bacterial endotoxin method for the testing of some biologically derived compounds during their early development phases.

REFERENCES

1. Seibert FB. The cause of many febrile reactions following intravenous injections. Am J Physiol 1925; 71:621.
2. Seibert FB, Mendel LB. Temperature variations in rabbits. Am J Physiol 1923; 67:83.
3. Cooper M. Quality Control in the Pharmaceutical Industry. New York: Academic Press, 1973:239.
4. Tui C, Schrift MH. A tentative test for pyrogen in infusion fluids. Proc Soc Exp Biol Med 1942; 49:320.
5. Welch H, Calvery HO, McClosky WT, Price CW. Method of preparation and test for bacterial pyrogens. J Am Pharm Assoc 1943; 32:65.

6. McClosky WT, Price CW, Van Winkle Jr W, Welch H, Calvery II O. Results of first U.S.P. collaborative study of pyrogens. J Am Pharm Assoc 1943; 32:69.
7. US Pharmacopeial Convention, Inc. US Pharmacopeia, Vol. XX. Easton: Mack Printing Co., 1979:902.
8. Greisman SE, Hornick RB. Comparative pyrogenic reactivity of rabbit and man to bacterial endotoxin. Proc Soc Exp Biol Med 1969; 131:1154.
9. Weary ME, Wallin RF. The rabbit pyrogen test. Lab Anim Sci 1973; 23:677.
10. Smith RT, Thomas L. Influence of age upon response to meningococcal endotoxin in rabbits. Proc Soc Exp Biol Med 1954; 86:806.
11. Tennant DM, Ott WH. Tolerance to bacterial pyrogens in the rabbit. J Am Pharm Assoc 1953; 42:614.
12. Probey TF, Pittman M. The pyrogenicity of bacterial contaminants found in biologic products. J Bacteriol 1945; 50:397.
13. Manning PJ, Ringler DH, Newcomer CE. The Biology of the Laboratory Rabbit. New York: Academic Press Inc., 1994; 12:261.
14. Personeus GR. Pyrogen testing of biologicals and small volume parenterals. Bull Parenter Drug Assoc 1969; 23:201.
15. Kobayashi M. Studies of pyrogens. II. Nippon Yakurigaku Zasshi 1951; 47:75.
16. Guide for the Care and Use of Laboratory Animals, Commission on Life Sciences, National Research Council, Institute of Laboratory Animal Resources. Washington, DC: National Academy Press, 1996.
17. Marcus S, Anselmo C, Luke J. Studies on bacterial pyrogenicity. II. A bacteriological test for pyrogens in parenteral solutions. J Am Pharm Assoc Sci Ed 1960; 49:616.
18. Braun HA, Klein VV. Some problems of pyrogen testing. Bull Parenter Drug Assoc 1960; 14:9.
19. Lamey RT, Weary ME, Murphy BF. Some aspects of the USP pyrogen test. Bull Parenter Drug Assoc 1969; 23:245.
20. Bennett IL, Cluff LE. Bacterial pyrogens. Pharmacol Rev 1957; 9:427.
21. Pharmaceutical Society of Great Britain. International Symposium on Pyrogens. St. Louis, Missouri: Mallinckrodt, Inc., 1975:22.
22. Grant R. Emotional hypothermia in rabbits. Am J Physiol 1950; 160:285.
23. Sheagren JN, Wolff SM. Demonstration of endogenous pyrogen in Afebrile rabbits. Nature 1966; 210:539.
24. Kass EH, Wolff, SM. Bacterial Lipopolysaccharides. Chicago: University of Chicago Press, 1973: 257.
25. Wolstenholme GEW, Birch J, eds. Pyrogens and Fever. London: Churchill Livingstone, 1971:207.
26. Varney RF. The intruders-pyrogens. Bull Parenter Drug Assoc 1962; 16:6.

13 Pyrogenicity Case Studies

James F. Cooper
Endotoxin Consulting Services, Greensboro, North Carolina, U.S.A.

Kevin L. Williams
Eli Lilly & Company, Indianapolis, Indiana, U.S.A.

The proverb "those ignorant of the past are doomed to repeat it," is not one that should apply to pharmaceutical manufacturing.

INTRODUCTION

Fortunately, or perhaps as a testament to the utility of the *Limulus* amebocyte lysate (LAL) test, there have been few significant[a] cases of pyrogenic responses to drugs manufactured in the United States after almost a century of parenteral therapy. When such adverse drug events (ADE) do occur they are usually complex and, should, rightfully, receive a great deal of attention. Such misadventures can be instructive from many perspectives. This chapter will describe three events and learning points from them. One event occurred at the beginning of the application of *Limulus* technology to pharmaceutical products. The two more recent events described appear to involve the presence of a nonendotoxin pyrogen that either contributed alone or in synergy with endotoxin. The proverb: those ignorant of the past are doomed to repeat is not one that should apply to pharmaceutical manufacturing. The events described include:

1. The demonstration in 1972 that aseptic meningitis (AM) is caused by endotoxin as administered via the intrathecal route during radionuclide cisternography (RC) (1).
2. A pyrogenic outbreak (2) resulted from an active pharmaceutical ingredient (API) supplied from a Chinese manufacturer (synergistic effect of lipopolysaccharide combined with nonendotoxin pyrogen at pyrogenic levels due partly to once-daily-dosing as allowed by the FDA's Modernization Act). The bulk supplier in question was later cited for significant current good manufacturing practices (cGMP) violations.
3. Following an outbreak of aseptic peritonitis, Baxter detected and subsequently precluded a nonendotoxin microbial contaminant in an icodextrin-containing dialysate.

    Given that many of the technical problems associated with LAL testing have been solved and that verification of in-process endotoxin reduction steps are commonplace,[b] one can see that when one does encounter a contamination problem it

---

[a] That is, involving a large number of people.
[b] By some estimates, the level of LAL in-process testing performed today is 60% to 70% and the use of validation is another 10%.

may be significant indeed. The following case studies represent such significant problems, how they occurred, potential causes, and the learning points derived from them.

CASE STUDY 1: DISCOVERY OF ENDOTOXIN AS A PYROGENIC CONTAMINANT OF INTRATHECALLY ADMINISTERED RADIONUCLIDES

At the dawn of LAL technology, little was known about the prevalence or significance of endotoxin in all but the most routine pharmaceutical drug applications. A specialized branch of medicine that utilizes radioisotopes to trace the flow of cerebrospinal fluid is called RC. RC required injection of 1 mL or less of radiotracer into the lumbar spinal canal; RC was superseded by more effective imaging modalities, such as computed axial tomography. RC had become known to physicians to be a significant risk of pyrogenic reactions and even AM in some instances documented to be up to 27% (3) for the former and 14% for the latter of intrathecal medicines administered (4). Furthermore, it was determined that combining intrathecally related tests (i.e., RC plus pneumoencephalograms), as is sometimes necessary in patients, could plague patient participants with an astonishing 41% (36/88) adverse drug reaction rate (3). Since the early days of intrathecal therapy and diagnostics, there have been significant additional therapies advanced via the intraspinal route (5), intractable pain, and spasticity are ameliorated by long-term intraspinal therapy delivered by an implanted spinal infusion pump. Given the extreme sensitivity of this route of administration for endotoxin,[c] as reviewed by Cooper and Thoma (5), it is prudent to take a zero endotoxin tolerance approach[d] to the bulk drug powders used by compounding pharmacies to prepare intraspinal medications.

Beginning in 1971, there were 39 AM reactions associated with RC over a 15-month period. Suspecting endotoxin, Cooper and Harbert (1) utilized the event to begin a study of the causation factors, especially suspecting endotoxin, by obtaining 10 lots specifically associated with 20 of the 39 adverse events. Early tracers of RC included ^{131}I-ISA or radioiodated human serum albumin and DTPA chelates of ^{111}In and [169]Yb. These radioisotopes could reveal cerebrospinal fluid dynamic abnormalities. Radioisotopes at this time were tested via the rabbit pyrogen test. When tested on a weight-dose basis the lots in question were all negative for pyrogenic activity.

Cooper, who first applied the LAL test [as developed by Levin and Bang (6)] to a pharmaceutical application (7) suspected endotoxin was the silent cause of these adverse events. Setting about to prove such a causation at this early date involved a "cradle to grave" preparation of both the test reagents (LAL) and standardization of the standard endotoxin to the "homemade" LAL reagent. The LAL was gathered and prepared by the Levin method from Limuli harvested from Chincoteague, VA, in 1971. One *Escherichia coli* endotoxin from Difco (026:B6) and one from *Klebsiella pneumoniae* (the FDA reference pyrogen at the time) were prepared in stock solutions and standardized to a sensitivity of

---

[c]100 to 1000 times more sensitive.

[d]A recommended 14 EU/day as endotoxin in this route is not cleared by the liver and occurs in only about 125 mL of total spinal fluid for an adult.

TABLE 1 Radionuclide Cisternography LAL Reaction Grades

Grade	Reaction conclusion	Sample/LAL attributes upon incubation (37°C)	Associated reaction times (min)
G	Strong positive	Firm gel when inverted 180°	<30
V	Positive	Increased viscosity, opacity and observance of gelatinous granules	30–60
NA	Trace	>60 min for V grade reaction	>60
N	Negative	No formation of opacity or gelatinous granules	>60

0.125 ng/mL [i.e., this is before the establishment of the "Endotoxin Unit (EU)" and a unit of pyrogenic activity]. In what can be viewed as an early indicator of kinetic assay quantitation (turbidimetric via spectroscopy), the RC samples were gauged according to the following reactions (Table 1).

In addition to the 100% association of the 10 implicated lots from the 39 ADE, an expanded study of 100 lots beginning in March of 1972 did not find evidence of a correlation of adverse events with any chemical or albumin found in the drug products.

The authors (1) suggested that endotoxin was the cause of the adverse AM events given the 100% correlation of the lots incurring symptomatic patients with strongly positive LAL results. Furthermore, as one might still conclude that endotoxin might be only one of several associated factors in AM inducement, a summary of Cooper and Harbert's thoughts on the matter are given below as evidence for endotoxin as the sole significant cause:

1. The positive LAL results of the 10 AM-associated lots
2. Same source of ^{131}I-IHSA associated with 24/25 reactions rules out significant differences in formulation as a cause of AM
3. AM reactions associated with (at least) two different radiotracers
4. For one LAL-positive test, a repeat pyrogen test at an increased dose revealed a positive rabbit pyrogen test
5. Endotoxin contamination was traced to production components (the anion-exchange resin used in radiochemical purification as provided by the manufacturer was found to be highly contaminated via LAL)
6. Significantly, enacted quality-assurance measures has reduced the incidence of adverse reactions

Learning points associated with this event include:

1. The necessity of depyrogenating ion exchange resins before use in pharmaceutical production.
2. The assignment of strict endotoxin limits for intrathecally administered products. Ultimately, the above study influenced United States Pharmacopeia (USP) Committee of Revision to adopt strict endotoxin tolerance limits for medications intended for injection into epidural or intrathecal spaces.

CASE STUDY 2: ENDOTOXIN/NONENDOTOXIN MICROBIAL CONTAMINANT SYNERGY

Perhaps the worst documented outbreak of pyrogenic parenteral product administered to patients in the United States occurred between April 1998 and August 1999.

Finished-product gentamicin from two different U.S. manufacturers, which used the same API supplier, contained a range of endotoxin activities up to the threshold pyrogenic response level ($\sim$5 EU/kg). Back testing of some of the lots revealed that "a significant number of patients developed pyrogenic reactions to doses as low as 2 EU/Kg" (8), thus it was suspected that, in addition to endotoxin, a nonendotoxin contaminant may also have been present and thus potentially acting synergistically.

Classified as an "aminoglycoside" antibiotic, gentamicin acts by binding to bacterial ribosomes thereby causing mistranslation (misreading of protein translation) errors and bacterial cell death (Fig. 1).

Gentamicin was isolated in 1963 by Weinstein and colleagues from the soil fungus *Micromonospora purpura* (of the Actinomycete group) (22). It was introduced in the United States in 1969. It is a "complex" of gentamicins C_1, C_{1a}, and C_2 and also gentamicin A which differs from the other members of the complex but is similar to kanamycin C (Merck, 1989). Within the aminoglycoside family the suffix "mycin" is used in the name when the antibiotic is produced by *Streptomyces* species and "micin," when produced by *Micromonospora* species (9).

The bulk supplier used the same process and process controls to supply both the dry and parenteral forms of the drug. Following are selected findings from an FDA inspection of the bulk supplier facilities that occurred after the outbreak (11):

1. Use of unsuitable water in final processing
2. No validation of the process when it was scaled-up years before
3. No second-person verification of batch action steps
4. Some records rewritten without explanation
5. No evaluation of the process step's ability to remove/reduce endotoxin
6. Composite testing of API revealed batches testing at the limit, but none over the limit

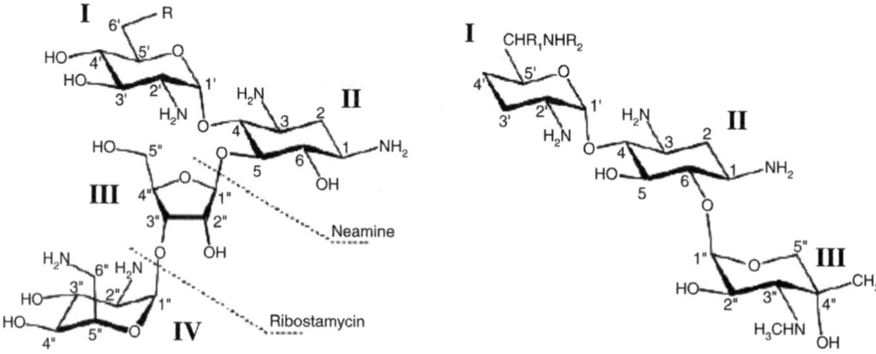

	R
Paromomycin	OH
Neomycin	NH$_2$
Ribostamycin	NH$_2$
Neamine	NH$_2$

	R$_1$	R$_2$
Gentamicin C1	CH$_3$	CH$_3$
Gentamicin C2	CH$_3$	H
Gentamicin C1a	H	H

FIGURE 1 Structures of the aminoglycoside antibiotics that bind in the A site of 16S rRNA. Comparison of the gentamicin components (4–6 ring II–ring I, ring II–ring III linkages) and the neomycin group (4–5 ring II–ring I, ring II–ring III linkages) of aminoglycosides. The neomycin group includes paromomycin, neomycin, ribostamycin, and neamine. Ribostamycin contains all rings except ring IV whereas neamine lacks both rings III and IV. *Source*: From Ref. 10.

7. Failure of the testing lab to perform control testing [as required by USP Bacterial Endotoxin Testing (BET)]
8. Water used for purification and final equipment rinses not tested for microbial total counts
9. No program to identify or gram-stain organisms
10. Postevent, no efforts were made to identify the root cause of the product safety problem and no subsequent CAPA plan was implemented

According to Friedman (11), the FDA placed the firm on import detention. Friedman attributed much of the problem to raw material variability, acknowledging the cGMP problems, but also implicating the "materials system" combined with the lack of process control. He cited the "intra-batch variability (i.e., drum-to-drum variability)" which was evidenced by the wide range of pyrogenicity of the associated batches, ranging from well below to equivalent to the threshold pyrogenic levels. Friedman also implicated the firm's investigational methods for using "composite" testing. The danger in this case was the mixing of suitable material with contaminated material, thereby producing a suitable material (i.e., diluted contaminant).

It is appropriate not to push all the responsibility for the event overseas to a substandard supplier. After all, it was American companies that accepted the bulk materials for use, even though endotoxin levels in the API were clearly out-of-trend. Another contributing factor was therapeutic utility of the "once-daily-dose" that had gained widespread acceptance given the kidney toxicity associated with the drug. The FDA Modernization Act of 1997 allowed doctors to use discretion in prescribing dosages for "off-label" uses. The Act allowed needed flexibility to provide individualized care but in the case of gentamicin allowed a drug contaminated near the limit to manifest pryogenic levels when the dose was effectively trebled.

> Traditionally, it has been given at a daily dose of 3–5 mg/kg in 3 divided doses. There has been a trend toward administering gentamicin in one daily dose (ODD) to minimize toxicity and simplify therapy; the infusion requires about one hour. Consequently, the USP reduced the allowable endotoxin from 1.7 to 0.7 EU/mg, effective January 2000. A cluster of pyrogenic reactions at a Los Angeles hospital prompted an investigation by the Center for Disease Control (CDC). They reviewed the records of 289 patients who received IV gentamicin prior to, during and after the study period. There was a 25% risk of reaction to ODD therapy and a much lower risk to the traditional therapy. Endotoxin assays found approximately 0.8 EU/mg, or half the limit of 1.7 EU/mg. The CDC concluded that the ODD regimen delivered sufficient endotoxin to match the tolerance limit, 5 EU/kg, and induce the reactions. In a worst-case scenario, a patient receiving 7 mg/kg of IV gentamicin having 0.8 EU/mg would receive 5.6 EU/kg (8).

Fanning et al. (12) reviewed the gentamicin ADEs and published their findings in a December 2000 issue of *NEJM*. There were 210 reactions[e] involving 155 patients (multiple reactions per patient), who experienced chills, fever, respiratory symptoms, and shivering within three hours after the start of infusion. Reactions were nine times more likely with ODD therapy. Most of the events caused no serious sequelae, but five (3%) were severe, requiring intensive-care support.

---

[e]A case of aseptic meningitis was reported following intrathecal administration of gentamicin in 1998. The role of endotoxin was not suspected, but the temporal relationship of the ADE and the contaminants of products in the marketplace could suggest pyrogenic contamination as a possible cause.

TABLE 2 Endoxin Levels (EU/mg) in Three Lots Determined as >1.7 EU/mg by the Food and Drug Administration

GS lot	FDA BET gel-clot	NIBSC gel-clot	GS vendor BET	Col. study KTA BET	Col. study KCA BET
G	1.5–12	0.75	1.0	0.6	0.4
D	0.15–1.8	0.75	0.6	0.6	0.4
J	2.3	0.75	0.7	0.6	0.4

Note: The FDA test lab reported that three lots from vendor A exceeded the endotoxin limit (EL) of 1.7 EU/mg. Subsequent tests by the collaborators did not reveal any lots that violated this limit. The FDA gel-clot results were highly variable. The principal difference in the FDA procedure was that the sample was buffered prior to testing rather than using buffered LAL reagent to resolve inhibition.

According to Fanning et al., the series of events leading to the exposure of the contamination may be summarized as follows:

1. Multiple problems in production of the API including endotoxin contamination
2. Use of once daily dosing effectively unmasked the API problem and lead to unexpected ADEs due to higher concentration of more than one impurity.

Cooper et al. (8) had the opportunity to study the lots in question as provided by the FDA. Cooper summarized their results in a presentation. Tables 2 and 3 are taken from that presentation as obtained from the collaborative effort.

The following overview points precede the collaboration investigation:

1. IV Gentamicin exhibits pH-related interference. It may be tested at 0.25 mg/mL or less with buffered LAL reagent to avoid test inhibition.
2. Vendor A used a USP kinetic turbidimetric assay for release of final products.
3. An FDA investigative lab used gel-clot LAL to test samples of API and final product.
4. Eleven lots were selected for additional testing by the collaborators based on BET results and capacity for inducing pyrogenic reactions. The lots were arbitrarily assigned an identity as samples A through K.

TABLE 3 Endoxin Levels (EU/mg) in 11 GS Lots by Kinetic Bacterial Endotoxin Testing with Reference Standard Endotoxin by Collaborators

GS Lot	KTA/A	KTA/B	KTA/C	KCA/B	KCA/C	KTA/W
A	NA	NA	<0.25	0.26	<0.25	0.02
B	NA	<0.25	<0.25	<0.25	<0.25	0.05
C	<0.25	0.32	<0.25	<0.25	<0.25	0.15
D	0.41	0.79	0.55	0.36	0.39	0.31
E	<0.25	0.27	<0.25	<0.25	<0.25	NA
F	0.43	0.84	0.57	0.38	0.36	NA
G	0.42	1.04	0.61	0.37	0.45	0.49
H	0.27	0.62	0.43	0.27	0.37	0.27
I	NA	NA	0.80	0.50	NA	NA
J	0.39	0.86	0.58	0.41	0.45	0.28
K	<0.25	<0.25	<0.25	<0.25	<0.25	NA

Note: All gentamicin samples were tested at 0.2 mg/mL, using a robust 0.05 to 5 EU/mL standard curve with reference standard endotoxin. These conditions produced a sensitivity of 0.25 EU/mg. Recovery of positive product controls was consistently in a range of 70% to 110%. The results generally agreed with the release-test results of gentamicin supplier A and showed only a slight reduction of endotoxin levels with time. There was less information available about bacterial endotoxin testing (BET) test results from supplier B, but there was less endotoxin in these samples as measured by BET methods.

TABLE 4 Summary of Pyrogen and Monocyte Activation Tests for Lots Associated with Pyrogenic Reactions

GS lot #	API lot #	Patient reactions	Study K-BET	Gel BET NIBSC	MAT rank NIBSC	MAT rank Novartis	Three rabbit pyrogen temp rise above baseline
G	213	15	0.6	0.75	7	9	1.24
D	213	3	0.5	0.75	9	3	1.36
J	213/533	1	0.5	0.75	10	5	0.89
C	533	2	<0.25	0.08	3	4	1.15
NA[a]	533	?	<0.25	NA[b]	NA[b]	NA[b]	0.25
I	533	?	0.7	0.75	11	8	1.87
F	533/229	3	0.6	0.75	8	6	0.96
H	229	1	0.3	0.75	4	7	0.28
E	?	24	<0.25	0.15	6	10	NA
A	?	7	<0.25	0.15	5	11	NA

Note: The lots of vendor A were rearranged by chronological order of production to reveal the relationship of active pharmaceutical ingredient (API) lot number with finished-product LAL and pyrogen tests; Lot C was an exception. The greatest number of patient reactions to medication from vendor A was associated with API No. 213, which had rabbit pyrogenicity and high ratings from the monocyte activation tests.
[a]Note assigned.
[b]Not available.

Collaborator testing via Kinetic BET and retests by vendor A found that lots related to ADEs (produced a range of 0.6–1 EU/mg) met the compendial endotoxin limit of 1.7 EU/kg. Rabbit pyrogen tests were conducted on eight of these lots, using a dose of 10 mg/kg. Therefore, rabbits received 6 to 10 EU/kg, based on BET results. Four lots failed the pyrogenicity test and two more were within 0.1°C of failing (Table 4).

A nonendotoxin contaminant from the cell walls of gram-positive organisms, peptidoglycan (PG), has been found to potentiate the endotoxin response. Co-administration of PG or its subunits caused elevated tumor necrosis factor and interleukin (IL)-6 levels in excess of either endotoxin or PG alone (13). Given this knowledge, the collaborators studied the nonendotoxin pyrogenic activity of the (A-K) samples by using the peripheral blood mononuclear cell (PBMNC)/IL-6 monocyte activation test. The PBMNC/IL-6 test utilizes the ability of the blood cell (monocyte) to detect structurally diverse pyrogens via the resultant production of a cytokine: IL-6 which has been shown to be more sensitive to diverse pyrogens than either TNF-α or IL-1β (14).

The laboratories of Stephen Poole, NIBSC, and Peter Brüegger, Novartis Basel, Switzerland used their capability for PBMNC/IL-6 testing. Given the suspicion of the presence of a nonendotoxin pyrogen or synergist activity, PG content was assayed via the silk worm (*Bombyx mori*) larvae plasma (SLP) test by Matsuura at Wako Diagnostics. No significant levels of PG were found. The impact of glucan levels (a nonendotoxin activator of the LAL alternate pathway) on endotoxin levels was also studied by Matsuura. The results of traditional LAL and endotoxin-specific LAL were the same, which is consistent with the absence of enhancement recorded with kinetic BET testing by the collaborators.

The lack of good agreement between LAL and in vitro pyrogen test data suggests the possibility that another entity was present and thus augmented the capacity of endotoxin to activate the cytokine system. For example, the higher level of impurities in this case may have synergized endotoxicity. The collaborators (8) summarized the conclusions of their study as follows:

> Nevertheless, it is unlikely that ADEs would have occurred if endotoxin had not been present. This outbreak suggests that a practice of using finished-product endotoxin limits for the API puts a significant number of patients at risk for adverse effects. It would seem prudent to reduce the API endotoxin limit to 25% for parenteral products that are produced by aseptic processing and are intended for IV or intrathecal route of administration. Hopefully, this reduction would minimize the risk of pyrogenic reactions to susceptible patients and neonates. The recently issued draft Guidance for Aseptic Processing[f] suggests lower limits as well for aseptic processing. We are excluding parenteral products from this API recommendation that are terminally sterilized because moist heat yields at least a 50-fold reduction of endotoxin in the final product. The intramuscular and subcutaneous routes are also excluded because they are at lesser risk for inducing pyrogenic reaction.

It is useful to generalize some situations that may require additional, nonendotoxin testing [i.e., monocyte activation tests (MAT), silkworm larvae plasma test (SLP)].

1. IV or IT drugs from fermentation or recombinant methods and produced via aseptic processing that may be subject to adventitious contamination
2. Complex proteins that may activate LAL by a nonendotoxin pathway (i.e., glucans)
3. Biological products currently screened with the rabbit pyrogen test.

In terms of "learning points" associated with the event, the pyrogenic reactions that occurred reveal a couple of salient points:

1. Synergistic contaminants pose a risk of potentially lowering the threshold pyrogenic response, K, if they occur.
2. There is apparently a wide range of responses associated with the human pyrogenic reaction (this can be seen in human Toll-like receptors polymorphisms as discussed in Chapters 6 and 19).
3. The threshold pyrogenic response may truly be viewed as a limit and not a worst-case level of pharmaceutical content as some reactions can indeed occur at or just below the 5 EU/kg level.
4. Accepting endotoxin levels which are clearly out-of-trend and near the endotoxin limit of the finished drug product should not be an acceptable practice.

CASE STUDY 3: NONENDOTOXIN MICROBIAL PYROGEN

Solutions of USP grade dialysis solution that had passed LAL testing for endotoxin showed pyrogenic activity when administered to patients between September 2001 and January 2003 (15,16). A global recall was issued by Baxter Healthcare in May of 2002. At this time, Martis et al. set out to determine the cause(s) of the pyrogenic activity. The final result would be a dose–response curve established between the drug solution containing PG and the peripheral blood mononuclear cell test which (also) utilized IL-6 as the cytokine of choice for detection purposes.

---

[f]http://www.fda.gov/cder/guidance/5882FNL.htm

In general terms, a peritoneal dialysis system and associated materials:

... is a device that is used as an artificial kidney system for the treatment of patients with renal failure or toxemic conditions, and that consists of a peritoneal access device, an administration set for peritoneal dialysis, a source of dialysate, and, in some cases, a water purification mechanism. After the dialysate is instilled into the patient's peritoneal cavity, it is allowed to dwell there so that undesirable substances from the patient's blood pass through the lining membrane of the peritoneal cavity into this dialysate ... The source of dialysate may be sterile prepackaged dialysate (for semiautomatic peritoneal dialysate delivery systems or "cycler systems") or dialysate prepared from dialysate concentrate and sterile purified water (for automatic peritoneal dialysate delivery systems or "reverse osmosis" systems). Prepackaged dialysate intended for use with either of the peritoneal dialysate delivery systems is regulated by FDA as a drug (17).

Peritonitis is a result of treatment due to either bacterial contamination or in the case of "aseptic" or "sterile" peritonitis due to microbial artifacts in the dialysis solution. Peritonitis manifests itself in symptoms including gastrointestinal disturbance (nausea, vomiting, and diarrhea) and fever and is typically bacterial in nature and evidenced by positive cultures of the dialysis solution; however, instances of nonmicrobial or aseptic peritonitis also occurs. Outbreaks of aseptic peritonitis occurred in 1977 and 1988 and were determined to be due to endotoxin contamination (18, 19). Icodextrin-containing peritoneal dialysate contains a polymer of glucose derived from the hydrolysis of corn-starch.

In the Martis et al. (16) investigation, the researchers followed "a standard aetiological approach" that included the following steps:

1. Verify and validate if common clinical materials, raw materials, or their handling was consistent with the cluster of complaints.
2. Establish whether the product or its raw materials for manufacture meet internal and external regulatory specifications.
3. Search for potential organisms or (bio)chemical contaminants that might be associated with or derived from the chemical components used in the product (i.e., extraordinary contaminants).
4. If a difference is identified, implement corrective and preventative action plan immediately.

Dialysate effluents were taken from patients after dialysate instillation and dwell: six using standard glucose-containing dialysis solutions (negative control) and two using icodextrin-containing solution associated with peritonitis. The resulting solutions were analyzed for icodextrin metabolites, total protein, PG, and pyrogenic cytokines: IL-6, IL-1β, and TNF-α.

Significant results, relative to this discussion, include:

1. Elevation in the IL-6 dialysate effluent from an afflicted patient (>5000 ng/L) versus a nonafflicted patient (59 ng/L).
2. No significant difference in IL-1β and TNF-α responses.
3. A rough doubling of the protein content in the complaint sample (23.6 vs. 12.5 g/L).
4. Endotoxin test results were within the allowed limit (<250 EU/L).
5. No increase in rabbit response in traditional rabbit testing.
6. The IL-6 results were not affected by pretreatment with endotoxin binding polymyxin B.
7. The activity was present in the raw material prior to product manufacture.

TABLE 5 Relation between Complaints per Million Units Sold and
Peptidoglycan Concentration in Icodextrin Solution

Determined PG concentration (μg/L)	Units sold	Complaints	Complaints per million units sold
$\leq$7.4	2,906,643	53	18.2
>7.4–15	835,539	10	12.0
>15–30	349,503	10	28.6
>30–60	231,330	8	34.6
>60	415,099	105	253.0

Subsequent analysis of 321 recalled batches of the drug revealed that 41% of the batches tested were positive for PG[g] as determined by the SLP.[h] See Chapter 16 for a discussion of the test. The investigators found that of the two raw material suppliers, all affected batches were from the same supplier. PG concentrations ranged from the 7.4 μg/L detection limit up to 303 μg/L. Absolute determination of PG was precluded by the low concentration and presence of large molecular weight glucose polymers (matrix) that proved to be interfering. However, the presence of muramyl dipeptide, the smallest polymeric subunits of PG, were identified. The authors state that "because β-glucan is positive in both the silkworm larvae plasma and *Limulus* amoebocyte lysate tests, and the dialysate contaminant was positive only in the silkworm larvae plasma test, β-glucan was probably not the immunological provocateur." However, it should be noted that LAL is a poor predictor of β-glucan content and β-glucan specific assays now exist.

Given the group's findings, they determined to identify the microbial culprits that caused the contamination. The production of icodextrin from cornstarch involves heat and acidification. Given such nonconventional culture conditions, the group was able to isolate a thermophilic, acidophilic, gram-positive organism: *Alicyclobacillus acidocaldarius* (previously *Bacillus acidocaldarius*). This is a common organism originally isolated from an acidic creek in Yellowstone National Park (20) and known to the food industry as a contaminant of orange and other juices and possessing a cell wall consisting of 40% PG. The vegetative cells are easily destroyed by pasteurization; however, they are spore formers and the spores persist (21). The group was also able to correlate the occurrence of pyrogenicity complaints with the PG content in μg/L as shown below in Table 5.

The supplier solved the contamination problem by cleansing the tanks and lines and implementing more robust filtration and carbon treatment steps, culturing samplings for thermophiles, and implementing the SLP test to monitor PG routinely at the test limit of detection.

The major learning points associated with Case Study 3 include:

1. If a pyrogenic reaction occurs clinically and it is suspected that a nonendotoxin microbial pyrogen may be involved, then a monocytic test using IL-6 may be necessary.

---

[g]The researchers state that they were looking for the following nonendotoxin microbial contaminants: peptidoglycan, exotoxins, protein A, lipoteichoic acid, glycoproteins, cell-surface polysaccharides, and DNA. "We made an a priori decision to investigate potential provocateurs on the basis of assay availability and assay performance when mixed with high concentrations of high molecular weight glucose polymers (icodextrin)" (15).
[h]SLP, Wako Pure Chemical Industries, Osaka, Japan.

2. The nonendotoxin microbial contaminant culprits may include a wide range of microorganism by-products including: PG, exotoxins, protein A, lipoteichoic acid, glycoproteins, cell-surface polysaccharides, and DNA.
3. Novel standards and assays may be employed to preclude contamination in specific manufacturing processes in conjunction with regulatory oversight.

REFERENCES

1. Cooper JF, Harbert JC. Endotoxin as a cause of aseptic meningitis after radionuclide cisternography. J Nucl Med 1975; 16(19):809–813.
2. Endotoxin-like reactions associated with intravenous Gentamicin–California, CDC. Morb Mortal Wkly Rep, 1998. www.cdc.gov/mmwrhtml/00055322.htm.
3. Banerji MA, Spencer RP. Febrile response to cerebrospinal fluid flow studies. J Nucl Med 1972; 13:655.
4. Messert B, Rieder MJ. RISA cisternography: study of spinal fluid changes associated with intrathecal RISA injection. Neurology 1972; 22:789–792.
5. Cooper J, Thoma LA. Screening extemporaneously compounded intraspinal injections with the bacterial endotoxin test. Am J Soc Health Syst Pharm 2002; 59:2426–2433.
6. Levin J, Bang FB. Clottalbe protein in *Limulus*: its localization and kinetics of its coagulation by endotoxin. Thromb Diath Haemorrh 1968; 19:186–197.
7. Cooper JF, et al. The *Limulus* test for endotoxin (pyrogen) in radiopharmaceuticals and biologicals. Bull Parenter Drug Assoc 1972; 26:153–162.
8. Cooper JF, Brugger P, Fanning M, Matsuura S, Poole S. Alert and Action Endotoxin Levels for APIs: A collaborative study of pyrogenic gentamicin. Parenteral Drug Association Annual Meeting, New Orleans, LA, December 11, 2002.
9. http://www.inchem.org.
10. Yoshizawa S, et al. Structural origins of gentamicin antibiotic action. EMBO J 1998; 17(22):6437–6448.
11. Friedman RL. Aseptic processing contamination case studies and the pharmaceutical quality system. PDA J Pharm Sci Technol 2005; 59(2):118–126.
12. Fanning et al. Pyrogenic reactions to gentamicin therapy. N Engl J Med 2000; 343(22):1658–1659.
13. Wang, et al. Shock 2001; 16(3):178–182.
14. Nakagawa, et al. Clin Diagn Lab Immunol 2002 May; 9(3): 588–597, doi: 10.1128/cdci9.3.588–597.2002.
15. Martis L, et al. Aseptic peritonitis due to peptidoglycan contamination of pharmacopoeia standard dialysis solution. Lancet 2005; 365(9459):588–594.
16. Martis L, et al. Aseptic peritonitis due to peptidoglycan. Lancet 2005; 366:289–290.
17. Code of Federal Regulations. Title 21, vol. 8, revised. April 1, 2005 (21CFR876.5630), Subchapter H- Medical Devices.
18. Karanicolas S, et al. Epidemic of aseptic peritonitis caused by endotoxin during chronic peritoneal dialysis. N Engl J Med 1977; 296:1336–1337.
19. Mangram AJ, et al. Outbreak of sterile peritonitis among continuous cycling peritoneal dialysis patients. Kidney Int 1988; 54:1367–1371.
20. Eckert K, Schneider E. A thermoacidophilic endoglucanase (CelB) from *Alicyclobacillus acidocaldarius* displays high sequence similarity to arabinofuranosidases belonging to family 51 of glycoside hydrolases. Eur J Biochem 2003; 270:3593–3602.
21. Alfredo P, et al. Heat resistance of *Alicyclobacillus acidocaldarius* in water, various buffers, and orange juice. J Food Protect 2000; 63(10):1377–1380.
22. Sande MA, Mandell GL. In: Rall TW, Murad F, eds. Antimicrobial Agents. The Pharmacological Basis of Therapeutics. 7th ed. New York: Macmillan Publishing Co., 1985: 1151–1169.

14

Developing Specifications for Active Pharmaceutical Ingredients, Excipients, Raw Materials, Sterile Pharmacy Compounds, and Nutritional Supplements

James F. Cooper
Endotoxin Consulting Services, Greensboro, North Carolina, U.S.A.

Kevin L. Williams
Eli Lilly & Company, Indianapolis, Indiana, U.S.A.

Recent endotoxin excipient testing references dictate limits for some parenteral excipients and, therefore, require the establishment of endotoxin quality control tests. However, the majority of parenteral excipients still do not have established endotoxin limits.

OVERVIEW

Williams (1) and Cooper (2) have published several methods for assigning endotoxin specifications to nonfinished drug ingredients. These methods will be detailed herein. The first method has been tagged a "control strategy" in that it seeks to estimate relevant limits by which to confine or control potential contaminants. There are cases, especially unique ingredients, that require one to develop relevant levels of endotoxin for targeting specifications. A second method, referred to here as the "strategic" method, is simpler, and may be preferable for well-characterized excipients.

DEVELOPING AN ENDOTOXIN CONTROL STRATEGY FOR DRUG SUBSTANCES/EXCIPIENTS

Finished products often contain ingredients in addition to the active drug substance. Excipients serve as solvents, solubilizing, suspending, thickening, and chelating agents; antioxidants and reducing agents, antimicrobial preservatives, buffers, pH adjusting agents, bulking agents, and special additives (3). Recent endotoxin excipient testing references (4,5) dictate limits for some parenteral excipients and, therefore, require the establishment of endotoxin quality control tests. However, the majority of parenteral excipients still do not have established endotoxin limits (EL). Nevertheless, for many the rationale for endotoxin testing is no different than for those that do. The FDA Guideline on Validation of the *Limulus* amebocyte lysate (LAL) Test (6), which outlines the determination of limits for "end product" testing, can be misapplied to drug substance and excipient testing. Relevant activities to be established to gain control over a given drug manufacturing process from an endotoxin control perspective include:

1. The formation of a comprehensive endotoxin control strategy by identifying the types of excipients used in various drug products;

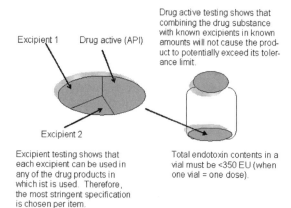

Excipient 1   Drug active (API)

Drug active testing shows that combining the drug substance with known excipients in known amounts will not cause the product to potentially exceed its tolerance limit.

Excipient 2

Excipient testing shows that each excipient can be used in any of the drug products in which ist is used. Therefore, the most stringent specification is chosen per item.

Total endotoxin contents in a vial must be <350 EU (when one vial = one dose).

FIGURE 1 The interrelationship of excipient, drug substance, and end product testing. *Abbreviation*: EU, endotoxin units.

2. The relative amounts of those excipients in each drug type;
3. The subsequent relevant tolerance limits (TL) for drug substances and excipients given [1] and [2].

Figure 1 shows the interrelationship of excipient, drug substance, and end product testing. This exercise should establish that proposed limits are appropriate and that existing excipient and drug substance limits used in the manufacturing process will not allow an associated drug product to fail its end product testing. Figure 2 gives an overview for the process as described here.

Every marketed product has a level of endotoxin safely tolerated, that is, an amount below the TL, which is defined as $TL = K/M$, where K is the threshold

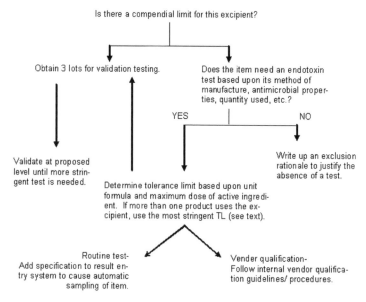

Is there a compendial limit for this excipient?

Obtain 3 lots for validation testing.

Does the item need an endotoxin test based upon its method of manufacture, antimicrobial properties, quantity used, etc.?

YES   NO

Validate at proposed level until more stringent test is needed.

Write up an exclusion rationale to justify the absence of a test.

Determine tolerance limit based upon unit formula and maximum dose of active ingredient. If more than one product uses the excipient, use the most stringent TL (see text).

Routine test-
Add specification to result entry system to cause automatic sampling of item.

Vender qualification-
Follow internal vendor qualification guidelines/ procedures.

FIGURE 2 Appraising an excipient for the necessity of inclusion in an endotoxin control strategy.

pyrogenic dose (TPD) constant in Endotoxin units (EU) per kilogram and M is the maximum human dose (MHD) in units per kg of body weight (70 kg /hour as per FDA Guideline). The TPD is the level of endotoxin capable of eliciting a pyrogenic response in a patient. The relevant dose is that to be administered in an hour. The TPD constant (K) differs depending upon the route of administration [parenteral or intrathecal (IT)]. The formula is straightforward except for the units, which vary from product to product depending upon the manner in which the product is administered. For drugs administered by weight, the weight is that of the active drug ingredient in milligrams or in units per milliliter. For drugs administered by volume, the potency is equal to 1.0 mL/mL (see Appendix D of the FDA Guideline for exceptions to the general formulae, including the use of radiopharmaceutical and IT doses and the use of pediatric weights).

The FDA's LAL Test Guideline (6) adjusts for a product's potency based upon either the weight of the active ingredient or the volume of the drug administered. It constitutes a package for answering the question: "how much can the product be diluted and still be able to detect the limit endotoxin concentration?" However, if the formulae are used to determine the drug substance or excipient TL or subsequent test dilution levels, they may not be appropriate if adjustments are not made to account for the relative amount of each ingredient as it occurs in the final product. To this end, an endotoxin control strategy is a tool to organize and facilitate laboratory testing of the drug substance and appropriate excipients at the appropriate TL (and test dilution) levels (1). Such a strategy as proposed involves the following steps:

1. Obtain the unit formula of a given drug product.
2. Determine the relative amounts of the drug substance and excipients contained in the unit formula.
3. Propose TL for each excipient (if no compendial limit).
4. Ensure that the final product will not exceed the TPD level based upon the proposed (or existing) TL for each relevant item.
5. Compare various product excipients to ensure that the most stringent excipient TL is chosen for validation and routine testing for each item; one does not want to have, for example, three different tests to meet three different specifications for endotoxin in lactose to meet the requirements for three different finished products.
6. Document the rationale for excluding from testing those excipients that are deemed not to require endotoxin testing and why.

DETAILING THE STRATEGY STEPS

1. Obtain the unit formula for a given drug product: The unit formula details the drug formulation contents.

Drug product constituent	Weight (mg)
Drug substance X	1
Mannitol	2.14
Sodium chloride	1.43
Polysorbate 80	2.5

2. Determine the relative amounts of the drug substance and excipients. The unit formula can be listed in a form that shows, based upon the maximum dose of the active ingredient, the corresponding amount of each excipient per dose:

Drug substance	Weight per dose (mg)
Drug substance X	35
Mannitol	75
Sodium chloride[a]	50
Polysorbate 80[b]	87.5

[a]See European Pharmacopeia (3rd ed., 1997) monograph for sodium chloride.
[b]No endotoxin limit in monographs.

3. Propose TL necessary to meet threshold pyrogenic response level:

Drug substance	Weight per dose	Proposed TL
Drug substance X	35 mg nmt[a]	7.0 EU/mg
Mannitol[b]	75 mg nmt	0.0025[c] EU/mg

[a]Not more than can be interpreted as less than since a test containing the limit concentration of endotoxin would be positive and hence fail the test.
[b]See European Pharmacopeia (3rd ed., 1997) monograph for mannitol.
[c]—.

TL for the given excipients may already exist, or prior to testing one can determine if a given product can "live" with the proposed limits. Existing or proposed TLs should subsequently be supported experimentally based upon the level of endotoxin detection that can be obtained and validated in the laboratory. Some limits may be dictated by regulatory bodies (i.e., sodium chloride has an EP monograph limit of not more than 5 EU or IU per gram or nmt 0.005 EU/mg).

4. Ensure that the final product cannot exceed the TPD level given the proposed (or existing) TLs for each relevant item:

Drug substance	Weight per dose	Proposed TL	EUs
Drug substance X	35 mg nmt	7.0 EU/mg	245 EU
Mannitol	75 mg nmt	0.0025 EU/mg	0.19 EU
Sodium chloride	50 mg nmt	0.005 EU/mg	0.25 EU
Polysorbate 80	87.5 mg nmt	1.0 EU/mg	87.5 EU
		Total EU in a dose = 332.94 EU	

The result of the values given earlier allows the user to view TPD in terms of total EUs delivered in a given dose. The 350 EU/dose limit comes from multiplying the value K (5.0 EU/kg for parenterals) by the average human weight as given by the FDA guideline (70 kg), which gives 350 EU; therefore, 350 EU is the total allowed in any given dose of parenteral end product. The formula may also be viewed as: TL = (5 EU/kg × 70 kg)/M, or TL = 350 EU/M where TL can be seen to be a function of the dose of the active ingredient or pyrogen dose. From the example we can see that the level of testing to be performed on the drug substance and excipients prior to drug product X manufacture is adequate to ensure (given passing results) that the TPD level of endotoxins (350 EU) cannot be exceeded during the final product manufacturing process. The goal of this exercise is to ensure that we set our drug substance and excipient specifications low enough to cover worst case scenarios of endotoxin content in any or all of the parts of the whole, equal to the level of their respective TL.

By this rationale our proposed drug substance specification may be set more stringently than the calculated value, (TL = K/M where M = 35 mg/70 kg) if one were to use the end product test limit (7.0 EU/mg vs 10 EU/mg). Such a specification will leave room for the combined EUs of all excipients (TL × weight of excipient per dose). This rationale for drug substances (active ingredient) or excipients has not been described in any guideline (in that the TL is based upon the active drug for end product testing only), but the necessity for such testing has become a clear expectation as evidenced by recent excipient TL requirements published in recent monographs for mannitol and sodium chloride by ongoing excipient harmonization efforts (7).

A formula to help determine more precisely a drug substance TL adjusted for excipients for an endotoxin control strategy can be constructed as follows:

$$\text{TL[drug substance with excipients (DSwe)]} = \frac{\left\{ \begin{array}{c} 350 - [(TLE_1 \times WE_1) \\ +(TLE_2 \times WE_2)\ldots] \end{array} \right\}}{W_{AD}}$$

where TLE_1 is the TL of excipient 1, WE_1 is the weight of excipient 1 per dose of active drug, and W_{AD} is the weight or units of active drug per dose. Note that the formula in (...) indicates all relevant excipients should be included in the calculation (i.e., all those that will not have an exclusion rationale).

For the example given earlier the formula would be filled in as follows:

$$TL_{(DSwe)} = \left\{ 350\,EU - \left[\frac{(0.0025\,EU/mg \times 75\,mg) + (0.005\,EU/mg \times 50\,mg) + (1.0\,EU/mg \times 87.5\,mg)}{35\,mg} \right] \right\}$$

$$TL_{(DSwe)} = \left\{ \frac{350\,EU - [(0.19\,EU) + (0.25\,EU) + (87.5\,EU)]}{35\,mg} \right\} = \left\{ \frac{350\,EU - 87.94\,EU}{35\,mg} \right\}$$

$$TL_{(DSwe)} = \frac{262.06\,EU}{35\,mg} = 7.48\,EU/mg$$

The drug substance TL for the drug adjusted given earlier for the given excipient types and amounts should not exceed 7.48 EU/mg. Again, compare this number to the "raw" TL given by TL = K/M; TL = 5.0 EU/kg/(35 mg/70 kg) = 10 EU/mg for the final drug product.

5. Compare various product excipients. To complicate matters, the interrelationship of various excipients used in numerous drug products should be considered, provided they are significant, as there can realistically be only one specification per item. This can be done by using the table arrived at, given in Subsection 4, in combination with tables created for other drug compounds and then comparing the proposed TL and excipient weights for their appropriateness. As an example of how an excipient TL may affect multiple products, compare the excipient TL proposed for drug product X (previously considered) to a newly created strategy for drug product Y (to be discussed later). The question to be answered when comparing tables is: do any of the proposed TL cause the number of EUs in the right hand column to exceed the 350 EU/dose limit for either of the existing product? If so, then that TL should be more strictly set and revalidated for routine testing. The vendor should be notified of the lower level requirement to allow the

appropriate preventive steps to ensure that their supply of excipient material can meet the new proposed limit.

Following is a comparison table for drug substance X and excipients with new product Y:

Weight per dose	Proposed TL	EUs
Drug substance Y 100 mg	nmt 3.0 EU/mg	300 EU
Polysorbate 80 87.5 mg	nmt 1.0 EU/mg	87.5 EU
Mannitol 100 mg	nmt 0.0025 EU/mg	0.25 EU
Sodium chloride 300 mg	nmt 0.005 EU/mg	1.5 EU
	Total EU in a dose = 389.25 EU	

The use of the old specification would allow the final product to theoretically exceeded the TPD of 350 EU/dose (given the unlikely occurrence that each excipient were contaminated at its proposed specification level). If the polysorbate limit is cut in half (if laboratory testing can support that level) given that the limits for sodium chloride and mannitol are given in the EP monograph and since they are already stringent limits, chances are that one will not want to validate sodium chloride or mannitol to lower levels. One can reexamine the polysorbate 80 level which currently has no pharmacopoeial endotoxin requirement.

The adjusted endotoxin control strategy for drug product Y will then be:

Drug substance	Weight per dose (mg)	Proposed tolerance limit	EUs
Drug substance Y	100	nmt 3.0 EU/mg	300 EU
Polysorbate 80	87.5	nmt 0.5 EU/mg	43.75 EU
Mzannitol	100	nmt 0.0025 EU/mg	0.25 EU
Sodium Chloride	300	nmt 0.005 EU/mg	1.5 EU
		Total EU in a dose = 345.5 EU	

The drug product TL calculation for product Y is: $TL = K/M$, 5.0 EU/kg/ (100 mg/70 kg) = $TL = 3.5$ EU/mg; therefore, the proposed specification of nmt 3.0 EU/mg is in the right neighborhood and will serve as a good place to begin specification determination given the earlier excipients. Note that the routine laboratory testing of Polysorbate 80 will be performed next to support a TL of nmt 0.5 EU/mg to accommodate the levels used in both product X and product Y. There should be only one TL (realistically) for Polysorbate 80, even though it may be used in many products (and therefore many tables). The table with the most stringent TL for polysorbate 80 will be used to set the routine testing specification. Next the proposed TL for the drug substance can be determined more exactly by using the formula given earlier. (If you use the formula for the drug substance TL you get 3.045 EU/mg.)

6. Document the rationale for excluding excipients from testing that are deemed not to require it.

Appendix E of the Guideline on Validation of the LAL Test (1) shows some products that do not contain excipients, or that only contain excipients in very small amounts, or with tight specifications (further research is necessary as the table, of course, does not list the excipients). For example, protamine sulfate has dose and TL values listed as: M = 0.71 mg/kg/hr and TL = 7.04 EU/kg. Looking at the package insert dosing information for Protamine Sulfate one can see that the maximum dose is 50 mg per patient. Therefore, this agrees with the values given in Appendix E (i.e., $50 \, mg/70 \, kg = 0.71 \, mg/kg/hr$). For this particular product the only excipient capable of adding endotoxin is sodium chloride. Since the sodium chloride limit is nmt $0.005 \, EU/mg$ and the sodium chloride content is 0.9% w/v (in this case), then the sodium chloride from a 5 mL injection (the maximum dose in mL of the 10 mg/mL solution) would be 45 mg sodium chloride $\times \, 0.005 \, EU/mg = 0.225 \, EU$ per dose (8); a negligible amount. Examples of drugs containing no excipients include vancomycin and vincristine sulfate.

An endotoxin control strategy, therefore, is most appropriate for drug products containing:

1. Numerous excipients
2. Significant (large amounts of one or more) excipients
3. Excipients with TL set with relatively high limits (perhaps due to difficult/incompatible laboratory tests or an ill-conceived historical method of determining its limit)
4. Drug substances and/or excipients with TL previously calculated using end product formulae
5. Excipients of natural (animal or plant) origin

In these cases, products may be more closely examined in light of an overall endotoxin control strategy.

Conversely, we can conclude that an endotoxin control strategy will be least necessary (or not necessary at all) for drug products containing:

1. Few to no excipients (drug substance = drug product)
2. Excipients in very small amounts
3. Excipients with very low TL (such as those with a compendial requirement)
4. Excipients incapable of adding appreciable endotoxin because they are antimicrobial and/or inhospitable to microbial life due to their method of manufacture, nature or origin, aseptic handling. For example, Cresol (hydroxytoluene), is an antimicrobial excipient that is obtained from either sulfonation or oxidation of toluene (9). The rationale for its exclusion from endotoxin testing would be that it is (*i*) manufactured from materials which cannot support microbial growth, (*ii*) at temperatures that are depyrogenating, and (*iii*) is unlikely to be postmanufacture contaminatable due to the lack of water that is needed to support microbial growth.

Although finished product testing is based upon the active ingredient calculations for drugs administered by weight per kg or by volume for drugs administered by volume with the potency equal to 1.0 mL/mL (as per the USP and FDA guideline), the end product test provides a test of the total contents of a given vial. The strategy given here is concerned with providing manufacturing with in-process testing that definitively demonstrates that when the tested parts are combined, they cannot cause the product to fail its endotoxin specification. One can demonstrate that the testing of end products provides assurance of the contents of the entire vial by performing some parallel maximum valid dilution (MVD) calculations using a simple example:

Drug substance	Weight per dose (mg)
Drug substance X	35
Mannitol	75
Polysorbate 80	87.5
	215

The MVD calculation based upon the dose of the active ingredient is as follows:

$$TL = 10\,EU/mg\{orTL = (5.0\,EU/kg)/(35\,mg/70\,kg)\}$$
$$PP = 10\,mg/mL$$
$$MVD = (10\,EU/mg \times 10\,mg/mL)/0.06\,EU/mL = 1{:}1666$$

The MVD calculation comes out the same if performed using the total weight in the vial instead as follows:

$$TL = 5.0\,EU/kg/(215\,mg/70\,kg) = 1.627\,EU/mg$$
$$PP = 215\,mg\ total\ weight/3.5\,mL\ (of\ 10\,mg/mL\ dose\ solution)$$
$$= 61.428\,mg/mL$$
$$MVD = (1.627\,EU/mg \times 61.428\,mg/mL)/0.06\,EU/mL = 1{:}1666$$

This example shows that the end product calculations do take into account the entire contents of the end product vial.

PROCESS DELIVERABLES

At the end of the "endotoxin control strategy" project, one has developed a list of excipients used in parenteral manufacturing, tables for drug product unit formulae that include the relative amounts per MHD, and TL of drug substances and excipients. Such a reference document will (eventually) become comprehensive for all organization's parenteral products and should be accessible to development scientists charged with providing new drug formulations of developmental [new chemical entities (NCE)] and clinical compounds. The document, therefore, will be dynamic to reflect new drug substances, new excipients, and new (more stringent) limits for old excipients used in new formulations. Such readily available information will provide a useful tool for setting appropriate and conservative TL for new drug compounds and will avoid potential critical errors in arriving at such limits. One may wonder at the utility of drug substance and excipient-endotoxin testing if the TL (and therefore both the validation and subsequent specifications and routine test levels) are not arrived at by using a valid rationale.

The trend in drug development is clearly toward greater product complexity. New biologically derived drugs often contain a number of unusual excipients in significant amounts (for example, new sustained release parenterals contain excipients not traditionally found in nonsustained released drugs (10) present in very large quantities). New drugs include never before tested formulations such as monoclonal antibodies, cell culture derived products, recombinant proteins, sustained release injections, etc. A frame of reference is needed to determine appropriate endotoxin TL for drug substances and excipients. An overall endotoxin control strategy can provide such a frame of reference.

While there are some safety factors included in EL calculations (11), it is still desirable to have a complete process whereby a drug's entire potential endotoxin contents are accounted for and appropriately tested, prior to as well as postmanufacture. Additionally, development scientists will not be faced with destroying a manufactured product that has failed its endotoxin end product specification due to the assignment of ill-conceived in-process specifications. An endotoxin control strategy will provide documented assurance that a drug product will meet its predetermined quality attributes and, more importantly, remove any doubt that the given product can deliver a deleterious amount of endotoxin contamination to a patient.

OVERVIEW OF COOPER'S STRATEGIC METHODS

The compendia prescribe ELs for finished injectable products, but there are few limits for active pharmaceutical ingredients (APIs) and excipients. This discussion proposes strategies for setting endotoxin specifications and suggests remedies for testing materials that interfere with the bacterial endotoxins test (BET) based on factors such as their relative purity, use in the industry, route of administration, and risk management.

REGULATORY DOCUMENTS FOR THE BACTERIAL ENDOTOXINS TEST

The FDA's LAL-Test Guideline (6) was the most influential document to emerge when the USP and pharmaceutical industry converted from the rabbit pyrogen test to endotoxin testing with LAL reagent tests. This Guideline encouraged the industry to use the new technology by defining requirements for rapid conversion to LAL methods. There was early concern that the new test might miss nonendotoxin pyrogen, but firm evidence to support the existence of nonendotoxin pyrogens or materials-mediated pyrogens in parenteral products did not materialize until recently (12). The Guideline introduced the concept of the EL, based on dose, to define a safe level of endotoxin. It also provided formulae for the use of dilution (MVD) or concentration [minimum valid concentration (MVC)] to overcome interfering test conditions. It described an assay to qualify analysts and reagents, a validation test to assure the absence of interference factors, and a limit (routine) LAL test to release parenterals by a validated method. Endotoxin test methods are discussed elsewhere in great detail. Although the Guideline is no longer the principal LAL document, it remains important because of extensive use. Also, it addressed current good manufacturing practices (cGMP) issues, such as sampling, retests, analyst qualification, and determination of reference standard endotoxin/ control standard endotoxin ratios, that are not found in the compendia. An improved, harmonized BET (HBET) became effective in 2001. The FDA Guide and new HBET have similar validation and end product release requirements, but the new chapter has simplified procedures, describes all LAL methods and allows for tests that exclude the influence of glucans. The HBET is now the most important regulatory document because it is more comprehensive, practical, and harmonizes the BET, globally.

ENDOTOXIN ALERT LEVEL FOR ACTIVE PHARMACEUTICAL INGREDIENTS

It is impossible to render materials absolutely pyrogen free because endotoxin is stable, highly potent, and ubiquitous in nature. Therefore, an EL represents the maximum safe amount of endotoxin that is allowed in a dose of a specific parenteral product. When a product contains endotoxin less than its EL, it may be labeled nonpyrogenic. The compendial EL for a product is calculated from the K/M formula where K, the tolerance limit, varies with the type of product and route of administration, as summarized in Table 1, and M is the maximum dose in units/kg. The occurrence of aseptic meningitis in patients receiving IT medications led to stringent limits for drugs administered by this route (13), as discussed in the previous chapter. The best sources for product-specific ELs are drug monographs and chapters in pharmacopoeia. Only a small number of APIs, such as human insulin and a few antibiotics, have a compendial limit for endotoxin. That leaves the choice of release limits for APIs and excipients to common sense. A strategy for assigning EL and test methods for noncompendial materials must account for their intended use, origin, and risk for potential endotoxin contamination. High risk for endotoxin is associated with materials that are derived from natural sources or processed in the presence of bioburden. An FDA surveillance study (14) found that 3% of samples had LAL-detectable endotoxin; all were products of natural origin. High risk is also assigned to materials that are intended for injection into a confined site, such as cerebral spinal or intraocular spaces. Low risk is associated with materials that are derived from a synthetic source and are available in pharmaceutical grade. The assignment of an end product EL to an API is risky; a failure might occur because of an unmasking effect induced by the end product formula or an additive effect of small amounts of endotoxin from excipients, water, and components. A suitable alert level for an API is a limit that is at least four times more stringent than the compendial EL. A high endotoxin risk is associated with APIs that are produced by fermentation or recombinant technology, filled by aseptic processing, and intended for intravenous or IT administration.

ENDOTOXIN LIMITS FOR INTRATHECAL DRUGS IN PHARMACY COMPOUNDING

Injectables prepared in compounding pharmacies are usually formulated from bulk nonsterile powders and are usually produced individually rather than in batches. It is difficult to assign an EL to compounded injectables because the pharmacy may not know the prescribed dose. There are safeguards that a pharmacy may

TABLE 1 Endotoxin Tolerance or Allowable Limit by Type of Parenteral Material

Parenteral type	Endotoxin tolerance limit (K)
Human or veterinary drugs and biologics	5 EU/kg
Parenterals by intrathecal injection	0.2 EU/kg
Radiophamaceuticals	175 EU/V[a]
Intrathecal radiopharmaceuticals	14 EU/V[a]
Continuous intraspinal infusion	14 EU/day[a,b]
Large-volume parenterals	0.5 EU/mL
Water for Injection	0.25 EU/mL
Medical devices by extraction	0.5 EU/mL up to 20 EU/device
Medical devices in intrathecal spaces	0.06 EU/mL up to 2.15 EU/device
Multiple ingredient small-volume parenteral	70 EU/V[a,b]
Excipient	3.5 EU per amount in 1 mL of SVP[b]
New chemical entity, preliminary	1 EU/mg[b] until human dose is known

[a]Maximum dose in volume (mL).
[b]Recommended limit by the author, not the Pharmacopeia.

take to reduce the risk of endotoxin contamination: (*i*) purchase materials from ethical suppliers that provide a Certificate of Analysis (CoA) for purity and endotoxin content, if available; (*ii*) screen and qualify incoming lots of drug substances with a validated BET; and (*iii*) apply aseptic technique and conduct an integrity test on every filter used for membrane sterilization.

Information about valid endotoxin test concentrations is difficult to find. A recent report addressed endotoxin testing of pain medications designed for intraspinal infusion (15). The report gave methods for determining a valid test concentration by gel-clot and kinetic turbidimetric LAL assays. Compounded pain medications were BET-compatible when an individual drug was diluted to 0.5 mg/mL, and the principal drug constituent of mixtures was diluted to 0.25 mg/mL. Table 2 summarizes compatibility and EL data. An EL of 14 EU/mL was recommended for intraspinal infusion solutions because of the potency of this route of administration and the fact that patient doses seldom exceed 1 mL per day when infused by implanted pump devices.

The procedures described for intraspinal medications are applicable for determining noninterfering BET test conditions, calculating ELs, and conducting appropriate validation for a broad range of sterile solutions that are compounded in the pharmacy.

ENDOTOXIN LIMITS FOR EXCIPIENTS

Excipients are essential components of small-volume parenterals (SVP). They serve a variety of functions, including stabilizing, preserving, and buffering. Mannitol and sodium chloride have both therapeutic and excipient applications. Therefore, an EL calculated for therapeutic use is inappropriately stringent for an excipient. A method for calculating an excipient EL is proposed based on its usual concentration in injectables.

The diversity in the use of excipients makes it a challenge to devise a uniform strategy for selection of limits and test protocols. One could simply set an arbitrary limit or assign limits based on their proportion in an SVP formulation, as previously discussed (1). However, excipients have a common attribute to exploit. An SVP is limited to 100 mL; this volume can represent the dose for calculating an EL. A compendium of excipients was published that details the range of concentrations for excipients in SVP formulations (16). A uniform way for calculating an excipient EL is proposed

TABLE 2 Recommended Bacterial Endotoxin Test Concentrations and Safety Data for Intraspinal Infusions Prepared from Bulk Powders

Bulk powder	LAL-Compatible TC[a] (mg/mL)	EL[b] (EU/mg)	LOD[c] (EU/mg)
Morphine	0.5	0.7	0.12
Baclofen	0.25	7.0	0.3
Bupivacaine	0.5	0.6	0.12
Clonidine	0.25	16.5	0.3
Fentanyl	0.5	14	0.12
Hydromorphone	0.5	1.2	0.12
Morphine mixture[d]	0.25	14 EU/day	0.3

[a]The highest test concentration (TC) that yielded valid recovery of endotoxin positive controls.
[b]The endotoxin limit where 14 EU is divided by the maximum dose per day.
[c]Limit of detection when reagent sensitivity, lambda, is 0.0625 EU/mL: LOD = Lambda/TC.
[d]Morphine mixed with baclofen, bupivacaine, or clonidine.

that is dependent on the maximum amount of excipient in 100 mL of an SVP:

$$\text{Excipient EL} = \frac{350\,\text{EU (Adult endotoxin tolerance limit)}}{\text{Maximum amount of excipient in } 100\,\text{mL}} = \frac{3.5\,\text{EU}}{1\,\text{mL}}$$

Table 3 is a list of commonly used excipients as well as a proposed endotoxin alert limit (EAL) and kinetic LAL test parameter for each. The EAL was determined by dividing the TL by the maximum concentration of an excipient. This number was then divided by 4 and rounded to assure a four-fold margin of safety. The

TABLE 3 Bacterial Endotoxin Test Information for Frequently Used Excipients

Pharmaceutical excipient	Concentration[a] (mg/mL)	Endotoxin alert level	LAL test concentration	LOD[b] ($\lambda = 0.05$)
Acetic acid	2–5	0.7 EU/mg	0.1 mg/mL	0.5 EU/mg
Benzyl alcohol	10–30	0.03 EU/mg	2 mg/mL	0.025 EU/mg
Carboxymethycellulose NA	8	1 EU/mg	1 mg/mL	0.05 EU/mg
Calcium chloride	0.1–1	0.2 EU/mg (USP)	1 mg/mL	0.05 EU/mg
Citric acid	0.1–1	0.5 EU/mg (EP)	0.25 mg/mL	0.2 EU/mg
Dextrose	10–50	10 EU/g (USP)	25 mg/mL	2 EU/g
Disodium EDTA	0.1	0.2 EU/mg (USP)	0.5 mg/mL	0.1 EU/mg
Ethanol	0.1 (v/v)	10 EU/mL	0.05 mL/mL	1 EU/mL
Gelatin	5	0.7 EU/mg	0.5 mg/mL	0.1 EU/mg
Glycerin	150	0.2 EU/mg	1.0 mg/mL	0.05 EU/mg
Glycine	10–24	0.15 EU/mg	2.5 mg/mL	0.02 EU/mg
Hydrochloric acid	Trace	NA	NA	NA
Lactose	10	0.35 EU/mg	1 mg/mL	0.05 EU/mg
Lactic acid	7.5	0.45 EU/mg	2.5 mg/mL	0.02 EU/mg
Magnesium sulfate	100	0.1 EU/mg (USP)	2.5 mg/mL	0.02 EU/mg
Mannitol	100	4 EU/g (EP)	50 mg/mL	1 EU/g
Methylparaben	1.8	1 EU/g	1 mg/mL	0.05 EU/mg
Phenol	5	0.7 EU/mg	0.25 mg/mL	0.2 EU/mg
Polyethylene glycol	500 (v/v)	0.007 EU/mL	20 mg/mL	0.0025 EU/mg
Polysorbate 80	10	0.1 EU/mg	2.5 mg/mL	0.02 EU/mg
Propylparaben	0.2	4.0 EU/mg	0.5 mg/mL	0.1 EU/mg
Sodium acetate	0.39	2.0 EU/mg	1 mg/mL	0.05 EU/mg
Sodium bisulfite	3.2	0.25 EU/mg	1 mg/mL	0.05 EU/mg
Sodium carbonate	1–33	0.025 EU/mg	2 mg/mL	0.025 EU/mg
Sodium chloride	9	5 EU/g (EP)	10 mg/mL	5 EU/g
Sodium citrate	10–28.5	1.2 EU/mg	2 mg/mL	0.025 EU/mg
Sodium hydroxide	Trace	Depyrogenating	NA	NA
Sodium lactate	10	0.1 EU/mg	1 mg/mL	0.05 EU/mg
Sodium metabisulfite	1–6.6	0.1 EU/mg	1 mg/mL	0.05 EU/mg
Sodium phosphate	1–10	0.1 EU/mg	1 mg/mL	0.05 EU/mg
Sorbitol	48	0.02 EU/mg	5 mg/mL	0.01 EU/mg
Sucrose	50–200	0.004 EU/mg	25 mg/mL	0.002 EU/mg
Thimerosal	0.1	10 EU/mg	0.1 mg/mL	0.5 EU/mg

[a]Excipient concentration source (10).
[b]LOD, Limit of Detection is lambda/TC where $\lambda = 0.05$ EU/mL for a kinetic turbidimetric analysis standard curve of 0.05–0.5 EU/mL.
Abbreviations: EDTA, ethylenediaminetetraacetic acid; LAL, *Limulus* amebocyte lysate; USP, United States Pharmacopeia.

TABLE 4 Bacterial Endotoxin Test Information for Nutritional Supplements

Nutritional supplement	Recommended daily dose (mg)	Endotoxin limit or alert level[a] (EU/mg)	MVC[b] (mg/mL)	LAL test concentration (mg/mL)	LOD (EU/mg) ($\lambda = 0.05$)
Ascorbic acid, Vitamin C	200	1.2 (USP)	0.027	1	0.05
Cyanocobalamin, B_{12}	0.005	400 (USP)	0.0001	0.1	0.5
Folic acid	0.6	357 (USP)	0.0001	0.1	0.5
Niacinamide	40	3.5 (USP)	0.01	1	0.05
Pyridoxine, B_6	6	0.4 (USP)	0.082	1	0.05
Riboflavin, B_2	3.6	7.1 (USP)	0.005	0.1	0.5
Thiamine, B_1	6	3.5 (USP)	0.01	1	0.05
Dexpanthenol	15	2.3	0.01	1	0.05
Retinol, Vitamin A	1	35	0.001	0.1	0.5
Ergocalciferol, Vitamin D	0.005	700	0.0001	0.1	0.5
Vitamin E	10	3.5	0.01	1	0.05
Phytonadione, Vitamin K	0.15	14	0.004	0.1	0.5
Biotin	0.06	580	0.0001	0.1	0.5

[a]Endotoxin alert level is calculated by dividing a tolerance limit of 35 EU by the dose.
[b]Minimum valid concentration (MVC) is calculated by dividing the lambda by the EL or EAL.
[c]LOD, limit of detection is lambda divided by the test concentration.
Abbreviations: EAL, endotoxin alert limit; EL, endotoxin unit; LAL, *Limulus* amebocyte lysate; USP, United States Pharmacopeia.

compendial limit is applied for those excipients that also have a therapeutic use, such as mannitol and sodium chloride. A test concentration is provided that is known to be noninterfering with at least one kinetic LAL reagent. Finally, the test sensitivity or limit of detection (LOD) is listed that is derived by dividing lambda by the test concentration. In each case, the LOD is more sensitive (lower value) than the highly conservative EAL, calculated by the formula given earlier. The proposed excipient EAL is conservative because the calculation assumes that an SVP is 100 mL, whereas volume of most SVPs is less than 10 mL. Test parameters presented in Table 4 were not designed to test an excipient with the greatest sensitivity; a more sensitive LAL method is always an option . Rather, the objective was to propose robust test conditions that were valid with most LAL reagents. The origin of an excipient is critical for achieving purity. Materials produced from natural sources such as mannitol or sucrose will likely have LAL reactive glucans (LRG) and endotoxin as contaminants. In contrast, mannitol produced by electrolytic reduction of mannose or dextrose is free of LRG. Gelatin is also contaminated with endotoxin to the extent that it may be necessary to screen multiple batches to find one that meets the suggested limit of 0.7 EU/mg. Finally, sodium carboxymethylcellulose is a glucan, so LRG blocking systems are needed to avoid a false-positive endotoxin result. With a few notable exceptions mentioned earlier, most excipients are available in a pharmaceutical grade with a CoA for absence of significant endotoxin levels. It is excessive to test all incoming excipients once the reliability of a supplier is established for a low-impact component. Also, there is no merit in testing sodium hydroxide pellets that are self-depyrogenating and used in trace concentrations. Sound scientific judgment should be used to establish a meaningful API or excipient BET procedures. Finally, interference screening is unnecessary for well-characterized excipients listed in Table 3, provided a suitability test [positive product control (PPC)] is used during routine testing.

INTERFERENCE TESTING FOR ACTIVE PHARMACEUTICAL INGREDIENTS AND EXCIPIENTS

The validation of BET methods for APIs and excipients is challenging because they are often presented in powder form, have solubility limitations, and may require neutralization. A common misconception about pH is that any LAL and sample mixture in the range of pH 6 to 8 is considered noninterfering. Actually, the reaction rate in kinetic BET systems is so pH dependent that recovery of the PPC will be altered if the pH of the LAL reagent and test samples are not within a few tenths of a pH unit. Excipients or APIs that are not pH neutral, such as phenol, acids, and weak bases, may require neutralization with dilute acid or base during the dissolution process, depending on the buffer capacity of the LAL reagent. Compatibility with LAL reagents is highly dependent on water solubility. Compounds that are poorly soluble in water may be dissolved in organic solvents that are miscible with water, and then diluted to a suitable test concentration that eliminates solvent interference. Most LAL reagents tolerate up to 5% of ethanol and 2% of dimethyl sulfoxide. If a precipitate begins to form in a kinetic BET study, there will be a progressive increase in the optical density that is readily distinguishable from an endotoxin reaction curve; more dilution is indicated in this case.

Endotoxin adsorption problems are often difficult to resolve. An analyst received a sample for qualification from a new API vendor. Even though a validated method was used, PPC recovery was zero. The analysts filtered the sample because it had an uncharacteristic haze; a retest gave normal recovery. It appears that the vendor had failed to filter the API after treating it with silica, a common absorber used to remove impurities; the vendor agreed to revise their process and remove the absorber. Finally, it is more efficient and informative to a test NCE at a robust, compatible LAL-test concentration than to attempt to develop a test method for an arbitrarily set, interfering test concentration. It is sufficient to test an NCE at a 1 EU/mg until clinical information has progressed to the point that an EL calculation becomes realistic.

ENDOTOXIN LIMITS FOR NUTRITIONAL SUPPLEMENTS

Injectable forms of vitamins, trace minerals, and related nutritional supplements are increasing in importance for managing patients who require extended care. Simplistic test methods are needed to conveniently screen incoming nutritional agents. Table 4 contains test information for commonly administered vitamins. When a compendial EL was not available, the recommended daily dosage for an ingredient was used to calculate a limit. Since incoming materials are seldom in solution MVC was calculated to determine a range of test concentrations that would yield a sufficiently sensitive result with a kinetic BET.

The EALs recommended in Table 4 are based on an allowed level of 35 EU per dose of ingredient, which is ten times more stringent than the USP tolerance level of 350 EU per dose. The table applied either the compendial EL or EAL calculated with the assumptions stated earlier. Then, the limits were used to calculate the MVC, which is the test sensitivity, lambda (λ), divided by the EL or EAL. A test concentration is provided by the author that is known to be compatible (noninterfering) with available gel-clot or kinetic LAL reagents. The strategy was to select a robust test condition rather than to use the most sensitive condition; convenient 1 or 0.1 mg/mL concentrations are recommended. Finally, the specific test sensitivity or LOD for each ingredient was calculated using lambda and the selected test concentration, such as a 0.05 to 5 EU/mL photometric standard curve. Note that the LOD for each ingredient in the table given is more sensitive than the limits presented in column three of the table.

Basically, the procedure for screening incoming ingredients is to weigh a sufficient amount to prepare the test concentration listed later in the chapter. Such solutions should be tested promptly to avoid development of bioburden. The fat-soluble vitamins (A, D, E, and K) may require water mixtures with additives such as polysorbate 80 or propylene glycol to yield a water-soluble test sample. Interference screening to establish test protocols is unnecessary for the well-characterized components listed in Table 4, provided a suitability test (PPC) is used during routine testing. Endotoxin testing of an ingredient may be skip tested if the vendor specifies an EL in the CoA and becomes a qualified vendor by consistently supplying materials that meet all specifications.

REFERENCES

1. Williams KL. Developing an endotoxin control strategy. Pharm Technol 1998; September:90–102.
2. Cooper JF. Screening active pharmaceutical ingredients and excipients for endotoxin. In: Williams KL, ed. Microbial Contamination Control in Parenteral Manufacturing. New York: Marcel Dekker, 2004:531–540.
3. Nema S, Washkuhn RJ, Brendel RJ. Excipients and their use in injectable products. PDA J Pharm Sci Technol 1997; 51(4):166–171.
4. European Pharmacopoeia. Monograph. 3rd ed, 1997.
5. Croes RV. Maltitol solution, mannitol, sorbitol, sorbitol solution, noncrystallizing sorbitol solution-suggested revisions for harmonization of pharmacopeial specifications and procedures. Pharmacopeial Forum 1998; 24(1).
6. U.S. Dept. of Health and Human Services. FDA Guideline on Validation of the *Limulus* Amebocyte Lysate Test as an End-Product Endotoxin Test for Human and Animal Parenteral Drugs, Biological Products, and Medical Devices. December, 1987.
7. Chowham ZT. The long, difficult, and frustrating process of harmonization of excipient standards. Pharm Technol 1997; March.
8. Stoklosa MJ, Ansel HC. Pharmaceutical Calculations. Philadelphia: Lea & Febiger, 1986.
9. Wade A, Weller PJ, eds. Handbook of Pharmaceutical Excipients. Washington and London: American Pharmaceutical Association and The Pharmaceutical Press, 1994.
10. Cleland JL, Imac A, Boyd B, et al. The stability of recombinant human growth hormone in Poly(lactic-co-glycolic acid) (PLGA) microspheres. Pharm Res 1997; 14(4):420–425.
11. Weary ME. Understanding and setting endotoxin limits. PDA J Pharm Sci Technol 1990; 44(1):16–18.
12. Cooper JF, Brügger P, Fanning M, Matsuura S, Poole S. Alert and action levels for APIs: A collaborative study of pyrogenic gentamicin. Parenteral Drug Association Annual Meeting. New Orleans, December, 2002.
13. Cooper JF, Harbert JC. Endotoxin as a cause of aseptic meningitis after radionuclide cisternography. J Nucl Med 1975; 16:809–813.
14. Twohy C, Duran AP, Munson TE. Endotoxin contamination of parenteral drugs as determined by the LAL method. J Parenter Sci Technol 1984; 30:190–201.
15. Cooper JF, Thoma LA. Screening extemporaneously compounded intraspinal injections with the bacterial endotoxins test. Am J Health Syst Pharm 2002; 59:2426–2433.
16. Powell MT, Nguyen T, Baloian L. Compendium of excipients for parenteral formulations. PDA J Pharm Sci Technol 1998; 52:238–311.

15 Depyrogenation Validation, Pyroburden, and Endotoxin Removal

Kevin L. Williams

Eli Lilly & Company, Indianapolis, Indiana, U.S.A.

Whereas sterilization processes are predictable, many depyrogenation procedures are purely empirical. Many specific instances of applying potent reagents to manufacturing equipment for the purpose of destroying applied endotoxin where one would predict that LPS would easily be demonstrated to be destroyed have only revealed that the LPS has hung on tenaciously defying the concepts of classical depyrogenation.

INTRODUCTION

This chapter discusses the depyrogenation (removal, reduction, or destruction) of endotoxin in regard to parenteral containers, container closures, and manufacturing processes. Often the depyrogenation of containers and container closures is believed to be governed by the treatment of medical devices, which is described in the 1985 FDA Guideline on Validation of the *Limulus* amebocyte lysate (LAL) test, however, the CFR Title 21 FDA Guidance (April 1, 2004) makes it clear that drug containers and drug container closures are not medical devices per se in regard to their treatment for depyrogenation. Subpart E Control of Components and Drug Product Containers and Closures 211.94 (c) states that "drug product containers and closures shall be clean and, where indicated by the nature of the drug, sterilized and processed to remove pyrogenic properties to assure that they are suitable for their intended use." Therefore, though some of the same principles of depyrogenation can apply, they do not govern how containers and closures should be tested.

HISTORICAL DEVELOPMENT OF DEPYROGENATION METHODS

Endotoxin is notoriously resistant to destruction by heat, desiccation, pH extremes, and various chemical treatments. The validation of endotoxin destruction or removal in the manufacture and packaging of parenteral drugs given its enduring nature and likelihood of occurrence is a critical concern to drug and device manufacturers. Lipopolysaccharide (LPS) requires dry heat of treatment around 250°C for half an hour to an hour to achieve destruction and standard autoclaving will not suffice. Many harsh chemicals that one might expect to be depyrogenating are not, and only pH adjustment as combined with heat effectively inactivates the LPS molecule. Whereas many sterilization processes are predictable, many depyrogenation procedures are purely empirical. Many specific instances of applying potent reagents to manufacturing equipment for the purpose of destroying applied endotoxin where one would predict that LPS would easily be demonstrated to be destroyed have only revealed that the LPS has hung on tenaciously defying reasoned predictions of its demise. Adding to the contribution of LAL in the historical development of pharmaceutical manufacturing processes is the fact that prior to the LAL assay there was no practical way to study the kinetics of depyrogenation processes.

Traditionally, depyrogenation is first thought of as the dry heat incineration of endotoxins from materials able to withstand the protracted dry-heat cycle needed to destroy the LPS molecule. Alternatively, the wash/rinse removal of endotoxin from items such as stoppers and plastic vials and alternative vial closures comes readily to mind when heat treatment is not an option. However, there are many additional and hybrid areas of depyrogenation that are less historically entrenched and which are subject to more complex validation support. The two broad classes of depyrogenation processes (Fig. 1) that may be applied to components, devices, articles coming into contact with parenteral drugs, and the drugs themselves include inactivation and removal. Specific methods that fall into the two categories include:

1. Inactivation
   - Heat, moist and dry
   - The use of ionizing radiation
   - Chemical inactivation (i.e., the use of strong acid/base solutions)
   - Oxidation (i.e., hydrogen peroxide)
   - Polymyxin B (PMB)
   - Biological inactivation
2. Removal
   - The use of physical size exclusion of endotoxin, (ultrafiltration, ion-exchange removal, or aggregation followed by filtration)
   - The use of charge differential (ion exchange)
   - Binding treatments (activated charcoal, LPS binding protein)

The last two decades of biotechnology [Lilly (Indianapolis, Indiana, U.S.A.) marketed Humulin™ in 1982] has brought about the concomitant necessity of

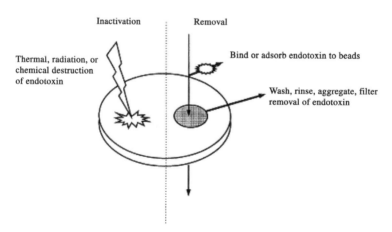

FIGURE 1 Inactivation and removal of bacterial endotoxins. Inactivation includes: Heat, moist, and dry, the use of ionizing radiation of components, chemical inactivation (i.e., strong acids/base solutions), oxidation (i.e., hydrogen peroxide), polymyxin B. Removal includes the use of physical size exclusion (ultrafiltration, ion-exchange removal) or aggregation followed by filtration, the use of charge differential (anion exchange), binding treatments (activated charcoal, lipopolysaccharide binding protein products, etc.).

removing large populations of endotoxin from products due to their manufacture in microbial-expression systems (especially *Escherichia coli*). Selected methods of depyrogenation mentioned earlier are employed to remove endotoxin from manufactured materials intended for parenteral use. A few of these methods will be examined. A recently described phenomenon has been put forward to describe a common and somewhat related occurrence in the clinical environment. The formation of "biofilms" [polysaccharide coatings formed from colonizing bacteria on invasive and medical devices of prolonged use such as catheters (1)] serves as an interesting examination of the dynamics of populations of bacteria and the problems associated with their removal and the demonstration and documentation thereof. Analogous to the realization that endotoxin is a dynamic part of the cell wall that is sloughed off via several natural processes (e.g., membrane vesicles), colonies of bacteria have been found to be more complex than previously assumed (2,3).

The oldest and simplest method of endotoxin removal from solid surfaces is rinsing with a nonpyrogenic solvent, usually Sterile Water for Injection. An example of such a validation process for large-volume parenteral glass containers was described by Feldstine et al. (4). Distillation is the oldest method known for effectively removing pyrogens from water. The mechanism of endotoxin removal is relatively simple. Because LPS is such a large molecule, it cannot accelerate as rapidly as water vapor and is left behind due to inertia.

Early investigators studying the thermostability of endotoxin concluded that moist heat supplied in conventional autoclaving was ineffective for depyrogenation. Hort and Penfold (5) reported that neither autoclaving nor boiling effectively destroyed pyrogens. Seibert (6) also found that only "long drastic heating" would destroy pyrogens. Although autoclave conditions for "normal sterilization" of solutions were ineffective for destruction of endotoxin, Banks (7) was able to demonstrate effective depyrogenation by autoclaving at 20 psi for five hours at a pH of 8.2, or for two hours at a pH of 3.8. More recent studies show that the action of certain depyrogenating agents can be enhanced by autoclaving. Cherkin (8) found that hydrogen peroxide was more effective in destroying pyrogen when the solution was autoclaved. Autoclaving also helped to eliminate residual H_2O_2. Similar findings have been reported for other solutions containing acid or base. Novitsky et al. (9) confirmed that autoclaving following conventional methods (121°C, 15 psi at near neutral pH for 20 minutes) was not sufficient to eliminate the pyrogenicity of 100 ng/mL of *E. coli* 055:B5. However, autoclaving for longer periods (180 minnutes) successfully reduced endotoxin levels to less than an LAL detectable limit of 0.01 ng/mL. Novitsky et al. also found that activated carbon treatment was more effective in removing endotoxin when solutions containing endotoxin and carbon were autoclaved.

The application of dry heat delivered through convection, conduction, or radiation (infrared) ovens has been the method of choice for depyrogenation of heat-resistant materials, such as glassware, metal equipment, and instruments, and of heat-stable chemicals, waxes, and oils. The standard method described in various national and international compendia and reference texts is an exposure of not less than 250°C for not less than 30 minutes and is based on the studies of Welch et al. (10) on the thermostability of pyrogens as measured with the rabbit pyrogen test. The mechanism of endotoxin inactivation is incineration. The development of the LAL has provided a more quantitative means of studying dry heat inactivation of endotoxin.

Tsuji and Lewis (12) discovered that the inactivation kinetics of LPS from *E. coli, Salmonella typhosa, Serratia marcescens,* and *Pseudomonas aeruginosa* was a nonlinear, second-order process in contrast to the inactivation of bacterial spores, which follow first order kinetics and that the LPS preparations from various organisms were almost identical in depyrogenation requirements (10–14). They compared the dry heat resistance of intact and purified LPS to that of spores with the greatest heat resistance. Purified LPS was shown to be twice as resistant as the native (whole-cell) endotoxin from which it was derived (14). Of greater importance was the author's convincing evidence that the general practice of increasing exposure time to compensate for lower process temperature is not supportable for LPS destruction, particularly at 175°C or less. Akers et al. (15,16) confirmed these findings and also determined the F-value requirements for destruction of 10 ng of *E. coli* 055:B5 endotoxin seeded into 50 mL glass vials, using both convection and radiant heat ovens. An F value[a] is the equivalent time at a given temperature delivered to a product to achieve sterilization or, in this case, depyrogenation. Linear relationships were established between oven temperatures and the logarithms of the endotoxin reduction times with both treatments. Before 1978, there were few studies addressing the destruction of endotoxin presumably due to the lack of a suitable quantitative method of measuring endotoxin reductions (17). Therefore, along with the LAL assay and the refinement of LPS standardization came a means of applying [as a biological indicator (BI) in a manner analogous to the use of sporeforming *Bacillus* species in sterilization studies], recovering, and detecting applied endotoxin.

DEPYROGENATION CONCEPTS BORROWED FROM STERILIZATION VALIDATION

Methods and mechanisms of proving the depyrogenation of various items have been largely borrowed from sterilization processes and modified to compensate for the thermal and chemical stability of LPS as compared to whole organisms. Depyrogenation processes (like sterilization methods) may involve the construction of D (death or destruction in the case of endotoxin since it is not alive) values but for regulatory purposes, the use of a three-log reduction validation serves as the official empirical demonstration of the "worst-case" destruction or removal of pyrogenic residues. When such a three-log reduction has been demonstrated, then it may be assumed that the process will remove any endogenous endotoxins that could be presented by any given component manufacturing process or subsequent (mis) handling events.

Again, the lack of transferability of linear assumptions of sterilization processes to depyrogenation processes has prompted many researchers to gather detailed data as it relates to endotoxin destruction. As described by Groves and Groves (14):

> ...although the spore destruction process is first-order, the nonlinear nature of the depyrogenation process invalidates for depyrogenation (but not for sterilization) the assumption that a longer time compensates for a lower temperature. Allowing a 50%

---

[a]F value, in sterilization terms, is the "time required to destroy all spores of a suspension when using a temperature of 121°C"(17).

safety margin, Akers et al. (16) suggest that the following conditions (minimum F_{170}) would be required to destroy *E. coli* (055 : B5) endotoxin:

1. 300°C, 118 minutes
2. 250°C, 750 minutes
3. 210°C, 1950 minutes
4. 175°C, 6000 minutes

It should be borne in mind that the time details given above represent the complete destruction of endotoxin as indicated by complete lack of reactivity with LAL, rather than multiple log reduction times as will be explored later in this chapter.

The definition of the death rate (D value) in sterilization technology is the "time for a 90% reduction in the microbial population exhibiting first order reaction kinetics" (18,19). Alternatively, the D value is "the negative reciprocal of the slope of the line" (20) constructed from the declining survival of organisms (LAL activity for endotoxin).

Death-rate curves in sterility validation can be constructed by graphing the number of organisms on the Y axis against the log of the heating time, exposure time (gas), or radiation dose on the X axis. Destruction curves similar to that seen in Figure 2A can be constructed using endotoxin data. However, the destruction of LPS has been demonstrated to be a second-order reaction as opposed to the first order. Figure 2B shows how the initial destruction occurs relatively rapidly whereas the remaining destruction is much more difficult to achieve. Tsuji and Harrison (13) demonstrated that a greater than two-log reduction of endotoxin can be achieved at 210°C in 150 minutes or in 130 minutes at 250°C in dry-heat depyrogenation. The comparison was made between the D values of spores of *Bacillus xerothermodurans*. Whereas the D value obtained for LPS was 170 minutes, that of *B. xerothermodurans* was less than 7 minutes. Ludwig and Avis (22) recently (1988 and 1991) verified the apparent biphasic nature of LPS thermal destruction observed by Tsuji et al. by applying LPS to glass capillary tubes. They noted, not a single linear line as observed in first-order kinetics (such as sterilization processes), but essentially two linear slopes that were associated with a high initial rate of decrease followed by a much more prolonged decline. While Ludwig and Avis reported the same type of biphasic curve as Tsuji and Lewis, they differed in the conclusion made previously that an infinite amount of time would be required to obtain greater than or equal to 4-log endotoxin reduction at 170°C. Ludwig and Avis obtained five logs of reduction between 1090 and 1237 minutes (approximately 16–20 hours) and a more p-ractical 3-log reduction in 100 minutes (again at 170°C) (22). They also demonstrated that LPS from rough strains could be depyrogenated by five logs in one-fourth the time it took to reduce LPS from smooth strains and they theorized that the core and O-antigen polysaccharides substantially aided in thermal resistance "perhaps by a physical shielding effect" (22). See Table 1 for a comparison of the Tsuji et al. and Ludwig and Avis studies. The data are from Ref. 23.

The references shown in Tables 1 and 2 are indicative of the lack of agreement in times and temperatures needed to achieve depyrogenation and hint at the plethora of conditions that can alter the time and temperature needed to bring about depyrogenation (load and type of material, oven tunnel speed, etc.). In common dry-heat depyrogenation practices involving oven tunnels that feed glass vials into pharmaceutical production lines to be filled with drug product, depyrogenation is achieved in an expedited manner (5–10 minutes) by using

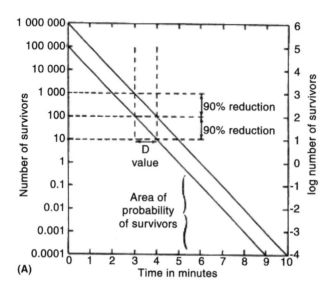

(A)

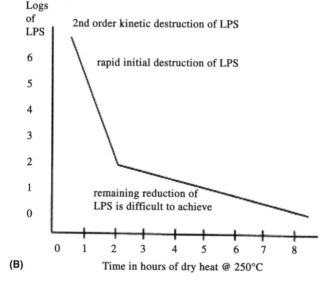

(B)

FIGURE 2 Microbial death-rate curves. (**A**) illustrates the concept of decimal reduction (D values) and probability of survivors. (**B**) hypothetically demonstrates the more difficult-to-achieve reduction of lipopolysaccharide after a relatively rapid initial reduction. *Source*: From Ref. 18.

temperatures well above 250°C to achieve F values equivalent to the targeted half hour at 250°C treatment ($F_{250} = 30$).

Such processes must be validated (and revalidated typically on an annual basis) they have the distinct advantage of the subsequent treatment of articles without the constant need for additional empirical data. A validated oven that reaches a given temperature (as per a given pattern load) for a determined time

TABLE 1 Time Required to Achieve Multiple Log Reductions

Log reduction	Temp °C	Tsuji et al. (1978–1979)[a] minutes	Ludwig and Avis (1990)[b] minutes
3	@210	13.6	7
	@300	0.089	<0.5
5	@210	Infinity[c]	19
	@300	0.19[c]	1
6	@300	0.27[c]	11

[a]Tsuji et al. used aluminum cups.
[b]Ludwig and Avis used glass.
[c]Extrapolated value.

TABLE 2 Time Required to Achieve Multiple Log Reductions Using Different Sources of Endotoxin

Log reduction	Temp °C	Bio Whittaker minutes	Difco minutes	ACC minutes
3	@225	5	5	5
	@250	<0.5	NA	2
5	@225	15	45	45
	@250	5	NA	19

Abbreviation: ACC, Associates of Cape Cod.

(belt speed) can be counted on, as governed by physical laws, to supply the appropriate thermal destruction. The concept of "overkill" destruction as described in the United State Pharmacopeia (USP) (Chapter 1211 "Sterilization and Sterility Assurance of Compendial Articles") states that "with heat-stable articles, the approach often is to considerably exceed the critical time necessary to achieve the 10^{-6} microbial survivor probability (i.e., overkill)" and is analogous to the 3-log reduction validation requirement for endotoxin destruction or removal.

WRITTEN REQUIREMENTS FOR DEPYROGENATION PROCESSES

The requirements for depyrogenation validation processes are somewhat vague and subject to interpretation. A short reference occurs in the USP, Chapter 1211 "Sterilization and Sterility Assurance of Compendial Articles," Dry-Heat Sterilization section as follows:

> Since dry heat is frequently employed to render glassware or other containers free from pyrogens as well as viable microbes, a pyrogen challenge, where necessary, should be an integral part of the validation program, for example, by inoculating one or more of the articles to be treated with 1000 or more USP Units of bacterial endotoxin. The test with Limulus lysate could be used to demonstrate that the endotoxic substance has been inactivated to not more than 1/1000 of the original amount (3-log cycle reduction). For the test to be valid, both the original amount and, after acceptable inactivation, the remaining amount of endotoxin should be measured.

The only other USP references to depyrogenation are in the Bacterial Endotoxins Test chapter (Chapter 85) and Pyrogen Test chapter (Chapter 151) which state that one should "treat any containers or utensils employed so as to destroy extraneous surface endotoxins that may be present, such as by heating in an oven at 250°C or above for sufficient time" and the references of the previous paragraph as a means of validating the oven referred to here and "render the syringes, needles, and glassware (to be used in the pyrogen test) free from pyrogens by heating at 250°C for not less than 30 minutes or by any other suitable method," respectively.

The USP/FDA "Guideline on Sterile Drug Products Produced by Aseptic Processing" (17) provides a review of the requirements for container/closure depyrogenation:

> It is critical to the integrity of the final product that containers and closures be rendered sterile and in the case of injectable products, pyrogen-free. The type of processes used to sterilize and depyrogenate will depend primarily on the nature of the material, which comprises the container/closure. Any properly validated process can be acceptable. Whatever depyrogenation method is used, the validation data should demonstrate that the process would reduce the endotoxin content by three logs. One method of assessing the adequacy of a depyrogenation process is to simulate the process using containers having known quantities of standardized endotoxins and measure the level of reduction … endotoxin challenges should not be easier to remove from the target surfaces than the endotoxin that may normally be present.

Rubber compound stoppers pose another potential source of microbial and (of concern for products intended to be pyrogen free) pyrogen contamination. They are usually cleaned by multiple cycles of washing and rinsing prior to final steam sterilization. The final rinse should be with USP water for injection. It is also important to minimize the lapsed time between washing and sterilizing because moisture on the stoppers can support microbiological growth and the generation of pyrogens. Because rubber is a poor conductor of heat, proper validation of processes to sterilize rubber stoppers is particularly important.

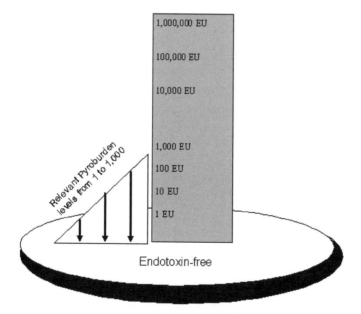

FIGURE 3 Pyroburden, endotoxin challenges, and three-log reduction levels. Munson's comments, and the USP and FDA aseptic guidelines state ≥3 logs reduced to pyrogen-free levels.

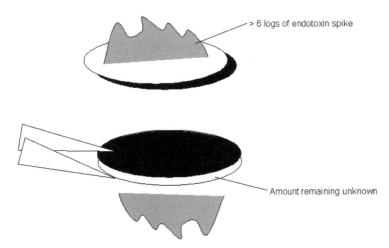

FIGURE 4 Is this validation? A mountain of applied spike is turned over (or washed) and the mountain of spike falls off. Has a >3 log reduction transpired? Increasing applied spikes to obtain better percent recovery (rather than developing better recovery methods) may result in spikes that are too easily removed, thereby revealing nothing about the depyrogenation process itself.

Helpful guidance on the topic of performing depyrogenation validation studies was provided by Munson, the former Chief of the Sterile Drug Branch of the FDA, in response to questions posed at several LAL User Group meetings in February 1991, May 1992, and January 1994. The LAL User's Group subsequently made Munson's comments available to participants in a printed form. Where the questions are contained within the answers, they are not repeated. Relevant Q&A include the following:

Q: Is it necessary to test for the absence of endotoxin on the final washed stoppers?
A: During the validation of the washing cycle, you must challenge the cycle with known endotoxin. The amount of endotoxin applied and the amount of endotoxin reduction achieved should be sufficient to demonstrate that the washing cycle will remove the amount of endotoxin coming in with your stoppers.
A: Endotoxin limits for components are very difficult to determine. The best way is to determine the pyroburden of the components, and if that pyroburden does not cause the finished product to exceed its limits, use the pyroburden values as the limits for the component.
A: If a 3-log reduction is impossible without destroying the properties of the material, then the alternative is to demonstrate what level of reduction can be achieved and that the pyroburden of the material does not exceed the reduction level.
A: Component pyroburden is important, even if the components are going to be depyrogenated, because you need to know how much endotoxin they are going to contribute to the final product. For components that are to be exposed to a validated depyrogenation process, you need assurance that the incoming component does not exceed the limit upon which the process was based.
Q: Is there a minimum number of endotoxin units that are permitted to be present on the stopper per FDA guidelines?

A: The minimum endotoxin units allowed is none detected. A 3-log reduction validation should be used. If the incoming stoppers have more than 3 logs of endotoxin, find a new vendor. The 3-log reduction is the safe, "no-questions-asked" way to validate depyrogenation. It is not the only way. If the data show that pyroburden on the incoming stoppers rarely exceeds 1 log, then a 2-log cycle may be acceptable. You must have data to support the process you are using.

By most accounts, the interpretation of the requirements listed (which are interpretations themselves) shows that the intention of the existing regulations are the performance and documentation of an overkill removal (for washed components) or destruction (for baked items) of the processing of incoming components. These guidelines may be misinterpreted leading to validation studies that can skirt the intention of the removal of endotoxin to low levels by applying levels of endotoxin that are not relevant to the demonstration of complete removal as depicted in Figures 3 and 4.

VALIDATION PHILOSOPHY AND ANCILLARY CONSIDERATIONS

Parenteral vials have been found to be a source of endotoxin contamination in the past but with the current use of shrink-wrapping instead of paper packaging this problem has largely disappeared. A team at Squibb (24) monitored 3200 incoming vials (prior to depyrogenation treatment) over an eight-month period and found only two that had responses at the detection limit of the lysate (nevertheless an unacceptable contamination rate). Furthermore, the demonstration that it rarely happens is not the same as the demonstration that it has not happened in a given instance. A delay in processing that allows pooled water to remain on stoppers combined with the exposure to nonsterile air invites the growth of bacteria regardless of the cleanliness of a stopper manufacturing process. The words "worst-case validation" are often used in the context of depyrogenation validation. The terms "worst case" and "validation" have been defined as follows:

> Worst case: "a set of conditions encompassing upper and lower processing limits and circumstances including those within standard operating procedures, which pose the greatest chance of process or product failure when compared to ideal conditions. Worst-case conditions do not however, necessarily induce product or process failure" (20).

> Validation: "establishing documented evidence which provides a high degree of assurance that a specific process will consistently produce a product meeting its predetermined specifications and quality attributes" (20).

Validation studies are governed by what could happen rather than the likelihood of their occurrence. New components made of new materials as well as new depyrogenation processes may bring erroneous assumptions if the data from existing studies are expected to extrapolate to the new items without rigorous validation (an early example being the attempted direct application of sterilization processes to achieve depyrogenation).

There should be awareness on the part of those charged with performing depyrogenation validation that there is a distinct difference between items that may be heat-treated and those that must be washed (inactivation vs. removal respectively) (18). The heat treatment of bottles and vials follows the more easily reasoned path that, given sufficient time and temperature, endotoxins will be destroyed. However, the wash removal of endotoxins is complicated by the tenacity

TABLE 3 Vial Closure and Container Materials

Elastomeric closures		Polymeric closures
Saturated	Unsaturated	
Polyisoprene	Butyl	Polyethelene
Styrene	Ethylene propylene	Polypropylene
Nitrile butadiene	Diene	Polyvinyl chloride
Polychloroprene	Silicone	Polystyrene

Source: From Ref. 25.

with which applied (CSE[b]-type or bulk) endotoxin sticks to rubber and other porous polymers (Table 3) that compose such materials. Endotoxin stuck to porous materials become entrenched and its removal is governed more by more difficult to quantify parameters including agitation and solubility. Thus, there are more variables involved than just heat and duration as in the case of heat inactivation (i.e., even the shape and size of a component being washed will affect the removal of endotoxin from it).

There is really no perfect way to verify that very low amounts of endotoxin, (i.e., ≤ 10 EU/stopper) given the adsorption into such porous materials, can be recovered. Therefore, often there is no perfect way to demonstrate that it has been removed. Common methods involving vigorous vortexing, sonication, or other means of agitation to dislodge it prior to testing are employed. While such methods conform to industry practices, they do not scientifically prove that a specific treatment, as in an hour of shaking (or five days for that matter) will dislodge any or all associated endotoxin from a given stopper. The selection of a vigorous method of dislodging of endotoxin is empirical (whatever works) and various labs have chosen to use either intense, short duration vortexing or prolonged but less vigorous mixing (such as shaking or sonication), or simply a wash with or without added surfactants. Agalloco has described the theoretical problem associated with cleaning validation studies that relate aptly to depyrogenation validation (endotoxin removal) studies when he characterized some inadequacies of cleaning validation in general by using a "tar baby" analogy:

> The cleanliness of the bath water may not necessarily relate directly to the cleanliness of the baby. If the contamination is not soluble in the cleaning agent, then the contamination will remain on the surface. If the contamination is not soluble in the final rinse, samples of the bath water will not detect the presence of residual contamination. The conclusion will be drawn that the baby is clean, when in fact both the cleaning and evaluation methods are inadequate (26).

In other words, if one determines the cleanliness of the baby (stopper) by measuring the "tar" (endotoxin) remaining in the bath water (laboratory rinse method), then one has to ensure that the method used does indeed remove the "tar." There must be some validation of the method to serve as a demonstration that the method removes endotoxin from "sticky" surfaces. At least in theory, endotoxin that clings tenaciously to a stopper (thereby escaping pyroburden detection) could be removed later by the surfactant action of a drug and become available for parenteral administration. For a number of years, the Lilly Laboratories (Indianapolis, Indiana,

---

[b]CSE, Control standard endotoxin.

U.S.A.) have been employing variations on a Pyrosperse™ solution soak method as a means of removing applied endotoxin for depyrogenation validations (27) from particularly sticky components.

The scenario of contaminated plastic molded components has not been typical of the pharmaceutical industy's experience given the molten formation of such devices from poured plastics, but when validating parenteral vial closures [nonbaked containers, and medical devices (tubing, etc.)] it should be borne in mind that it is the nature of new components and processes to change the circumstances to which users have grown accustomed. It is more desirable to begin with the end in mind. For example, "How can I prove that this item (stopper) is not (grossly) contaminated given the underlying assumption of extreme adsorption?" One is really trying to prove wrong the assumption that the items are grossly contaminated. The problem becomes increasingly difficult with the increasing complexity of the depyrogenation process. The simplest depyrogenation to demonstrate is the traditional dry-heat incineration. Did the oven reach the required temperature for the required time? Sufficient historical data exist to support the conclusion that such a time and temperature is indeed depyrogenating and is typically verified via a periodic revalidation.

Characterization of commercial concentrated endotoxin used for such spike studies has greatly aided in "getting back" numerical values that are very close to the theoretical value (i.e., 48,800 EU/component of a 50,000 EU/component spike application). The characterization of the spike together with the application and recovery of a "lower" level (i.e., the 3-log reduction amount) spike recovery (i.e., 50 EU/component) during the method validation for a given component ensures that the method developed is sensitive and, therefore, that the washed stoppers returned from manufacturing and tested by the QC lab are not analogous to the "tar baby bath water." Alternatively, one is really only proving that one's method of recovery is grossly inadequate and may cause one to wonder what is being proved by such a study (Fig. 5).

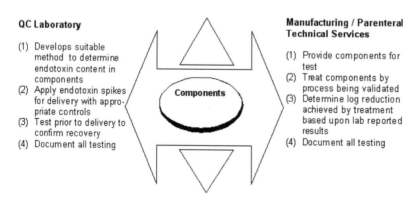

FIGURE 5   Manufacturing and quality control support depyrogenation validation activities.

DEVELOPING A PROCESS FOR TRADITIONAL DEPYROGENATION VALIDATION ACTIVITIES (DRY HEAT AND WASHING)

It is instructive to separate out manufacturing and QC laboratory division of labor in the fragmented depyrogenation validation process. Regardless of how specific companies have organized such activities, practically speaking, a natural division exists between the manufacturing and QC functions in the depyrogenation validation process. The manufacturing area may have a validation group that runs the studies to document that their processes comply with current good manufacturing practices requirements including depyrogenation validation. QC laboratories support these efforts in supplying the expertise in the specific endotoxin application. Therefore, the coordination of activities involves manufacturing and lab support. The manufacturing group determines and documents the depyrogenation treatment process (oven or washer) and the laboratory supplies inoculated components, performs before and after depyrogenation treatment LAL testing with accompanying controls, documents and reports the results.

There are typically two sets of activities occurring together in such studies: (*i*) the laboratory needs validation documentation that the lab bacterial endotoxin testing method to be used is valid for a given specific article that the manufacturing will depyrogenate and (*ii*) manufacturing will prove that a given process (oven tunnel, stopper washer, etc.) will perform as purported (i.e., will remove >3 logs of applied endotoxin). The typical activities to be performed are shown in Figure 5.

Pyroburden Testing

Since the CFR states[c] that it is the independent QC laboratory's responsibility to decide the suitability of depyrogenation of components, the user must recognize differences existing in the activities and requirements of laboratory validation to support pyroburden methods and depyrogenation validation processes (3-log reduction validation) though they are highly similar in many respects. A difference in the two lies in the fact that pyroburden is a release test for components to allow them to be used in marketed products whereas the 3-log reduction test is part of the validation of a manufacturing process. Often they have already undergone a validated depyrogenation process at the supplier's facility and therefore testing at the user facility serves as a "spot check" of that process's efficacy.

When testing is used as basis for lot acceptance, the number of components to be tested should be derived from a statistical (or at least reasoned) sampling of a given lot of components based upon the lot size and the data generated should involve individual testing, not an average or composite test of an arbitrary number of components pooled together. Given the statistically determined number of stoppers of a lot (e.g., 100,000 stopper) that needs to be tested to assure compliance to a given specification, the laboratory should not pool the stoppers for test (21 CFR subpart E 211.84). One needs to determine if individual member stoppers of the sample group exceeds the limit specification. The pooling of samples for test will result in an average value that will not reveal the number of EU/component for individual components.

---

[c]CFR 211.22 states "there shall be a quality control unit that shall have the responsibility to approve or reject all components, drug product containers, closures, in-process materials, packaging material, labeling and drug products states. . . ."

DEPYROGENATION INDICATOR AND RECOVERY VARIABILITY

It is common knowledge in the endotoxin-testing lab that depyrogenation validation recoveries of applied endotoxin is a highly variable process dependent
upon many difficult to control variables. An analogous variability in sterilization
validation BI recovery has been reported by Shintani and Akers (28). They list
several BI variables including carrier material, primary packaging material,
culture medium, different sport suspensions (but not BI resistance), retrieval technique, and population variability in purchased BI suspensions. For depyrogenation
studies, a number of variables can affect the demonstration of the reduction of
applied endotoxin:

1. Type of endotxoin applied (vendor source and presentation, that is, those
    applied by the manufacturer or by the user, different application methods
    employed).
2. Amount of endotoxin applied (common application amounts range from 1000
    to 100,000 EU per component).
3. The type of material to which the endotoxin is to be applied (the smoothness or
    roughness of rubber or alternative polymer vial closures, glass, etc.)
4. The extraction method chosen to recover the applied endotoxin before and after
    depyrogenation treatment.
5. The potency variability inherent in highly concentrated endotoxin spike
    solutions.
6. The effects of assay interference that may come from leaching or detergent are a
    possibility with rubber or polymer and also with glass after heating (interfer-
    ence controls are included to gauge this variable).
7. Process treatments contain many variables in vial oven tunnel or stopper
    washer facilities and affect the mix of recoveries in such studies (the large
    number of such process variables is the reason endotoxin is used as an indicator
    rather than simply relying on physical measurements of time and temperature
    applied).

Due to the variables mentioned earlier in this section and particularly the last
item on the list, such activities are empirical in nature and the simplicity of the 3-log
reduction criteria is sometimes in vivid contrast to the plethora of different means of
demonstrating that the criteria had been met. The concentrated endotoxin standard
challenge is the empirical indicator that determines the suitability of a depyrogenation process whereas the physical process parameters may serve as supporting data
(F, D, and Z values) and used as gauges of the mechanical working order of the
process.

NONHEAT INACTIVATION METHODS
Acid-Base Hydrolysis
Depyrogenation utilizing acid or alkaline hydrolysis reduces or eliminates the biological activity of bacterial LPS by deactivating lipid A. Lipid A is linked to core
polysaccharide by 2-keto-3-deoxyoctonic acid (KDO), an eight-carbon sugar acid
unique to bacterial LPS. Acid hydrolysis acts upon this acid-labile ketosidic
linkage to separate lipid A from the remainder of the LPS molecule. Because the
released KDO and its attached core polysaccharides act as solute carriers for the
lipid portion of the molecule, the free lipid A is insoluble in aqueous systems

and its pyrogenic activity is reduced or eliminated. However, Galanos et al. (29) demonstrated that, when free lipid A was combined with bovine serum albumin, pyrogenicity was equal to that of intact endotoxin. Further, acid hydrolysis may act upon the lipid A fraction, altering conformation of the molecule and masking necessary functional sites; alternatively, it may cleave off fatty acid molecules at different rates, further effecting lipid solubility and thereby pyrogenicity. Acid hydrolysis, using 0.05 N HCl for 30 mm at 100°C (30) or 1.0% glacial acetic acid for two to three hours at 100°C (31) has been used for depyrogenation.

Alkylation Including Ethylene Oxide
Unlike acid hydrolysis, alkaline hydrolysis does not involve the loss of pyrogenic activity through the loss of KDO or fatty acids; instead, major chemical and biological alterations of the degraded molecule result from saponification of fatty acids (32). In 1956, Neter et al. (33) reported that neither heat alone (100°C, 24 hour, pH 7.2) nor hydrolysis in 0.25 N NaOH at 56°C for six minutes appreciably reduced pyrogenicity of *E. coli* and *Salmonella abortus equi* LPSs. However, exposure to 0.25 N NaOH at 56°C for one hour produced a moderate loss of pyrogenicity for the *E. coli* LPS and a marked reduction for the *Salmonella* LPS. Niwa et al. (32) reported that depyrogenation is enhanced when LPS is subjected to alkaline hydrolysis with 0.1 N NaOH in either 95% ethanol or 80% dimethylsulfoxide.

   Several authors have reported that treating endotoxin with alkylating agents decreases pyrogenicity. Schenck et al. (34) demonstrated a 100-fold decrease in pyrogenicity when endotoxin was treated with acetic anhydride. The same group reported a 100- to 1000-fold decrease when endotoxin was treated with succinic anhydride. The mechanism behind this reduction was thought to be acetylation and succinylation, respectively. However, even though succinylation caused a marked decrease in pyrogenicity, the endotoxin adjuvanicity was not abrogated. Further studies demonstrated that treatment with phthalic anhydride, a strong alkylating agent, caused a 10,000-fold reduction in pyrogenicity and a 1000-fold decrease in lethality in mice; however, the ability of treated endotoxin to induce nonspecific resistance was not altered. Alkylation was thought to occur through nucleophilic substitution in the glucosamine linkage of lipid A and/or in the ethanolamine of the core. There is conflicting evidence concerning the ability of succinylation to decrease the pyrogenicity of endotoxin. Westphal concluded that succinylation did not alter the pyrogenicity of endotoxin by reaction with OH groups available on the KDO disaccharide (35).

   Ethylene oxide (EtO) is also a strong alkylating agent. A study published by Tsuji and Harrison (13) showed a 94% reduction following EtO sterilization of *E. coli* 0127:B8 endotoxin inoculated onto aluminum or glass. The EtO sterilization cycle used involved 12% EtO and 88% Freon, 50% relative humidity, and 3.5 psig for 6.5 hours. Additional work on this method should be encouraged because it could have widespread application for depyrogenation of heat-labile substances and EtO-sterilized medical devices.

Oxidation
Knowledge of oxidative inactivation of endotoxins can be traced to the beginning of the century, when Hort and Penfold (36) reported that *Salmonella typhosa* cells lost fever-producing capacity when washed in hydrogen peroxide. Although, the

mechanism of action of H_2O_2 on LPS is unknown, the peroxidation of the fatty acids present in the lipid A region of LPS has been suggested.

Taub and Hart (37) utilized H_2O_2 to detoxify pyrogens in Sterile Water for Injection USP, normal saline, and dextrose-saline solutions. They found that the most effective treatment was boiling in the presence of 0.1% H_2O_2 for two hours. Under these conditions, the final solution was also free of peroxide. An adaptation of this procedure was successfully applied by Menczel (38) to large-scale depyrogenation of infusion solutions at a Tel Aviv hospital. DeRenzis (39) described the endotoxin inactivation capacity of H_2O_2 as measured by a cell-growth indicator. When 3% H_2O_2 was added to equal parts of cell-growth medium that was then incubated at room temperature for 24 hours and subsequently dialyzed, the ability of endotoxin to inhibit cell growth was substantially reduced. Case and Novitsky (40) clearly demonstrated that the inactivation of endotoxin by H_2O_2 is dependent on time, pH, and concentration. Using as little as 2.7% H_2O_2 at 65°C for 1 hour, these authors observed an approximately 90% reduction of endotoxin. When the H_2O_2 was increased to 27%, virtually 100% destruction was achieved within one hour. Oxidative depyrogenation using hydrogen peroxide offers several advantages over other methods. H_2O_2 is safe to handle, can be easily eliminated from solution, and appears to inactivate endotoxin under nonextreme conditions (i.e., low concentration of H_2O_2 and low temperature). Its chief disadvantage is that H_2O_2 may adulterate a solution or product. Methods of oxidative depyrogenation using agents other than H_2O_2 exist and may offer advantages for specific applications. These include treatment with molecular O_2 (41), hypochlorous acid or hypochlorite (42,43), periodic acid or sodium periodate (33,44), dilute potassium permanganate (45), acidic alkaline, neutral permanganate, nitric acid, dichromate, and selenium dioxide (46).

Ionizing Radiation (Gamma Radiation)

Several studies have been reported in which ionizing radiation with ^{60}Co was utilized to reduce the toxicity of bacterial endotoxin. Bertok and Szeberenyi (47) describe the use of a ^{60}Co-irradiated endotoxin preparation, TOLERIN that significantly decreased the endotoxin's lethal and hypotensive effects in a dose-related manner. Endotoxin's ability to activate the complement system was also affected, and immunoadjuvant properties and ability to stimulate nonspecific resistance were retained. Csako et al. (48) investigated the physical and biological properties of ^{60}Co ionizing radiation. Physical and biological changes were reported to be dose dependent. A gradual loss of the polysaccharide components (O side chain and R core) was observed, and activity tests suggested that destruction of lipid A was dose related. Both pyrogenicity and LAL reactivity of the endotoxin were destroyed by increasing the doses of radiation. However, because it increases the possibility of unknown chemical changes to drugs and parenteral solutions, the use of the ionizing radiation in depyrogenating these materials is unlikely. Ionizing radiation would be of far greater use in producing endotoxin that has lost its harmful pyrogenic and toxic properties but retained beneficial properties, such as adjuvanicity, that increase the body's natural defense.

Gamma irradiation has proven capable of reducing endotoxin loads and is currently used in sterilization and is notable for its ability to penetrate medical devices (49), raw materials, excipients, new drug delivery systems includes liposomes and monoclonal antibodies (50). The ease of validation has been described by Reid as being dependent upon a single variable: time:

> Gamma radiation processing with its single variable, time, makes validation very easy. Time is the only variable as Co^{60} (cobalt 60) decays at a fixed rate. Once the total number of curies installed and the required dose is known, only the time, which control the dwell time of the carrier/tote at each position around the source rack, need to be set. This is in direct contrast to gas and steam sterilization where a vacuum system, gas/steam mixture and the uniformity of the heat/gas within the sterilization chamber must be monitored. Similarly for electron beam, the power variables (i.e., current, voltage) and the rate of movement of the transport system must be strictly controlled and monitored throughout the radiation process.

Csako et al. also studied the effects of gamma radiation (Co^{60}) on standard endotoxin preparations and found that a dose of 1 Mrad brought about a reduction of about 200X in the pyrogenicity of LPS, however, only an "eight-fold decrease in the titer of LAL activity was found." Their study demonstrated a dose dependent, exponential destruction of LPS via irradiation. In summary they state:

> At higher doses of radiation, a direct relation was observed between the degradation of the molecular and supramolecular structure and the loss of biologic function. At lower doses of radiation, however, there was variability among the functional assays in their rate of change with progressive irradiation of the RSE. The results suggest that the carbohydrate moiety plays an important role both in determining the supramolecular structure and in modulating certain biologic activities of bacterial endotoxins (51).

Biological Inactivation Methods
Polymyxin B
Several studies have showed that the cationic antibiotic PMB can abrogate the biological activity of LPS (52,53). Morrison and Jacobs (54) described the mechanism of endotoxin inactivation as a stoichiometric binding of PMB to the lipid A region of LPS. Although these authors claim a 1:1 molar binding between PMB and LPS, in a study by Cooperstock (55), 100 to 200 times more PMB were required to inactivate LPS as measured by the LAL test. Novitsky and Case (56) recently reviewed this controversy. Using a turbidimetric adaptation of the LAL test, Novitsky and Case (56) found no inhibition of LPS in the LAL test at levels to 3.4 mg/mL of PMB sulfate. They concluded that the observed inhibition of LPS in the LAL test was due not only to the binding of PMB to LPS but also to the interaction of PMB and LAL. They also suggested that the type of endotoxin used could influence the amount of PMB-LAL inhibition observed and that the effects of PMB on LAL may be unrelated to its effects on other biological entities. Until further studies are carried out, caution should be exercised in interpreting LAL test results involving PMB inactivation of LPS. However, removal of endotoxin from solution based on its PMB-binding characteristics was recently achieved by Issekutz (57), who coupled PMB to Sepharose affinity columns and successfully removed nearly 1 to 10 μg/mL of several endotoxins from various solutions. The columns retained their binding capacity for at least 18 months and could be regenerated by eluting desorbed endotoxin from the columns with 1% sodium deoxycholate.

LAL
The mechanism of depyrogenation by LAL is uncertain. It was suggested by Rickles et al. (58) that LAL was capable of removing endotoxin from concanavalin A and

erythropoietin by adsorption. Simultaneously, another independent report by Nachum et al. (59) appeared, presumably describing the same phenomenon, but suggesting that the mechanism of depyrogenation was the inactivation due to the enzymatic action of LAL. Nachum et al. (59) found that the enzyme-inactivating fraction of LAL could be obtained by heating LAL to 60°C for 20 mm. The LAL was then centrifuged at 5000 x g for 6 mm at 5°C to remove the precipitate. The supernatant, which contained the inactivating factor(s), was successfully used to inactivate 80% of several endotoxins tested at 500 ng/mL. Treatment was for 30 mm at 37°C. Although the method is very interesting, it is reported to be quite costly and difficult to control.

More recently, a highly selective method to remove (not an inactivation method) endotoxin from small volumes of contaminated solutions has been developed from another blood product of the horseshoe crab called endotoxin neutralizing protein (ENP) as described in this chapter in the section entitled "Nonheat Inactivation Methods."

DEPYROGENATION BY ENDOTOXIN REMOVAL
Rinsing
The oldest and simplest method of endotoxin removal of solid surface contaminants is rinsing with a nonpyrogenic solvent, usually Sterile Water for Injection USP. Low levels of surface endotoxin can be effectively removed from glassware, device components, and stoppers, for example, with an appropriate washing procedure. Rinse water can be monitored throughout the process with LAL to validate endotoxin removal. An example of such a validation process for large-volume parenteral glass containers was described by Feldstine et al. (4).

Distillation
Distillation is the oldest method known for effectively removing pyrogens from water. The mechanism of endotoxin removal is relatively simple. Water is forced to undergo two-phase changes, from liquid to vapor and from vapor to liquid. During the first phase, rapid boiling in the still causes the water to evaporate and the water vapor to accelerate. Because LPS is such a large molecule, it cannot accelerate as rapidly as water vapor and is left behind due to inertia. Those LPS molecules remaining in water droplets carried in the steam are dropped by gravity due to their high molecular weight. It has long been known that freshly distilled water collected and maintained in sterile depyrogenated containers is nonpyrogenic. It was the application of this knowledge that allowed initiation of commercial large-volume parenteral production in the United States in the years preceding World War II.

Ultrafiltration
Ultrafilters are rated based upon the molecular weight cutoff (MWCO) or the so-called nominal molecular weight limit (NMWL) rather than by the size of the filtration pores. Genovesi (60) describes the so-called "cutoff" as the molecular weight of the smallest molecule that will be at least 95% excluded by the filter from the passing solute. The basic subunit size of LPS (the monomeric LPS molecule) is about 10,000 to 20,000. It can, therefore, be effectively removed from solution by a 10,000 molecular weight ultrafilter. However, the unaggregated

TABLE 4 Removal of *E. coli* Endotoxin from Various Solutions by Ultrafiltration

Solution	Endotoxin conc. (g/mL)	Endotoxin (g/mL) recovered in filtrate form				
		0.2 μm	0.25 μm	$10^{5\text{MWCO}}$	$10^{6\text{MWCO}}$	$10^{4\text{MWCO}}$
Water	10^{-6}	10^{-6}	10^{-10}	10^{-10}	10^{-10}	10^{-10}
0.9% NaCl	10^{-6}	10^{-6}	10^{-10}	10^{-10}	10^{-10}	10^{-10}
5 mM MgCl$_2$	10^{-6}	10^{-6}	10^{-10}	10^{-10}	10^{-10}	
5 mM EDTA	10^{-6}		10^{-6}	10^{-10}	10^{-10}	
0.5% Na cholate	10^{-5}			10^{-10}	10^{-7}	10^{-10}
1.0% Na cholate	10^{-5}			10^{-6}	10^{-7}	10^{-10}
2% Na cholate[a]	10^{-5}			10^{-5}	10^{-5}	10^{-10}
1% Deoxycholate	10^{-5}			10^{-5}	10^{-5}	10^{-10}

[a]With 5 mM EDTA.
Abbreviations: EDTA, ethylenediaminetetraacetic acid; MWCO, molecular weight cut off.
Source: From Ref. 62.

monomeric form of LPS is seldom, if ever, found in aqueous solutions. Normally, LPS molecules aggregate into vesicles ranging in molecular weight from 300,000 to 1 million. Therefore, endotoxin in aqueous solutions can sometimes be removed by ultrafilters rated at 100,000 molecular weight or even higher (61), though that size of filters would not be expected to yield a completely depyrogenated solution. Ultrafiltration as a method for removing pyrogens has been successfully applied to a large number of low- to medium-molecular-weight drugs and solutions. Endotoxin-contaminated antibiotics have been successfully depyrogenated without significant loss of the antibiotic (56), and the process has also been utilized for large-scale production of electrolyte solutions (57). Higher molecular weight solutions contaminated with aggregated endotoxin of a similar size may also be successfully ultrafiltered if the endotoxin can be disaggregated through the use of such agents as chelators or surface-active detergents (62). Large NMWL filters can be used to sometimes remove highly aggregated endotoxin (as is often the case in aqueous solutions) via 100,000 to 500,000-MWCO filters (60). These effects can be manipulated to achieve aggregation and subsequent filtration removal (Table 4). The aggregate size of a solution can be determined by filtration with progressively smaller NMWL filters until endotoxin activity is no longer seen in the filtrate.

A more difficult situation arises when the endotoxin aggregates and the solute is of a similar molecular size. In such cases the two may still be separated by ultra-filtration if a means of manipulating the endotoxin aggregation size can be found via the removal of factors that decrease aggregate size such as cations, detergents, and chelators. Whereas in the LAL test one is concerned with supplying such factors to bring about the dispersion of the purified LPS to gain full recovery, alternatively for depyrogenation purposes the very same principles may be employed in reverse that were described in Chapter 11 to aid in the dispersion of CSE.

Reverse Osmosis

Reverse osmosis membranes consist of cellulose acetate or polyamide materials with pores small enough to exclude ions. Such semipermeable filters are termed "reverse osmosis" membranes, if they can retain large amounts of salts under pressure-filtration conditions. Conventional reverse osmosis membranes (nominally rated at pore sizes around 10 Angstroms) remove endotoxins by simple size exclusion-the pores in the membrane are far too small to pass the pyrogens (62). At intermediate pore sizes, the ability of these filters to retain pyrogens has been poorly documented and reports have been contradictory. Nevertheless, conventional reverse osmosis membranes are extremely effective for removing endotoxin from water. Their use for depyrogenation has been limited, however, because very few molecules other than water can pass through the pore structure of the reverse osmosis membrane. In practical operation, a well-maintained reverse osmosis membrane of high integrity routinely removes 99.5% to 99.9% of the pyrogen load to the system in a single pass, even when the challenge levels are as high as a microgram of endotoxin per milliliter.

Activated Carbon

Depyrogenation of solutions based upon the physical adsorption of endotoxin to charcoal, particularly activated charcoal, has had a long history and is well documented in the literature (64–66). Most commonly, charcoal is added to a solution, the solution is agitated, and, finally, the carbon is removed via filtration or precipitation. The method has been successfully used to treat a wide range of pharmaceuticals, including saline, dextrose solutions, and antibiotics (64). However, activated charcoal has a great affinity for high-molecular-weight, nonionized substances, which in certain situations may limit its application (65). Although activated charcoal can be applied over a broad pH range and is not affected by electrolyte concentrations, its use with solutions containing low concentrations of active agents is limited. Adsorption of active ingredients may also occur. Its principal limitation is the difficulty of completely removing all traces of the charcoal. Reinhardt describes the use of a sintered activated charcoal filter for use in depyrogenation that lessens the problem of charcoal removal (64–66). The filter allows continuous processing of solutions by means of a design that combines adsorption and entrapment (via pore size). The filter can also be depyrogenated by dry heat and reused. However, with the exception of water and physiological electrolyte solutions, only concentrated solutions of raw materials and intermediates are recommended for filtration, due to possible loss by adsorption.

Electrostatic Attraction Including Charge-Modified Media

Depth filtration using asbestos-containing filters has also long been used in pyrogen removal (67,68), but has since been banned by the FDA due to concerns over some studies indicating asbestos carcinogenicity. Depth filters from materials other than asbestos are available for commercial use in removing large amounts of endotoxin not possible with membrane filters, which can rather quickly become clogged. Charge-modified depth (CMD) filters of "cellulose and modified inorganic filter aids" have been fashioned in a manner to mimic the efficiency of asbestos filters (60). The drawbacks associated with such filters include (*i*) requirement of a positive charge on the medium, (*ii*) coupled with a negative charge on the endotoxin (in the pH range of 4.5–8), (*iii*) nonendotoxin negatively charged particles can over-run the binding capacity of the filter, and (*iv*) the solutions being filtered must be fairly stable in that changes in pH, organic content, and cations can limit the adsorption of endotoxin onto the CMD matrix (60).

Membranes produced from polyamides (nylon), or with amines covalently bonded to their surfaces, exhibit overall net positive charges in aqueous solutions with a pH below 9 and adsorb negatively charged endotoxins. Charge-modified microporous depyrogenation products utilizing positive ζ-potential (zeta) membranes have been available for years and have been used successfully for depyrogenating a wide range of pharmaceutical solutions (69). The chemical structure of biologically active pyrogens and the effect of the suspending media on their activity necessitate designing charge-modified filters specifically tailored for the product involved.

The removal of endotoxin by electrostatic attraction to other cationically charged adsorbents is also well documented. Barium sulfate and ion-exchange resins have been reported to be effective for reducing pyrogens (70–72). However, their performance seems to be highly dependent on the concentration of pyrogens found in the solutions.

Hydrophobic Attraction to Hydrophobic Media

Aliphatic polymers, such as polypropylene, polyethylene, polyvinylidene fluoride, and polytetrafluoroethylene have a unique specific affinity for binding endotoxin. This property was utilized by Harris and Feinstein (73) to prepare an LAL propylene bead assay to detect endotoxins in materials considered to be inhibitory to the gel-clot LAB assay. However, the electrostatic mechanism does not explain why endotoxin is adsorbed to these polymers, because the polymers lack hydrophilic ionizable groups capable of interacting with the anionic endotoxins. Instead, the nonpolar groups common to these polymers give the membrane surface a hydrophobic quality. And, given that all endotoxins have both a hydrophilic polysaccharide tail and a hydrophobic lipid A core, hydrophobic interaction between the membrane polymer and the lipid A core region is probably responsible for the adsorption of LPS. Robinson et al. (74) describe a microfiltration process using microporous membrane filters made from hydrophobic materials that provides effective microfiltration in a range extending from that of ultrafiltration to the upper boundary of reverse osmosis. According to these authors, a 0.1 μm polypropylene membrane was capable of adsorbing greater than 10 μg of LPS per square centimeter of filter area, over a broad pH range, with a log reduction value of 3 to 4. Minobe et al. (75) examined a series of compounds used in the preparation of column chromatography absorbents with a high affinity for pyrogen. Of the materials that proved successful in this application, the absorbent prepared by immobilizing histamine on aminohexyl-Sepharose CL4B with glutaraldehyde treatment had the highest affinity for pyrogen. Studies to determine the mechanism of action suggested that both ionic and hydrophobic interactions contributed to endotoxin adsorption. It was suggested that affinity chromatography with immobilized histamine could be utilized to remove endotoxins from relatively unstable macromolecular substances, such as enzymes, hormones, and antibodies-substances that are difficult to depyrogenate by more conventional methods.

LABORATORY DEPYROGENATION

The endotoxin quality control lab is routinely involved in a couple of depyrogenation processes for internal purposes including the depyrogenation of labware (utensils, tubes, containers, etc.) and the removal of endogenous endotoxin for product validation, as required by the USP. The first method is very well characterized and involves cooking utensils in a validated oven according to the pattern load and time/temperature parameters established in-house (generally, 250°C for 30 minutes to 2 hours). In the latter instance, the USP requires that samples to be used for Inhibition/Enhancement validation testing must be endotoxin free (at least within the relevant quantification range).

The validation of an endotoxin testing method for compounds that turns out to contain endotoxin poses somewhat of a time-consuming obstacle. Presumably, the initial unspiked test is positive at some level and one does not know at this point whether it is interference (enhancement) or endotoxin. Therefore, two choices of action remain. Repeat the development study again by another proposed method (if enhancement is suspected), or by first treating the sample by a depyrogenation method that does not change the sample prior to testing it again (if contamination is suspected). If ultrafiltration is the treatment chosen, it may be accomplished by one of several commercially available methods (i.e., Sartorius 20,000 dalton cut-off filter), the molecular weight of the product will have to be verified or, alternatively, the potency of the product in the filtrate will have to be demonstrated post filtration. It would not be appropriate to remove the product along with the endotoxin and then demonstrate the lack of interference of the filtrate (basically only the solvent and dissolved excipients). Therefore, the molecular weight of the product will have to be less than 20,000 daltons or other relevant molecular weight based upon the filtration device.

Given a macromolecule, a charge binding filter or, a commercial resin affinity bead, developed and commercialized by a LAL manufacturer, can be used. The affinity beads, End-X™ (Associates of Cape Cod) are coated with ENP (another natural blood-product of the horseshoe crab: anti-LPS) (76,77). One to two milliliters of sample is mixed with the End-X coated beads in the pyrogen-free container supplied, gently shaken for 4 to 24 hours, depending upon the level of contamination to be removed, and allowed to settle or centrifuged prior to pouring off the sample. Up to 50 ng of endotoxin (corresponding to about 500 EU of *E. coli* endotoxin) can be removed per tube treatment. The ENP binds endotoxin, which in turn settles to the bottom of the tube given the 65 μm bead attached to it. The method works for a variety of endotoxin from gram-negative organisms but, interestingly, not for *Vibrio* spp., which was the very species that lead Bang to begin his studies into the clotting of the crab's blood. Profos' Endotrap® is another method that has become available recently and in effect serves as a miniature chromatography column through which the sample is poured once it is "primed" by rinsing with buffers. Repeated passes through the plastic column will cumulatively remove endotoxin from a variety of solutions.

ENDOTOXIN REMOVAL CASE STUDIES

Modern techniques used to remove endotoxins from drugs during parenteral manufacturing in many cases involves the combination of several of the methods discussed earlier in this chapter. Macromolecules cannot be removed by simple ultrafiltration given that their size may be similar to endotoxin aggregates. Three case studies will be reviewed in which endotoxin removal processes were devised for (*i*) a 32 Kda enzyme [superoxide dismutase (SOD)], (*ii*) a high MW α-1,6 branched a-1,4 glucan (Amylopectin) derived from corn or potato starch and used as an encapsulation matrix for pharmaceutical products, and (*iii*) another protein derived from *E. coli* fermentation process that, like endotoxin, possesses an anionic charge, thus making removal difficult. The latter product contained, before endotoxin removal, on a higher range of 500,000 EU/mL and was reduced to less than 50 EU/mL by the method devised.

Case Study 1: In what researchers at Sigma Chemical called "Case Study 1," endotoxin removal to meet a proposed specification level of <0.25 EU/mg of protein (78). Held et al. designed the initial purification of the protein to achieve >99% purity using "extraction, heat treatment, clarification, and ammonium sulfate fractionation of bovine liver" followed by three chromographic steps which removed the majority of endotoxins. At this stage the product yielded endotoxin values between 0.16 and 0.72 EU/mg, which provided no consistency in meeting the necessary specification (nmt 0.25 EU/mg). The authors, therefore, employed a "polishing step" to perform the remaining three-fold reduction of endotoxin with an eye on adding only a minimal additional cost to the process. They used a positively charged, 1 ft^2, 0.2 μm disposable Posidyne filter (Pall) to achieve the required reduction of endotoxin with no loss of product. The natural negative charge of LPS above a pH of 2.0 allowed the use of ion exchange as a means of binding the endotoxin to the filter matrix while the protein solution passed.

Case Study 2: The same Sigma Chemical group (75) had a formidable task of reducing up to approximately 500 EU/g to <20 EU/g. The low solubility and viscosity of the amylopectin prevented the filtration removal of endotoxin. First they added 400 gm of food-grade amylopectin to 20 L of 2 mM ethylenediaminetetraacetic acid to reduce the aggregate size of the endotoxins. They heated to 85°C to 90°C and stirred the mix for one hour. After cooling to 54°C–56°C they added sodium hydroxide to a final concentration of 0.25 M and stirred for another hour to hydrolyze the endotoxin base labile bonds (i.e., lipid A-KDO). The solution was neutralized using HCl and cooled to room temperature. Repeated ultrafiltration with 300,000 MW cutoff filters was used to remove salts and endotoxin. Upon concentration to 10 L, the solution was diluted to 30 L with endotoxin-free water. This was followed by repeated reconcentration to 10 L followed by redilution in endotoxin-free water for a total of nine times. The final solution was filtered through a 0.45 μm Posidyne filter, frozen, lyophilized and stored overnight under vacuum. Thus, the group combined three different, well-known mechanisms to remove the endotoxin in stages: treatment with moderate heat and alkali, filtration separation by molecular weight cuttoff filters, and ion exchange binding to the 0.45 μm filter. They quantitated the endotoxin removed by each of the processing steps to find that the reduction factors achieved were 20, 5, and 2, respectively. The final filtration resulted in a solution of <1 EU/gram. The authors point out that, "even water with endotoxin levels that are below the detection limit can become a major contributor to endotoxins when large volumes are used for repeated cycles of diluiton and concentration of a product" (78).

Case Study 3: A group from Applied Genetics found that they could use anion-exchange filtration to bind a DNA repair enzyme (photolyase) with an anionic charge while passing LPS (also with an anionic charge and thus the added degree of difficulty) via manipulation of the pH and salt concentrations of the filtrate (79):

> The key is finding conditions under which the endotoxin quantitatively binds to the membrane anion-exchange filter while the target protein passes through. This can be

accomplished in many cases by careful selection of pH and salt concentrations. Under the proper conditions, the endotoxin and some charged protein components are released on the filter, resulting in not only removal of endotoxin but also partial protein purification ... Endotoxin removal from this target protein is a particularly challenging task because photolyase is a DNA-binding protein and therefore also binds to anion exchangers (79).

The group used Sartorious (Sartobind^{TM}) Q-MA filters for both small-scale (Q-100MA) and large-scale filtration (total of ten, Q-550; 293 mm diameter filters). Both filters are made of cross-linked regenerated cellulose membranes with quaternary ammonium functional groups in a polysulfone housing. The working surface area of the small and large-scale filters respectively was 100 cm^2 and 5500 cm^2 (10 linked filters × 550 cm^2) for the large-scale application.

The series of experiments employed bacterial extracts of 500,000 to 10 million EU/mL to challenge the filters. The first pass through the filters obtained a log reduction of endotoxin levels as measured by LAL. The second pass obtained a total of three logs of reduction (to 100 EU/mL) followed by a final pass that further cut the endotoxin level by half (to 50 EU/mL). Importantly the selection of the ionic strength of the buffer rinses for the membrane absorption application selected did not bind the product to the filter, thus the authors obtained the added benefit of "12-fold increase in specific activity of photolyase in the extract." The scale up of the process allowed for a 100-fold increase in the capacity (volume) with a concomitant increase of only 55-fold increase of absorption area. A demonstration of the binding capacity for endotoxin (Cap$_E$) was given in the formula:

$$Cap_E = [(E_0 - E_1) \times V_1]/Q_{abs}$$

where

E$_0$ is the endotoxin concentration of the starting material
E$_1$ is the endotoxin concentration after the first pass
V$_1$ as the volume (mL) in the first pass between regeneration steps
Q$_{abs}$ is the effective absorption area in cm^2 of the Q-MA filter

Using the combined results from the small-scale and large-scale experiments, Belanich et al. obtained an average endotoxin binding capacity of 2.25 million EU/cm^2 of filter area. They described the project's success in terms of the creation of "a multiplier in the preferentially absorbing endotoxin from the sample ... (thus allowing a) competitive binding advantage to the anion-exchange membrane compared with protein" (79). This case study demonstrates the project-specific nature of ion-binding applications in that each drug, diluent, and process used will require extensive work in determining the conditions that will allow the capture of endotoxin while allowing the elution of the product to be depyrogenated.

REFERENCES

1. Wellman N, Fortun S, McLeod B. Bacterial biofilms and the bioelectric effect, antimicrob. Agents Chemother 1996; 40(9):2012–2014.
2. Costerton JW, et al. Biofilms, the customized microniche. J Bacteriol 1994; 176(8): 2137–2142.
3. Watnick P, Kolter R. Biofilm, city of microbes. J Bacteriol 2000; 182(10):2675–2679.
4. Feldstine P, et al. A concept in glassware depyrogenation process validation. Parenter Drug Assoc 1979; 33(3):125.

5. Hort EC, Penfold WJ. Br Med J 1911; 2(3):1510.
6. Seibert FB. Fever-producing substance found in some distilled waters. Am J Physiol 1923; 67:90.
7. Banks HM. A study of hyperpyrexia reaction following intravenous therapy. Am J Clin Pathol 1934; 4:260.
8. Cherkin A. Destruction of bacterial endotoxin pyrogenicity by hydrogen peroxide. Biochemistry 1975; 12:625.
9. Novitsky TJ, Ryther SS, Case MJ. Depyrogenation by moist heat. PDA Technical Report No. 7: Depyrogenation, 1985:109–112.
10. Welch H, et al. The thermostabiity of pyrogens and their removal from penicillin. J Am Pharm Assoc 1945; 34:114.
11. Robertson JH, Gleason D, Tsuji K. Dry-heat destruction of lipopolysaccharide: design and construction of dry-heat destruction apparatus. Appl Environ Microbiol 1978; 36:705.
12. Tsuji K, Lewis AR. Dry-heat destruction of lipopolysaccharide: mathematical approach to process evaluation. Appl Environ Microbiol 1978; 36:710.
13. Tsuji K, Harrison SJ. *Limulus* amebocyte lysate-a means to monitor inactivation of lipopolysaccharide. In: Cohen E, ed. Biomedical Appzications of the Horseshoe Crab (Limulidae). New York: Alan R. Liss, 1979:367–378.
14. Groves FM, Groves MJ. Dry Heat Sterilization and Depyrogenation, in Encyclopedia of Pharmaceutical Technology, Swarbrick J, Boylan JC, eds. New York: Marcel Dekker Inc., 1991:447–484.
15. Akers MJ, Avis KE, Thompson B. Validation studies of the Fostoria infrared tunnel sterilizer. J Parenter Drug Assoc 1980; 34:330.
16. Akers MJ, Ketron KM, Thompson BR. F-value requirements for the destruc-tion of endotoxin in the valida-tion of dry heat terilization/depyrogenation cycles. J Parenter Drug Assoc 1982; 36:23.
17. Sweet BH, Huxsoll JF. Depyrogenation by Dry Heat. Parenteral Drug Association, Inc., PDA Technical Report No. 7 (chapter 12), 1985.
18. Brusch CW. Quality assurance for medical devices. In: Avis KE, Lieberman HA, Lachman L, eds. Pharmaceutical Dosage Forms, Parenteral Medications. New York: Dekker, 1993:487–526.
19. Berger TJ, et al. Biological indicator comparative analysis in various product formulations and closure sites. PDA J Pharm Sci Technol 2000; 54(2):101–109.
20. Finocchario CJ. The use of biological indicators as an affirmation of sterilization process effectiveness. Pharm Eng 1993; Jan/Feb:26–30.
21. Leahy TJ. Microbiology of sterilization processes. In: Carleton FJ, Agalloco JP, eds. Validation of Aseptic Pharmaceutical Processes. New York: Marcel Dekker Inc., 1999, 253–277.
22. Ludwig JD, Avis KE. Validation of a heating cell for precisely controlled studies on the thermal destruction of endotoxin in glass. J Parent Sci Techol 1988; 42(1):9–40.
23. Ludwig JD, Avis KE. Dry heat inactivation of endotoxin on the surface of glass. J Parent Sci Techol 1990; 44(1):4–12.
24. Berman D, et al. Cycle development criteria for removal of endotoxin by dilution from glassware. J Parent Sci Techol 1987; 41(5):158–163.
25. Hanna S. Quality assurance. In: Avis K, Lieberman H, Lachman L, eds. Pharmaceutical Dosage Forms: Parenteral Medications. New York: Marcel Dekker Inc., 19–16.
26. Agalloco J. Points to consider in the validation of equipment cleaning procedures. J Parent Sci Tech 1992; 46(5):163–168.
27. Berzofsky R, Scheible LS, Williams KL. Validation of endotoxin removal from parenteral vial *closures*. BioPharm 1994; June:58–66.
28. Shintani H, Akers J. On the cause of performance variation of biological indicators used for sterility assurance. PDA J Pharm Sci Techol 2000; 54(4):332–342.
29. Galanos C, et al. Biological activities of lipid A complexed with bovine serum albumins. Eur J Biochem 1972; 31:230.
30. Tripodi D, Nowotny A. Relative structures and functions in bacterial 0-antigens. V. Nature of active sites in endotoxin lipopolysaccharides of Serratia marcescens. Ann N Y Acad Sci 1966; 133:604.

31. Luderitz, et al. Lipid chemical structure and biologic activity. In: Kass EH, Wolff SM, eds. Bacterial Lipopolysaccharides. Chicago: University of Chicago Press, 1973.

32. Niwa M, et al. Alteration of physical, chemical, and biological properties of endotoxin by treatment with mild alkali. J Bacteriol 1969; 97:1069.

33. Neter E, et al. Studies of enterobacterial lipopoly-saccharides; effects of heat and chemicals on erythrocyte modifying antigenic, toxic and pyrogenic properties. J Immunol 1956; 76:377.

34. Schenck JR, et al. The enhancement of anti-body formation by *E. coli* lipopolysaccharide and detoxified derivative. J Immunol 1969; 102:1411.

35. Westphal O. Bacterial endotoxins. Int Arch Allergol Appl Immunol 1978; 74:1985.

36. Hort EC, Penfold WJ. Microorganisms and their relation to fever. J Hyg (Lond) 1912; 12:361.

37. Taub A, Hart F. Detoxification of pyrogens by hydrogen peroxide in some USP injections. J Am Pharm Assoc 1948; 37:246.

38. Menczel E. A note on the depyrogenation of infusion solutions by hydrogen peroxide. J Am Pharm Assoc 1951; 40:175.

39. DeRenzis FA. Endotoxin-inactivating potency of hydrogen peroxide: Effect on cell growth. J Dent Res 1981; 60:933.

40. Case MJ, Novitsky TJ. Depyrogenation by Hydrogen Peroxide. PDA Technical Report No. 7: Depyrogenation, 1985:84–92.

41. DeRenzis FA. Endotoxin-inactivating potency of molecular oxygen: Effect on cell growth. J Dent Res 1980; 59:1521.

42. Dean HR, Adamson RS. A method for the preparation of a nontoxic dysentery vaccine. B Med J 1916; 1:611.

43. Charomat R, Leehat P. Preparation of nonpyrogenic solutions. Ann Pharm Fr 1950; 8:171.

44. Goebel W. Studies on the Flexner group of dysentery bacilli. VI. The detoxification of Shigella paradysenteriae by means of periodic acid. J Exp Med 1947; 85:499.

45. Carter EB. A proposed chemical test for pyrogen in distilled water for intravenous injections. J Lab Clin Med 1930; 16:289.

46. Suzuki S. Preparation of nonpyrogenic drugs for injection. I. Removal of substances having positive reaction to tetrabromophenolphthalein ethyl ester by the usual re-fining process. J Pharm Soc Jpn 73:615.

47. Bertok L, Szeberenyi S. Effect of radiodetoxified endotoxin on the liver microsomal drug metabolizing enzyme system in rats. Immunopharmacol 1983; 6:1.

48. Csako G, et al. Physical and biological properties of U. S. Standard Endotoxin EC after exposure to ionizing radiation. Infect. Immunol 1983; 41:190.

49. Guyomard S, et al. Defining the pyrogenic assurance level (PAL) of irradiated medical devices. Int J Pharm 1987; 40:173–174.

50. Reid BD. Gamma processing technology: an alternative technology for terminal sterilization of parenterals, PDA J Pharm Sci Technol 1995; 49(2):83–89.

51. Csako G, Suba EA, Ahlgren A, Tsai CM, Elin RJ. Relation of structure to function for the U. S. reference standard endotoxin after exposure to 60Co radiation. J Infect Dis 1986; 153(1):98–108.

52. Butler T, Moller G. Mitogenic response of mouse spleen cells and gelation of Limulus lysate by lipopolysaccharide of Yersinia pestis and evidence for neutralization of the lipopolysaccharide by polymyxin B Infect Immunol 1977; 18:400.

53. Morrison DC, Curry BJ. The use of polymyxin B and C3H /HEJ mouse spleen cells as criteria for endotoxin contamination. J Immunol Methods 1979; 27:83.

54. Morrison DC, Jacobs DM. Binding of polymyxin B to the lipid A portion of bacterial lipopolysaccharides. Immunochem 1976; 13:813.

55. Cooperstock MS. Inactivation of endotoxin by polymyxin B. Antimicrob Agents Chemother 1974; 6:422.

56. Novitsky TJ, Case MJ. Inactivation of endotoxin by polymyxin B. PDA Technical Report No. 7: Depyrogenation, 1985:93–97.

57. Issekutz AC. Removal of Gram-negative endotoxin from solutions by affinity chromatography. J Immunol Methods 1983; 61:275.

58. Rickles FR, et al. Endotoxin contamination of biological reagents; detection and removal of endotoxin with Limulus amebocyte lysate. In: Cohen E, ed. Biomedical Applications of the Horseshoe Crab (Limulidae). New York: Alan R. Liss, 1979:203–207.
59. Nachum R, et al. Inactivation of endotoxin by Limulus amebocyte lysate. J Invert Pathol 1978; 32:51.
60. Genovesi CS. Validation of unique filtration processes. In: Carleton FJ, Agalloco JP, eds. Validation of Aseptic Pharmaceutical Processes. New York: Marcel Dekker Inc., 473–506.
61. Nelson LL. Removal of pyrogens from parenteral solutions by ultrafiltration. Pharm Technol 1978; 2(5):46.
62. Sweadner KJ, Forte M, Nelson LL. Filtration removal of endotoxin (pyrogens) in solution in different states of aggregation. Appl Environ Microbiol 1977; 34:382.
63. Henderson LW, Beans E. Successful production of sterile pyrogen-free electrolyte solution by ultrafiltration. Kindey Int 1978; 14:522.
64. Berger A, Ellenbogen GD, Ginger L. Pyrogens. Adv Chem 1956; 16:168.
65. Gemmell DH, Todd JP. Activated carbon for pharmaceutical purposes. Pharm J 1945; 154:126.
66. Brindle H, Rigby G. Preparation of nonpyrogenic water and infusion fluids, using activated charcoal. Pharm J 1946; 157:85.
67. Kaden H. The use of asbestos filter beds in the production of sterile and pyrogen-free solutions. Pharmazie 1975; 30:752.
68. Koppensteiner G, et al. An experimental investigation of the elimination of pyrogens from parenteral medicines. Drugs Made Ger 1976; 19:113.
69. Gerba CP, et al. Pyrogen control by depth filtration. Pharm Technol 1980; 83:83–88.
70. Reichelderfer PS, et al. Reduction of endotoxin levels in influenza virus vaccines by barium sulfate adsorption-elution. Appl Environ Microbiol 1975; 30:892.
71. Nolan JP, McDevitt JJ, Goldmann GS. Endotoxin binding by charged and uncharged resins. Proc Soc Exp Biol Med 1975; 149:766.
72. Polmer CHR, Whittet TD. The removal of pyrogenicity from solutions of purified pyrogens and tap waters using ion exchange resins. Chem Ind 1971; (341).
73. Harris NS, Feinstein R. The LAL bead asay for endotoxin. In: Cohen E, ed. Biomedical Application of the Horseshoe Crab (Limulidae). New York: Alan R. Liss, 1979:265–274.
74. Robinson JR, et al. Depyrogenation by microporous membrane filters. PDA Monograph on Depyrogenation, 1985.
75. Minobe S, et al. Characteristics of immobilized histamine for pyrogen adsorption. J Chromatogr 1983; 262:193–198.
76. Alpert G, et al. Limulus antilipopolysaccharide factor protects rabbits from meningococcal endotoxin shock. J Infect Dis 1992; 165:494–500.
77. Wainwright NR, et al. Endotoxin Binding and neutralizing activity by a protein from Limulus polyphemus. In: Nowotny A, Spitzer JJ, Ziegler EJ, eds. Cellular and Molecular Aspects of Endotoxin Reactions. Amsterdam: Elsevier Science Publishers, 1990:315–325.
78. Held DD, et al. Endotoxin reduction in macromolecular solutions: two case studies. BioPharm 1977; March:32–37.
79. Belanich M, et al. Reduction of endotoxin in a protein mixture using strong anion-exchange membrane absorption. Pharm Technol 1996; March:142–150.
80. Williams KL. Differentiating endotoxin removal from inactivation in vial component depyrogenation validation. Pharm Technol 1995; 19(10):72–84.

16

Automation, Process Analytical Technology, and Prospective Testing

Kevin L. Williams

Eli Lilly & Company, Indianapolis, Indiana, U.S.A.

The simply stated solution [to] most assay related problems is to build better assays from the beginning. The question is: how does one achieve better assays without a concomitant increase in time and cost of repeat testing?

OVERVIEW

Automation of the bacterial endotoxin test (BET) may allow for the reduction of the variability associated with the kinetic *Limulus* amebocyte lysate (LAL) test. The gel-clot assay, though it has been automated in some past efforts, remains for most practical purposes, like *Limulus* itself, unchanged. However, from another vantage, one can see that the kinetic and end point tests are really semi-automated extensions of the original gel-clot assay. Automation removes many common operator associated real-world challenges faced by analysts in preparing products for test via robotic preparation. Automation should provide answers to users common concerns such as:

1. Did I add the spike?
2. Did I vortex that tube?
3. (phone rings . . .) Where was I? Diluting the second or third standard?

Automation may add complexity or induce the possibility of mechanical error. The user's questions may become:

1. What was that noise? (e.g., collision error)
2. Who is going to perform the preventative maintenance (PM) this quarter and what tests should be used to gauge potentially complex systems?
3. Is it worth running those five samples robotically (high test process threshold)?

Process analytical technology (PAT) has been embraced by the Food and Drug Administration (FDA) as a means of assuring the quality of manufacturing processes and decreasing reliance on end product testing, which is statistically less likely to detect defects, in this case a loss of endotoxin control. A couple of PAT test systems have been introduced recently which seek to address water testing for endotoxin control at the source of its preparation.

BACTERIAL ENDOTOXIN TEST AUTOMATION GOALS AND PROCESS
Goals

The goal of automation is to reduce assay variability and to free users for other tasks, including supervising the robotic operation and ensuring the proper documentation and reporting of the test results. A benefit can also be expected in removing users from the hazards of repetitive motion stress injury. It is commonly believed that automated methods should increase the test's sensitivity and provide faster results, whereas in truth, automated assays are limited by the same method mechanism as their manual counterparts (1). However, automation may:

1. reduce variability associated with multiple users,
2. consolidate test equipment and consumables, thereby increasing user control over these items from a variability and qualification/maintenance perspective (e.g., a robot may replace the use of a dozen or so manual pipettes which each require their own PM procedures and associated documentation),
3. consolidate test result documentation and reporting,
4. remove users from potential long-term repetitive motion injury hazards such as carpel tunnel syndrome associated with manual tasks. Carpal tunnel has proven to be a significant problem associated with the use of manual pipettes.

Perhaps, the most persuasive driver of automation is the elimination of reruns due to failed system suitability parameters (not an out of specification result) such as standard curve, sample percent coefficient of variation (%CVs), curve linearity, or slope recoveries, or those due to extraneous user or environmental contamination (hot wells). In the latter case, the robotic preparation removes the user (a microbiological unknown) and substitutes a controlled environment around the instrument (i.e., via filtered air and wiping down the area regularly with a bleach solution). Because LAL reagents are expensive, the cost of rerunning an entire plate can be substantial if it happens on a regular basis. A qualified robot should avoid such reruns.

Viewing Variability in Process

It is interesting to view the entire LAL test system as a process whether looking to automate or not. The variability associated with the kinetic BET can be a cause of frustration. Generally, the source of variability resides:

1. in assays for substances that retain a degree of interference that has not been eliminated by the method developed,
2. inherently in the LAL test method including reagents, pipettes, labware, etc.,
3. and in the linear regression (LR) standard curve plot and resultant sample extrapolation.

McCullough and Weidner-Loeven (2) list four common sources of variability in the LAL test: reagent, method, product, and laboratory. LAL extraction procedures, although similar, are proprietary but can be expected to differ in buffering capacity and divalent cation content. Such formulation differences are a source of variability, particularly when comparisons are made between different manufacturers. It is common for users to validate an alternate test if the positive product control (PPC) recoveries begin to fail their system suitability requirements, presumably due to lot-to-lot changes in LAL over time. McCullough gives examples of gel-clot 2λ (two lambda) spike recoveries of "product X" in different noninhibitory concentration (NIC) assays using different manufacturer's LAL reagents. The test shows a >100-fold difference in the dilution required to overcome interference (i.e., one recovered at 1:10, whereas the other did not recover even at 1:1000).

There is no claim to comparability of interference patterns between LAL methods (gel-clot vs. kinetic chromogenic, for instance).

Product variability, of course, will depend upon the quality of the assay developed given the specific interference problem(s). Indicative of the quality of the assay developed is the recovery of the 2λ spike in the gel-clot assay and the difference from 100% recovery in the kinetic assays. Ultimately, the recovery of the product spike will depend upon the degree to which interference factor(s) have been overcome. The *United States Pharmacopoeia* (USP)/FDA Guideline three-lot validation requirement may not always demonstrate that a method is inadequate, and it is prudent to test additional validation lots where interference is suspected to be lurking in valid recoveries. Evidence of lurking interference may be seen in the form of (*i*) recoveries at the edge of the allowable range (50% and 200%), (*ii*) in divergent recoveries (>25% difference), or (*iii*) in cases where one lot shows significant but acceptable interference when compared with the others.

Lot-to-lot variability in a parenteral product, active pharmaceutical ingredient, or excipient (salt or cation content, etc.) and even container presentation are causes of lot-to-lot assay variability. Lab variability is introduced by minute differences in analyst technique (pipetting), dilution schemes (with the recommended dilutions each being 1:10 or less), labware (consumables), sample storage, spiking method (plate vs. tube), or water quality [particularly with lower lambda tests as USP rated water is labeled <0.25 endotoxin unit (EU)/mL whereas lambda may be as low as <0.005 EU/mL].

Deming, an expert whose work has been credited with much of Japan's quality improvements in the 1980s, demonstrates the importance of an overall process in determining the results that come from that process (3). Addressing the variability of a given system, Deming uses an enacted skit shown below to make a point about variability as it relates to a process. In his seminars, Deming would use the "red bead" demonstration to show that systems, not individual workers, produce products and services and that the individuals can only produce as desired in tandem with the system of which they are a part. Gabor (3) describes the red bead demonstration that Deming often gave in his quality seminars:

> A vessel contains a total of 4000 beads, 3200 white and 800 red. Deming in his new role as foreman explains how the work (of producing only white beads) is done, using a paddle with 50 depressions in it. "Why are there fifty holes in the paddle?" he asks. "One for each bead," volunteers one of the Willing Workers (from the audience). "There's a better reason," says Deming sternly. "Why are there fifty holes in the paddle? Because there are five in one direction and ten in the other." (The audience laughs loudly.) "We understand our business here. We know what it is. Our procedures are absolutely fixed, no departures."
>
> Deming demonstrates the (worker's) procedure. When he pulls the paddle out of the bin, there are some red beads mixed in with the white. Says the guru. "I've purposely drawn some red beads so you'll know what they look like." (Again, loud laughter from the audience.) "You'll carry them over to inspector number one, who will make a count in silence and record it on paper. Next, inspector number two will count and put it on paper. The chief inspector is responsible for the count. If they differ, there may be a mistake. If they agree there must be a mistake. The chief inspector is responsible." Twice during the exercise, the "inspectors" fail to agree on the count, demonstrating the folly of relying on inspection as a means of quality control.
>
> When "production begins, worker after worker is derided for getting red beads mixed in with the white beads (using the demonstrated paddle method). Those who do

best (five reds) are rewarded with merit increases, and those who do worst (eleven reds) are dismissed. When the workers fail in their task. Deming (in his role) always has an answer as to what they did wrong: "you didn't agitate for five seconds, axis horizontal, forty-four degrees, follow the procedures." Willing Worker attrition is high as, naturally, workers are unable to get out only white beads by the prescribed method.

At the end of the production run, Deming plots the results of the process control chart. Low and behold, the system is in control; that is, the system is functioning in a stable manner, given the materials, tools, and procedures that define the process. The reason for the defects is inherent to the process: they have nothing to do with external circumstances (worker's technique).

There are a number of ways the production of red beads could be minimized, but none of them is within the control of the Willing Workers. One way would be to make sure that there are fewer red beads (or defectives) coming from the supplier in the first place. Only management can change that by either switching suppliers or working with the existing supplier to improve the quality of its production. Another way would be to give each worker a pair of tweezers to systematically pick out only the white beads. Again, its up to the management to furnish the tweezers and the new work rules.

In the spirit of Deming, the BET assay may be viewed as a system with isolated subsystems, some of which the users have control over and some over which they do not (Fig. 1). Deming's summary of a poor test system may be read in a humorous light, but to those who have been trained in the LAL gel-clot and kinetic methods (to a lesser degree the kinetic assay) for components, and in-process samples, the story is somewhat less humorous.

A robot can aid in reducing assay variability by standardizing the 1000 small things a user does (often unconsciously) in preparing an assay.

1. Glass and plastic consumables used by the robot are often limited by what fits, thereby reducing what can be used to one or at best a couple of acceptable versions of troughs, reagent containers, tips, etc.

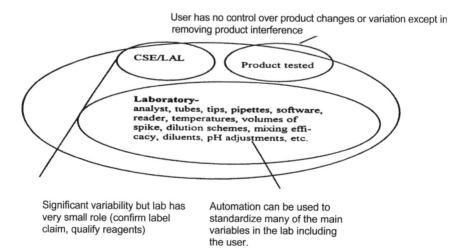

FIGURE 1 Known bacterial endotoxin test (kinetic) universe. User has no control over product changes or variation except in removing product interference.

2. Spiking and mixing, the robot is programmed to do it the same way again and again.
3. Programmed dilution schemes will not vary.
4. Timing of LAL addition, plate to reader addition, and assay initiation are constant.
5. Pipette tools are the same as is the method of dispensation (blowout, to contain, or to deliver).
6. Tips are prewetted (as needed)
7. "Total test variability is additive and may be the result of a number of subtle differences in reagent formulation and use, test method, product specifications, or laboratory procedures. Laboratory analysts, supervisors, and managers must be aware of these variables" (2).

It stands to reason that small labs may actually have an advantage in controlling assay variability due to fewer users, limited use of equipment, etc.

Bacterial Endotoxin Test Automation Shortcomings

The problems associated with automating the test often lies in the difficulty in obtaining an adequate mix of the control standard endotoxin (CSE), which is manually achieved by vortexing. Aspiration is used in lieu of vortexing, which requires the user to show that an adequate mix is achieved. The CSE in water constantly clings to the glass or plastic container or aggregates due to its hydrophobic nature. The following is a list of automation caveats, some of which have been partially or completely overcome since 2001 when the 2nd edition of this book was published.

1. Lack of "wildcard" software capability with available instruments was a problem when the previous edition of this book was written. However, now there are several commercial systems on the market that have addressed it, albeit with "custom" fitting of the software to the user's particular dilution scheme required. The wildcard problem as an "out-of-the-box" solution can be described as the capability to program an instrument to perform specific dilutions by the user simply by adding the appropriate dilution factor for each sample.
2. Lack of good manufacturing practices (GMPs) quality control related issues has similarly been overcome in the past five years, including password protection and suitable out-of-the-box robotic user interface for GMP applications. The necessity of addressing the FDA CFR Part 11 requirements have brought pressure to bear in meeting the software security challenges.
3. The more complete the automation solution, the more difficult the timing issues become: the pre-incubation of plates, LAL addition (especially in light of the fact that it must be reconstituted and refrigerated prior to use), and assay initiation must be rapid. Since the LAL/endotoxin reaction is optimum at 37°C and the fact that the temperature must be strictly maintained ($\pm 1^\circ$C) at that temperature, robotic activities must occur in a manner to prevent cooling of pre-incubated plates (i.e., the LAL must be added and the plate initiated in a time comparable to hand addition). Developers are limited by the fact that the reaction begins when the LAL contacts the sample and any associated delay will reduce the reaction times obtained for samples and standards. Any great disparity created between the addition of LAL to the initial wells (typically the standards) and the later wells (typically samples) may skew the results if the samples contain endotoxin and may affect the spike recoveries even if they do not.

4. User acceptance: people are always behind robotic activities; the manufacturer, user, or application developer bears the responsibility for robotic malfunction. Presumably, points of consideration that may appear relatively small to a developer may be viewed as critical omissions in the overall acceptance of the tool for everyday use (1). Therefore, if the developer and the end user are not the same group (in-house), then the users should be consulted as to the proposed automated process design. Some sticking points may include containers and racks to house samples, CSE, and LAL preparations and, importantly, the user-friendliness of the robotic user interface. The documentation requirements should ideally be simplified by the employment of a robotic system but in reality may create additional documentation layers as redundant precautions are enacted.
5. The availability of appropriate consumables: (endotoxin-free, noninterfering plastic, etc.) also may frustrate efforts to develop an optimum system if a dependable supply of such tools cannot be relied upon. Custom or unusual containers may require custom robotic holders be created. A complete listing and discussion of such potential problems may be found in Craig and Hoheisel's (4). The authors discuss in detail the documentation, user expectations, errors, resources, metrics, personnel concerns, etc., and remind the reader that the expectation that automated systems offer the advantage of greater precision and accuracy than manual systems is a misconception (p. 129). What automated systems are designed to bring about is the reduction of variability associated with interoperator assay performance. The discussion is refreshing in its candor and the fact that it addresses the most complex interface of the robotic user.
6. A rarely explored area of opportunity in automation involves the use of "robot-ready" sample collection. The difficulty arises if the submitting area and the testing area are different groups of individuals/departments. Great gains could be realized if sampling vessels could be used directly on the robot. However, often the area that realizes the gain is not the area that feels the pain of the sampling container change and or sampling change.
7. PAT, as discussed subsequently, can address this latter point in that the most efficient test is that performed at the sampling site. The FDA has encouraged the development of such "rapid methods" in their GMPs for the 21st Century document.

Computer System Validation Overview

The necessity of computer system validation (CSV) was brought about by the FDA's August 1997 electronic record and signature regulation in 21 CFR Part 11. CSV was already an expectation before that time but the scope of the 1997 requirements caught many by surprise in that they went far beyond what was previously required (5). At this time, much of the industry was focussed on the so-called Y2K problem. This was followed by the September 2001 draft outline on FDA expectations in regard to 21 CFR Part 11 for computer system and software validation. According to Huber (5), a "system" combines components such as a computer and a method. This is true in kinetic BET testing. The validation of the system is required even though each component had some in-house validation or may come with validation documentation from the vendor. The proper installation and suitable interaction of the system components (with the user's method) is

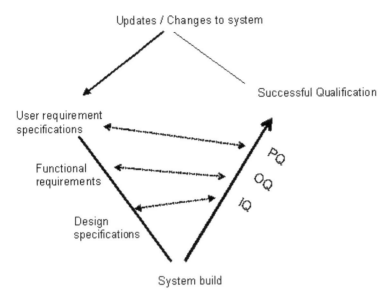

FIGURE 2 Life cycle model. Horizontal lines indicate relationships. *Abbreviations*: IQ, installation qualification; OQ, operational qualification; PQ, performance qualification. *Source*: From Ref. 5.

typically performed and documented in an installation qualification, operational qualification, and performance qualification [see Fig. 2 derived from Huber's book (p. 37)]. The diagram shows the inter-relationship of CSV (not a typical lab function) to 3Q testing which is typically performed by the lab users. Note that the left side of the chart is largely set by the software manufacturers and understood and documented subsequently by the installer's CSV, whereas the right side is more familiar to users as more related to the application as it is used. Fortunately, for GMP users, manufacturers have built-in 21 CFR Part 11 compliance in the software applications with appropriate security measures including extensive password protections, different user access levels, data archiving, and auditing capabilities. The software and hardware also include built-in tests to check the suitability of the mechanical operation (uniformity, system self-test, etc.). Additional complexity has been added recently with the advent of "networkable" software [e.g., ACC's (East Falmouth, Massachusetts, USA) KC4[TM] Signature software[a] or Cambrex's (East Rutherford, New Jersey, USA) WinKQCL[TM] ver. 3.0] in which a copy resides on the server and each client PC with attached reader also contains a copy of the software. The data generated at the client PCs can be accessed from any computer with access to the server for viewing the data generated, second person verification, e-signature release, and printing. The CSV complexities multiply with the addition of the server application.

COMMERCIALLY AVAILABLE UNITS

Most of the published BET automation projects in the past 20 years involve some common activities. Typically, either the kinetic turbidimetric or the chromogenic assays are automated due to the advantages associated with them. The activities

---

[a]Trademark of Bio-Tek Instruments, Inc.

common to modern LAL automation instrumentation provided by Charles River Laboratories (CRL) and Cambrex include the following robotic functions. In this regard they closely mimic what is performed by hand during kinetic testing.

1. Serial dilution of a standard curve from a CSE solution (lyophilized and mixed or as liquid CSE not requiring mixing as in the case of Cambrex's Pyrosense™ rFC robot).
2. Serial dilution of test samples from liquid or reconstituted solid samples or testing undiluted samples (e.g., water).
3. Direct robotic spiking of endotoxin standard into the microtiter plate(s) (PPCs).
4. The plated samples are preincubated (37°C) and lysate is added robotically at the end of the ten-minute incubation period.
5. The data are recorded by the analyzing software for LR or other analysis and data reporting.

The Cambrex LAL system, called Auto-LAL™, was developed using the Biomek 2000™ platform with a BioTek™ reader attached to the workstation (6). The two proprietary programs developed by Cambrex, the kinetic reader software WinKQCL (used also in a stand-alone fashion with a typical plate reader) and the Beach™ program which serves as the user's interface with the robot were the software used. The microtiter plate is filled with sample dilutions, spike, and LAL reagent while residing in the plate reader. The door automatically responds as needed to aid in maintaining the desired plate temperature (37°C) prior to assay incubation. The Biomek 2000 platform is particularly well suited for multiple sample testing that does not require a wide variety of dilution factors and diluents in that it automates the route tasks of sample addition, spiking, curve preparation, and plating, thus reducing the most common causes of retesting samples (i.e., system suitability failures). The CRL employs two different Tecan™ robots to provide varying degrees of automation and customization as determined by the user's needs.

A Custom-Fitted Application Example

The Lilly laboratory has a history of automation efforts using the Beckman-Coulter (Fullerton, California, USA) Biomek 2000 platform (7,8). The most recent application is a simplistic robot employing "robot-ready" testing of water samples in the same containers in which they arrive (Fig. 3). This application design simply seeks high throughput and low user interaction due to the large quantity of water samples received. Sampling sites could not send capped tubes due to the size of the sampling spigots; the robot, therefore, was customized with holders for the water containers they were sent in, specifically the 25 cm^2 Corning culture flasks (item number 430168) which come depyrogenated and are made of nonreactive polystyrene. Forty-four of the flasks fit on the workstation per run and are added to two 96 well plates with standard curve and spikes in duplicate. The run takes approximately 15 minutes and during this time the user may be creating the reader template necessary when the plates are ready.

Perhaps, the most critical aspect of automating the kinetic LAL assay is found in obtaining a good mix of the CSE. The Beckman-Coulter platform is well suited for the degree of liquid mixing needed to adequately prepare the CSE due to (*i*) the velocity of the air displacement, (*ii*) the large volumes it is capable of

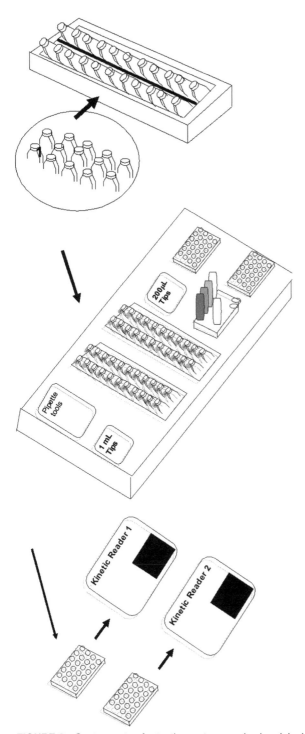

FIGURE 3 Custom setup for testing water samples in original containers.

aspirating and dispensing (up to 1000 μL), and (*iii*) the very small opening in the tip that the liquid is forced through (~1 mm). The coefficients of correlation for the robotic assays are almost invariably −1.000. Beckman-Coulter also makes available the tips, troughs, and other consumables needed with a certificate of analysis certifying that they are endotoxin-free, which is an essential convenience.

VIEWING KINETIC DATA

Similar to automation is the activity of developing alternative ways to view kinetic data (i.e., use of alternative software to view data, for instance) or software customization utilized to process data.

The Bow in the Curve

The use of polynomial regression (PR) analysis has gained a foothold recently in LAL testing due to a general sense that the error associated with the %PPC in many instances can be great (i.e., when $r = <1.0$). Given that the line created and used as a reference to extrapolate unknown values from may not touch the actual data points generated, the phenomenon has been described as the "bow" in the LR curve (Fig. 4). A statistician who examined some kinetic data casually believed that the data may actually be better observed as two separate linear lines (H. Du, personal communication, 2000); however, such a prospect would have no current acceptable application due to FDA linear or PR requirements.

The best LR lines are, of course, linear ($r = -1.000$) and have steep slopes (i.e., are more negative as -0.220 is steeper than -0.180). The slope of the standard curve affects the precision of the assay in that small variations in kinetic reaction times

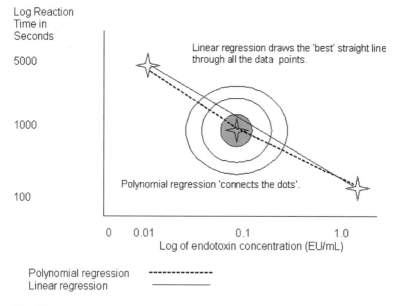

FIGURE 4   Diagram of the phenomenon referred to as the "bow in the curve."

(on the Y-axis) become large variations in predicted EUs on the X-axis if the slope of the line is not sufficiently steep (R. Berzofsky, personal communication, 1995). Also affecting the apparent %CV of results is the software method used to calculate those %CVs. At least two different methods are currently employed in kinetic software. One method examines the differences in the raw optical density values obtained and the other uses the data after it has been extrapolated against the standard curve. The latter method results in %CV values that are much larger (i.e., more variable) than the former. Users should be aware of these differences when setting %CV specifications for standards and samples and in comparing manual to robotic variation, particularly when comparing data generated by readers that differ in the means of determining the %CV. In cases where both methods are used in a lab, (or between labs) it can create the illusion that one set of data is better or "tighter" than the other.

Polynomial Regression

The ability to readily develop an endotoxin assay can be punctuated with a variety of confounding factors including drug compound interference, method variability, instrument problems, operator problems, reagent problems or significant common cause, and/or special cause variability of both known and unknown origin. Today's development compounds run the gamut from biological compounds that have some ability to mimic endotoxin activity in the LAL assay to extremely "chemical" substances affectionately known in the lab as "gasoline."

LAL manufacturers have done an excellent job of controlling the variability associated with endotoxin (the proverbial "can of worms") standard curves and the LAL material as a crab blood derivative, but the basic math (LR) behind the kinetic standard curve contains inherent variability. Consider the following couple of scenarios as examples of inherently poor data to (standard) curve correlation:

Scenario 1

An analyst runs a standard curve in LAL reagent water (LRW) and runs a LRW "sample" with an associated PPC spike. The analyst gets a good coefficient of correlation of 0.998 and excellent %CVs of <1.0% for all standards and samples, but the %PPC recovery of the LRW "sample" is 122%, which seems poor given that this is the same CSE and sterile water as is used to make the standard curve.

Question

Why does the midpoint of the standard curve (MPSC) value differs from the same endotoxin in the same water by 22%?

Answer

Let us say the MPSC for Scenario 1 is 0.5 EU/mL and the associated reaction time is 1200 seconds. The LRW sample average spike reaction time is also 1200 seconds. There is a seeming contradiction: 1200 seconds equals 1200 seconds but 100% does not equal 122%. There must be an error in the software calculations. Unfortunately, there is not: 100 may indeed equal 122 by LR. Remember, in this example, there is no TRUE inhibition or enhancement because the sample and standard are the same thing (CSE in water).

Perhaps, a development compound was tested by a method that perfectly matched in reaction time the recovery of the 0.5 EU/mL standard and PPC, but is still being penalized (in this example, by 22%) because: LR does not draw a straight line through the MPSC. This is common knowledge to most analysts, but seldom are we confronted with such a stark example of what the "bow in the curve" means. After all, what more can a method developer do than perfectly match the sample recovery to CSE recovery in LRW? Indeed, the only way to improve Scenario 1 would be to introduce some interference into the sample test in order to cancel out the error of the LR line (which would certainly come back to haunt one later).

A formula should be developed that forces the plot through the all important MPSC. And indeed it has been. Simply stated, PR draws the standard curve line through the dots formed by the standard curve points rather than forming a "best fit" straight line through the dots. Each vendor supplies software now that contains a PR analysis capability along with appropriate software precautions to prevent its misuse (i.e., an internal software requirement that the FDA requirement for linearity is met prior to the use of any gathered data for the purpose of drawing a PR curve).

Scenario 2

An analyst tests development compound "X" by a kinetic assay and again gets a good coefficient of correlation (0.998) and excellent %CVs (<1.0%) for all standards and samples, but the %PPC recovery of the sample is only 45%. Making the appropriate sample treatment adjustments, the analyst returns to the reader and obtains a spike recovery value of 65% the second time around.

Questions

Has the method adjustment made by the analyst (*i*) helped the sample spike recovery effort, (*ii*) hurt the sample spike recovery effort, or (*iii*) provided enough relevant information to determine if the method has really been incrementally improved by the given sample treatment?

Answer

Given the error associated with the sterile water assay in Scenario 1, it becomes obvious that in the situation posed by Scenario 2 few conclusions can be drawn as to the "better" PPC recovery (i.e., 45% or 65%).

The uninspiring results in Scenario 2 raise perhaps a more relevant method development question when using LR: How close in seconds is the PPC recovery to the sample irrespective of the "best fit" curve? Is there an easy way to know if the 65% recovery is indeed any better than the 45% recovery[b]? Given the availability of the PR, one need not rely on "eyeballing" the values obtained by LR. PR performs the math and readily answers the question in a scientific and systematic way. PR removes the bow from the curve and, therefore, draws the standard curve line directly through the MPSC.

Polynomial Regression Caveats

There are some issues remaining to be addressed with the use of PR for end product release testing that may limit its use, including

1. the views of various international regulatory bodies on the use of PR, as no mention of it is made in the harmonized chapter,
2. internal corporate issues: policy and procedures must be defined as a lab cannot have it both ways and only use the PR model if it helps bring the %PPC for a given sample closer to 100% recovery,
3. the incorporation of PR may increase or even decrease the % recovery of items historically validated and successfully tested by LR.

---

[b]Before deciding upon the next assay attempt, it is helpful to determine whether there has been an incremental improvement in what has already been done (i.e., are we going in the right direction?) or if the two results are really mathematically indistinguishable given the limitations of linear regression.

For domestic end product testing (PR has been approved for use by the FDA), method development work, water testing, in-process testing, and component testing, the use of PR is helpful and provides, in some cases, a more meaningful way to view the data. The utility of the PR of course will diminish with increasing linearity of the standard curve, but seemingly small variations from complete linearity can produce exaggerated effects on the stated %PPC recovery (as seen in Scenario 1).

PR provides a method development tool to help determine when interference has been overcome completely (i.e., the variability that remains is inherent in the LR standard curve). In Scenario 1, it would be wise to accept the 22% variability rather than trying to improve on an assay that, in reality, neither inhibits nor enhances the recovery of CSE. Conversely, PR also reveals when a method is dependent upon the nonlinear (LR) curve to achieve the desired spike recovery range (i.e., poor recovery is being made to look better than it is by the error in the standard curve), thus alerting an analyst that perhaps the assay should be improved upon [for another discussion on "Curved versus Straight" standard curves, see (9)].

Given Scenarios #1 and #2, the most basic method development question asked as the test began was: "What is the %PPC recovery?" but has now ended up being: "Does the sample interfere with the absolute recovery of sample spike as determined by comparing the sample spike recovery to the middle standard curve point (not line)?" or more simply stated: "What is the PR %PPC recovery?"

At the risk of belaboring the point, the LR line begs the question: What is the sample PPC trying to prove? Namely, that the sample containing 0.5 EU/mL actually recovers 0.5 EU/mL. Why have an entire curve at all if one is only going to reference the one midpoint? Any given answer must be extrapolated over an established range that can only be of value if the range is linear or "extrapolatable." The regulatory answer is two-fold in that (*i*) the requirement for linearity of the standard curve that brackets every log increase in the curve requires at least three points (as per FDA Guideline) to be a valid curve and only then can the data be viewed in a polynomial light within a valid perspective and (*ii*) the opposite is also true in that if consistency of standard curves is demonstrated, then standard curves may be archived (not run but recalled from a previous assay) and a single point included as a control (as per the 1987 FDA Guideline).

In-Plate Spike Caveat

A caveat may be inserted here concerning the use of spikes directly added to a plate. If the prediluted samples are subjected to harsh conditions (chemical or physical), then the validation should include spikes that have been subjected to the same conditions as the samples. In this manner, if CSE is reduced by the harsh treatment, then the method may be destroying endotoxin as a function of the method. This situation must be addressed, as the goal of testing is to detect endotoxin and not treat the sample so that endogenous endotoxin cannot be recovered. Spiking directly into the plate will not provide a test of such conditions.

DEVELOPING A BETTER TOOLBOX

Given the increasing availability of laboratory robotics for BET, it is useful to discuss the potential benefits that robotic assay development may provide over the traditional assay development process. Typically, method development of a

BET for a novel development compound proceeds in a trial error fashion by the parameters outlined in the FDA's Guideline on Validation of the *Limulus* Amebocyte Lysate Test as an End Product Endotoxin Test for Human and Animal Parenteral Drugs, Biological Products, and Medical Devices (1). "Trial and error" here means testing a compound based upon some preliminary observations such as solubility and pH characteristics. A product will be reconstituted if it is a solid and diluted in a series of two-fold dilutions in water if it is water soluble and tested in a NIC test to determine an appropriate dilution for inhibition/enhancement testing given the maximum valid dilution (MVD) restraints with a chosen LAL sensitivity. Enhancement occurs if the PPCs recover significantly more endotoxin than that has been added; inhibition occurs when an analyst cannot recover the (2λ gel-clot or, alternatively, the MPSC spikes for kinetic) spikes added to the product dilution series within a reasonable level, $\pm 50\%$ at a dilution relevant to the MVD. Note that the harmonized BET chapter now allows for a 50% to 200% range. If the product contains endotoxin, it may be advantageous to remove it for validation purposes prior to validation, and if the product is small enough, it can be passed through a filter or otherwise it may be removed by a binding removal method. This discussion provides the background for follow up by the PAT section.

With interfering compounds, the process must be repeated until sufficient parameter changes (diluent type, LAL/CSE type, LAL lambda, dilution factor, etc.) allow good recovery of the spikes without recovery in the nonspiked serial dilutions. In simpler terms: a good assay is one that gives back no more or no less CSE than that has been added. Such testing proceeds step by step, chronologically, until an acceptable test is obtained. In small labs with few parenteral products, the proposal to automate the development of the BET may appear to be a great luxury, almost superfluous; however, in a lab with many compounds and a very active development program (i.e., compounds always in flux), testing the many drug candidates (many which will not survive to market) in a timely manner can be taxing given that many of the compounds have never been tested before and may have (several) interference problems to be resolved.

The development of a new assay for the BET for a given compound may be as simple as:

1. calculating the new product's proposed tolerance limit and MVD based upon the clinical dose of the material,
2. diluting the material in sterile reagent water, and
3. testing it by either the gel-clot, end point, or kinetic (turbidimetric or chromogenic) method at a dilution below the MVD.

However, it seems that the days of simplistic validations have passed given the complex nature of modern drugs (i.e., Biologics). More and more compounds have complex mitigating factors seemingly designed to frustrate assay development efforts. Such factors may include:

i.   products with poor solubility in water (the LAL reaction is a water based reaction); including time release parenteral formulations (10),
ii. prospective products that are so expensive that product development scientists are reluctant to supply sufficient quantities for protracted method development and validation,
iii. products with multiple interference properties not overcome by simple dilution,

iv. products with tiny MVDs that do not allow for significant dilution as a means of overcoming interference,

v. products that either contain (low) levels of endotoxin or that have the ability to mimic endotoxin in the LAL reaction,

vi. products that once validated do not stay validated; i.e., the lot-to-lot variability (of either the product or the LAL reagent) of the reaction with the LAL assay is not sufficiently resolved with the requisite three validation lots.

The simply stated solution to most assay-related problems is to build better assays from the beginning. The question is: How does one achieve better assays without a concomitant increase in time and cost of repeat testing?

Most laboratories have a reserve of development "tools" in their "toolbox" that they use over and over in somewhat of a hopscotch manner to arrive at an acceptable LAL test. The choice of the tool to use next is subject to an educated guess based upon past experience or, at worst, a random selection given a lack of understanding of a product's particular characteristics and/or a lack of previous test history. Therefore, there is an art to assay development. In order to treat assay development as a science, to save on assay costs, and to cut the time needed to develop an assay, development scientists should gain as much information about a given product prior to testing it, particularly development compounds that have not been characterized as marketed products. Robotic method development could achieve, in theory, the systematic application of one's available tools to overcome inevitable interference problems due to a number of mechanisms (pH, insolubility, cation depletion, etc.). Given that the attempt to predict interference effects are often spotty at best due to the complex interaction of sample, CSE, and LAL, making sample treatment predictions difficult, one must learn to apply the best tools to give the best assay possible. Cooper's paper (11) on the causes of endotoxin recovery interference mechanisms is must reading and serves to demonstrate the complexity, multiplicity, and confounding nature of factors that may be encountered.

Experimental design has been widely used to reveal the best method for subsequent development by combining the extreme ends (high and low) of a given method to predict trends and test a wider range of possibilities than traditional trial and error testing. The goal in any initial testing is the same: to collect information-rich data (1). The same principles can be loosely applied to LAL assay development in an effort to find the best assay given the use of a wide number of readily available tools. For example, if compound X is tested in three different diluents with the third test giving acceptable results, then one is tempted to stop and validate two more lots to meet the FDA requirements on LAL Validation (12). However, since one has only tried methods A, B, and C, one does not know that a much better method does not lie down the road (for instance, at K). An assumption of prospective assay development of a robotic method development screening assay is that a detailed preliminary screening assay can be performed, then one may start with a better method than one ended with by the traditional method development process. This is not an approach that uses experimental design, but it is an attempt as Haaland (1) says to "increase the information content of the data." Haaland calls the nonstatistical experimental approach the "one-variable-at-a-time" approach and "if there are interactions among the variables the 'one-at-a-time' method may miss the solution because it doesn't thoroughly explore the space of possible solutions." The interrelation of LAL screening, verification of the method found (i.e., seemingly best method can be reproduced), and validation [three exemplary tests as per FDA Guideline (13)] can be seen in his mountain-climbing analogy.

> A useful analogy to the idea of iterative problem solving is climbing a mountain. For example, we don't want to expend most of our resources just getting to the base camp. At timely intervals, we want to evaluate whether or not the current direction is leading us toward the summit. Different climbing strategies are required for the final ascent to the summit than for earlier stages of the climb. In this context, screening experiments help us identify plausible directions to climb in order to reach the summit, optimization experiments are the ascent to the summit, and verification experiments prove we were there (1).

The goal in developing a robotic screening assay for (particularly development) parenteral drug compounds then becomes the creation of an automated assay that, with some of the following characteristics:

1. Offers a wide range of dilution factors,
2. Accesses a wide variety of interchangeable diluents for each sample to be tested,
3. Creates robotic programs with the flexibility to test several different user-defined parameters for multiple samples (i.e., perhaps a program for "insolubles" and another for acidic or basic compounds, etc.).

Admittedly, these are ambitious goals given the variability that can occur in an already developed method. But the rewards to the area can be envisioned to include:

1. Compiling method development tests into a single (or double) assay report from which a validation test may be selected. Previously, for products that are difficult to validate, one may end up with a thick and confusing file
2. Providing faster turn around (throughput) of development compound assay validation
3. Providing more rugged assays by revealing the most promising method(s) sooner
4. Reducing user judgment (the art) in developing such assays by systematically applying the lab's available tools
5. Reducing costs by reducing multiple trial and error testing and the necessity of revalidation, and
6. Perhaps, also cutting costs by reducing LAL reagent use by employing $\frac{1}{2}$ area 96 well plates or some other adaptation.

PROCESS ANALYTICAL TECHNOLOGY FOR BACTERIAL ENDOTOXIN TEST

Two platforms have recently been introduced or are in the process of being introduced that have the potential to significantly impact PAT for bacterial endotoxin water testing. The first is a point-of-use hand-held device called PTS™ by its creator Charles River LABs (CRL). The second is in the manufacturer qualification stage as an automated in-line test device utilizing Cambrex's new r-factor C reagent, PyroGene®, and is called PyroSense.

PTS™ Hand-Held Device

The PTS hand-held point-of-use system (approximately 9″ long × 5′ wide × 2.5″ tall) consists of a plastic-housed spectrophotometer containing a small slit opening in the front for consumable card insertion. The cards about the size and shape of traditional gram-stain slides are clear plastic and contain channels for samples to be drawn into the reaction wells by capillary action (similar to Vitek™ microbial ID cards). Once, in the wells, the samples interact with colyophilized buffer and LAL (and CSE for spiked wells) where the conventional kinetic chromogenic reaction occurs and is monitored for yellow color formation over time. The system has found utility in both the pharmaceutical manufacturing/research environments and also in the testing of short-lived radioactive isotopes used for diagnostic, clinical purposes. The unit also doubles as a gram-stain determination device (PTS Gram ID™) based on the time it takes for a sample to react with LAL: quickly for gram negatives, less quickly for mold and yeast which contain reactive β-glucans, and much more slowly for gram positives which do not have significant LAL-reactive artifacts. All results are obtained within three minutes.

The manufacturer has a platform to add various ingredients to monitor changes which could revolutionize method development work using preformulated solutions for different types of interference problems, be it solubility, pH range, or chelators (i.e., refer to the previous toolbox discussion). CRL has already expanded the use of the instrument to a second instrument, the PTS BCA™, that can detect protein in sample solutions. The reaction utilizes the protein bicinchoninic acid interaction (biuret reaction) with protein to cause the formation of a purple color that is read at 562 nm. The archived standard curve uses bovine serum albumin or bovine gamma globulin.

PyroSense™ rFC Robot

A PAT system being developed by Cambrex is an in-line BET of water for injection and other clean water systems. The unit is "piped" into designated control points in the water loop and monitors the flow through the system. This is accomplished via internal robotic movement of consumables (reagents), which are compartmentalized into disposable cartridges consisting of three 96 well plates and sufficient tips and reagents to perform the associated standard curve and samples for each run. The system would make human sampling acts and infrastructure (i.e., containers and transportation) obsolete, including (*i*) pulling the sample, (*ii*) running the samples, (*iii*) reporting the samples, and (*iv*) flagging the samples that are out of alert limits. The unit is currently undergoing testing at various sites in the United States and Europe. Presumably, results obtained would avoid the error associated with bacterial growth that can occur with samples that are taken and held over time, thus giving a "truer" result and saving valuable manufacturing time, effort, and potentially product by allowing manufacturers to correct excursions as they occur.

PROSPECTIVE TESTS FOR MICROBIAL ARTIFACTS

Two important re-occurring themes in this chapter that may help form a view of the future direction of parenteral contamination testing are: (*i*) endotoxin is the major residual survivor in the realm of microbial cell envelope materials, but it is not the only important cellular artifact[c] and (*ii*) although endotoxin is generally the most potent of such modulins,[d] it is not the only one or the only potent one. Several general questions form the broad outline for this section:

1. What are some likely paths to prospective tests for endotoxin?
2. Might such prospective tests be expanded to include nonendotoxin parenteral contaminants?
3. What are the implications if these changes are implemented in analytical testing?
4. What are the critical drivers of such changes?

Historically, endotoxin testing has progressed from a fairly insensitive but broadly inclusive pyrogen method to the exquisitely sensitive but narrow LAL methodology. From this history, one may extrapolate characteristics to be desired for a new assay not only for bacterial endotoxin but also for some other potentially deleterious host active microbial substances. A desirable futuristic test would be more inclusive than LAL (reminiscent of the pyrogen test) but would retain the sensitivity and specificity advantages of LAL. Given the decline of the horseshoe crab populations in many parts of the world (13) and the recent advances in molecular biology, the successor to the LAL test may be another LAL test of a recombinant nature (recently made available commercially) or perhaps a miniaturized derivative of today's test(s) (or both).

If one were to make a wish list of assay capabilities to associate with a futuristic assay for bacterial endotoxins such a test might end up not being an endotoxin test at all. Considering the modern expansion of microbial constituents (modulins) at a cellular level and the ever accumulating knowledge of the importance of the molecular action of such substances in terms of the host response, it may prove desirable to screen drug products for as many microbial contaminants as possible simultaneously with a single test [i.e., subplanting sterility, bioburden, indicator organism recovery (microbial purity), fungi (β-glucan), mycoplasma, endotoxin, and other microbial by-product detection, such as enterotoxins and superantigens] or, more realistically perhaps one test for living organisms and another for relevant microbial artifacts. The justification for such testing would be driven by either:

1. Product-specific (indication-specific) concerns of nonendotoxin artifact contamination
2. The potency (relative biological activity) of some nonendotoxin modulins
3. The emerging technology itself
4. An increase in the likelihood of nonendotoxin contamination given an increase in manufacturing methods sensitive to alternative (nongram-negative) contamination
5. Necessity—as would occur in the case that LAL became unavailable[e] and would therefore have to be supplanted with a new technology, potentially with multiple artifact detecting capabilities.

---

[c]The term artifact emphasizes the nonliving nature of this type of residual contamination.
[d]The term modulin emphasizes the capacity of (deleterious) host activity by a given artifact, microbe, or microbial by-product.
[e]Unlikely, if not impossible, now with the availability of a recombinant version of factor C.

The PDA Journal of Pharmaceutical Science and Technology technical report No. 33 describes three broad categories of microbiological testing technologies including (*i*) viability-based, (*ii*) artifact-based, and (*iii*) nucleic acid-based technologies. Clearly, the concern for endotoxin as a contaminant lies in its occurrence as an artifact. It is in this capacity that the three paths of future testing are being explored. It is the enduring potent biological activity of endotoxin as an artifact coupled with its almost indestructible nature that separates it from other host artifacts and modulins that are both less biologically active and less resistant to inactivation by heat, chemical, and other common pharmaceutical manufacturing treatments. Therefore, the viability-based[f] and nucleic acid-based[g] technologies can be viewed as less relevant as proposed tests to any eventual replacement of LAL, although they could and do currently find utility in relevant applications such as clinical detection in blood plasma or the examination of complex media used in cell culture (14,15). According to the PDA report (14), artifact-based technologies that may prove relevant to the detection and quantification of microbial constituents include (*i*) the use of fatty acid profiles [gathered by gas chromatography-mass spectrometry (GC-MS)], (*ii*) florescence antibody techniques, (*iii*) enzyme-linked immunosorbent assay (ELISA), and (*iv*) latex agglutination (as well as the continued reliance on LAL).

Given the genesis of microarrays[h] (16,17), instrumental biosensors (18,19), and polymerase chain reaction (PCR) (20,21) using probes that are capable of detecting femtogram levels (10^{-15}) of DNA, mRNA, or rRNA, some have noted a paradigm shift from the detection of gene products such as proteins and contaminating antigens (endotoxin) to genome fragments, especially given the sequencing of the whole genomes of organisms (20). DiPaolo et al. (21) relate the current importance of monitoring for potential bacterial contamination in the production of drugs using recombinant methods:

> The use of recombinant DNA technology and continuous cell lines in the manufacture of biopharmaceuticals has raised the possibility of introducing potentially oncogenic or transforming DNA into the product as an impurity. Although the actual risk of incorporating tumorigenic sequences into the recipient's DNA is negligible, the FDA continues to require lot-to-lot testing for residual host cell DNA, recommending that the final product should contain no more than 100 pg cellular DNA per dose, as determined by a method with a sensitivity of 10 pg (22). These recommendations have resulted in a significant scientific challenge to develop sensitive and robuts assays that can meet the criteria with samples typically containing milligram amounts of biotherapeutic protein.

As an example of a DNA-based detection system is the Isis TIGER[TM] (Triangulation Identification for Genetic Evaluation of Risks) biosensor system. This is an automated microbial identification system with the capability of probing solutions for up to 5000 different microorganisms and viruses simultaneously and telling the user ALL[i] of the types of bacteria and viruses that are present.

---

[f]Including solid-phase cytometry and flow fluorescence cytometry.

[g]Including DNA hybridization probes and ribotyping/molecular typing and PCR.

[h]"When gene sequence information is available, oligonucleotides can be synthesized to hybridize specifically to each gene. Oligonucleotides can be synthesized *in situ*, directly on the surface of a chip, or can be pre-synthesised and then deposited on to the chip"(17).

[i]"... including those that are newly-emerging, genetically altered and unculturable" – from Commercialization Plans for Isis' TIGER Biosensor System, Monday, May 23, 2005 via www.Isis.com.

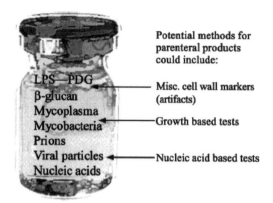

Potential methods for
parenteral products
could include:

LPS—PDG —————— Misc. cell wall markers
β-glucan   (artifacts)
Mycoplasma
Mycobacteria ◄————Growth based tests
Prions
Viral particles ◄————Nucleic acid based tests
Nucleic acids

FIGURE 5 Microbial detection and characterization of potential parenteral contaminants.

Complementary and/or Prospective Methods Overview
β-Glucan-Insensitive LAL and
Endotoxin-Insensitive LAL

Many investigators have made modifications of the traditional gel-clot and kinetic LAL methods for various purposes, usually to overcome interference with specific products or to omit the possibility of false-positive recovery due to specific LAL reactive material [e.g., β-glucan (23)]. Many modified LAL tests have little practical utility and only a handful of prospective non-LAL assays really have any hope in supplanting or even complementing the LAL test. There is not really a method on the horizon that is an obvious replacement for the LAL test. In Pearson's first edition of this book, many of the potential methods described have not been utilized in the past two decades. This is a testimony to the suitability and practicality of the current LAL tests. Another testimony to the BET test is the lack of adverse events associated with pharmaceutical or medical device contamination since the use of LAL. The difficulty in replacing LAL lies in its extreme ease of use, sensitivity, and specificity, which in turn is also a testament to the crab's defense system.

A number of researchers have been able to remove the factor G biosensor contained within the LAL reagent by separating out the individual enzyme and protein constituents (removing factor G) and recombining the remaining constituents to create an endotoxin-specific LAL reagent for both gel-clot and kinetic assays (24,25). The more easily applied solution to the presence of β-glucans in pharmaceutical testing applicatioins is the use of glucan-blocking buffers made from concentrated β-glucans (laminaran and curdlan). The alternative task of removing the factor C pathway enzymes has also been achieved to obtain reagents insensitive to endotoxin and specific to various β-glucans including curdlan, pachyman, laminaran, and lichenan (26). Kitagawa et al. (23) reported that the sensitivity toward curdlan was approximately 10^{-10} g/mL.

Non-LAL Tests for Endotoxin and Other Artifacts

Some non-LAL assays have served in some instances to complement the LAL and pyrogen tests and some may hold potential as eventual alternative tests as they have already served as complementary or confirmatory tests to the use of LAL testing in specific applications:

1. ELISA with monoclonal antibody (MAb) against *Limulus* Peptide C (27)
2. Gas chromatography-mass spectrometry (GC-MS) of 3-hydroxy fatty acids (28,29)
3. Cultured human mononuclear cells (MNC) followed by pyrogen testing (human leukocytic pyrogen test (LPT) or thymocyte proliferation (TP) assay (26,30,31)
4. Polymyxin B stoichiometric binding of lipopolysaccharide (LPS) (26)
5. Silk worm larvae plasma (SLP) test (32)
6. PCR test for specific fragments of bacterial DNA that should not be present: Dussurget and Roulland-Dussoix, at the Institut Pasteur, amplified DNA fragments of mycoplasmas to act as probes and detected as little as 10 fg of specific mycoplasma DNA sequences (not a test for endotoxin) (33).

Some non-LAL assays such as GC-MS or polymyxin B binding may achieve a stoichiometric determination of LPS content that is not a measure of the relative biological responsiveness of a given endotoxin solution. Although this may seem at first glance to be an ideal advantage in providing a truer means of LPS quantitation, it is the biological responsiveness of the LAL test that provides the current basis for regulatory acceptability and is one that is strictly enforced (and historically is the result of much effort to achieve) through the establishment of reference standards, controls standards, LAL standardization, and the relationship of LPS activity to the threshold pyrogenic response in both man and rabbits. In other words, the biological responsiveness of LPS as a means of quantification will not only go away, presumably it will have to be correlated to any truly quantitative nonbiological measure (i.e., non-LAL or nonpyrogen method) developed.

Gas Chromatography-Mass Spectrometry

A quantitative method for determining the lipid A (fatty acid) content of endotoxin has been reported by Maitra et al. (34). The procedure combines GC with an MS detector and is predicated on the detection of β-hydroxymyristic acid, the amide-linked long-chain fatty acid most frequently associated with gram-negative bacterial endotoxin, particularly of the family Enterobacteriaceae. *Salmonella minnesota* Re 595 was used as a standard, and selected ion monitoring at an atomic mass unit of 315.4 was employed. The fatty acid hydrolytic products of LPS were converted to methyl esters. Silica gel chromatography was used to separate methyl esters of hydroxy fatty acids from other fatty acid methyl esters. Trimethylsilyl ether derivatives of the hydroxy fatty acid methyl ester were determined. As little as 200 fmol of β-hydroxymyristic acid could be detected, and the assay is sensitive to that and other fragments of endotoxin. However, the method cannot distinguish bioactive markers from those that have been deactivated, as in residues left from a depyrogenation process, and therefore may be prone to false-positive detection. To increase the likelihood of a relevant match, several such fatty acid markers present increases the likelihood that the sample does indeed contain fatty acids derived from the lipid A moeity. Successful variations on the mass spectrometric detection have also been reported (29).

The GC-MS method allows for quantification of endotoxin by relating (integrating) the (triangular) area in the marker fatty acid recovered (β-hydroxymyristic) to the areas obtained for standards added and recovered by the method. There are some current commercial efforts to apply the technology to endotoxin detection. Quantifying endotoxin content in a manner analogous to the qualitative identification of bacterial isolates using GC (which has reached the routine testing laboratory) coupled with MS is probably the most readily foreseeable prospective method for endotoxin detection. The microbial ID GC is coupled to an extensive computer database to reference chromatograms for standard (ATCC) organisms as well as a variety of environmental and clinical isolates (28). Given that the biochemical and GC methods now work side by side in some microbial identifications laboratories, it is not hard to envision different methods of endotoxin quantification existing for specific applications.

Clinical researchers have been able to correlate the quantification of Meningococcal endotoxin in septic shock patients with LAL test results (35). Brandtzaeg et al. concede that the utility of the LAL assay in measuring plasma LPS activity is still debatable and that in most cases the use of GC-MS is not feasible due to the low levels of gram-negative endotoxins present. However, they were able to correlate their own LAL assay results with their GC-MS measurements due to the high endotoxin plasma concentrations associated with patients afflicted with the deadly *Neisseria meningitidis* infection. The team was able to show that the bioactive endotoxin was associated with *N. meningitidis* infection and not another source (such as from the gut) by identifying the 3-hydroxy lauric acid (3-OH-12:0), which is characterized as a neisserial lipid A marker not found in *Enterobactereaceae*. *Neisseria meningitidis* LPS is very potent from an endotoxin perspective due to its active production of excess outer membrane material called "blebs"(36).

The GC-MS method has been used to confirm the suspected presence of false-positive endotoxin reactions occurring in LAL assays. Maitra et al. (34) used GC-MS to test hemodialyzer rinses containing up to 4800 ng of endotoxin equivalents per milliliter to reveal that the solutions did not contain any measurable $\beta(OH)$ C_{12}, C_{14}, or C_{16} fatty acids. The authors used a chemical method to show that a cellulose derivative caused the nonspecific LAL activation, thereby confirming the utility of the GC-MS results in an application supporting the use of LAL. It is incumbent on users claiming that LAL activity is not due to endotoxin (such as with β-glucans) to have an independent method to prove such a contention. GC-MS has also found utility in detecting and sometimes quantifying markers of contaminants in environmental studies in which allergic and respiratory symptoms have been associated with microbe-contaminated air and in monitoring environments for the presence of fungal (via ergosterol detection) and gram-negative (via lipid A fatty acid detection) biomass. Saraf et al. (37) correlated the sensitive determination of the two markers with the total culturable fungi and LAL assay respectively in organic dust samples and found a good correlation, particularly in fatty acids of 10 to 14 carbon chain lengths (as opposed to hydroxy acids of 16 to 18 carbons).

In addition to the detection of endotoxin by GC-MS, the method has been used to aid the clinical determination of other markers present in septic synovial fluid and septic arthritic joints via the identification of levels of gram-positive markers, namely muramic acid (a component of peptidoglycan) (38). The method used "in tandem MS (MS-MS)" to screen out background peaks thereby allowing the researchers to detect 30 ng/mL (a 1000-fold increase in sensitivity over their previous attempts) of muramic acid.

The variety of these studies demonstrates an apparent strength of the GC-MS method in that multiple markers can be investigated, whereas specific methods,

TABLE 1 Microbial Contamination Marker Detection by Gas Chromatography-Mass Spectrometry

Marker	Indicates the presence of	Non-GC assays
3-OH fatty acids (lipid A)	Endotoxin (gram-negative organisms)	LAL, pyrogen
β-Glucans[a]	Yeast and fungi	SLP
Ergosterol	Yeast and fungi	Liquid chromatography
Muramic acid	Peptidoglycan (gram-positive organisms) SLP	
Long-chain fatty acids	Mycobacteria	Acid fast stain
Unique lipopeptides	Mycoplasma (and other Mollicutes)	Broth[b] or agar culture,[c] PCR

[a]Detectable by endotoxin insensitive LAL and LC-MS.
[b]Broth culture: 5% CO_2 up to six weeks—sediment and pH change (39).
[c]Agar culture: inverted microscopic observation—"fried egg" appearance (39,40).
Abbreviations: GC, gas chromatography; LAL, *Limulus* amebocyte lysate; LC, liquid chromatography; MS, mass spectrometry; PCR, polymerase chain reaction; SLP, silk worm larvae plasma.

such as LAL or SLP, are limited to the detection of, at most, a couple of microbial substances (i.e., endotoxin and β-glucan) (See Table 1 for a list of microbial markers that may be applicable to the GC-MS method of detection).

Cultured Human Mononuclear Cell Tests (Monocyte-Dependent Tests)
Methods employing the production of cytokines in vitro (via human macrophages) have been devised. The human LPT was used to detect lipopolysaccharide (LPS) in a contaminated clinical drug lot that could not be detected by the LAL or conventional pyrogen method (30). This instance was described in Chapter 13. The in vitro pyrogen test (IPT) developed as an alternate method (to the pyrogen assay) is such a method and is discussed in the next section. Biotechnology-based methods have been used to confirm the production of cytokines as a response to various pyrogens (26). Though elaborate, expensive, and time-consuming by LAL testing standards (as well as being coupled with a monocyte culture procedure requiring human blood), some have proven useful in instances of suspected nonendotoxin pyrogen contamination or in suspected human-specific pyrogenic activity due to drug product modification of an endotoxin conaminant, thus necessitating such a heroic effort to demonstrate the mechanism of host bioactivity. In vitro exposure of human cultured MNC to pyrogenic materials causes them to secrete specific inflammatory cytokines such as interleukin (IL)-1β, IL-6, tumor necrosis factor (TNF)-α, and IL-1α. Some such methods are briefly described in Table 2. All employ the cultivation of suspected pyrogens with human MNC; however, the methods may vary in the particular MNC used, the cytokines produced, and therefore detected, as well as the means of detection.

A method called the LP by Dinarello et al. (30) used the conventional pyrogen assay (with all its associated difficulties; see Chapter 12) to detect the cytokines generated in human blood MNC, whereas another method described by Hansen and Christensen (31) later used a TP assay to detect the "IL-1-like activity" generated from MNCs. The use of MNCs for LP testing obtained sensitivities in the range of the rabbit pyrogen test (500 pg/mL) and was as much as 40-fold less sensitive than the LAL test. The minimal stated level of detection of LPS in the MNC TP assay was 200 pg/mL of test solution, whereas LAL reacts with endotoxin at a level of 5 pg/mL (and 0.5 ng/mL for pyrogen testing). The only

TABLE 2 Mononuclear Cell Cytokine Tests for Endotoxin

Method/cytokine[m]	Application	Pros/cons[n]	Reference
Human leukocytic pyrogen test/cytokines not characterized	Used to detect an atypical product endotoxin contamination	Uses the rabbit pyrogen test to detect pyrogenicity of generated cytokines	(39)
Human monocytoid cell lines (Mono Mac 6)/TNF production	Applied to several parenteral blood products including: IgG for i.v., albumin, and fetal calf serum	Appears to eliminate some false-positives associated with LAL and achieves sub-ng/mL levels of sensitivity	(58)
Human monocytoid cell lines (Mono Mac 6)/ interleukin-6 production	Study performed to determine the utility of the method to detect a wide variety of inactivated microbes (see pros/cons)	LPS, *S. aureus* and *S. typhimurium* showed significant activity. Organisms studied: *S. aureus* (G + B), *S. Typhimurium* (G − B), *C. albicans* (yeast), *Aspergillus niger* (fungi), *Influenza* virus, LPS	(49)
Human mononuclear cells/ thymocyte-proliferation assay detects IL-1-like activity	Studied as an in vitro alternative to the rabbit pyrogen test (especially for nonendotoxin pyrogens)	20 hr incubation of monocytes in blood; TPA requires preparation from C3H/HeJ mice; 40 times less sensitive than LAL (200 pg/mL vs. 5 pg/mL)	(49)

Note: Eperon et al. state: "Since macrophages are exquisitely sensitive to endotoxin, they can be regarded as functional analogues of *Limulus* amoebocytes..."
[m]Method of detection typically via cytokine detection.
[n]MNC tests require human blood, "before the assays can be widespread, human monocytes must be substituted with monocytes from other sources, for example, rabbits or a convenient cell line" (31).
Abbreviations: IL, interleukin; LAL, *Limulus* amebocyte lysate; LPS, lipopolysaccharide; TNF, tumor necrosis factor.
Source: From Ref. 57.

obvious advantage to MNC testing appears to be the potential detection of gram-positive, fungal and viral contaminants in addition to LPS. See Table 3 for an overview of some MNC tests developed for endotoxin detection and not for quality control purposes.

Polymyxin B Stoichiometric Binding of Lipopolysaccharide

Wilson and Harvey (41) explored the practicality of using the well-known ability of polymyxin B to bind stoichiometrically (1:1) to lipid A to quantitate lipopolysaccharides (LPS). Polymyxin B has been used for some time to remove LPS from various solutions (42). Wilson and Harvey bound polymyxin B covalently to Sepharose beads and the LPS-binding capability of the resulting gel was found by incubating with standard amounts of radiolabeled ^{14}C-LPS. Though the assay demonstrated the ability to detect LPS in this mannner, quantiation was only achieved in the microgram range. The low sensitivity of the stoichiometric assay was stated to be due to the low specific activity of the biosynthetically prepared ^{14}C-LPS as measured in dpm/μg of LPS. The authors predicted (but did not demonstrate) that the sensitivity could be increased by alternate (nonradioactive) enzyme-linked (ELISA) methods of labeling.

TABLE 3 *Limulus* Immunological Tests for Endotoxin

Method	Application	Pros/cons	Reference
Immunohistochemical	Research method for the visual identification/localization of endotoxin in tissues via factor C and a rabbit antibody against it[o]	in vivo method; qualitative only	(59)
Immunolimulus	Detects O-antigen serotypes of *Escherichia coli, Salmonella, Shigella,* etc.	Detects only smooth bacterial LPS for which MAbs[p] can be made; uses *Limulus* test (cLAL) to detect MAb captured LPS	Serotype-specific and cross-reactive antibodies used (60)
Whole-blood agglutination test	Endotoxemia detection; polymyxin B "conjugated to the Fab fragment of antibody 1C3/86" (35). Antibody binds to erythrocytes of all blood groups while polymyxin B binds LPS	Sensitivity comparable to LAL test (35)	(61)

[o]Rabbit antifactor C IgG.
[p]MAb, Monoclonal antibody.
Abbreviations: LPS, lipopolysaccharide; LAL, *Limulus* amebocyte lysate; MAb, monoclonal antibody.

Silk Worm Larvae Plasma

A novel mechanism of detecting specific non-LPS microbial components including β-glucan (βG) and peptidoglycan (PG) (contained within gram-positive and in lesser amounts in gram-negative bacteria) has been described (43,44) and is available in a commercial form (45) for experimental purposes. In a method reminiscent of the early LAL test, the SLP test makes use of another primitive blood-based host defense system, namely that of the SLP. Melanin, a black-pigmented protein, serves as a self-defense molecule in insect hemolymph and is the end product of a cascade-type reaction utilizing multiple serine proteases called the prophenoloxidase (proPO) cascade. The reagent commercialized by Wako Pure Chemical Industries, Ltd.[j] contains all the components of the proPO cascade just as LAL contains the components of the factor C and G cascades. SLP reacts with both peptidoglycan and β-glucan.

The method has been applied to gram-negative and gram-positive bacterial detection as both types contain peptidoglycan. An initial experimental application of the method has been examined for its utility as a supplementary tool in the detection of bacterial meningitis (which was also one of the first clinical applications of the early LAL test. The rapid determination of the nature of the infection is critical to the patient's treatment. Of the 215 test samples from

[j]Osaka, Japan.

172 patient cerebrospinal fluid (CSF) first taps and 43 "up" taps, initial taps were 18% (31) positive with SLP correlating 100% with the obtained culture results which included 21 *Hemophilus influenza*, 2 *N. meningitides* (gram-negative), 6 *Streptococcus pneumonococcus*, and 2 *Staphylococcus aureus* (both gram-positives). The subsequent up taps were 10% positive (four responses) all containing *H. influenza* (46). The author concludes that a "combination of SLP and LAL may work for the best" given that 85% of bacterial meningitis cases are from gram negatives and 15% from gram positives. The author used the SLP in a visual determination mode and stated that the kinetic colorimetric method (also melanin detection-based) is being pursued. Note that both methods are applicable using the reagents supplied from Wako (for research purposes only). Since the reagent detects both peptidoglycan and β-glucan, standards are available in the form of peptidoglycan (*Micrococcus luteus*, 1 μg/mL) and curdlan, which is a form of β-1, 3-glucan (a water-insoluble polysaccharide produced by *Alcaligenes faecalis* var. *myxogenes*). Curdlan is solubilized by the addition of water and 5 N NaOH at 37°C for 30 minutes. Another set of researchers used LAL and SLP to show that not only is endotoxin a concern in dialysate contamination, but also peptidoglycan may be a pyrogen as per their measurements of both made on 54 dialysate samples from 9 dialysate facilities (43). Evidence of the effects of muramyl dipeptide (MDP is a peptidoglycan subunit) on human peripheral blood MNC (PBMNC) included increased cytokine production (IL-1β and TNF-α) in association with increased concentrations of MDP. They showed that the presence of both endotoxin and MDP resulted in 5 to 10 times the cytokine production that comes from either contaminant alone.

The In Vitro Pyrogen Test (Whole-Blood Pyrogen Test)

The concept of an in vitro "human pyrogen test" that utilizes whole-blood [and the underlying physiological basis of the fever reaction: the activation of blood monocytes by exogenous pyrogens to produce endogenous pyrogens (cytokines)] has gained support recently with the commission of the Hartung group (University of Konstanz) by the European Commission to investigate the development of such a test with an eye toward eventual compendial inclusion (47–49). The use of isolated monocytes/leukocytes has proved to be highly variable, and therefore Hartung et al. have evaluated tests that employ diluted, fresh, whole-blood in a procedure that involves sample incubation and subsequent ELISA detection of immunoreactive monophage-secreted cytokines (IL-h, IL-6, and TNF-α). The former two cytokines are largely intracellular as opposed to the latter, which is secreted into the incubated medium (blood) and, therefore, perhaps more amenable to assay. Additionally, IL-6 has been purported to be the principal endogenous precursor to fever and, therefore, the most accurate predictor of the pyrogenic response. Hartung et al. collaborated with the European Centre for the Evaluation of Alternative Methods (ECVAM) beginning in 1999 to propose and perform tests needed to eventually establish such a human pyrogen test. The test participants summarized their discussions from the ECVAM Workshop 43 in ATLA/2001 and claimed a test sensitivity of 0.03 to 0.1 IU/mL when compared with the BET limit of detection given as 0.03 IU/mL.[k] The authors address the need for nonendotoxin

---

[k] Kinetic chromogenic assays can be as sensitive as 0.005 EU/mL.

TABLE 4 Whole-Blood Assay (In Vitro Pyrogen Test) Claims

Need	Advantage
For nonendotoxin pyrogens	Lists 13 exogenous microbial pyrogen and two exogenous nonmicrobial pyrogen classes (the two nonmicrobial classes are drugs and devices/plastics)
Instances of nonendotoxin contamination	Cites events associated with parenterally manufactured biologicals (most referenced by the group members's own experiences), including immunoglobulins, human serum albumin, hepatitis B vaccine, pertussis vaccine, influenza vaccine, tick-borne-encephalitis vaccine, gentamycin (actually contaminated below or near the limit but given at elevated, off-label dose)
"Comparison of testability"	A range of sample types according to rabbit, LAL, or IPT test and lists only recombinant proteins as being questionably tested via the IPT
"Special problems with biological products …"	Notes that vaccines raise both pyrogen- and LAL-related problems, such as when vaccines derived from GNB contain endotoxin as a component, are inherently pyrogenic although LAL nonreactive, or that contain aluminum hydroxide, which interferes with the LAL test, and finally, the fact that many blood products are incompatable with LAL testing
Medical devices	Adherant pyrogens could be incubated in IPT without the need for elution which is notably inefficient and potentially may affect biocompatibility (i.e., rejection by local inflammatory reaction)
r-DNA used for biologicals	New expression systems (GNB, GPB, fungi, mammalian, and insect cells) may be contaminted by expression organisms without LAL detection

pyrogen testing in several instances (Table 4). Table 5 lists items that cannot be tested via IPT.

Hartung et al. state that the European Pharmacopoeia Commission should examine each monograph individually to determine if replacement of the rabbit pyrogen test requirement should be done by means of LAL or IPT. One LAL supplier, CRL, has marketed a commercial kit for investigational purposes. Some industry debate has begun on the utility of the test and some have called into question the relevance of nonendotoxin pyrogens under any circumstances. Novitsky [Associates of Cape Cod (ACC)] asserts: "many microbial components once thought to be pyrogens have since been shown to be contaminated with endotoxin. A recent example is lipoteichoic acid (LTA)"(50). He cites a study by Gao et al. (51) that found contaminating endotoxin in commercial preparations of LTA and another by Morath et al. (52) (that includes Hartung as a co-author) suggesting that crude preparations of LTA are not suitable for use as indicators of immune cell activation.

TABLE 5 Materials that Cannot be Tested with In Vitro Pyrogen Test

Drugs that interact with monocytes	IL-1, receptor antagonists, nonphysiological solutions, cytotoxic agents, r-proteins with cytokine activity (i.e., INF-γ), or cytokine detection such as rheumatic factors

Abbreviations: IL-1, interleukin-1; INF-γ, interferon-γ.

However, pointing to the lack of general agreement, Novitsky maintains that β-glucans "represent a clear case of an adulterated (i.e., contaminated product when present in an otherwise current GMP-prepared pharmaceutical drug or device" and suggests differentiating and quantifying such contamination using ACC's glucan-specific LAL products. Elsewhere, he details ACC's current thinking on a particular nonendotoxin "pyrogen": "it has been our policy to treat glucans as 'bioactive' molecules and as 'foreign substances' when present in pharmaceutical preparations" (53). In the ACC technical report, Novitsky prescribes caution in moving too quickly to IPT and details perceived shortcoming on several fronts.

1. IPT is not adequately characterized or validated.
2. Lack of a valid nonendotoxin pyrogen standard.
3. The requirement for fresh, whole human blood.
4. The variability associated with donor blood in that some contain endotoxin.
5. Twelve to 24 hours incubation for cytokine expression; assay of up to four hours for cytokine assay.

More recently, a United States counterpart of the Hartung study has been proposed by National Toxicology Program (NTP), NTP Interagency Center for the Evaluation of Alternative Toxicological Methods, in collaboration with the Interagency Coordinating Committee on the Validation of Alternative Methods (see *Federal Register*/Vol. 70, No. 241/Friday, December 16, 2005/Notices, pp. 74833–74834) in that they are considering convening an independent peer review panel to evaluate the validation of five IPT methods including:

1. Human PBMNC/IL–6 IPT (PBMNC/IL–6),
2. Human whole-blood/IL–1 IPT (WB/IL–1),
3. Human whole-blood/IL–1IPT: application of cryopreserved human whole-blood cryo (WB/IL–1),
4. The human whole-blood/IL–6 IPT (WB/IL–6),
5. An alternative IPT using the human monocytoid cell line MONO MAC–6 (MM6/IL6).

It should be remembered that these proposals are to explore the replacement of the rabbit pyrogen test and not the LAL assay.

Other Immunological Tests for Endotoxin

There are a number of specialized immunological tests (some used experimentally in conjunction with LAL) developed for clinical applications such as the detection of endotoxemia in blood plasma and other investigational applications. The effect of blood plasma on LAL tests has made the quantification of endotoxin in blood less than consistent [See Hurley's paper (54) for a detailed discussion of methods of endotoxemia detection]. Several highly specialized immunological assays involving LAL have been described. Many of the methods employ MAbs against LPS or LOS by the continuous culture method originally developed by Kohler and Milstein (55) for MAb production in the mid-1970s. Immunological assays derive their specificity from their interaction with the polysaccharide (O-antigen) moiety of LPS. Given that the polysaccharide portion is the most variable part of the molecule, the specificity is often limited to specific serotypes. A short mention of selected types of MAb and Immuno *Limulus* methods that have been developed with relevant references are shown in Table 3.

The Mother of Invention

At an AAPS meeting (56), Gordon Binder (former Amgen CEO) gave a rousing talk in which he described the need for better use of existing technology in lieu of the development of new technology. His point being that there is much more that can be done to improve the technology that currently exists (Bang spoke similarly in his talk on serendipity). Binder's contention was that, in general, the industry is not making use of the information already possessed to anywhere near its full potential. The example he used concerned the looming crisis that Amgen faced in losing Government reimbursement for a lead product. The government proposed limiting reimbursement where blood levels were not considered in the low range (thus arguably not requiring therapy). However, when Amgen scientists studied the accuracy and variability inherent in the instruments used for such measurements, they showed that the government's proposed restrictions were not scientifically justified given the amount of variability inherent in the analytical instrumentation employed (i.e., the "good" vs. "bad" blood levels considered therapeutic were statistically indeterminate by the current instrumentation). Binder seemed incredulous that decisions of this magnitude (i.e., hundreds of millions to billions of dollars not to mention the personal cost of loss or reduction of a valuable therapy) could be made based upon erroneous assumptions and/or insufficient data gathering.

Significant changes in LAL testing probably will not occur until a driving event such as the (near) extinction of horseshoe crabs on the Atlantic seaboard transpires. Perhaps, then there will be a urgency in looking to cut the use of LAL material and/or a wholesale sea change to the use of the recombinant factor C product(s). One wonders if additional crab blood,[1] or a myriad of other potential host-derived biosensor markers will be found, as the unique utility of the horseshoe crab blood is largely removed by any recombinant test (i.e., the huge volume of liquid blood and the ease of harvest of that blood, etc., become irrelevant). As in the case of PyroGene that employs the 33 amino acid base pairs from *Carcinoscropius* (99 DNA base pairs to clone), any creature with a blood or immunity system (from spiders to oysters to plants, etc.) has biosensors galore for everything from endotoxin to peptidoglycan to β-glucans. Indeed, this would be a "brave new world" for microbial artifact testing. Presumably, any artifact that a creature is found to have innate immunity against (perhaps even prions) can be copied and developed in a recombinant form with an indicator attached (chromophore, etc.) to provide novel methods. As the saying goes "necessity is the mother of invention," necessity brings about opportunities that do not seem possible in the present setting. In many respects, the development of the LAL test was accompanied by the desire, if not necessity, of better monitoring (quantification) of parenteral manufacturing processes that have grown in complexity with the rapid rise of biotechnology (which roughly parallels the rise of the use of LAL).

Product or Indication Specific Drivers of Analytical Change

Lastly and relevant to parenteral manufacturing in the consideration of potential drivers of change in analytical testing for contamination control is the ever-accumulating knowledge of the interrelationship of microbes, their by-products,

---

[1]Patent law not withstanding.

and human disease states. Two disease states relevant to such a discussion include systemic fungal infection and sepsis.

β-Glucan is a fungal (or cellulosic breakdown) artifact well known to the bacterial endotoxin lab due to the discovery of its LAL reactivity. Although the substance is not forbidden from being present in parenteral products, neither is it tested for (other than accidentally if the LAL used should happen to be sensitive to it, as some LAL formulations are and some are not) nor has it been found to be a common contaminant. However, since it is used as a diagnostic marker for systemic fungal infections, it is not hard to envision that those who manufacture parenteral drugs to treat such infections could realistically be expected to preclude the possibility of β-glucan contamination.

A second, more complex indication and thus a more speculative proposition would be the association of minute amounts of nonendotoxin contaminantion with the occurrence of sepsis. In a similar manner, as gram-negative organisms (and thus the endotoxin they produce) have been correlated with gram-negative sepsis, gram-positive organisms have been implicated with approximately 50% of the instances of sepsis. What is not known is whether the possibility exists that minute amounts of gram-positive cellular artifacts introduced from medical devices, infusion solutions, or even parenteral drugs could be relevant contributing factors to this disease state. What is also documented is the correlation of the historical rise of sepsis with the use of antibiotics and medical intervention (see Chapter 18).

REFERENCES

1. Haaland PD. Experimental Design in Biotechnology. Vol. 105. New York: Marcel Dekker, 1989.
2. McCullough KZ, Weidner-Loeven C. Variability in the LAL test: comparison of three kinetic methods for the testing of pharmaceutical products. J Parenter Sci Technol 1992; 44(1):69–72.
3. Gabor A. The Man who Discovered Quality. How W. Edwards Deming Brought the Quality Revolution to America. Penguin, 1992:326.
4. Craig AG, Hoheisel JD. Automation: Genomic & Functional Analyses, Methods in Microbiology. Vol. 28. Academic Press, 109–130.
5. Huber L. Validation of Computerized Analytical and Networked Systems Englewood: Interpharm Press, 2002:228.
6. Blumenthal R. Automating kinetic LAL testing. LAL Rev 1999; 1–2.
7. Williams KL. Complete automation of the bacterial endotoxin assay. Biopharm 1994.
8. Williams KL. Robotic screening for optimum endotoxin assays. Pharm Technol 2000; 24(5):46–54.
9. Novitsky TJ. Curved vs. Straight standard curves. LAL Update 1998; December.
10. Cleland JL, et al. The stability of recombinant human growth hormone in poly(lactic-coglycolic acid) (PLGA) Microspheres. Pharm Res 1997; 14(4):420–425.
11. Cooper JF. Resolving LAL test interferences. J Parneter Sci Technol 1990; 44(1):13–15.
12. FDA Guideline on Validation of the *Limulus* Amebocyte Lysate test as an End-Product Test for Human and Animal Drugs. Biological Products, and Medical Devices. U.S. Dept. Health and Human Services. 1987.
13. Clines FX. Acts to Protect Embattled Horseshoe Crab. In New York on the web, 2000.
14. PDA. Evaluation, Validation and Implementation of New Microbiological Testing Methods. PDA J Pharm Sci Technol 2000; 54:1–39.
15. Watson A, et al. Technology for microarray analysis of gene expression. Curr Opin Biotechnol 1998; 9:609–614.
16. Braxton S, Bedilion T. The integration of microarray information in the drug development process. Curr Opin Biotechnol 1998; 9:643–649.

17. Gingeras TR. Studying microbial genomes with high-density oligonucleotide arrays. ASM News 2000; 66(8):463–469.
18. Nice EC, Catimel B. Instrumental biosensors: new perspectives for the analysis of biomolecular ineractions. BioEssays 1999; 21:339–352.
19. Briggs J. Sensor-Based system for rapid and sensitive measurement of contaminating DNA and other analytes in biopharmaceutical development and manufacturing. J Parenter Sci Technol 1991; 45(1):7–12.
20. Swarbrick J, Boyan Jc, eds. DNA probes for the identification of microbes. Encyclopedia Pharm Technol, 19.
21. DiPaolo B, et al. Monitoring impurities in biopharmaceuticals produced by recombinant technology. PSTT 1999; 2(2):70–82.
22. Points to Consider in the Manufacture and Testing of Monoclonal Antibodies Products for Human Use Food and Drug Administration. Bethesda: The Center for Biologics Evaluation and Research, 1997.
23. Kitagawa T, et al. Rapid method for preparing a b-glucan-specific sensitive fraction from *Limulus* (*Tachypleus tridentatus*) amebocyte. J Chromatogr 1991; 567:267–273.
24. Tamura H, et al. A new test for endotoxin specific assay using recombined *Limulus* coagulation enzymes. Jpn J Med Sci Biol 1985; 38:256–273.
25. Obayashi T, et al. A new chromogenic endotoxin-specific assay using recombined *Limulus* coagulation enzymes and its clinical applications. Clin Chim Acta 1985; 149:55–65.
26. Novitsky TJ. Endotoxin detection in body fluids: chemical versus biochemical methodology. In: Brade H, et al. eds. Endotoxin in Health and Disease. New York: Marcel Dekker, 2000, 831–839.
27. Zhang G-H, et al. Sensitive quantitation of endotoxin by enzyme-linked immunosorbent assay with monoclonal antibody against *Limulus* peptide C. J Clin Microbiol 1994; 32(2):416–422.
28. Olson WP, Groves MJ, Klegerman ME. Identifying bacterial contaminants in a pharmaceutical manufacturing facility by gas chromatographic fatty acid analysis. Pharm Technol 1990; February: 32–36.
29. Sonesson A, et al. Determination of endotoxins by gas chromatography: evaluation of electron-capture and negative-ion chemical-ionization mass spectrometric detection of halogenated derivatives of B-hydroxymyristic acid. J Chromatogr 1987; 417:11–25.
30. Dinarello CA, et al. Human leukocytic pyrogen test for detection of pyrogenic material in growth hormone produced by recombinant *Escherichia coli*. J Clin Microbiol 1984; 20(3):323–329.
31. Hansen EW, Christensen JD. comparison of cultured human mononuclear cells, *Limulus* amebocyte lysate and rabbits in the detection of pyrogens. J Clin Pharm Ther 1990; 15:425–433.
32. Tuchiya M, et al. Detection of peptidoglycan and b-glucan with silkworm larvae plasma test. FEMS Immunol Med Microbiol 1996; 15:129–134.
33. Dussurget O, Roulland-Dussoix D. Rapid, sensitive PCR-based detection of mycoplasmas in simulated samples of animal sera. Appl Environ Microbiol 1994; 60(3):953–959.
34. Maitra SK, Nachum R, Pearson FC. Establishment of beta-hydroxy fatty acids as chemical marker molecules for bacterial endotoxin by gas chromatography-mass spectrometry. Appl Environ Microbiol 1986; 52(3):510–514.
35. Brandtzaeg P, et al. Meningococcal Endotoxin in lethal septic shock plasma studied by gas chromatography, mass-spectrometry, ultracentrifugation, and electron microscopy. J Clin Invest 1992; 89:816–823.
36. DeVoe IW, Gilchrist JE. Release of endotoxin in the form of cell wall blebs during in vitro growth of *Neisseria meningitidis*. J Exp Med 1973; 138:1156–1167.
37. Saraf A, et al. Quantification of ergosterol and 3-hydroxy fatty acids in settled house dust by gas chromatography-mass spectrometry: comparison with fungal culture and determination of endotoxin by a *Limulus* amebocyte lysate test. Appl Environ Microbiol 1997; 63(7):2554–2559.

38. Fox A, et al. Absolute identification of muramic acid at trace levels, in human septic synovial fluids in vivo and absence in aseptic fluids. Infect Immun 1996; 64(9):3911–3915.
39. Kenny GE. Mycoplasmas. In: Lennette EH, ed. Manual of Clinical Microbiology. Washington: ASM, 1985:407–411.
40. Waris ME, et al. Diagnosis of *Mycoplasma pneumoniae* Pneumonia in children. J Clin Microbiol 1998; 36:3155–3159.
41. Wilson M, Harvey W. A new assay for bacterial lipopolysaccharides. Curr Microbiol 1990; 21:91–94.
42. Issekutz AC. Removal of gram-negative endotoxin from solutions by affinity chromatography. J Immunol Methods 1983; 61:275–281.
43. Tsuchida K, et al. Detection of peptidoglycan and endotoxin in dialysate, using silkworm larvae plasma and *Limulus* amebocyte lysate methods. Nephron 1997; 75(4):438–443.
44. Ashida M, Yamazaki HI. Molting and metamorphosis. In: Onishi O, Ishizaki H, eds. Biochemistry of the Phonoloxidase System in Insects: with Special Reference to its Activation. Tokyo: Japan Sci Soc Press, 1990:239–265.
45. Wako Pure Chemical Industries. Package Insert, Osaka, 1999.
46. Kahn W. New rapid test for diagnosing bacterial meningitis. ASM 1996.
47. Hartung T, Wendel A. Detection of pyrogens using human whole blood. In Vitro Toxicol 1996; 9:353–359.
48. Hartung T, Fennrich S, Wendel A. Detection of endotoxins and other pyrogens by human whole blood. J Endotoxin Res 2000; 6:184.
49. Hartung T, et al. Novel pyrogen tests based on the human fever reaction (The Report and Recommendations of ECVAM Workshop 43). ATLA 2001; 29:99–123.
50. Novitsky TJ. BET vs. PT non-endotoxin pyrogens. LAL Update 2002; 20(2).
51. Gao JJ, Xue Q, Zuvanich EG, Haghi KR, Morrison DC. Commercial preparations of lipoteichoic acid contain endotoxin that contributes to activation of mouse macrophages in vitro. Infect Immun 2001; 69:751–757.
52. Morath S, Geyer A, Spreitzer I, Hermann C, Hartung T. Structural decomposition and heterogeneity of commercial lipoteichoic acid preparations. Infect Immun 2002; 70:938–944.
53. Novitsky T. Letter from the president. LAL Update 2002; 20(3), Associates of Cape Cod.
54. Hurley JC. Endotoxemia: methods of detection and clinical correlates. Microbiol Rev 1995; 8(2):268–292.
55. Kohler G, Milstein C. Continuous cultures of fused cells secreting antibody of predefined specificity. Nature 1975; 256:495–497.
56. Binder G. AAPS Conference. 2000.
57. Eperon S, et al. Human monocytoid cell lines as indicators of endotoxin: comparison with rabbit pyrogen and *Limulus* amoebocyte lysate assay. J Immunol Methods 1997; 207: 135–145.
58. Lloyd AW, Hunter AC. A Comparative study of mono mac 6 cells, isolated mononuclear cells and *Limulus* amoebocyte lysate assay in pyrogen testing. Pharm Sci Technol Today 2000; 3:106–110.
59. Uragoh K, et al. A Novel immunohistochemical method for in vivo detection of endotoxin using horseshoe crab factor C. J Histochem Cytochem 1988; 36(10):1275–1283.
60. Hansen EJ, et al. Detection of *Haemophilus ducreyi* lipooligosaccharide by means of an immunolimulus assay. J Immunol Methods 1995; 185(2):225–235.
61. Rylatt DB, et al. A Rapid whole-blood immunoassay system. Med J Aust 1990; 152: 75–77.

17 | *Limulus* Amebocyte Lysate Testing of Medical Devices

Peter S. Lee

Baxter Healthcare Corporation, Round Lake, Illinois, U.S.A.

Risk assessment tools can be utilized to identify potential risk associated with bacterial endotoxin contamination in a medical device manufacturing operation.

HISTORICAL BACKGROUND

In the mid 1970s, a number of medical device manufacturers began using the *Limulus* amebocyte lysate (LAL) test as an alternative to the *United States Pharmacopeia* (USP) rabbit test for pyrogen (bacteria endotoxins) testing of medical devices and administrative sets (1). The United States Food and Drug Administration (FDA) then provided conditions for the use of the LAL test as a sensitive indicator for the presence of bacterial endotoxins and as an alternative to the USP rabbit pyrogen test for medical devices in November 4, 1977 (2). Medical device manufacturers had to submit adequate data establishing equivalency of the USP rabbit test and the LAL test used. These data were then submitted to the FDA to obtain approval to use the LAL test. A key study reported by Mascoli in 1978 provided the answer to the question of nonendotoxin pyrogens (3). This study data confirmed that all pyrogens in fluids and devices were indeed bacterial endotoxins based on 28,410 rabbits tested and 143,196 LAL tests performed. The same study also concluded that there were no incidents of unexplained false negative LAL test results, that the LAL test was more sensitive in detecting endotoxins then the rabbit test, and that the LAL test was also equally reproducible to the USP rabbit test.

A Health Industry Manufacturers Association (HIMA) collaborative study conducted in 1979 provided clarification with regard to finding a suitable pass/fail point for the LAL testing of medical devices that was comparable to the USP rabbit test (4,5). If the LAL test used can be performed to demonstrate a test failure rate significantly greater than 50% at 0.1 ng/mL of the standard endotoxin used, the test would be considered qualified under the conditions of the evaluation to be equivalent to the USP rabbit test. This study established the level of 0.1 ng/mL to be the release limit for the LAL test for medical devices. Following receipt of the 1979 HIMA report, the FDA issued a draft guideline in 1979. This draft guideline required the submission of three types of data to be generated by the medical device manufacturer using the LAL test. The three data types required were the sensitivity and reproducibility data, the inhibition test data, and the parallel test data between the USP rabbit pyrogen test and the LAL test method used (6). A release limit of 0.04 ng/mL was also established for intrathecal devices used in contact with the cerebrospinal fluid (7). More medical device manufacturers could now seek product clearance and approval to use the LAL test in place of the USP rabbit test for bacteria endotoxin testing of medical devices. These medical device products represented many general classes of devices including transfusion and infusion assemblies (8,9).

On March 29, 1983, the FDA announced in the *Federal Register* that a revision of the draft guideline for medical devices was now available as part of the draft guideline covering parenteral drugs for animal and human use (10). The significant changes made to this 1983 draft guidelines specific to LAL testing of medical devices were (i) the adoption of the USP endotoxin reference standard, (ii) the expression of endotoxin limits (ELs) in endotoxin unit or EU/mL, (iii) instead of ng/mL and the equivalency of ELs to those for drug for a 70 kg human adult at 0.5 EU/mL for medical devices except for medical devices in contact with the cerebrospinal fluid where the EL was set at 0.06 EU/mL (11,12).

Another HIMA Collaborative Study provided the comparison needed between the endotoxin standard used in the previous HIMA report to the USP reference standard (13). The study concluded that the previously reported pass/fail EL for medical devices of 0.1 ng/mL (or 1.0 ng/kg when injected into rabbits at 10 ml/kg) is approximately the same as the 5.0 EU/kg EL established for drugs and biological products in the 1983 FDA draft guideline, that is, 1.0 ng is equal to 5 EU of USP Reference Standard Endotoxin (RSE) or 0.5 EU/mL.

The FDA finally published the "Guideline of Validation of the LAL Test as an End Product Endotoxin Test for Human and Animal Parenteral Drugs Biological Products, and Medical Devices" on December 1987 (14). The LAL test method can now be used as an end product test for medical devices and is at least equivalent to the USP rabbit test if the LAL test is validated according to the 1987 FDA Guideline on the Validation of the LAL Test.

The last in-process revision to the USP <161> medical device chapter was presented in 1994 and was eventually updated in the First Supplement to USP 23 in 1995 (15). The USP chapter title was changed from "Transfusion and Infusion Assemblies" to "Transfusion and Infusion Assemblies and Similar Medical Devices." Other changes included the way the medical device ELs were expressed and the elimination of discrepancies between extraction procedures for different types of medical devices.

In 2002, the Association for the Advancement of Medical Instrumentation (AAMI) provided an updated standard document to provide general criteria to be applied to the determination of bacterial endotoxins on or in medical devices, components, or raw materials using the bacterial endotoxins test (BET) methodologies or LAL test methods (16). Most medical device manufacturers have now switched to using the established cost-effective LAL test in place of the USP rabbit test.

REGULATORY AND COMPENDIA CONSIDERATIONS

FDA requires that a medical device manufacture labeling a device as nonpyrogenic must validate the LAL test for that medical device in the laboratory to be used for end product testing before using the LAL test as an end product endotoxin test for any medical device. No preclearance prior to the use of the LAL test as an end product test is required if it is used according to the "FDA Guideline on the Validation of the LAL Test." Any significant deviations from "FDA Guideline on the Validation of the LAL Test" would require a premarket notification under section 510(k) (14). If a sterile end product medical device is labeled pyrogen free, a description of the method used to make that determination is also required such as the use of the LAL test (17). A sterile device can also be labeled with only the fluid path of the sterile device as sterile and nonpyrogenic (18).

The USP <161> compendia requirements apply to sterile and nonpyrogenic assemblies or devices in direct or indirect product contact with cardiovascular system, lymphatic system, or cerebrospinal fluid. The medical devices exempted were orthopedic products, latex gloves, or wound dressings (19).

PREPARATION OF MEDICAL DEVICES TEST SAMPLES

Sampling

The sampling criteria for selection of medical device end product units for bacterial endotoxin testing using the LAL tests are based on the premise that the medical device manufacturing process is in control and in compliance with the medical devices Quality System Regulation (QSR) requirements. The selection of medical device end product or finished units for testing shall be based on criteria defined in a predetermined sampling plan. The sampling plan should specify the device sample size, the group or family from which the device samples are to be taken, and other key device sampling criteria.

Sample size shall be based on a rationale specified in the sampling plan. This rationale may be based on applicable regulatory requirements, drawn from published guidelines, or based on manufacturing operation validations. Medical device sampling is conducted in terms of the number of device units randomly sampled per batch or lot of device produced. This device test sampling can be based on batch or lot size according to the 1987 "FDA Guideline on the Validation of the LAL Test" (14):

- 2 devices = Lot sizes < 30 devices
- 3 devices = Lot sizes 30 to 100
- 3% of the lot up to a maximum of 10 devices per lot = Lot sizes >100

Device sampling per USP <161> allows the number of device test samples selected to be between three to ten devices (19). The number of medical device sampled per batch or lot manufactured can vary from two to not more than ten devices. The medical device test samples should also be manufactured and selected for testing in the finished or end product form. The sampling group is generally defined as the product batch or lot. Device sample selection may be based on a sampling group other than the production batch if there are established data and associated risk assessment done to support a different device selection basis.

Medical device test samples may be obtained prior to (pre-) sterilization or after (post-) sterilization of the finished medical devices (16). Post-sterilization device samples covers all factors that may affect the device product tested or the LAL test used. If pre-sterilization device samples are selected for testing, the acceptability of this sampling shall be documented. Pre-sterilization device test samples rationale may include the device manufacturer's knowledge of the device product manufacturing process that may contribute to the bioburden of the device product. It was previously reported that it would require an administration of at least 1000 microorganisms per mL of most gram-negative bacteria to cause a pyrogenic reaction in rabbits (20). An equivalent of 40,000 gram-negative bacteria would be needed per device tested to fail the LAL testing if 40 mLs of volume extracting solution was used on a single device unit. A similar number of microorganisms are therefore needed before the LAL test will detect the endotoxins associated with whole bacterial cells. The device tested may then be sampled prior to sterilization if it contains little or no bioburden. For medical device end products or finished products that support microbial growth, the choice of pre-sterilization sampling may not be appropriate. This is particularly observed with devices containing solutions that may provide moisture and nutrient needed for promotion of microbial growth. Medical devices test samples can also be any device units tested after primary packaging pre- or post-sterilization. Any device batch or lot that required rework where the rework compromises the integrity of the device test sample prior to repackaging would require additional device test samples after repackaging. The program for ongoing routine LAL testing should consistently reflect either pre or poststerilization device sampled.

In the testing of multicomponent kit products, either the individual components or the entire kit may be considered as a device entity. Standard LAL testing procedures should be applied in the case of individual component qualifications. The same consideration of a kit as a single unit shall address sample preparation in adherence to LAL testing requirements and the applicable device product ELs. Additional information with regards to the selection of components related to device kits and sets for LAL testing are provided in the Association for the Advancement of Medical Instrumentation (AAMI) 2002 standard document (16).

Extraction Solutions

Prepare the device test sample solutions by extracting the selected medical devices using an extracting solution according to the extraction parameters recommended by the FDA and the USP (14,19). The extracting solutions can be LAL Reagent Water or nonpyrogenic water and in some instances nonpyrogenic normal saline is used. LAL reagent water can be sterile water for injection or other water that show reaction with the specific LAL reagent with which it can be used, at the limit of the sensitivity of such reagent. The quality of the LAL reagent water used for rinsing the medical devices is critical. It was reported that the presence of 10 μmol/L of aluminum chloride present in LAL reagent water used for the LAL testing totally inhibited the recovery of added USP RSE (21). Medical devices can either be rinsed or soaked (immersed) in extraction solution to obtain a device test sample extraction. The selected medical device(s) test samples may be cut or disassembled by using depyrogenated instruments or scissors.

The soaked or immersed extraction method is the choice for devices labeled sterile, nonpyrogenic or pyrogen free. The device should be soaked or immersed if the exterior surface of the device test sample contacts the cardiovascular system or contact membranes that may allow the transfer of endotoxins to the cardiovascular system. This particular extraction method can be considered worst case as either the whole or parts of the whole medical device claimed to be nonpyrogenic is completely soaked or immersed in the extracting solution in a depyrogenated container.

The rinse method is done by filling the fluid pathway with the extraction solution and used for medical devices labeled nonpyrogenic fluid pathway. The rinsing method has taken into account the cumulative endotoxins that may be present throughout the entire length of the internal surface area that make up the nonpyrogenic fluid path for the device tested. The extracted solution is therefore reflective of the maximum potential for bacterial endotoxins from all internal surfaces of the nonpyrogenic fluid path of the device that the administered fluid will pass through to reach the end-user patient.

The extraction methods (rinse or soaked) used depend on the specific nonpyrogenic label claim for the medical device tested or the directions for end use of the device. The rationale for either rinsing or soaking the medical device test sampled should be documented.

The temperature of the extraction solution has to be heated to 37°C +/− 1°C prior to device extraction (19). Hold the extraction solutions in contact with the relevant pathway or in contact with the soaked device or devices during the predetermined time of extraction. The minimum extraction time for the rinsed fluid pathway is not less than one hour at controlled temperature (typically between 18°C to 25°C), or other demonstrated equivalent conditions (14). The minimum extraction time for soaked devices should be from 15 minutes at 37°C or one hour at controlled room temperatures (typically between 18°C to 25°C), or other demonstrated equivalent conditions (14). The extracted solutions can either be tested individually for a single device or combined (pooled) extract from a predetermined number of devices using the LAL test.

An AAMI Task Group reported that the validation of the current extraction recovery efficiency for LAL testing of medical devices was not recommended (22). The extraction parameters recommended by the FDA and USP for medical device had proven through the years of LAL testing based on regulatory evidences, to be sufficient in assuring the nonpyrogenicity of medical devices at the specified ELs tested. The ELs established for medical devices by the FDA and USP also have a margin of safety incorporated to account for the less than 100% extraction recovery efficiency which was further supported by the limited number of available literature that referenced this concern (12, 23–26).

ENDOTOXIN LIMITS FOR MEDICAL DEVICES

For medical devices the endotoxin limit (EL) is not more than 20 EU per device except for those used in intrathecal devices that are in contact with the cerebrospinal fluid is not more than 2.15 EU per device (19). The EL for the rinsing and extracting solution is calculated by the formula (note that one USP EU is now equal to one International Unit (IU) of endotoxin:

$$EL = \frac{(K \times N)}{V}$$

where K is equal to the amount of endotoxin allowed per device, N is equal to the number of devices tested, and V is equal to the total volume of the extract or rinse.

For example,

$$EL = \frac{20\,EU \times 1\,device}{40\,mL}$$
$$= 0.5\,EU/mL$$

The above formula also takes into account that different extraction solution volumes may be appropriate for different medical devices. This would be extremely helpful for unusually small or large devices that come into contact with the end-user patient by adjusting the extraction volume as needed.

The following equation is used to calculate the volume of extraction solution:

$$V = \frac{(K \times N)}{EL}$$

where K is equal to the amount of endotoxin allowed per device, N is equal to the number of devices tested, EL is equal to the EL for the rinsing or extracting solution. For example,

$$K = 20\,\text{EU/device}$$
$$N = 3\,\text{devices}$$
$$EL = 0.125\,\text{EU/mL}$$

The total volume of the extract or rinse solution (V) is equal to 480 mLs.

$$V = \frac{20 \times 3}{0.125}$$
$$= 480\,\text{mLs}$$

Therefore the device EL can now change as the extracting solution volume is changed for the different medical devices. The previous standard extract of 40 mL/device would have the device EL set at 0.5 EU/mL for general medical devices. The EL established by the FDA and the USP also has a substantial safety margin built in based on less than 100% extraction recovery efficiency. FDA has therefore assigned a tighter limit for medical devices than for drugs at 200 EU versus 350 EU for a 70 kg adult human person (14). Intrathecal devices with direct contact with the cerebrospinal fluid has a tighter EL of 2.15 EU per device. This EL would also apply to intrathecal device tray components having components that can also come into direct contact with the cerebrospinal fluid. Dura substitute devices that are final sterilized devices are also tested for nonpyrogenicity with the tighter EL of 0.06 EU/mL (27). There is also no requirement to adjust the EL for a pooled medical device extracted solutions. The 1987 FDA Guideline on the Validation of the LAL Test (page 2, paragraph D) states that the EL accounts for the affect of the pooling of extracted solutions (14). The calculated medical device EL will be only limited to the sensitivity of the LAL reagent used for the LAL testing.

Additional questions that may be asked to facilitate the EL calculations for the medical devices test sampled are as follows:

1. Is the final product a medical device or combination of both medical device and drug solution (product family or group)?
2. What are the regulatory submission based on and the labeled claims for non-pyrogenicity (fluid pathway or whole exterior surface)?
3. What materials are used (specifically the device components contents in a set or tray and each component chemical composition)?
4. Is there any schematic diagram or detailed description of the final medical device (include manufacturing process flow and number of components making up the final assembled finished device)?

The Maximum Valid Dilution (MVD) is the maximum allowable dilution of a test sample where the EL can be determined.

$$MVD = \frac{\text{Endotoxin limit (EU/ML)}}{\lambda \text{ or Lysate sensitivity (EU/ML)}}$$

For example,

$$MVD = \frac{0.5\,\text{EU/mL}}{0.125\,\text{EU/mL}}$$
$$= 4$$

The maximum allowable dilution of the extract solution where the EL can be determined in this example is 4 or by a dilution factor of 1:4.

LAL TEST METHOD VALIDATION FOR MEDICAL DEVICES
General Requirements
No pre-clearance is needed prior to use of the LAL test as an end product test (routine testing) if it is used according to the FDA Guideline on the Validation of the LAL Test. LAL test method validation requirements are listed in the FDA Guideline on the Validation of the LAL Test (14):

1. Use of FDA licensed LAL reagent in all validation—Including in-process and end product LAL testing.
2. Initial qualification of the LAL laboratory analyst—Each analyst using a single lot of LAL and a single lot of endotoxin should perform the test for confirmation of labeled LAL reagent sensitivity or of performance criteria. The procedures and criteria used for initial qualification and re-qualification of the LAL analysts in the laboratory is found in appendix A of the Guideline on the Validation of the LAL Test.
3. Demonstrate sensitivity and reproducibility of the LAL test used—A Control Standard Endotoxin (CSE) can be used if a reproducible correlation between the CSE and the USP RSE has been demonstrated. The determination of the relationship between the CSE and RSE can be found in appendix C of the FDA Guideline on the Validation of the LAL Test. Sensitivity of the LAL test method must be at least 0.5 EU/mL. Sensitivity is determined by the procedure and criteria found in appendix A of the FDA Guideline on the Validation of the LAL Test. Include negative control and standards (in duplicate). Also consider the stability and storage condition of the endotoxin standards used.
4. Inhibition/Enhancement testing of the LAL test method used—Lack of product interference of the LAL test must be demonstrated for each type of devices before routine use of the LAL test method. The two types of product interference are inhibition and enhancement. Each product line of devices utilizing different materials or methods of manufacturer should be checked for inhibition and enhancement of the LAL test method used.

Inhibition/Enhancement Testing
For the medical devices test sampled, each product line of devices utilizing different material or method of manufacture must be checked for inhibition or enhancement

TABLE 1 Harmonized LAL Test Methods

United States Pharmacopeia (USP) LAL techniques	Japanese Pharmacopeia (JP) LAL techniques	European Pharmacopeia (EP) LAL test methods
Gel-clot techniques	Gel-clot techniques	Gel-clot methods
Limit test	Limit test	Limit test
Assay test	Assay	Semi-quantitative test
Photometric techniques	Photometric techniques	Turbidimetric end point method
Turbidimetric technique	Turbidimetric technique	Chromogenic kinetic method
End point-turbidmetric	End point-turbidimetric	Chromogenic end point method
Kinetic-turbidimetric	Kinetic-turbidimetric	Turbidimetric kinetic method
Chromogenic technique	Chromogenic technique	
End point-chromogenic	End point-chromogenic	
Kinetic-chromogenic	Kinetic-chromogenic	

of the recognized LAL test methods or BET for bacterial endotoxins testing. See Table 1 for the LAL test methods recognized as the harmonized bacterial endotoxins tests in the USP <85> BETs that become official as of January 1, 2001(28–30). The requirements associated with conducting the inhibition and enhancement test or interfering factors test for these LAL test methods are covered in the FDA Guideline on the Validation of the LAL Test and in the USP/European Pharmacopeia/ Japanese Pharmacopeia (14,28–30).

A medical device manufacturer may provide technical rationale or justification for dividing its medical device products into groups of products (families) according to common chemical formulation (material of device and device components), and may qualify only a representative product from each similar group or family of medical device products. The representative product chosen from each group must be the one that with the largest surface area contacting body or fluid administration to a patient end user.

At least three production batches or lots of each product type must be tested for inhibition/enhancement (14). If one product batch or lot is manufactured only once a year, validate and release each batch or lot concurrently until all three batches or lots are completely validated for the LAL test method used. Once again, it is important to know that LAL testing prior to sterilization is permitted for dry medical devices only. Dry medical devices are devices that are manufactured without exposure to water through the entire manufacturing process. Medical devices that are exposed to water during the manufacturing process or contain solutions are considered wet devices. These wet devices have a higher risk of providing moisture and potential nutrition that can support microbial growth and may not be appropriate for pre-sterilization sampling.

If undiluted rinsing or extracting solution cause test interference to the LAL test method used, repeat the inhibition/enhancement testing after neutralizing and removing the inhibiting substance, or after the solution has been diluted by a factor not to exceed the MVD.

LAL Test Method Interferences

LAL test method interferences is a test method condition that causes a significant difference between the end points of a positive water control and positive product control (PPC) series using a standard endotoxin (gel clot LAL test method) or where your positive product recovery must be within 50% to 200% of the known concentration of endotoxin added to the product (chromogenic or turbidimetric LAL test methods). If the product tested causes the endotoxin recovery to be less than expected, the product is inhibitory to the LAL test method used. If the product tested causes the endotoxin recovery to be higher than expected, the product is enhancing the LAL test method used (14,19,28).

LAL test method interfering conditions are highly variable, and the true nature of the underlying mechanisms for the cause of the interference may be difficult to define. However, principal LAL test interferences would include the following (31):

1. Sub-optimal pH conditions—A pH of 6.4 to 8.0 is said to be optimal and a pH requirement of 6.0 to 8.0 taken on a given test sample and LAL lysate mixture prior to testing is required (28).
2. Aggregation or adsorption of control endotoxin spikes—Strong salts solutions can cause a large increase in the LAL test sample ionic strength that will cause endotoxin aggregation and poor endotoxin spike recovery.
3. Unsuitable cation concentrations—This LAL test method interference can occur due to organic chelators or citrate containing solutions like the anticoagulant solutions. Heparin has also been reported to be inhibitory to the LAL test (32,33).
4. Inhibitory enzyme or protein modification—This LAL test method interference occurs when enzymes necessary to complete the LAL reaction are denatured by strong chemical such as alcohols or phenols. It was also reported that drinking water treatment oxidants such as chlorine, monochloroamine and potassium permanganate were able to inactive endotoxin but at a relatively slow rate with the concentration of oxidants used for the study (34).
5. Nonspecific LAL activation—This LAL test method interference includes the detection of LAL-reactive materials or drugs that mimic endotoxins such as those containing serine proteases. The LAL-reactive materials or activators were β-D-glucans in nature and interferes with the LAL test through the factor G enzymatic cascade pathway (35–37). Glucan interference of LAL test methods can be tackled using either one of the two following approaches (37). The first approach is to identify the source of the glucan contamination with the intent of removing or eliminating the source of glucan from the product or process. The second approach is to use glucan-blocking reagents for routine LAL release testing of products such as medical devices with known background glucan coming from cellulosic-based components so that the LAL test can still be specific for bacteria endotoxins (38,39). This can be achieved by validating the various commercially available glucan-blocking reagents with the LAL test methods used. The purpose of this validation is to ensure that the glucan-blocking reagents do not interfere with the LAL test method used and to verify the effectiveness of the glucan-blocking reagent from triggering the LAL test used. USP also noted that LAL reagent reacts with some β-glucans in addition to bacterial endotoxins and as such suggest that those LAL reagent preparations be treated to not react with β-glucans and must be used for samples that contain glucans (28). LAL-reactive materials may impact the LAL test method validation for device products such as cellulosic hemodialyzers (40–43), cellulosic filters used as a device component or a part of the manufacturing processing step (44–47), and wound dressings made from biomaterials (48).

6. Solubility and viscosity of products tested—This LAL test interference is due to LAL test samples that are insoluble or have the inability to form true aqueous solution such as lipid based product such as liposomal delivery systems. The insolubility of these LAL test samples causes refractive scattering of the light signal that interferes with the chromogenic quantitative LAL test method by preventing the light signal's proper detection. Moderately viscous LAL test solutions can cause LAL test interference by preventing cofactors and enzymes in the LAL reagent from reacting at the proper rate and thus effectively reducing the rate of reaction of the lysate enzyme reaction cascade (49–51).

However, over 90% of LAL test method interferences are solved by simple dilution up to a dilution factor of 1:40 with LAL reagent water (52). You can always decrease the endotoxin sensitivity of your assay with corresponding increase in your dilution as long as your dilution factor does not exceed the calculated MVD for that product.

For medical devices that cannot be tested by any of the recognized LAL test methods due to nonremovable inhibition or enhancement, the USP pyrogen rabbit test <151> is applied as the last resort (53).

LAL TEST METHOD RE-VALIDATION

Reasons for LAL test method re-validation as part of laboratory testing change control that may impact the current validated LAL test method are as follows:

1. Change in the product itself or product label or product use direction
2. Change in the LAL test method used
3. Change in the LAL test method parameters (e.g., sample extraction parameters)
4. Change in medical device manufacturing process
5. Change in sources of device raw materials

The level of significance and risk assessment of the above changes would dictate whether there is a need to re-validate the LAL test method and should be an integral part of the medical device manufacturer change control system. The FDA has also recognized the differences in the LAL test methods by requiring that inhibition/enhancement testing or test for noninterference be repeated on three lots of finished product whenever a change in LAL test method to be used. The FDA also allows pre-treatment of products or extracted test solutions to render them testable. As long as it can be demonstrated that the pre-treatment allows for the PPC recovery of the added bacteria endotoxins to be within the acceptable limits of the LAL test methods being used, the pre-treatment will be acceptable to the FDA (14).

The LAL test method validation data may be expressed graphically or in a tabular form or in a format most meaningful for the product. For each group of devices, protocols, test results and other relevant information from the LAL test method validation should be compiled, documented and on file at the manufacturing site (14). Cooper had provided a practical example of the planning and execution of the LAL test method validation for end product testing as well as the contents that goes into a comprehensive LAL test method validation report. It was also suggested to validate multiple LAL test methods at the same time because of the resource and cost associated with the validations (54,55).

ROUTINE LAL TESTING OF MEDICAL DEVICES
Routine Sampling
LAL testing should be conducted under similar requirements for selecting device test samples, preparation of extraction solutions and specific pre-treatment of extraction solutions as for the inhibition/enhancement testing. This includes performing the routine LAL test with the same dilution used for the validation. The extracted solutions can either be tested individually for a single device or combined (pooled) extract from a pre-determined number of devices using the LAL test. The extracted solution should be kept under appropriate holding conditions and length of time for endotoxin stability until it is LAL tested in duplicate with appropriate negative control and PPC in place. Standard series for the photometric LAL test methods is recommended. Standard series for the first gel clot test for the day can be used provided that consistency has been observed and trended in the LAL testing laboratory conducting the LAL gel clot test.

Measurement of pH on routine LAL testing is not required for a validated LAL test method unless the device manufacturer had committed to such testing. It was also noted that the PPC used in routine LAL testing would fail unless the test sample and LAL reagent mixture is neutral (56). Medical device extract solutions are typically within the pH range of 6.0 to 8.0 for LAL testing.

For device product release, end product batch or lot testing is generally used to confirm product nonpyrogenicity. An example of a sampling plan in terms of sample size per batch or lot for a minimum of three device test samples to a maximum of ten device test samples per USP is shown in Table 2

Frequency
The frequency of routine LAL testing of medical devices should be based on prior regulatory commitments, historical data trends and defined routine sampling plan. The frequency of LAL testing for routine production in most instances is for every batch or lot of finished medical device product manufactured. For LAL test frequency other than every batch or lot, the potential for pyrogenicity to occur for each device manufacturing process may be assessed for potential endotoxin contamination risk to determine an alternate frequency of LAL testing needed. For example, well controlled device manufacturing process and materials with an established history of low risk of endotoxin contamination, capable of producing finished products with endotoxin levels that consistently meet the specified limits (57).

Repeat LAL Amebocyte Lysate Testing
The routine LAL test is valid if it meets the acceptance criteria for the validated LAL test method used. The device tested is acceptable if the level of endotoxin

TABLE 2 Routine LAL Testing of Each Batch or Lot of Finished Device Products

Total number of device test samples per batch/ lot for routine LAL testing	First of batch or lot no. of units	Middle of batch or lot no. of units	End of batch or lot no. of units	Random from batch or lot no. of units
Three (3)	1	1	1	0
Ten (10)	3	3	3	1

determined by LAL testing is less than the limit determined for the medical device. If the endotoxin level exceeds the medical device specification, the device is considered out-of-specification (OOS), further investigation would follow in accordance to documented procedures. The LAL test is invalid if it does not meet the acceptance criteria for the validated LAL test method used and would need to be handled according to documented procedures for it.

The LAL test may not be repeated no more than twice (14). The first repeat test consists of twice the initial number of replicates of the device sample in question, to examine the possibility that an extrinsic occurred in the initial LAL test. The second repeat consists of an additional ten units. The USP states that if the test sample fails the LAL test, it can be retested once by another LAL test method (19). False positive LAL test results due to β-D-glucans in medical devices may potentially occur during routine LAL testing and must be addressed accordingly on a case-by-case basis according to the FDA memo provided by Munson (58). It would be useful for each LAL testing laboratory conducting routine LAL testing to have an OOS or out-of-limits (OOL) investigation plan in place.

To help investigate LAL test OOS or OOL in the LAL testing laboratory or impacted device manufacturing site, the cause and effect investigative approach is one of many investigational techniques or tools that can be used to identify potential causes of the bacterial endotoxin OOS or OOL LAL test results. The cause-and-effect diagram also known as the fishbone diagram or Ishikawa diagram seen in Figure 1 can be used to systematically list the different causes that can be attributed to an effect or to a problem (59). The list of potential causes is by no means limited to the causes listed, additional causes can be further identified by each laboratory or manufacturing site conducting the investigation of the LAL testing laboratory or

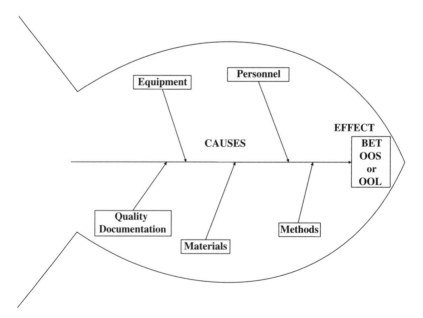

FIGURE 1 Identification of potential causes of LAL testing out-of-limits using the cause-and-effect fishbone diagram.

device manufacturing process implicated. The five primary categories of potential causes of the LAL test OOS or OOL effect are personnel, equipment, materials, method, and quality documentation. All LAL test OOS or OOL investigations should be thorough, timely, unbiased, well documented and scientifically defensible. Further confirmation of the root cause analysis and any Corrective Action & Preventative Action associated with the LAL test OOL or OOS will have to be completed for each investigation initiated and checked for effectiveness. The FDA has also provided the draft guidance on investigating OOS test results for pharmaceutical production to further add to any OOS or OOL investigations conducted at your laboratory and/or manufacturing site (60).

A rationale for routine LAL sampling and testing plan is essential to demonstrate that the LAL testing of these finished medical devices (manufacturing process), are capable of producing finished products with endotoxin levels that consistently meet specified limits. The FDA can collect bacterial endotoxins samples during an inspection of a medical device manufacturer only when endotoxin control is necessary for the device and when on review of the manufacturer's test methodology is led to the believe that the manufacturer's test results may be unrealistically low. Ten device units are collected and analyzed using the LAL test methods or BET methods found in the USP (61).

ALTERNATE BATCH RELEASE TESTING
General Considerations
Alternatives to device batch or lot testing may be used if it has been demonstrated that the medical device manufacturing processes and materials are well controlled (in a state of control) and are capable of producing products with endotoxin levels that consistently meet specified limits (historical trends). Sufficient data from batch or lot testing should demonstrate the acceptable endotoxin levels for the routine release LAL testing for the finished device. Alternatives to batch or lot testing may not be allowed, where specific regulation/compendia require every batch or lot to be LAL tested. The every batch or lot testing requirements may exist for the following: products used for infusion or transfusion, wound or tissue irrigation, and/or products that contain biological ingredients/components or water excluding water for injection or inhalation (16). Batch or lot testing alternatives may include one or more logical alternatives. These can be demonstrated by either reducing the test sample numbers, reducing the test sampling frequency, using sampling based on product grouping, or testing of raw materials may be chosen as an alternative.

In establishing an alternative to batch or lot testing, the rationale and sampling plan shall need to be documented. This documentation should contain the necessary information regarding manufacturing design, validation and control. The risk associated with the reduction in the ability to detect an inadvertent manufacturing process change leading to a product not meeting the specified EL should be evaluated within this document.

Manufacturing Process Qualification (Design, Validation and Change Control)
The manufacturing operation being evaluated for alternative to batch testing should ideally be designed to minimize the presence of bacterial endotoxin on

the product. The manufacturing design should take into consideration material selection and suppliers as well as controlling material and component handling and product water contact. Water and packaging components used in the manufacturing process are some of the major sources of bacterial endotoxin contamination (62–64). Incoming raw water supply to the manufacturing facility can be also potential sources of bacterial and cyanobacterial endotoxins (65,66). LAL testing is therefore routinely conducted on water used in the manufacturing process (67–69). The manufacturing validation procedure of the manufacturing operation should be documented with the records of the validation retained. The validation should include:

1. Process Qualification (PQ)—Installation qualification or IQ, operational qualification or OQ, and performance qualification or PQ
2. Process Risk Assessment—Key process elements noted by a risk assessment tool involving a detailed schematic of the process

The process risk assessment may include raw materials, extrusion operations, aqueous washing and drying processes (wet versus dry processes), product/component handling, and manual versus automated assembly. For nonpyrogenic products, any change that would likely affect the bacterial endotoxin level on the product must be included.

The process should have well-established operating specifications and exist as a process operating in a state of control. This manufacturing operation must be evaluated for variables that could lead to endotoxin contamination. Failure Mode and Effects Analysis (FMEA) can be used as a risk assessment tool to identify potential risk associated with bacterial endotoxin contamination in a medical device manufacturing operation. The FMEA evaluation should list potential key process steps and control points for endotoxin introduction. A study by Lee used this approach to enable medical device manufacturers to successfully conduct a FMEA for bacterial endotoxin risk for dry medical device manufacturing process (70). Table 3 indicates an example of a partially completed FMEA for a step involving injection molding of device component. The risk level of each potential cause of failure is obtained by multiplying the likelihood of Occurrence (O), the Severity level (S), and the likelihood of Detection (D) to give you the Risk Priority Number (RPN) or RPN = O × S × D. This should be performed after all the key steps/functions have been identified and analyzed. The FMEA team can now determine the minimum RPN at which corrective action or justification is required. See Figure 2 for a summarized flowchart that will enable medical device manufacturers to successfully conduct a FMEA for bacterial endotoxin contamination risk for dry medical device manufacturing operation.

For each key control point of the manufacturing process identified within the risk assessment:

1. Justify the step of the process is under control (list controlling equipment or procedures).
2. Explain if current monitoring performed at this step of the process is sufficient (specify monitoring method, monitoring frequency and specification limits).
3. Determine if new testing is needed at this step of the process (define frequency, specification limits and Out-of-Specifications actions).

TABLE 3 A Partial Example of the Failure Mode and Effects Analysis for Bacterial Endotoxin Contamination Risk for an Identified Injection Molding Step

Process step	Process function	Potential failure mode	Potential effect of failure	Potential cause of failure	O	S	D	RPN
1.0 Injection molding	1.1 Transfer of molded components to inspection sites	Bacterial endotoxin cross contamination of molded components during transfer to inspection sites	Bacterial endotoxin cross contamination onto molded components	Bacterial endotoxin transferred from equipment surfaces	1	3	3	9
	1.2 Inspection sites	Manual handling of molded components	Bacterial endotoxin cross contamination onto molded components	Improper personnel cleanliness (wet hands)				

O = Occurrence rating.
S = Severity rating.
D = Detection rating.
RPN = OxSxD = Risk priority number.

Change control to the manufacturing process needs to be implemented. The endotoxin level of the product and/or manufacturing operation qualification can be impacted by process changes and deviations. These changes should be assessed to determine the impact and the extent of qualification and document the rationale for the decision made. Process change control system needs to be established for the medical device manufacturing process evaluated to include the following:

1. Develop a change control system for the process or reference the established change control system.
2. Ensure that any process changes that could potentially affect the bacterial endotoxin level of the product be evaluated.
3. Consider the degree of the change to determine the extent of the operational re-qualification.
4. Document all the above change control system including the rationale for the decisions reached.

MAINTENANCE OF PROCESS QUALIFICATION

The alternate batch testing documentation shall be reviewed and evaluated on a periodic basis to assess the continued validity of the manufacturing operation, as well as the total effects of all minor and major changes on the product endotoxin level. This review is an overall evaluation of the entire alternate batch testing validation and manufacturing operation qualification package and validation re-qualification should be performed as needed.

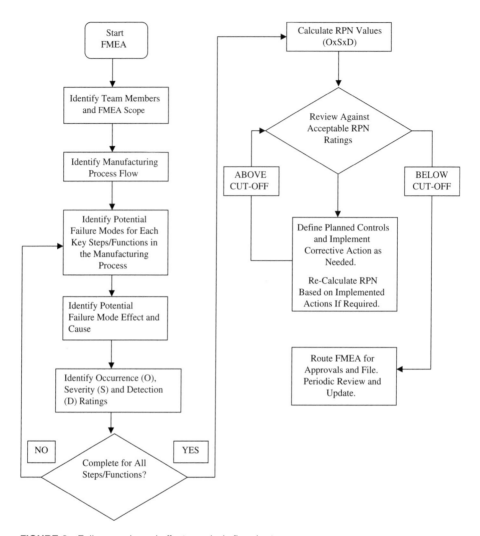

FIGURE 2 Failure mode and effects analysis flowchart.

Other Medical Device Considerations

Sterile medical or surgical latex gloves can now be tested for bacterial endotoxins using the LAL test methods following the recently published D7102-04 ASTM Standard (71). Finished sterile medical or surgical gloves shall be considered nonpyrogenic if the EL use is equal or below the EL of 20 EU per pair of gloves tested using the LAL test methods. A number of other studies also had indicated the presence of bacteria endotoxins in sterile surgical gloves including one study that reported that endotoxin was the factor in causing adverse reaction to nonsterile latex examination gloves (72–74).

Surgical mesh for general surgical uses such as implantation to reinforce areas of weakened soft tissue can also be LAL tested for pyrogenicity. If a surgical mesh is labeled pyrogen free or nonpyrogenic, the USP rabbit test or an equivalent test (i.e., LAL test) is performed on the final end product and lot release based on satisfactory results meeting specified endotoxin release limits (75).

Sterile ophthalmic viscosurgical devices were also tested for bacterial endotoxins using the gel clot LAL test method to potentially avoid pyrogenic levels that may cause post-operative inflammatory reaction related to the human eye (76). Presence of β-D-glucans were also observed for the ophthalmic viscosurgical devices that contains hyaluronic acid and hydroxypropylmethylcellulose that may interfere with the LAL test method used for testing such devices. Other similar devices that may be impacted by β-D-glucans are device products such as cellulosic hemodialyzers (40–43), cellulosic filters used as a device component or a part of the manufacturing processing step (44–47), and wound dressings made from biomaterials (48).

Reprocessed single-use medical devices that come into direct or indirect contact with blood should be assessed for residual bacterial endotoxins after reprocessing the devices for reuse (77). There has also been concerns of bacterial endotoxins released by bacterial biofilm formed on reprocessed medical devices (78), biofilm formed in components associated with portable water used for haemodialysis (79, 80) and biofilm formed in sterilizer water reservoirs (81, 82). A summary of the LAL testing conducted during the reprocessing validation and routine monitoring to be conducted with a validated LAL test method should be established to ensure that the reprocessed devices do not cause pyrogenic reaction in end-patient use (83).

SUMMARY

A search of the FDA medical device recall database was conducted using the key words "endotoxin" and "pyrogen" as the search criteria. The results from the recall database search generated a number of recalled medical devices or medical device components that exceeded the specified ELs or pyrogen levels. These recalled medical devices included a catheter component, a stent delivery component, disposable sets and temperature probes. Another search of the FDA Manufacturer and User Facility Device Experience database for reported adverse events between 2004 and 2005 led to eight reports on endotoxin and 151 reports on pyrogen. In almost all instances, each device manufacturer had listed LAL testing as one of the identified test that either had to be verified to meet the LAL test method acceptance criteria for endotoxin determination or verified to meet the specified endotoxins limits as part of the device manufacturer's investigation of the reported adverse event. A similar search of FDA warning letters issued to medical device manufacturers led to a number of endotoxins or pyrogen related observation items not in conformance with the medical devices QSR(21 CFR 820) (84). Some of the observation items were related to failure to meet production and process controls (21 CFR 820.70); process validation (21 CFR 820.75); receiving, in-process, and finished device acceptance (21 CFR 820.80); as well as corrective and preventative action (21 CFR 820.100) requirements. LAL testing of medical devices with a validated LAL test method will continue to be used for medical device end product testing and to be used to provide the assurance that the LAL tested device end product do not exceed the specified EL.

REFERENCES

1. Weary M, Baker B. Utilization of the *Limulus* amebocyte lysate test for pyrogen testing large volume parenterals, administration sets, and medical devices. Bull Parenter Drug Assoc 1977; 31(3):127–133.

2. Federal Register. 1977; 42:57749–57750.
3. Mascoli CC, Weary ME. *Limulus* amebocyte lysate (LAL) test for detecting pyrogens in parenteral injectable products and medical devices: advantages to manufacturers and regulatory officials. J Parenter Drug Assoc 1979; 33(2):81–95.
4. Health Industry Manufacturers Association, HIMA Collaborative Study for the Pyrogenicity Collaborative Study for the Pyrogenicity Evaluation of a Reference Endotoxin by the USP Rabbit Test. Vol.1. HIMA Document Series, 1979 No.7.
5. Dabbah R, Ferry Jr. E, Gunther DA, et al. Pyrogenicity of *E. Coli* O55: B5 endotoxin by the USP rabbit test- a HIMA collaborative study. J Parenter Drug Assoc 1980; 34(3):212–216.
6. Weary M, Pearson F. Pyrogen testing with *Limulus* amebocyte lysate. Med Device Diagn Ind 1980; 2(11):35–39.
7. Ross VC, Bruch CW. Endotoxin testing of medical devices with LAL: FDA requirements. In: Watson SW, et al. eds. Endotoxins and Their Detection with the *Limulus* Amebocyte Lysate Test. New York: Alan R. Liss, 1982, 39–48.
8. Pearson FC, Weary ME, Dabbah R. A corporate approach to in-process and end-product testing with the LAL assay for endotoxin. In: Watson SW, et al. eds. Endotoxins and Their Detection with the *Limulus* Amebocyte Lysate Test. New York: Alan R. Liss, 1982:231–246.
9. Marlys W. Pyrogen testing of parenteral products- status report. J Parenter Sci Technol 1984; 38(1):20–23.
10. Federal Register. 1983; 48:13096–13098.
11. Ross VC. LAL testing of medical devices: a regulatory update. Med Device Diagn Ind 1984; March:35–40.
12. Ross VC, Twohy CW. Endotoxin testing of medical devices with LAL: FDA requirements. In: Cohen E ed. Bacterial Endotoxins Structure, Biomedical Significance, and Detection with the *Limulus* Amebocyte Lysate Test. New York: Alan R. Liss, 1985, 267–280.
13. Pearson FC, Weary ME, Sargent HE, et al. Comparison of several control standard endotoxins to the national reference standard endotoxin- an HIMA collaborative study. Appl Environ Microbiol 1985; 50(1):91–93.
14. FDA. Guideline on validation of the *Limulus* amebocyte lysate assay as an end-product endotoxin test for human and parenteral drugs, biological products, and medical devices. DHHS, 1987.
15. USP. Biological test and assays: <161> transfusion and infusion assemblies. Pharmacopeial Forum 1994; 20(1):6894–6896.
16. AAMI. Bacterial endotoxins- test methodologies, routine monitoring, and alternatives to batch testing. Assoc Adv Med Instrum 2002: ANSI/AAMI ST72.
17. FDA CDRH. Updated 510(k) sterility review guidance K90-1; guidance for industry and FDA. DHHS 2002; August:5.
18. FDA CDRH. Labeling regulatory for medical devices. DHHS 1989; August:23.
19. USP. Biological test and assays: <161> transfusion and infusion assemblies and similar medical devices, USP29-NF24 2006:2547.
20. Weary M. Pyrogens and pyrogen testing. In: Swabrick E, Boyan JC, eds. Encyclopedia of Pharmaceutical Technology. New York: Marcel Dekker, Inc., 1988:185.
21. Duner KI. The importance of the quality of water in *Limulus* amebocyte lysate tests. J Parenter Sci Technol 1995; 49(3):119–121.
22. Bryans TD, Braithwaite C, Broad J, et al. Bacterial endotoxin testing: a report on the methods, background, data, and regulatory history of extraction recovery efficiency. Biomed Instrum Technol 2004; 38(1):73–78.
23. Twohy CW, Duran AP. Extraction of bacterial endotoxins from medical devices. J Parenter Sci Technol 1986; 40(6):287–291.
24. Roslansky PF, Dawson ME, Novitsky TJ. Plastics, endotoxins and the *Limulus* amebocyte lysate test. J Parenter Sci Technol 1991; 45(2):83–87.
25. Berzofsky R, Scheible L, Williams KL. Validation of endotoxin removal from parenteral vial closures. Biopharm 1994; June:58–66.
26. Ragab AA, Motter RVD, Lavish SA, et al. Measurement and removal of adherent endotoxin from titanium particles and implant surfaces. J Orthop Res 1999; 17(6):803–809.

27. FDA CDRH. guidance document for dura substitute devices; guidance for industry. DHHS 2000; November:4.
28. USP. Biological test and assays: <85> bacterial endotoxins test. USP29-NF24 2006:2521.
29. EP. 2.6.14. Bacterial Endotoxins. EP 5.0. 2005:161.
30. JP. 6. Bacterial Endotoxins Test. JP XIV. 2001:20.
31. Cooper J. Resolving LAL test interference. J Parenter Sci Technol 1990; 44(1):14–15.
32. Sullivan JD, Watson SW. Inhibitory effect of heparin on the *Limulus* test for endotoxin. J Clin Microbiol 1975; 2(2):151.
33. Marcum JA, Levin J. Heparin inhibition of endotoxin- dependent *Limulus* amebocyte lysate coagulation. Thromb Haemost 1989; 62(2):294–297.
34. Anderson WB, Mayfield CI, Dixon DG, Huck PM. Endotoxin inactivation by selected drinking water treatment oxidants. Water Res 2003; 37: 4553–4560.
35. Morita T, Tanaka S, Nakamura T, Iwanaga S. A new $(1 \rightarrow 3)$-β-D-glucan-mediated coagulation pathway found in *Limulus* amebocytes. FEBS Lett 1981; 129(2):318–321.
36. Roslansky PF, Novitsky TJ. Sensitivity of *Limulus* amebocyte lysate (LAL) to LAL-reactive glucans. J Clin Microbiol 1991; 29(11):2477–2483.
37. Cooper JF, Weary ME, Jordan FT, et al. The impact of non-endotoxin LAL-reactive materials on *Limulus* amebocyte lysate analysis. J Pharm Sci Technol 1997; 51(1):2–6.
38. Tanaka S, Aketagawa J, Takahashi S, et al. Inhibition of high-molecular-weight-$(1 \rightarrow 3)$-β-D-glucan-dependent activation of a *Limulus* coagulation factor G by laminaran oligosaccharides and curdlan degradation products. Carbohydr Res 1993; 244:115–127.
39. Zhang G, Baek L, Burchardt O, Koch C. Differential blocking of coagulation-activating pathways of *Limulus* amebocyte lysate. J Clin Microbiol 1994; 32(6):1537–1541.
40. Pearson FC, Bohon J, Lee W, et al. Characterization of *Limulus* amebocyte lysate-reactive material from hollow-fiber dialyzers. Appl Environ Microbiol 1984; 48(6):1189–1196.
41. Pearson FC, Bohon J, Lee W, et al. Comparison of chemical analyses of hollow-fiber dialyzer extracts. Artif Organs 1984; 8(3):291–298.
42. Pearson FC. The possible role of *Limulus*– amebocyte-lysate-reactive material in hemodialysis. Blood Purif 1987; 5:115–122.
43. Pearson FC, Dubczak J, Weary M, Anderson J. Determination of endotoxin levels and their impact on interleukin-1 generation in continuous ambulatory peritoneal dialysis and hemodialysis. Blood Purif 1988; 6:207–212.
44. Anderson J, Eller M, Finkelman M, et al. False positive endotoxin results in a dc product caused by $(1 \rightarrow 3)$-β-D-glucans acquired from a sterilizing cellulosic filter. Cytotherapy 2002; 4(6):557–559.
45. Usami M, Ohata A, Horiuchi T, et al. Positive $(1 \rightarrow 3)$-β-D-glucan in blood components and release of $(1 \rightarrow 3)$-β-d-glucan from a depth-type membrane filters for blood processing. Transfusion 2002; 42:1189–1195.
46. Ohata A, Usami M, Horiuchi T, Nagasawa K, Kinosbita K. Release of $(1 \rightarrow 3)$-β-D-glucan from depth-type membrane filters and their in vitro effects on proinflammatory cytokine production. Artif Organs 2003; 27(8):728–735.
47. Nagasawa K, Yano T, Kitabayashi G, et al. Experimental proof of contamination of blood components by $(1 \rightarrow 3)$-β-D-glucan caused by filtration with cellulosic filters in the manufacturing process. J Artif Organs 2003; 6:49–54.
48. Nagakawa Y, Murai T, Hasegawa C, et al. Endotoxin contamination in wound dressings made of natural biomaterials. J Biomed Mater Res Part B Appl Biomater 2003; 66B: 347–355.
49. Harmon P, Cabral-Lilly D, Reed RA, et al. The release and detection of endotoxin from liposomes. Anal Biochem 1997; 250:139–146.
50. Piluso LG, Martinez MY. Resolving liposomal inhibition of quantitative LAL methods. J Pharm Sci Technol 1999; 53(5):260–263.
51. Sakai H, Hisamoto S, Fukutomi I, et al. Detection of lipopolysaccharide in hemoglobin-vesicles by *Limulus* amebocyte lysate test with kinetic-turbidimetric gel clotting analysis and pretreatment of surfactant. J Pharm Sci 2004; 93(2):310–321.
52. Guifoyle DE, Munson T. Procedure for improving detection of endotoxin in products found incompatible for direct analysis with *Limulus* amebocyte lysate. In: Watson SW,

et al. eds. Endotoxin and Their Detection With the *Limulus* Amebocyte Lysate Test. New York: Alan R. Liss, 1982:79–90.

53. USP. Biological test and assays: <151> pyrogen test. USP29-NF24 2005:2546.
54. Cooper JF. Validation of bacterial endotoxins test methods. LAL Times 1999; 6(2):1–4.
55. Cooper JF. Documenting validation of a BET application. LAL Times 1999; 6(3): 1–4.
56. FDA. Human drug CGMP notes. DHHS 1996; March:3.
57. Pfeiffer M. Testing medical disposables using the *Limulus* ameboecyte lysate (LAL) test. Med Device Technol 1990; 37:37–51.
58. Munson T E. Memo: statement concerning glucans and LAL-reactive material in pharmaceuticals and medical devices. DHHS, 1992.
59. ASQ. 6. Cause and effect diagrams. In: Russell JR, ed. The Quality Audit Handbook-Principles, Implementation and Use. 2nd ed. Milwaukee: ASQ Quality Press, 2000: 216.
60. FDA. Draft guidance- investigating out of specification (OOS) test results for pharmaceutical production. DHHS, 1998.
61. FDA CRDH. Inspection of medical device manufacturers final guidance for industry and FDA. DHHS, 2001.
62. FDA. ITG subject: pyrogens, still a danger. Inspectional Technical Guide No. 32. DHHS, 1979.
63. FDA. ITG subject: bacterial endotoxins/pyrogens. Inspectional Technical Guide No. 40. DHHS 1985.
64. Sykora JL, Keleti G, Roche R, et al. Endotoxins. Algae and *Limulus* amebocyte lysate test in drinking water. Water Res 1980; 14: 829–839.
65. Anderson WB, Slawson RM, Mayfield CI. A review of drinking -water -associated endotoxin, including potential routes of human exposure. Can J Microbiol 2002; 48:567–587.
66. Hunter PR. Cyanobacterial toxins and human health. J Appl Symp 1998; 84(Suppl): 35S–40S.
67. Novitsky TJ. Monitoring and validation of high purity water system with the *Limulus* amebocyte lysate test for pyrogens. Pharm Eng 1984; 4(2):21–23.
68. Dawson ME. Microbes, endotoxins and water. Pharm Eng 1988; 8(2):9–12.
69. Gould MJ. Microorganisms- evaluation of microbial/endotoxin contamination using the LAL test. Ultrapure Water 1993; September:43–47.
70. Lee PS, Plumlee B, Rymer T, Schwabe R, Hansen J. Using FMEA to develop alternatives to batch testing. Med Device Diagn Ind 2004; January:148–154.
71. ASTM Standard. D7102-04 Standard Guide for the Determination of Endotoxins on Sterile Medical Gloves. PA: ASTM International, 2005.
72. Holmdahl L, Nasser C. Endotoxin and particulate matter on surgical gloves. J Long-Term Eff Med Implants 1977; 7 (3&4):225–234.
73. Peiro SA, Kulander L, Eriksson O. Quantitative determination of endotoxins on surgical gloves. J Hosp Infect 1990; 16:167–172.
74. Williams PB, Halsey JF. Endotoxin as a factor in adverse reactions to latex gloves. Ann Allergy Asthma Immunol 1997; 79:303–309.
75. FDA CDRH. Guidance for the preparation of a premarket notification approval for a surgical mesh. DHHS 1999; March:5.
76. Dick HB, Agustin AJ, Pakula T, Pfeiffer N. Endotoxins in ophthalmic viscosurgical devices. Eur J Ophthalmol 2003; 13(2):176–184.
77. Dunn D. Reprocessing single-use devices- the equipment connection. AORN J 2002; 75(6):1143–1158.
78. Rioufol C, Devys C, Meunier G, Perraud M, Goullet D. Quantitative Determination of endotoxins released by bacterial biofilms. J Hosp Infect 1999; 43:203–209.
79. Morin P. Identification of the bacteriological contamination of a water treatment line used for haemodialysis and its disinfection. J Hosp Infect 2000; 45:218–224.
80. Marion-Ferey K, Pasmore M, Stoodley P, et al. Biofilm removal from silicone tubing: an assessment of the efficacy of dialysis machine decontamination procedures using an in vitro model. J Hosp Infect 2003; 53:64–71.
81. Holland SP, Mathias RG, Morck DW, Chiu J, Slade SG. Diffuse lamellar keratitis related to endotoxins released from sterilizer reservoir biofilms. Ophthalmology 2000; 107(7): 1227–1234.

82. Martin MV, Dailey Y. A preliminary investigation of the microbiology and endotoxin content in the water reservoirs of benchtop non-vacuum autoclaves. Br Dent J 2001; 191(11):622–624.

83. FDA CDRH. Guidance for industry and FDA staff- medical device user fee and modernization act of 2002, validation data in premarket notification submissions (510(k)s) for reprocessed single-use medical devices. DHHS. 2003 July:19.

84. Code of Federal Regulations. Title 21 Food and Drugs, Chapter I Food and Drug Administration DHHS, Subchapter H Medical Devices, Part 820 Quality System Regulation. Title 21, Vol. 8, Revised as of April 1, 2005.

Receptors, Mediators, and Mechanisms Involved in Bacterial Sepsis and Septic Shock

Edwin S. Van Amersfoort and Johan Kuiper
Division of Biopharmaceutics, Leiden/Amsterdam Center of Drug Research, Leiden University, Leiden, The Netherlands

INTRODUCTION

Under normal circumstances, many bacteria live in coexistence with humans. The skin, digestive tract, upper respiratory tract, external urogenital organs, and conjunctiva all contain bacteria and many of them are commensal and do not cause disease. The presence of bacteria on or in these organs is not a threat to the body because the lumen of nasal and oral cavity, airway, digestive tract, and urogenital organs are connected to the "external environment" and are thus secluded from the normally sterile "internal environment."

Pathogenic as well as commensal microorganisms evoke an immune response if they, or their constituents, pass the barrier between the external and internal environment. After recognition of the bacteria or products thereof, the body launches an attack, kills the bacteria, and repairs putative damage. This sequence of events is highly regulated, enabling the body to combat infection by a tailor-made attack that is fierce enough to eradicate the bacteria, but not so fierce that unnecessary damage to the body is caused.

Bacteria evolved as some of the first living organisms on earth and have been endowed with an enormous capacity to adapt to changes in environment. The building plan of bacteria is the result of millions of years of evolution and is, despite its simplicity compared to multicellular organisms, highly refined. The bacteria commensal and pathogenic to humans and animals belong to the gram-positive bacteria, gram-negative bacteria, *Rickettsia*, *Chlamydia*, and *Mycoplasma*. The groups of gram-positive and gram-negative bacteria comprise most species. Differentiation between these two groups is based on a characteristic difference in appearance after staining with the gram-stain, corresponding to differences in cell wall architecture.

A large number of gram-positive and gram-negative bacteria are pathogenic to humans. Some of these, along with the diseases that they may cause, are listed in Table 1. The symptoms caused by an infection with these bacteria ranges from almost none in the case of small lesions to severe illness and even death in the case of a generalized, systemic infection (bacteremia or sepsis). The character of the symptoms depends largely on the pathogenic species and the immunological condition of the host.

SEPSIS AND SEPTIC SHOCK

Sepsis and septic shock, caused by gram-negative and gram-positive bacteria, fungi, viruses, and parasites, have become increasingly important over the past decades (1). In the United States, the septicemia rates more than doubled

TABLE 1   Gram-Negative and Gram-Positive Pathogenic Bacteria

Gram-negative bacteria	Gram-positive bacteria
E. coli (urinary tract infections)	*S. aureus* (e.g., hospital-acquired infections)
S. typhi (typhoid fever)	*S. epidermidis* (e.g., hospital-acquired infections)
Klebsiella pneumoniae (e.g., pneumonia)	*S. saprophyticus* (urinary tract infections)
Vibrio cholerae (cholera)	*Streptococcus pyogenes* (scarlet fever)
Helicobacter pylorus (gastritis, stomach ulcer)	*S. pneumoniae* (pneumonia)
Shigella dysenteriae (dysentery)	*Corynebacterium diphtheriae* (diphtheria)
N. meningitides (meningitis)	

between 1979 and 1987 causing up to 250,000 deaths annually (2,3) The percentage of gram-negative infections varies between 30% and 80% and that of gram-positive infections between 6% to more than 50% of all cases of septicemia in the early 1990s (4,5). The increasing septicemia rates result probably from the increasing use of catheters and other invasive equipment, by chemotherapy, and by immunosuppression in patients with organ transplants or inflammatory diseases (6,7).

In many cases of sepsis, the presence of microorganisms (bacteremia) or lipopolysaccharide (LPS) (endotoxemia) cannot be detected in blood, which has prompted the adaptation of the definitions of sepsis and septic shock (Table 2) (6,8,9).

The clinical phenomena of sepsis and septic shock are highly complex (Fig. 1). Paradoxically a weakened immune system may contribute to the development of

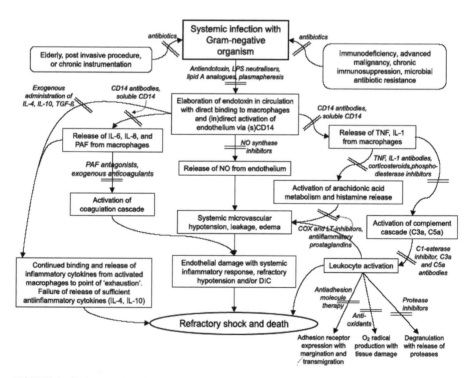

FIGURE 1   Pathogenesis of sepsis. The double lines indicate potential therapeutic intervention points. *Abbreviations*: DIC, disseminated intravascular coagulation; IL, interleukin; NO, nitric oxide; PAF, platelet-activating factor; TNF, tumor necrosis factor. *Source*: From Ref. 17.

TABLE 2 Definitions of Sepsis and Septic Shock

Bacteremia	Positive blood cultures
Sepsis	Clinical evidence of infection, tachypnea (>20 breaths/min), tachycardia (>90 beats/min), hyperthermia, or hypothermia
Sepsis syndrome	Sepsis plus hypoxaemia or elevated plasma lactate or oliguria
Septic shock	Sepsis syndrome plus hypotension (despite adequate volume resuscitation)

sepsis, but the detrimental processes that may ultimately lead to death are caused by an exaggerated, systemic response to an infection. The widespread activation of cells responsive to bacteria or bacterial components results in the release of an array of inflammatory mediators (cytokines) that induce vasodilatation and upregulation of adhesion molecules, and this results in the extravasation of neutrophils and monocytes, activation of leukocytes, lymphocytes, and endothelial cells, and myocardial suppression (Fig. 1) (3,10,11). Besides stimulation of coagulation by cytokines, bacterial components may directly interact with the coagulation system. The resulting disseminated intravascular coagulation (DIC) causes hypoperfusion and hypoxia. Together with the damage caused by the intra and extravascular phagocytic cells, organ failure develops (12,13). This may initiate the often lethal stage of sepsis, in which multiple organ failure (MOF) mostly involving lungs, liver, and kidneys develops (3,6,14). In addition, the hypoperfusion caused by DIC may impair the gut mucosal barrier with translocation of bacteria to the mesenteric lymph nodes and, under conditions of ongoing stress, to several organs and the circulation. The released bacteria will "feed" the MOF and significantly worsen the prognosis (15).

There are marked differences in the response to gram-positive and gram-negative bacteria. The immunological response to gram-negative bacteria mainly involves leukocytes and production of cytokines such as tumor necrosis factor-α (TNF)-α, interleukin (IL)-1, and IL-6. The release of exotoxins by gram-positive bacteria, many of which are superantigens, activates T cells and, as a result, a different cellular response and different cytokine profile, with relatively low amounts of TNF-α, IL-1, and IL-6, and increased amounts of IL-8 (2,7,16).

Bacterial Cell Wall Architecture: Lipopolysaccharide and Lipoteichoic Acid
LPS and lipoteichoic acid (LTA) are the main building blocks of the outer leaflets of the bacterial cell wall membranes and as such contribute to and are essential for stability and growth. Often they are not directly exposed to the external environment because many naturally occurring gram-positive and gram-negative bacteria are fitted with a thick polysaccharide capsule (18). A schematic representation of the gram-positive and gram-negative cell wall is shown in Figure 2.

Lipopolysaccharide
LPS is a major constituent of the outer membrane of gram-negative bacteria, which also contains (glycerol)phospholipids and proteins [e.g., OmpA (19)]. LPS is a prerequisite for bacterial viability and LPS is only toxic after release from the bacterial wall and exposing its toxic moiety, lipid A, to immune cells, thus evoking an inflammatory response. LPS is released from the bacterial cells when they multiply, but also when bacteria die or lyse (20,21).

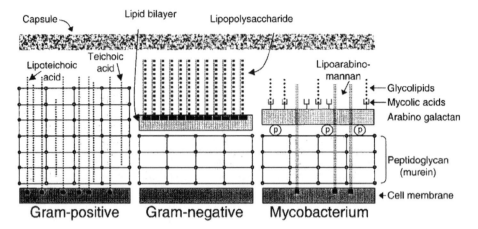

FIGURE 2   Cell wall structure of bacteria. All types of bacteria contain a cell membrane surrounded by a peptidoglycan-containing layer. Lipoteichoic acid and LAM are inserted into the cell membrane of gram-positive bacteria. Lipopolysaccharide forms the outer layer of the outer membrane of gram-negative bacteria. The mycobacteria also contain a carbohydrate shell but not all bacteria contain a capsule.

The LPS molecule consists of four different parts (21–23). The first and the most essential part is lipid A: the covalently linked lipid component of LPS. Six or more fatty acid residues are linked to two phosphorylated glucosamine sugars. All bacterial species carry a unique LPS and some of the variations reside in the lipid A moiety and lipid A represents the toxic moiety (24). The second part of the LPS molecule consists of the inner core. It consists of two or more KDO (2-keto-3-deoxyoctonic acid) sugars, linked to the lipid A glucosamine, and two or three heptose (L-glycero-D-manno-heptose) sugars linked to the KDO. Both sugars are specific to bacteria. The outer core, the third part of the LPS molecule, consists of common sugars and is more variable than the inner core. The fourth moiety of the LPS molecule is the O-antigen. This part of the LPS molecule is attached to the terminal sugar of the outer core. It extends from the surface of the bacteria and is highly immunogenic. It is composed of units of common sugars, but there is a huge interspecies and interstrain variation in the composition and length. In a single LPS preparation, the length of the O-antigen may vary from 0 to as much as 40 repeating units, but generally consists of 20 to 40 repeating units. Each unit is composed of three sugars with a single sugar connected to the first and third sugar of the unit. LPS molecules with O-antigen are denoted as S-LPS. Colonies from bacteria with O-antigen-containing LPS have a smooth (S) appearance on the plate, whereas bacteria that express an O-antigen-lacking LPS have a rough (R) appearance.

Lipoteichoic Acid

LTA resembles in certain respects LPS and can therefore be considered the gram-positive counterpart of LPS. LTA contains a diacylglycerol lipid moiety instead of a phospholipid-like structure and LTA contains highly charged glycerophosphate repeating units in contrast to the oligosaccharide repeating units in LPS. LTA is, like LPS, essential for the growth of the bacteria (25). The architecture of gram-positive cell wall is markedly different from that of gram-negative bacteria, since it contains only a single cell membrane in which LTA molecules are inserted. The outside of the gram-positive cell wall is covered with a thick layer consisting of peptidoglycan (PGN) and teichoic acid (Fig. 2) (26).

The gram-positive bacterial cell membrane contains in addition to LTA other lipid constituents such as diglucosyldiacylglycerol, phoshatidylglycerol, diacylglycerol, and lysylphosphatidylglycerol (25,27). A long tail of repeating 1,3-linked glycerophosphate units is connected to the glucoside moiety (25,27,28). The number of repeating units varies widely, depending on species, strains, and growth conditions, but for *Staphylococcus aureus* generally ranges between 4 and 30. D-alanine may be incorporated at the 2 position of the glycerophosphate tail, but the extent of alanine substitution depends not only on factors such as species and strain, but also on growth conditions and growth stage (25).

THE HOST RESPONSE TO LIPOPOLYSACCHARIDE AND LIPOTEICHOIC ACID

As soon as a bacterium enters the body, it is confronted with two lines of defense: a humoral and a cellular line. The humoral factors comprise complement, antibodies, and acute phase proteins. The other line of defense is the cellular line. Especially the mononuclear cells (monocytes and macrophages) and the neutrophils are of high relevance since these cells may recognize LPS and LTA directly, or indirectly after complement and antibody binding to bacterium and its constituents.

Under physiological conditions, the immune cells are continuously exposed to low levels of LPS derived from gastrointestinal bacteria that enter the body via the portal vein. This LPS is taken up by macrophages and may be essential to maintain a basal level of attentiveness of the immune system (Table 3).

Cellular Defense

LPS and other bacterial (surface) components are recognized by complement and antibodies, leading to opsonization and lysis of the bacterium. Phagocytes (monocytes, macrophages, and PMN) are able to recognize opsonized bacterial components by complement receptors (CRs) and Fc-receptors (bind IgG antibodies) (30). Furthermore, they express receptors that recognize the bacterial components. In the host response to bacteria, the mononuclear phagocytes (monocytes and macrophages) are of major importance. Recognition of LPS or other bacterial components by these cells leads to the initiation of a cascade of release of inflammatory mediators, vascular and physiological changes, and recruitment of immune cells

TABLE 3 Beneficial and Toxic Effects of Endotoxin

Beneficial effects	Toxic effects
Increased resistance to infection and malignancy	Fever
Protection from lethal irradiation	Hypoglycemia
Adjuvanticity	Hypotension
Normal development of lymphoid organs	Diarrhea/weight loss
	Disseminated intravascular coagulation
	Abortion
	Shock/death

Source: From Ref. 29.

(Fig. 3). This was first recognized in a mouse strain unresponsive to LPS: C3H/HeJ mice. When macrophages from the LPS responsive C3H/HeN strain were transferred to C3H/HeJ mice, a normal reaction to LPS could be elicited.

An LPS-activated macrophage becomes metabolically active and produces intracellular stores of oxygen free radicals and other microbicidal agents (lysozyme, cationic proteins, acid hydrolases, lactoferrin) and secretes inflammatory mediators (31–33). One of the key mediators is TNF-α (6). After exposure to LPS, TNF-α is the first cytokine released by the macrophages. TNF-α mRNA is constitutively transcribed in Kupffer cells, allowing rapid release of TNF-α after an inflammatory challenge. IL-1 and IL-6 are not constitutively expressed, but the mRNAs of these cytokines, as well as those of TNF-α, are immediately transcribed after a challenge and maximum mRNA levels have been found 40 minutes postchallenge in mouse liver macrophages.

The release of TNF-α, IL-1, IL-6, IL-8, IL-12, platelet-activating factor (PAF), chemokines, and eicosanoids has profound effects on the surrounding tissue (34–37). In concert with the complement pathway derived anaphylatoxins C3a and C5a, they attract PMN from the circulation and activate them. The extravasation of PMN is enabled by vasodilatation and upregulation of adhesion molecules on endothelial cells, PMN, and macrophages. The PMN react to these stimuli by intravascular aggregation, adherence to the endothelium, diapedesis, and by the production of inflammatory mediators like TNF-α, leukotriene B$_4$, and PAF (38). The (activated) PMN express CD14, CD11/CD18, and several complement and Fc-receptors and are thus able to recognize and phagocytose LPS, bacterial fragments, and whole bacteria. As specialized phagocytes, PMN produce an impressive series of microbicidal agents, such as lysozyme, bactericidal/permeability-increasing

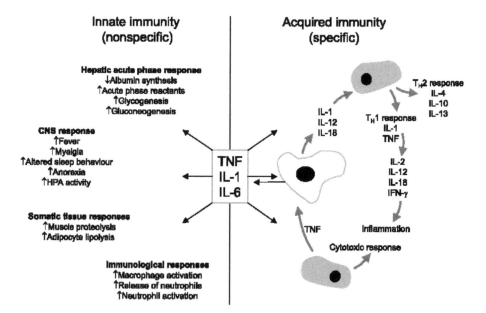

FIGURE 3 The cellular responses to Lipopolysaccharide (LPS). The responses of innate and acquired immunity. *Abbreviations*: HPA, hypothalamus-pituitary–adrenal; IL, interleukin; TNF, tumor necrosis factor. *Source*: From Ref. 40.

protein (BPI), enzymes, and oxygen free radicals. These agents are mainly used for lysosomal killing of microorganisms. However, adherence of the PMN to endothelial cells and the presence of high concentrations of stimuli may also result in the release of microbicidal agents and much of the endothelial damage observed in sepsis is caused by these agents (6). The endothelial cells respond to LPS (via sCD14) and to the circulating cytokines by the release of IL-1, IL-6, eicosanoids, the vasoactive agents endothelium-derived relaxation factor, and endothelin-1, chemokines, and colony-stimulating factors (39). The inflammatory mediators secreted by the different cell populations attract and activate B and T-lymphocytes. In return, the latter release mediators such as IL-2, IFN-γ, and GM-CSF (6). IL-2 and GM-CSF are involved in proliferation and activation of PMN and mononuclear cells, whereas IFN-γ enhances the effects of LPS on mononuclear cells (6). The actions of the activated immune cells combined with the effects of the inflammatory mediators cause symptoms such as fever, endothelial damage, capillary leakage, peripheral vascular dilatation, coagulation disorders, microembolization, and myocardial depression (Fig. 3). These phenomena may finally result in multiple organ dysfunction, shock, and death (6).

Compared with LPS, relatively little is known about the actions of LTA in vivo and in vitro. In contrast to gram-negative bacteria in which LPS is the major biologically active moiety, in gram-positive bacteria LTA, PGNs, and exotoxins are highly relevant with respect to the immunological response (2). LTA and PGN are able to induce the release of nitric oxide (NO), IL-1, IL-6, and TNF-α by macrophages and to activate the oxidative burst in vitro (41). Furthermore, the effects of LTA and PGN may be synergistic (42). Like LPS, the bacterial species largely determines the potency of the biological actions of LTA (41). In vivo both LTA and PGN cause the release of NO, TNF-α, IFN-γ, and induction of circulatory failure (42), which indicates that the gram-positive bacterial components induce similar effects as LPS both in vitro and in vivo.

In vivo challenges with viable and killed bacteria reveal marked differences between gram-positive and gram-negative bacteria in the kinetics of bacteria-induced TNF-α release, and similar differences were observed in vitro (33,43). In contrast, LPS and LTA exhibit similar kinetics of TNF release in vivo (42) Despite the differences between bacteria and LPS, it has recently been shown that *Salmonella typhimurium* and the LPS thereof induce similar changes in macrophage-gene expression in vitro, confirming the early observations that LPS mimics whole gram-negative bacteria in many respects (45).

Humoral Defense

Bacteria activate both complement pathways: *Escherichia coli* polysaccharide surface components (O-antigen, capsule, and LPS) trigger the alternative pathway by binding to complement factor 3 (C3) (46). Lipid A binds C1q and activates the classical pathway. The classical complement pathway is also activated in the presence of specific antibodies (IgG and IgM) against gram-negative bacterial constituents. In all three cases, C3b is deposited on the molecule or cell surface, which promotes phagocytosis by macrophages and neutrophils, and leads to insertion of complement factors C5 to C9 [membrane attack complex (MAC)] into the cell surface in many cases leading to lysis of the bacterium. Similar to LPS, LTA activates the classical pathway by interacting with C1 and C1q (47). In addition, erythrocyte-bound LTA activates the alternative complement pathway resulting in lysis of the erythrocytes (48,49).

With the cleavage of C3 and C5, the chemo-attractive and vasoactive agents C3a and C5a are released. They cause increased vascular permeability, upregulate adhesion molecule expression on endothelial cells and neutrophils, and attract and activate these phagocytes. Furthermore, they activate basophilic granulocytes and mast cells. These cells release a variety of vasoactive compounds (such as histamin), facilitating the invasion of phagocytes.

During infection, liver parenchymal cells are stimulated by TNF-α, IL-1, and IL-6 to produce "acute phase proteins." These comprise C-reactive protein (CRP), serum amyloid A, lipopolysaccharide-binding protein (LBP), serum amyloid P, hemopexin, haptoglobin, complement factors C3 and C9, α_1-acid glycoprotein, α_2-macroglobulin (α_2M), and some proteinase inhibitors. The expression is differentially upregulated from several fold (C3 and C9) to even 1000-fold (CRP) (50). Albumin is a so-called negative acute-phase protein since its production is down regulated during inflammation (50).

The Liver

The liver is the largest solid organ in the body, constituting 2% to 5% of the body weight in adults and is considered to be of major importance in the body's defense mechanism against bacteria and foreign macromolecules derived from bacteria and microorganisms (51). The liver consists of various cell types: liver parenchymal cells (hepatocytes), endothelial cells, and Kupffer cells. The liver parenchymal cells represent 60% of the liver cells. Liver parenchymal cells are main producers of plasma proteins (e.g., albumin) and acute-phase proteins. Liver endothelial cells exhibit several receptors that allow endocytosis of (foreign) ligands such as LPS and LTA (52). Kupffer cells are the liver macrophages, which constitute 805 to 90% of the fixed tissue macrophages [reticuloendothelial system (RES)]. Kupffer cells remove all kinds of old, unnecessary and damaged material from the circulation (immune complexes, erythrocytes, tumor cells, cellular debris, and apoptotic cells) (52). In addition, these cells remove with high efficacy the foreign materials from the blood (51). In relation to the defense against bacteria and bacterial components, Kupffer cells are highly relevant cells. They play a major role in both clearance and detoxification of LPS from the circulation (especially the portal vein) and the production of inflammatory mediators in response to LPS (53).

The liver plays a major role in removal and degradation of bacteria and bacterial compounds. Eighty percent of intravenously injected bacteria is rapidly taken up by the liver, whereas the rest of the bacteria is found in lungs and spleen (52). The clearance of bacteria is species- and strain-specific with generally higher residual levels for virulent strains compared with avirulent strains (54). Electron microscopy reveals that radioactive S-LPS rapidly associates with Kupffer cells followed by association with liver parenchymal cells and excretion of radioactivity into the bile (52,53).

Macrophages and the Response to Lipopolysaccharide
and Lipoteichoic Acid

Macrophages have been shown to play a pivotal role in the cellular response to LPS. The RES consists of specialized tissue macrophages (mainly Kupffer cells in the liver) responsible for the primary response to microorganisms in most tissues. Macrophages remove endotoxin and bacteria from the lymph and blood circulation and respond to the binding of LPS by the production of inflammatory mediators. Upon challenge with LPS, LTA, or other bacterial compounds, the Kupffer cells release a series of inflammatory mediators like TNF-α, IL-1, IL-6, eicosanoids, PAF, NO, and reactive oxygen. Not only free LPS and LTA, but also live and killed bacteria can elicit the release of TNF-α. The last group of products released in response to LPS are the reactive oxygen species. Activation of the Kupffer cells and infiltrating PMN by LPS, TNF-α, and other inflammatory mediators induce intracellular production of O_2^-, H_2O_2, and other potent microbicidal products. Although these compounds are responsible for killing of phagocytosed microorganisms, they are released at high concentrations of activators and cause extensive tissue damage. NO is a microbicidal product that may cause vasodilation, endothelial damage, damage to hepatocytes, and inhibition of acute-phase protein production and adhesion molecule expression in liver and lungs (55,56).

Detoxification of Lipopolysaccharide

LPS is processed after uptake by macrophages and PMN. This is confirmed by the observations that LPS or LPS metabolites are excreted in bile and feces (57). One of the intracellular degradation pathways may be the removal of fatty acids by acyloxyacyl hydrolase, and deacylated LPS probably has decreased biological activity. A second way of processing may be digestion of the O-antigen. LPS released by Kupffer cells showed a decreased sugar/lipid ratio compared with native LPS (57). Like deacylated LPS, dephosphorylated LPS appears to have a decreased biological activity.

LIPOPOLYSACCHARIDE AND LIPOTEICHOIC ACID RECEPTORS

Over the past 20 years, one of the major aims in LPS research has been the elucidation of the sequence of events between binding of LPS to a cell and the response of the cell. The first LPS receptor identified was the CD11b/CD18 or CR3 receptor. It has been shown that the binding of LPS-coated erythrocytes to PMN is mediated through this receptor. However, it turned out that the cells were not sufficiently activated through the CD11b/CD18 receptor and the quest for identification of the cell-activating LPS receptor was continued. In 1990, CD14, previously only known as a monocyte specific antigen, was identified as the receptor involved in cellular activation. However, due to the fact that CD14 lacks a transmembrane signaling domain, the involvement of an accessory receptor was proposed. Subsequently, the Toll-like receptors (TLRs) were identified as signaling receptor for LPS, LTA, and a variety of other microbial constituents (Table 4).

Lipopolysaccharide-Binding Protein

LBP is an acute phase protein (58) and is induced by IL-6 and IL-1. The serum levels of LBP increase strongly during infection (58). LBP is in serum associated with lipoproteins (59). LBP binds to LPS varying from smooth LPS to rough LPS, lipid A and lipid IV_A with a Kd of 1 to 58 nM for binding of LBP to lipid A (60). The binding site for lipid A is situated in the N-terminal part between amino acids (aa) 91 to 108, with the positively charged arginine residues within this region fulfilling an essential role. The C-terminal part of the LBP molecule, however, mediates the transfer of LPS to CD14.

TABLE 4 Lipopolysaccharide and Lipoteichoic Acid Receptors and Some of Their Ligands

Receptor	Ligands
LBP	LPS, LTA
CD14 and TLR	LPS, LTA, other microbial constituents, apoptotic cells
β_2-integrins	C3bi, C3b, ICAM-1, LPS
SR-A	Oxidized LDL, apoptotic cells, LPS, LTA
MARCO	Bacteria
L-selectin	GlyCAM-1, CD34, MAdCAM-1, Sgp200, LPS, LTA
P-selectin	PSGL-1 (Sialyl Lewis^X moiety), LPS
Heptose receptor	LPS

Abbreviations: LBP, lipopolysaccharide-binding protein; LDL, low-density lipoprotein; LPS, lipopolysaccharide; LTA, lipoteichoic acid; MARCO, macrophage receptor with collagenous structure; SR-A, class A scavenger receptor.

LBP catalyzes the transfer of LPS to CD14, thus enhancing the LPS-induced activation of monocytes, macrophages, and PMN by 100 to 1000-fold (58). The CD14-mediated activation of peritoneal macrophages by heat killed *S. aureus* bacteria, LTA, cell wall PGN, or mycobacterial lipoproteins is not enhanced by LBP. Application of anti-LBP antibodies together with LPS protected D-galactosamine sensitized mice from death (61).

Besides its pro-inflammatory role, LBP may also have anti-inflammatory actions, such as the LBP-mediated catalysis of LPS and LTA transfer to high-density lipoprotein (HDL) and other lipoproteins (See section on lipoproteins) (62). LBP was shown to be involved in the neutralization of LTA by HDL, extending the anti-inflammatory role of LBP to gram-positive organisms (62).

CD14

Since the addition of anti-CD14 antibodies decreases LPS-induced TNF-α release and transfection of CD14-negative Chinese Hamster Ovary cells with CD14, conferred responsiveness to LPS CD14 has been identified as an important LPS receptor with a binding affinity of 4×10^{-8} M. The mechanism of LPS binding to CD14 is shown in Figure 4.

In addition, CD14 transgenic mice are more sensitive to LPS, whereas CD14-deficient mice are highly resistant to LPS (63). CD14-deficient mice were less sensitive to a challenge with live gram-negative bacteria, due to the accelerated clearance of bacteria (63). The clearance of live *S. aureus* and the TNF-α levels were even higher in CD14-deficient compared with wild-type mice. CD14 may be important for the response to S-LPS rather than other types of LPS (A).

CD14 is a glycosyl phosphatidyl inositol (GPI)-linked receptor that lacks a transmembrane domain; it was rapidly identified that an accessory molecule is needed for signal transduction, which was later on identified as the TLR.

Although LPS was the first CD14 ligand discovered, later many other microbial ligands for CD14 were identified, but these are also ligands for the TLRs. Molecular cloning of the CD14 gene revealed a 1.4 kb transcript encoding a 356 amino acid protein (64). CD14 is GPI-linked and has a high leucine content (17.7% human CD14, 15.5% murine CD14) (65). A repeating leucine-rich, 24-residue motif (LxxLxLx) can be recognized (65). The LPS-binding site and the sites involved in the interaction of CD14 with the putative accessory receptors have been identified in the N-terminal part of CD14. Two putative LPS binding

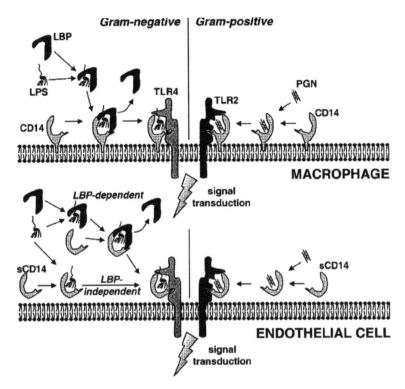

FIGURE 4 Binding of bacterial ligands to CD14 and sCD14. The involvement of LBP, (s)CD14, and TLR2 and TLR4 in the activation of CD14-expressing cells (e.g., macrophages) and of cells that do not express CD14 (e.g., endothelial cells). LPS (*left*) and PGN (*right*) represent TLR4- and TLR2-specific ligands, respectively. *Abbreviations*: LBP, lipopolysaccharide-binding protein; LPS, lipopolysaccharide; PGN, peptidoglycan; TLR, Toll-like receptor.

sites were mentioned: aa 39 to 44 and aa 57 to 64. CD14 is expressed by cells of the myeloid lineage (monocytes, macrophages, and PMN), B-cells, liver parenchymal cells, gingival fibroblasts, and microglial cells.

A soluble form of CD14, sCD14, is released by mononuclear cells and is dose dependently induced by LPS and TNF-α, whereas IFN-γ and IL-4 inhibit the release of sCD14 (66). In septic shock patients, sCD14 levels are increased and the levels have been found to correlate with mortality. The sCD14 may also transfer LPS sensitivity to cells such as endothelial and epithelial cells that do not express membrane bound CD14

Toll-like Receptors

Because of the absence of a transmembrane signaling domain in CD14, the presence of an LPS signaling receptor was expected. The receptor was found after the cloning of the defective gene in the LPS-unresponsive C3 h/HeJ and C57Bl6/10ScCr mice (67–69): TLR4, named after the homologous Toll protein in *Drosophila melanogaster*. The signaling pathway components in mammals (top row) and *Drosophila* (bottom row) are given in the following.

Signaling Pathways of TLRs

By now, TLR1 to 10 have been identified, all are (likely) involved in immune responses. The TLRs, the IL-1 receptor, the IL-18 receptor, and a number of mammalian and nonmammalian proteins exhibit a striking similarity with respect to the Toll/IL-1 receptor domain (TIR); hence, this family of receptors is called the TIR superfamily. Three major groups can be determined: (*i*) the immunoglobulin domain sub-group, containing the IL-1RI and the IL-18R; (*ii*) the leucine-rich-repeat subgroup, containing the TLRs; (*iii*) the adaptor subgroup, which includes the MyD88 protein that is essential for TLR2- and TLR4-mediated signaling (380).

So far, the specificities of TLR2, TLR3, TLR4, TLR5, and TLR9 (partially) have been revealed. A substantial amount of data now suggest that TLR4 is mainly involved in the recognition of LPS from gram-negative bacteria, whereas TLR2 recognizes not only gram-positive cell wall constituents such as PGN and LTA, but also microbial lipoproteins and lipopeptides and yeasts. In addition, TLR3 recognizes viral dsRNA, TLR5 recognizes bacterial flagellin, and TLR9 recognizes bacterial CpG DNA. Of the remaining TLRs identified, TLR1 may function as an accessory receptor for TLR2 in the recognition of *Neisseria meningitidis* cell wall components, whereas other investigators observed the heterodimerization of the signaling domain of TLR2 with either TLR1 or TLR6 enabling recognition of zymosan, Group B Streptococci-soluble factor, or gram-positive lipopeptides and lipoproteins. In response to *S. aureus* modulin, however, TLR1 inhibited and TLR6 enhanced the TLR2-mediated response, indicating a modulatory role for these proteins. This is confirmed by the findings of Spitzer et al. who observed inhibition of TLR4-mediated responses by TLR1 in endothelial cells. A similar role could be envisioned for some other TLRs of which no microbial specificity has been determined.

The expression patterns of the TLRs vary widely; whereas TLR1 is expressed on almost all myeloid and lymphoid cells, so far the TLR3 has only been shown to be expressed on dendritic cells. TLR2 and TLR4 exhibit comparable expression patterns and in steady state are mainly represented on PMN, monocytes, macrophages, and dendritic cells. However, both receptors are also present on various other cell types including epithelial and endothelial cells. In comparison to CD14, the number of TLR4 molecules on monocytes is small: CD14 is expressed at approximately 115,000 molecules, whereas TLR4 is present at $\pm$1300 molecules per monocyte, which has led some investigators to propose that TLR4 expression may be a limiting factor in the response to LPS. The expression levels of TLR2 and TLR4 have been shown to be modulated by LPS and other microbial components. During infection, TLR2 and TLR4 are expressed on cells otherwise expressing very low levels of these receptors.

β_2-Integrins

The CD18 antigens or β_2-integrins comprise a family of three closely related cell-surface glycoproteins with a varying CD11 α-chain and an equal CD18 β-chain: (*i*) $\alpha_1\beta_2$-integrin: LFA-1 or CD11a/CD18; (*ii*) $\alpha_2\beta_2$-integrin: CR3, MAC-1, or CD11b/CD18; (*iii*) $\alpha_3\beta_2$-integrin: CR4, p150,95, or CD11c/CD18. LFA-1 is expressed on all leukocytes, CR3 is expressed on monocytes, macrophages, PMN, and lymphocytes, whereas CR4 is expressed abundantly on monocytes and macrophages (70). LFA-1 recognizes the adhesion molecules ICAM-1 and ICAM-2, CR3 recognizes surface-bound C3bi and surface-bound fibrinogen, and CR4 binds surface-bound fibrinogen as well (70).

Many strains of *E. coli* are recognized by macrophages without the intervention of antibodies and complement. All three members of the CD18 family are capable of binding LPS. The part of the LPS recognized by CD18 resides in the lipid A region (72).

Selectins
The β_2-integrins are not the only adhesion molecules involved in the binding of LPS. Recently, Malhotra et al. (73) showed that P-selectin and L-selectin are able to bind LPS. In addition, L-selectin also mediated binding of LTA (73). It was proposed that L-selectin may represent the low-affinity serum-independent signaling receptor involved in the response to high concentrations of LPS.

Scavenger Receptors
Hampton et al. demonstrated that lipid IV_A can bind to a class A scavenger receptor (SR-A). Binding to the SR-A resulted in uptake but not in activation of the cells and uptake was followed by dephosphorylation, which renders the lipid IV_A less toxic (74). The scavenger receptor competitor polyinosinic acid (polyI) reduced liver uptake of lipid IV_A by approximately 35%, indicating a considerable scavenger receptor-mediated binding to the liver (74). Besides LPS and the gram-negative bacterium *E. coli*, SR-A also binds LTA and whole gram-positive bacteria such as *S. aureus*, *Listeria monocytogenes*, and *Mycobacterium tuberculosis* (74). The MARCO scavenger receptor (Macrophage Receptor with Collagenous structure), which also belongs to the SR-A, recognizes gram-negative and gram-positive bacteria.

Besides the bacteria and bacterial components, SR-A recognizes a broad range of ligands, among which acetylated low-density lipoproteins (LDLs), oxidized LDL, maleylated BSA, polyI, and polyG (75,76). MARCO is very similar to SR-AI, and hence its designation as an SR-A.

Cross-competition studies with LPS and several other scavenger receptor ligands have shown that there are also other scavenger receptors, expressed on Kupffer cells and liver sinusoidal endothelial cells, involved in the binding of LPS (77,78). The in vitro binding of LPS to Kupffer cells, liver sinusoidal endothelial cells, and peritoneal macrophages from SR-A-deficient mice is significantly reduced compared with cells from wild-type mice, which shows that the SR-A does recognize LPS and does contribute to the binding and uptake of LPS (78). Binding by scavenger receptors may actually form a protective mechanism by removing excess microorganisms or components thereof, thus preventing binding to the highly sensitive CD14 receptor and the development of septic shock. Based on the available data, the SR-A can be considered anti-inflammatory due to the uptake of LPS or other bacterial compounds, circumventing the CD14-TLR signaling pathway.

LIPOPOLYSACCHARIDE AND LIPOTEICHOIC ACID-BINDING PROTEINS
Neutrophilic Lipopolysaccharide-Binding Molecules
Bactericidal/Permeability Increasing Protein
BPI is a cationic 55 kDa protein that binds specifically to gram-negative bacteria and kills bacteria by increasing the permeability (79,80). Binding of BPI to LPS neutralizes the biological activity of LPS in vitro (79,80). In vivo, BPI or rBPI$_{23}$ reduced LPS

or bacteria-induced TNF release, liver damage, NO production, mortality, and protected against cardiovascular depression (81). In healthy volunteers, BPI causes a significant reduction in serum LPS, TNF, IL-6, IL-8, IL-10 levels, and several other parameters (82). The results of a clinical study in children with meningococcal sepsis were promising: of the 26 patients, only 1 died (4%) (83). However, in a larger placebo-controlled study, the mortality in the rBPI$_{21}$-treated patients was not significantly reduced, although there was a trend towards improved outcome in the primary outcome variables (84). The feasibility of the use of BPI for the treatment of sepsis and septic shock in humans may be restricted due to the limited half-life of approximately 10 minutes in vivo (85).

Lactoferrin
Lactoferrin is an 80 kDa glycoprotein that is present in neutrophilic granules, milk, and mucosal secretions (86). Lactoferrin has been shown to bind LPS and to be bacteriostatic to bacteria, indirectly through chelation of iron ions and directly through destabilization of the gram-negative bacterial cell membrane (86). Lactoferrin is a major LPS-neutralizing compound produced and excreted by stimulated PMN. Lactoferrin peptides containing the LPS-binding site have been shown to prevent the LBP-mediated binding of LPS to CD14, which results in a reduction of TNF and IL-6 release by THP-1 cells in vitro. Germ-free piglets that were fed lactoferrin were less sensitive to LPS, as shown by reduced mortality and hypothermia (87).

LIPOPROTEINS
Lipoprotein Metabolism
In human blood, four major lipoprotein classes can be distinguished according to their density: chylomicrons, very low-density lipoproteins (VLDLs), LDLs, and HDLs. These lipoprotein classes differ with respect to size, electrophoretic mobility, and lipid and apolipoprotein composition.

Apolipoprotein E
Apolipoprotein E (apoE) is an arginine-rich protein with a molecular weight of 34.2 kDa. ApoE is synthesized in a wide variety of tissues, including the liver, central nervous system, kidneys, adrenal glands, testes, and ovaries, but not the intestines (88). However, the highest levels of apoE mRNA are found in the liver parenchymal cells and it is also produced by macrophages from the liver, lungs, and spleen (88).

Several physiological and pathological functions for apoE have been proposed. These include the role of apoE in lipid metabolism (as described earlier), intracellular lipid redistribution, atherogenesis, neurobiology (nerve regeneration, association of the apoE4 serotype with neuropathologic lesions in Alzheimer's disease) (89), and immunomodulation (inhibition of proliferation of peripheral blood mononuclear cells and lymphocyte activation; inhibition of TNF secretion by glial cells) .

The Anti-Inflammatory Role of Lipoproteins
Ulevitch et al. were the first to observe that if LPS is mixed with serum or plasma, a decrease in buoyant density results. Pre-incubation of the LPS with the plasma decreased the ability of LPS to induce neutropenia and a pyrogenic response in

rabbits. Further investigations showed that the LPS was bound to HDL and that a plasma protein aided in the binding. In rabbits, the uptake of LPS by the adrenal glands was increased after LPS binding to HDL, which indicates that binding of LPS to HDL results in a decreased recognition by LPS receptors. Since then, in vivo and in vitro experiments have shown that LPS and LTA bind to and are neutralized by lipid emulsions (90), chylomicrons (91), VLDL (92), LDL (92), 0HDL (92), apoAI (93), apob (93), and apoE (94).

In vivo experiments have shown that the injection of LPS–HDL complexes may affect the serum decay of LPS and inhibits the LPS-induced release of cytokines when compared with LPS alone (91). In addition, in several experiments, the infusion of recombinant HDL (rHDL), VLDL, or lymph-derived chylomicrons and lipid emulsion also resulted in inhibition of LPS-induced physiological changes (95). Pajkrt et al. (96), in an experimental setting, infused rHDL into humans who were subsequently challenged with a low dose of LPS and observed a significant reduction in the release of proinflammatory cytokines and a partial reduction in the activation and/or release of components involved in coagulation. LDL receptor knockout mice, with cholesterol levels twice those in C57Bl6 mice, are less susceptible to LPS than wild-type mice, as shown by decreased mortality and reduced release of TNF, IL-1, and IL-6 (97). In contrast, the severely hypercholesterolemic apoE-knockout mice are more sensitive to LPS (98).

So far, only the binding of LPS to lipoproteins was discussed, but binding to apolipoproteins has also been reported. Emancipator et al. (93) and Usynin et al. have shown that both apob and apoAI are able to bind and neutralize LPS. Our group has shown that LPS binds apoE and causes a redistribution in vivo, reducing the uptake by Kupffer cells and promoting the binding to liver parenchymal cells (94). In addition, we have also shown that apoE binds LTA resulting in a similar redistribution from Kupffer cells to liver parenchymal cells and in a strongly decreased TNF release in vivo (94).

CLINICAL AND EXPERIMENTAL SEPSIS THERAPIES

Because of the complexity of immunological defense and sepsis, the development of pharmacological interventions is difficult (17,99). One approach would be to prevent infection in patients at high risk (Fig. 5). However, timely treatment to prevent sepsis or septic shock is often not possible or the prevention of infection is simply insufficient. The standard treatment often consists of administration of fluid and vasopressors to restore blood pressure and organ blood flow, oxygenation, and administration of antibiotics (100–102). Although the eradication of the microbial organism and fighting the pathophysiological changes are highly desirable, alternative approaches actively suppressing the deleterious effects of inflammation, while retaining the antimicrobial defense, are needed (Fig. 1).

The first alternative approach to treatment of sepsis was through antibody preparations to LPS. Three antilipid A IgM preparations were used, HA-1A and E5, and a polyclonal antiserum against the LPS core of *E. coli* J5. The human anti-*E. coli* J5 (Re-LPS) antiserum was first used to treat a small group of patients with septic shock. This cross-reactive antiserum barely significantly improved overall prognosis in septic shock, but it was not possible to determine whether the antibodies or other compounds (e.g., inflammatory mediators) from the donor conferred protection (103). E5 decreased mortality in a first trial, but provided no protection in successive trials (104,105). HA-1A (Centoxin™) was protective in

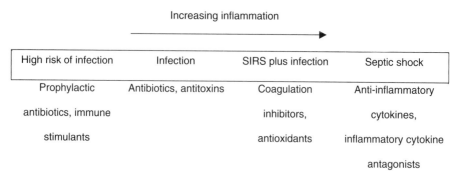

FIGURE 5   Scheme for preventing and treating sepsis. *Abbreviation*: SIRS, systemic inflammation response syndrome. *Source*: From Ref. 102.

one trial, whereas it had no effect in a second and tended to increase mortality in a subgroup of patients in a third trial (106). Very little is known about the mechanism of protection of these antibodies. Although it was expected that the HA-1A antibody recognized lipid A specifically, later it was discovered that it bound rather unspecific to hydrophobic substances (106). Other attempts to treat patients with an anti-LPS antibody have also failed (17). As listed in Table 5, a substantial number of patients have been treated with the various preparations, but no overall benefit was observed.

Also the recombinant 23 kDa N-terminal part of BPI, which is a powerful LPS-neutralizing agent, has been used to treat septic patients. Although the initial results of a small trial in children with meningococcal sepsis were promising, a larger trial showed no real benefit (83,84). In addition to the disappointing results of these trials, the use of therapeutics only effective against gram-negative organisms may not be desirable due to the delay caused by the time-consuming identification of the pathogenic organism.

Both in vitro studies with whole-blood from septic patients and in vivo studies in healthy volunteers challenged with LPS indicate that treatment with rHDL could be effective in septic shock. However, as yet no data are available from clinical trials with recombinant HDL (96,107).

Immunosuppression and Neutralization of Pro-Inflammatory Cytokines

Although general immunosuppression seems to be an obvious choice in the treatment of sepsis, the overall mortality increased (108). Similarly, nonsteroidal anti-inflammatory drugs that suppress the COX-enzymes were also proven ineffective. Since TNF has been shown to be a key mediator in the pathogenesis of sepsis, a recombinant humanized murine anti-TNF antibody preparation (Remicade™ or infliximab) and a TNF-R:Fc fusion protein (Enbrel™ or etanercept) have been tested for the treatment of sepsis (109,110). In the clinical trials, these preparations proved ineffective. Paradoxically, these TNF antagonists are very effective against Crohn's disease (inflammatory bowel disease) and rheumatoid arthritis, while infection and sepsis are contraindicated. Another important cytokine in inflammation and sepsis is IL-1. A recombinant IL-1 receptor antagonist has been tested in two large Phase III trials, but was not effective (111). In healthy human volunteers, LPS tolerance could be induced by the infusion of monophosphoryl lipid

TABLE 5 Randomized Controlled Trials of Immunotherapy in Sepsis and Septic Shock

Study	Agent	Primary end point	Active drug		Placebo		P-value	Comments
			N	% Mortality	N	% Mortality		
Root et al. (92)	rhGCSF	29-day mortality	348	29	353	25.5	0.38	rhGCSF increased leukocytes
Abraham et al. (93)	MAB-T88	28-day mortality	413	37	413	34	0.36	More adverse events in MAB-T88 group
Abraham et al. (100)	TFPI	28-day mortality	880	34.2	874	33.9	0.88	More bleeding in TFPI arm
Abraham et al. (102)	LY315920Na/ S-5960	28-day mortality	LD: 196	37.2	196	33.2	0.53	Favorable dose-dependent effect if treated within 18 hours
Schuster et al. (103)	rhPAF-AH	28-day mortality	HD: 194 LD: 45	36.4 21	43	44	0.07	Trend for reduced multiple organ failure
Opel et al. (104)	rhPAF-AH	28-day mortality	HD: 39 643	28 25	618	24	0.80	Well tolerated
Bakker et al. (107)	546C88	Shock resolution, 72 hours	161	40	161	24[xx]	0.004[xx]	No difference in survival
Lopez et al. (105)	546C88	28-day mortality	439	59	358	49	0.001	Stopped early by the Data and Safety Monitoring Board

Source: From Ref. 117.

A, but no clinical trials in septic patients have been performed (112). Interestingly, cross-tolerance to gram-positive infection could be induced in mice, indicating that this therapy might be effective in gram-negative and gram-positive sepsis (112).

The use of corticosteroids has been a subject of debate for many years. Corticosteroids are known to regulate a number of immune responses. Glucocorticoids inhibit a number of inflammatory processes, such as leukocyte infiltration and cytokine production, whereas glucocorticoids have a positive effect on cardiac output by a blockade of NO synthesis (113,114). On the basis of these effects, patients have been treated in two large clinical trials using corticoids in the early phase of sepsis (115). The results of these trials indicated eventually that there were no benefical effects of corticoids in the early phase of sepsis. More recently, it was observed that patients with a so-called adrenocortical insufficiency may have a poor prognosis (108). On the basis of this hypothesis, trials were started in which patients were treated with a lower dose of corticosteroids (300 mg of hydrocortisone per day) for a number of days at a later stage in sepsis. The outcome of this lower dose of steroids seems to be more promising than the higher dose of steroids in the early phase of sepsis, and more recent trials (1998–2002) using glucocorticoids for the treatment of sepsis have been more encouraging than the trials from before 1988 (108).

The latest success in the treatment of sepsis in adults was the PROWESS study (Human Activated Protein C Worldwide Evaluation in Severe Sepsis) (116). In this large double-blind study, the effect of activated protein C was studied. After the treatment of 1520 patients, the study was abrogated because of the significant survival advantage in the actively treated group (mortality 24.7% vs. 30.8% for placebo, $P = 0.005$). The mode of action of activated protein C is most probably based on its ability to inhibit both thrombosis (lower levels of D-dimer) and inflammation (as seen in a reduced level of IL-6), whereas fibrinolysis is promoted. Bleeding is the most frequent and serious adverse event that may be induced by rhAPC treatment and discussion is ongoing on the effect of heparin on activated protein C therapy. Drotrecogin alfa (activated) (Xigris—Eli Lilly), the commercially available recombinant human activated protein C, is now licensed for treating adults who have severe sepsis with MOF. Therapies with other agents that address the coagulation pathway, such as TFPI and antithrombin III, were not effective.

Although the blocking or modulation of a number of other targets, including complement and coagulation factors, neutrophil adherence, and NO release, has been shown to be promising in animals, it remains to be determined whether these therapeutic approaches will be effective in humans (17,99).

REFERENCES

1. Glauser MP, et al. Septic shock: pathogenesis. Lancet 1991; 338:732–736.
2. Opal SM, Cohen J. Clinical gram-positive sepsis: does it fundamentally differ from gram- negative bacterial sepsis? Crit Care Med 1999; 27:1608–1616.
3. Parillo JE. Pathogenetic mechanisms of septic shock. N Engl J Med 1993; 328:1471–1477.
4. Basu SK, et al. Mouse macrophages synthesize and secrete a protein resembling apolipoprotein E. Proc Natl Acad Sci USA 1981; 78:7545–7549.
5. Geerdes HF, et al. Septicemia in 980 patients at a university hospital in Berlin: prospective studies during 4 selected years between 1979 and 1989. Clin Infect Dis 1992; 15:991–1002.
6. Bone RC. The pathogenesis of sepsis. Ann Intern Med 1991; 115:457–469.
7. Bone RC. Gram-positive organisms and sepsis. Arch Intern Med 1994; 154:26–34.
8. Bone RC. Why new definitions of sepsis are needed. Am J Med 1993; 95:348–350.

9. Venet C, et al. Endotoxaemia in patients with severe sepsis or septic shock. Intensive Care Med 2000; 26:538–544.

10. Karima R, et al. The molecular pathogenesis of endotoxic shock and organ failure. Mol Med Today 1999; 5:123–132.

11. Wagner JG, Roth RA. Neutrophil migration during endotoxemia. J Leukoc Biol 1999; 66:10–24.

12. Mammen EF. The haematological manifestations of sepsis. J Antimicrob Chemother 1998; 41(suppl A):17–24.

13. van Gorp EC, et al. Review: infectious diseases and coagulation disorders. J Infect Dis 1999; 180:176–186.

14. Werb Z, Chin JR. Endotoxin suppresses expression of apoprotein E by mouse macrophages in vivo and in culture. A biochemical and genetic study. J Biol Chem 1983; 258:10642–10648.

15. Yao YM, et al. The inflammatory basis of trauma/shock-associated multiple organ failure. Inflamm Res 1998; 47:201–210.

16. Sriskandan S, Cohen J. Gram-positive sepsis. Mechanisms and differences from gram-negative sepsis. Infect Dis Clin North Am 1999; 13:397–412.

17. Horn KD. Evolving strategies in the treatment of sepsis and systemic inflammatory response syndrome (SIRS). QJM 1998; 91:265–277.

18. Roberts IS. The biochemistry and genetics of capsular polysaccharide production in bacteria. Annu Rev Microbiol 1996; 50:285–315.

19. Manthey CL, et al. Endotoxin-induced early gene expression in C3H/HeJ (Lpsd) macrophages. J Immunol 1994; 153:2653–2663.

20. Hubsch AP, et al. Protective effects of reconstituted high-density lipoprotein in rabbit gram-negative bacteremia models. J Lab Clin Med 1995; 126:548–558.

21. Rietschel ET, et al. Bacterial endotoxin: molecular relationships of structure to activity and function. FASEB J 1994; 8:217-225.

22. Lugtenberg B, Van Alphen L. Molecular architecture and functioning of the outer membrane of *Escherichia coli* and other Gram-negative bacteria. Biochim Biophys Acta 1983; 737:1–115.

23. Raetz CRH. Biochemistry of endotoxins. Annu Rev Biochem 1990; 59:129–170.

24. Kotani S, et al. Synthetic lipid A with endotoxic and related biological activities comparable to those of a natural lipid A from an *Escherichia coli* Re-mutant. Infect Immun 1985; 49:225–237.

25. Fischer W. Lipoteichoic acid and lipids in the membrane of *Staphylococcus aureus*. Med Microbiol Immunol (Berl) 1994; 183:61–76.

26. Dmitriev BA, et al. Layered murein revisited: a fundamentally new concept of bacterial cell wall structure, biogenesis and function. Med Microbiol Immunol (Berl) 1999; 187:173–181.

27. Fischer W, Koch HU. Alanyl lipoteichoic acid of *Staphylococcus aureus*: functional and dynamic aspects. Biochem Soc Trans 1985; 13:984–986.

28. Fischer W, et al. On the basic structure of poly(glycerophosphate) lipoteichoic acids. Biochem Cell Biol 1990; 68:33–43.

29. Vogel SN, Hogan MM. Role of cytokines in endotoxin-mediated host responses. In: Oppenheim JJ, Shevach EM, eds. Immunophysiology. The Role of Cells and Cytokines in Immunity and Inflammation. New York, Oxford: Oxford University Press, 1990: 238–258.

30. Frank MM, Fries LF. The role of complement in inflammation and phagocytosis. Immunol Today 1991; 12:322–331.

31. Hiemstra PS, et al. Antimicrobial proteins of murine macrophages. Infect Immun 1993; 61:3038–3046.

32. Mayer AMS, Spitzer JA. Continuous infusion of *Escherichia coli* endotoxin in vivo primes superoxide anion release in rat polymorphonuclear leukocytes and Kupffer cells in a time-dependent manner. Infect Immun 1991; 59:4590–4598.

33. Roitt IM. Immunity to infection. In: Roitt IM, ed. Essential Immunology. Oxford: Blackwell Scientific Publications, 1994: 243–271.

34. Hack CE, et al. Role of cytokines in sepsis. Adv Immunol 1997; 66:101–195.

35. Katori M, Majima M. Cyclooxygenase-2: its rich diversity of roles and possible application of its selective inhibitors. Inflamm Res 2000; 49:367–392.
36. Malhotra R, et al. Role for L-selectin in lipopolysaccharide-induced activation of neutrophils. Biochem J 1996; 320:589–593.
37. Qureshi N, et al. Location of fatty acids in lipid A obtained from lipopolysaccharide of Rhodopseudomonas sphaeroides ATCC 17023. J Biol Chem 1988; 263:5502–5504.
38. Van Epps DE, et al. Relationship of C5a receptor modulation to the functional responsiveness of human polymorphonuclear leukocytes to C5a. J Immunol 1993; 150:246–252.
39. Mahalingam S, Karupiah G. Chemokines and chemokine receptors in infectious diseases. Immunol Cell Biol 1999; 77:469–475.
40. Dinarello CA, Moldawer LL. Proinflammatory and anti-inflammatory cytokines in rheumatoid arthritis. A Primer for Clinicians. 2001
41. Bhakdi S, et al. Stimulation of monokine production by lipoteichoic acids. Infect Immun 1991; 59:4614–4620.
42. De Kimpe, et al. The cell wall components peptidoglycan and lipoteichoic acid from Staphylococcus aureus act in synergy to cause shock and multiple organ failure. Proc Natl Acad Sci USA 1995; 92:10359–10363.
43. Cui W, et al. Differential tumor necrosis factor alpha expression and release from peritoneal mouse macrophages In vitro in response to proliferating gram-positive versus gram-negative bacteria. Infect Immun 2000; 68:4422–4429.
44. Silverstein R, et al. Differential host inflammatory responses to viable versus antibiotic-killed bacteria in experimental microbial sepsis. Infect Immun 2000; 68:2301–2308.
45. Rosenberger, et al. Salmonella typhimurium infection and lipopolysaccharide stimulation induce similar changes in macrophage gene expression. J Immunol 2000; 164:5894–5904.
46. Joiner K, et al. A quantitative analysis of C3 binding to O-antigen capsule, lipopolysaccharide, and outer membrane protein of E. coli O111B4. J Immunol 1984; 132:369–375.
47. Loos M, Clas F, Fischer W. Interaction of purified lipoteichoic acid with the classical complement pathway. Infect Immun 1986; 53:595–599.
48. Hummell DS, Swift AJ, Tomasz A, Winkelstein JA. Activation of the alternative complement pathway by pneumococcal lipoteichoic acid. Infect Immun 1985; 47:384–387.
49. Weinreb, et al. The ability to sensitize host cells for destruction by autologous complement is a general property of lipoteichoic acid. Infect Immun 1986; 54:494–499.
50. Fey GH, et al. Cytokines and the acute phase response of the liver. In: Arias IM, Boyer JL, Fausto N, Jakoby WB, Schachter DA, Shafritz DA, eds. The Liver: Biology and Pathobiology. New York: Raven Press, Ltd, 1994: 113–143.
51. Desmet VJ. Introduction. Organizational principles. In: Arias IM, Boyer JL, Fausto N, Jakoby WB, Schachter DA, Shafritz DA, eds. The Liver: Biology and Pathobiology. New York: Raven Press, Ltd, 1994:3–14.
52. Kuiper J, et al. Kupffer and sinusoidal endothelial cells. In: Arias IM, Boyer JL, Fausto N, Jakoby WB, Schachter DA, Shafritz DA, eds. The Liver: Biology and Pathobiology. Raven Press, Ltd., New York1994:791–818.
53. Decker K. Biologically active products of stimulated liver macrophages (Kupffer cells). Eur J Biochem 1990; 192:245–261.
54. Biozzi G, et al. The kinetics of blood clearance of isotopically abeled Salmonella enteritidis by the reticulo-endothelial system in mice. Immunology 1960; 3:74–89.
55. Aono K, et al. Kupffer cells cytotoxicity against hepatoma cells is related to nitric oxide. Biochem Biophys Res Commun 1994; 201:1175–1181.
56. Bankey, et al. Sequential insult enhances liver macrophage-signaled hepatocyte dysfunction. J Surg Res 1994; 57:185–191.
57. Fox ES, et al. Uptake and modification of [125] I-lipopolysaccharide by isolated rat Kupffer cells. Hepatology 1988; 8:1550–1554.
58. Schumann RR, et al. Lipopolysaccharide binding protein: its role and therapeutical potential in inflammation and sepsis. Biochem Soc Trans 1994; 22:80–82.

59. Park CT, Wright SD. Plasma lipopolysaccharide-binding protein is found associated with a particle containing apolipoprotein A-I, phospholipid, and factor H-related proteins. J Biol Chem 1996; 271:18054–18060.
60. Gazzano-Santoro H, et al. Competition between rBPI23, a recombinant fragment of bactericidal/permeability-increasing protein, and lipopolysaccharide (LPS)-binding protein for binding to LPS and Gram-negative bacteria. Infect Immun 1994; 62:1185–1191.
61. Gallay P, et al. Mode of action of anti-lipopolysaccharide-binding protein antibodies for prevention of endotoxemic shock in mice. Proc Natl Acad Sci USA 1994; 91:7922–7926.
62. Grunfeld C, et al. Lipoproteins inhibit macrophage activation by lipoteichoic acid. J Lipid Res 1999; 40:245–252.
63. Haziot A, et al. Resistance to endotoxic shock and reduced dissemination of Gram-negative bacteria in CD14-deficient mice. Immunity 1996; 4:407–414.
64. Ferrero E, Goyert SM. Nucleotide sequence of the gene encoding the monocyte differentiation antigen, CD14. Nucleic Acids Res 1988; 16:4173.
65. Setoguchi M, et al. Mouse and human CD14 (myeloid cell-specific leucine-rich glycoprotein) primary structure deduced from cDNA clones. Biochim Biophys Acta 1989; 1008:213–222.
66. Schütt C, et al. Endotoxin-neutralizing capacity of soluble CD14. Res Immunol 1992; 143:71–78.
67. Poltorak A, et al. Defective LPS signaling in C3H/HeJ and C57BL/10ScCr mice: mutations in Tlr4 gene. Science 1998; 282:2085–2088.
68. Poltorak A, et al. Genetic and physical mapping of the Lps locus: identification of the toll-4 receptor as a candidate gene in the critical region. Blood Cells Mol Dis 1998; 24,:340–355.
69. Qureshi ST, et al. Endotoxin-tolerant mice have mutations in Toll-like receptor 4 (TLR4) J Exp Med 1999; 189:615–625.
70. Wright SD. Multiple receptors for endotoxin. Curr Opin Immunol 1991; 3:83–90.
71. Wright SD, Jong MTC. Adhesion-promoting receptors on human macrophages recognize *Escherichia coli* by binding to lipopolysaccharide. J Exp Med 1986; 164:1876–1888.
72. Malhotra R, Bird MI. L-selectin—a signalling receptor for lipopolysaccharide. Chem Biol 1997; 4:543–547.
73. Hampton RY, et al. Recognition and plasma clearance of endotoxin by scavenger receptors. Nature 1991; 352:342–352.
74. Dunne DW, et al. The type I macrophage scavenger receptor binds to Gram-positive bacteria and recognizes lipoteichoic acid. Proc Natl Acad Sci USA 1994; 91:1863–1867.
75. Krieger M, Herz J. Structures and functions of multiligand lipoprotein receptors: macrophage scavenger receptors and LDL receptor-related protein (LRP). Annu Rev Biochem 1994; 63:601–637.
76. Terpstra V, et al. Hepatic and extrahepatic scavenger receptors: function in relation to disease. Arterioscler Thromb Vasc Biol 2000; 20:1860–1872.
77. Shnyra A, Lindberg AA. Scavenger receptor pathway for lipopolysaccharide binding to Kupffer and endothelial liver cells in vitro. Infect Immun 1995; 63:865–873.
78. Van Oosten M, et al. New scavenger receptor-like receptors for the binding of lipopolysaccharide to liver endothelial and Kupffer cells. Infect Immun 1998; 66:5107-5112.
79. Elsbach P, et al. Separation and purification of a potent bactericidal/permeability-increasing protein and a closely associated phospholipase A2 from rabbit polymorphonuclear leukocytes. J Biol Chem 1979; 254:11000–11009.
80. Weiss J, et al. Purification and characterization of a potent bactericidal and membrane active protein from the granules of human polymorphonuclear leukocytes. J Biol Chem 1978; 253:2664–2672.
81. Ammons WS, et al. Protective effects of an N-terminal fragment of bactericidal/permeability-increasing protein in rodent models of Gram-negative sepsis: role of bactericidal properties. J Infect Dis 1994; 170:1473–1482.
82. von der Mohlen MA, et al. Inhibition of endotoxin-induced cytokine release and neutrophil activation in humans by use of recombinant bactericidal/permeability- increasing protein. J Infect Dis 1995; 172:144–151.

83. Giroir BP, et al. Preliminary evaluation of recombinant amino-terminal fragment of human bactericidal/permeability-increasing protein in children with severe meningococcal sepsis. Lancet 1997; 350:1439–1443.

84. Levin M, et al. Recombinant bactericidal/permeability-increasing protein (rBPI21) as adjunctive treatment for children with severe meningococcal sepsis: a randomised trial. rBPI21 Meningococcal Sepsis Study Group. Lancet 2000; 356:961–967.

85. Bauer RJ, et al. A phase I safety and pharmacokinetic study of a recombinant amino terminal fragment of bactericidal/permeability-increasing protein in healthy male volunteers. Shock 1996; 5:91–96.

86. Baveye S, Elass E, Mazurier J, Spik G, Legrand D. Lactoferrin: a multifunctional glycoprotein involved in the modulation of the inflammatory process. Clin Chem Lab Med 1999; 37:281–286.

87. Lee WJ, et al. The protective effects of lactoferrin feeding against endotoxin lethal shock in germfree piglets. Infect Immun 1998; 66:1421–1426.

88. Elshourbagy NA, et al. Apolipoprotein E mRNA is abundant in the brain and adrenals, as well as in the liver, and is present in other peripheral tissues of rats and marmosets. Proc Natl Acad Sci USA 1985; 82:203–207.

89. Marin DB, et al. The relationship between apolipoprotein E, dementia, and vascular illness. Atherosclerosis 1998; 140:173–180.

90. Grunfeld C, et al. Lipoproteins inhibit macrophage activation by lipoteichoic acid. J Lipid Res 1999; 40:245–252.

91. Harris HW, et al. Human very low density lipoproteins and chylomicrons can protect against endotoxin-induced death in mice. J Clin Invest 1990; 86:696–702.

92. Eggesbo JB, Lyberg T, Aspelin T, Hjermann I, Kierulf P. Different binding of 125I-LPS to plasma proteins from persons with high or low HDL. Scand J Clin Lab Invest 1996; 56:533–543.

93. Emancipator K, et al. In vitro inactivation of bacterial endotoxin by human lipoproteins and apolipoproteins. Infect Immun 1992; 60:596–601.

94. Rensen PCN, et al. Human recombinant apolipoprotein E redirects lipopolysaccharide from Kupffer cells to liver parenchymal cells in rats in vivo. J Clin Invest 1997; 99: 2438–2445.

95. Feingold KR, et al. Role for circulating lipoproteins in protection from endotoxin toxicity. Infect Immun 1995; 63:2041–2046.

96. Pajkrt D, et al. Anti-inflammatory effects of reconstituted high-density lipoprotein during human endotoxemia. J Exp Med 1996; 184:1601–1608.

97. Netea MG, et al. Low-density lipoprotein receptor-deficient mice are protected against lethal endotoxemia and severe Gram-negative infections. J Clin Invest 1996; 97:1366–1372.

98. de Bont N, et al. Apolipoprotein E knock-out mice are highly susceptible to endotoxemia and *Klebsiella pneumoniae* infection. J Lipid Res 1999; 40:680–685.

99. Abraham E. Why immunomodulatory therapies have not worked in sepsis. Intensive Care Med 1999; 25:556–566.

100. Cohen J, Glauser MP. Septic shock: treatment. Lancet 1991; 338:736–739.

101. Rackow EC, Astiz ME. Pathophysiology and treatment of septic shock. JAMA 1991; 266:548–554.

102. Wheeler AP, Bernard GR. Treating patients with severe sepsis. N Engl J Med 1999; 340:207–214.

103. Ziegler EJ, et al. Treatment of Gram-negative bacteremia and shock with human antiserum to a mutant *Escherichia coli*. N Engl J Med 1982; 307:225–1230.

104. Greenman RL, et al. XOMA sepsis, a controlled clinical trial of E5 murine monoclonal IgM antibody to endotoxin in the treatment of Gram-negative sepsis. JAMA 1991; 266:1097–1102.

105. Angus DC, et al. E5 murine monoclonal antiendotoxin antibody in gram-negative sepsis: a randomized controlled trial. E5 Study Investigators. JAMA 2000; 283: 1723–1730.

106. Baumberger C, et al. Modulation of endotoxic activity of lipopolysaccharide by high-density lipoprotein. Pathobiology 1991; 59:378–383.

107. Gordon BR, et al. Low lipid concentrations in critical illness: implications for preventing and treating endotoxemia. Crit Care Med 1996; 24:584–589.
108. Cronin L, et al. Corticosteroid treatment for sepsis: a critical appraisal and meta-analysis of the literature. Crit Care Med 1995; 23:1430–1439.
109. Clark MA, et al. Effect of a chimeric antibody to tumor necrosis factor-alpha on cytokine and physiologic responses in patients with severe sepsis—a randomized, clinical trial. Crit Care Med 1998; 26:1650–1659.
110. Fisher CJ, et al. Treatment of septic shock with the tumor necrosis factor receptor:Fc fusion protein. The Soluble TNF Receptor Sepsis Study Group. N Engl J Med 1996; 334:1697–1702.
111. Opal SM, et al. Confirmatory interleukin-1 receptor antagonist trial in severe sepsis: a phase III, randomized, double-blind, placebo-controlled, multicenter trial. The Interleukin-1 Receptor Antagonist Sepsis Investigator Group [see comments]. Crit Care Med 1997; 25:1115–1124.
112. Astiz ME, et al. Pretreatment of normal humans with monophosphoryl lipid A induces tolerance to endotoxin: a prospective, double-blind, randomized, controlled trial. Crit Care Med 1995; 23:9–17.
113. Boumpas DT, et al. Glucocorticoid therapy for immune-mediated diseases: basic and clinical correlates. Ann Intern Med 1993; 119:1198–1208.
114. Munford RS, Dietschy JM. Effects of specific antibodies, hormones, and lipoproteins on bacterial lipopolysaccharides injected into the rat. J Infect Dis 1985; 152:177–184.
115. Lucas CE, Ledgerwood AM. The cardiopulmonary response to massive doses of steroids in patients with septic shock. Arch Surg 1984; 119:537–541.
116. Bernard GR, et al. Efficacy and safety of recombinant human activated protein C for severe sepsis. N Engl J Med 2001; 344:699–709.
117. Astiz ME, Rackow EC. Septic shock. Lancet 1998; 351:1501–1505.

Index